Frans C. Stades
Milton Wyman · Michael H. Boevé · Willy Neumann · Bernhard Spiess

Ophthalmology for the Veterinary Practitioner

Frans C. Stades
Milton Wyman · Michael H. Boevé · Willy Neumann · Bernhard Spiess

Ophthalmology for the Veterinary Practitioner

Second, revised and expanded edition

schlütersche

1. English Edition 1996   1. Dutch Edition 1996
2. English Edition 2007   1. Spanish Edition 1998
1. German Edition 1996   1. Portuguese Edition 1998
2. German Edition 1998   1. Italian Edition 2000
3. German Edition 2006   1. Japanese Edition 2000

© 2007, Schlütersche Verlagsgesellschaft mbH & Co. KG, Hans-Böckler-Allee 7, 30173 Hannover
E-mail: info@schluetersche.de

Printed in Germany

ISBN 978-3-89993-011-5

Bibliographic information published by Die Deutsche Nationalbibliothek

Die Deutsche Nationalbibliothek lists this publication in the Deutsche Nationalbibliografie; detailed bibliographic data are available in the Internet at http://dnb.ddb.de.

The authors assume no responsibility and make no guarantee for the use of drugs listed in this book. The authors / publisher shall not be held responsible for any damages that might be incurred by the recommended use of drugs or dosages contained within this textbook. In many cases controlled research concerning the use of a given drug in animals is lacking. This book makes no attempt to validate claims made by authors of reports for off-label use of drugs. Practitioners are urged to follow manufacturers' recommendations for the use of any drug.

All rights reserved. The contents of this book, both photographic and textual, may not be reproduced in any form, by print, photoprint, phototransparency, microfilm, video, video disc, microfiche, or any other means, nor may it be included in any computer retrieval system, without written permission from the publisher.

Any person who does any unauthorised act in relation to this publication may be liable to criminal prosecution and civil claims for damages.

Contents

Authors X

Abbreviations XI

Origin of Plates and Figures XII

1	**Introduction**	1
2	**Clinical and Differential Diagnostic Procedures**	
2.1	Description of the patient	5
2.2	Patient history	5
2.3	Animal handling, equipment, and instruments	8
2.3.1	Restraint and sedation	8
2.3.2	Materials and instruments	8
2.4	Examination of the eye and its adnexa .	8
2.4.1	Head, skull, and orbital area	8
2.4.2	Tear film and tear production	9
2.4.3	Ocular discharge	10
2.4.4	Eyelids (palpebrae)	10
2.4.5	Conjunctiva	11
2.4.6	Globe (bulbus)	12
2.4.7	Sclera	13
2.4.8	Cornea	13
2.4.9	Anterior and posterior chambers	13
2.4.10	Pupil and iris	14
2.4.11	Lens	14
2.4.12	Vitreous	14
2.4.13	Fundus	14
2.4.14	Additional and specific examinations	15
2.5	Differential diagnosis	16
2.5.1	Introduction	16
2.5.2	The "red" eye	16
2.5.3	Epiphora without distinct blepharospasm . . .	16
2.5.4	Blepharospastic / painful eye (Schirmer tear test not decreased)	16
2.5.5	Protrusion of the nictitating membrane with enophthalmos	16
2.5.6	Exophthalmos	16
2.5.7	The "blue-white" cornea	17
2.5.8	The "pigmented" eye	17
2.5.9	The "blind" eye	17
3	**Diagnostics and Therapeutics for Eye Diseases**	
3.1	Introduction	19
3.1.1	Into the conjunctival sac	19
3.1.2	Subconjunctival	21
3.1.3	Retrobulbar	21
3.1.4	Intraocular	21
3.1.5	General rules	22
3.2	Ocular therapeutic agents	22
3.2.1	Vasoconstrictors	22
3.2.2	Antihistamines (nowadays mostly replaced by corticosteroids)	22
3.2.3	Antiglaucoma agents	23
3.2.3.1	Miotics. Facilitating drainage of aqueous	23
3.2.3.2	Moderating production of aqueous: carbonic anhydrase inhibitors	23
3.2.3.3	Osmotic agents	23
3.2.3.4	Other agents used to reduce ocular pressure	23
3.2.4.	Mydriatics	23
3.2.5	Antimicrobial agents	24
3.2.5.1	"Initial choice" antibacterials	24
3.2.5.2	Antimycotics	25
3.2.5.3	Antiviral drugs: DNA-synthesis inhibitors . . .	25
3.2.6	Corticosteroids	25
3.2.6.1	Topical, into the conjunctival sac	25
3.2.6.2	Subconjunctival	25
3.2.6.3	Oral	25
3.2.7	Non-steroidal anti-inflammatory drugs (NSAIDs)	25
3.2.7.1	Prostaglandin synthesis inhibitors	25
3.2.8	Local anesthetics	26
3.2.9	Vitamins, epithelializing agents, and neutral agents	26
3.2.10	Collyria	26
3.2.11	Other "drugs" for ocular use	26
3.2.11.1	Diagnostic agents	26
3.2.11.2	Chemical cauterizing agents	27
3.2.11.3	(Discharge-)dissolving agents	27
3.2.11.4	Anti-hypertensive agents (in secondary retinopathy)	27
3.2.11.5	Other drugs used on the eye	27
3.2.12	Radiation	27
3.2.13	Protective devices	27
3.3	Surgical possibilities	27
3.3.1	Anesthesia	27
3.3.2	Preparation of the operative field	28
3.3.3	Positioning on the operating table	28
3.3.4	Draping	28
3.3.5	Magnification equipment	28
3.3.6	Surgical equipment	28
3.3.7	Suture material	28
3.3.8	Hemostasis	29
3.3.9	Cryosurgery	29
3.3.10	Laser techniques	29

4	**Ocular Emergencies**		**7**	**Eyelids**	
4.1	Introduction	31	7.1	Introduction	73
4.2	Luxation or proptosis of the globe	31	7.2	Ankyloblepharon	74
4.3	Chemical burns	34	7.3	Aplasia palpebrae	74
4.4	Blunt trauma	34	7.4	Dermoids / dysplasia of the lid	76
4.4.1	Orbital fractures	34	7.5	Distichiasis	76
4.4.2	Contusion of the globe	35	7.6	Entropion	78
4.4.2.1	Suffusion (hyposphagma)	35	7.6.1	Entropion in sheep and horses	86
4.4.2.2	Traumatic corneal edema	35	7.7	Ectropion and / or oversized palpebral fissure (macroblepharon) (Ect / OPF)	86
4.4.2.3	Hyphema	35			
4.4.2.4	Trauma with deeper penetration	36			
4.5	Penetrating or perforating trauma	37	7.7.1	Shortening of the lower palpebral conjunctiva	87
4.5.1	Lid lacerations and conjunctival sac wounds	37			
			7.7.2	V-Y Method	87
4.5.1.1	Lacerations of the lid edge including the lacrimal canaliculus	39	7.7.3	Simple wedge resection	87
			7.7.4	Kuhnt-Szymanowski method, Blaskovic's modification	87
4.5.1.2	Lacerations with loss of tissue	39			
4.5.2	Conjunctival lacerations	39	7.7.5	Kuhnt-Szymanowski method	87
4.5.3	Corneal lacerations	40	7.7.6	Z-plasty / free transplants	88
4.5.3.1	General rules of treatment	40	7.7.7.	Total fissure shortening methods	88
4.5.3.2	Non-perforating corneal wounds	40	7.8	Trichiasis	89
4.5.3.3	Perforating corneal defects	43	7.8.1	Nasal fold trichiasis	89
			7.8.1.1	Removal of nasal folds	89
			7.8.1.2	Medial canthoplasty	90
5	**Orbital and Periorbital Structures**		7.8.2	Upper eyelid trichiasis	90
5.1	Introduction	47	7.8.3	Caruncle trichiasis and trichiasis in other locations	91
5.2	Congenital abnormalities	48			
5.3	Trauma	48	7.9	Blepharophimosis	94
5.4	Enophthalmos	48	7.10	Oversized / overlong palpebral fissure	94
5.4.1	Enophthalmos due to loss of support	48			
5.4.2	Enophthalmos due to Horner's syndrome	49	7.11	Injuries	94
5.5	Exophthalmos	49	7.12	Ptosis	94
5.5.1	Exophthalmos due to swelling of the temporal muscles	50	7.13	Lagophthalmos	95
			7.13.1	Medial canthoplasty	95
5.5.2	Exophthalmos due to retrobulbar processes	50	7.13.2	Lateral canthoplasty	95
			7.14	Blepharitis	95
5.6	Enucleation of the globe including the conjunctiva	53	7.14.1	Non-specific blepharitis	95
			7.14.2	Chronic blepharitis	95
5.7	Evisceration of the globe	56	7.14.3	Specific blepharitis	96
5.8	Enucleation of the globe	56	7.14.3.1	Chalazion / hordeolum	96
5.9	Exenteration of the orbit	56	7.14.3.2	Blepharitis adenomatosa (meibomianitis)	96
5.10	Orbitotomy	56			
			7.14.3.3	Juxtapalpebral defects / granulomatous changes	96
6	**Lacrimal Apparatus**				
6.1	Introduction	59	7.14.3.4	Eosinophilic granuloma	96
6.2	Keratoconjunctivitis sicca (KCS)	61	7.14.3.5	Blepharitis in birds	99
6.3	(Sialo)dacryoadenitis	64	7.14.3.6	Blepharitis in horses	99
6.4	Tear stripe formation	65	7.15	Neoplasia of the eyelids	99
6.4.1	Micropunctum or stenosis of the lacrimal punctum	65	7.15.1	Sarcoids in horses	103
6.4.2	Atresia and secondary closure of the punctum	66	**8**	**Conjunctiva and Nictitating Membrane**	
			8.1	Introduction	105
6.5	Dacryocystitis	67	8.2	Non-pigmented margin of the nictitating membrane	106
6.6	Lacerations	70			
6.7	Cysts and neoplasia	70	8.3	Dermoid	106
			8.4	Ectopic cilia	106

8.5	Protrusion of the nictitating membrane 107		10.6.1.1	Chronic superficial keratitis (Überreiter) / pannus / keratitis pannosa / photoallergic keratitis / vascular and pigmentary keratitis / German Shepherd dog keratitis 135	
8.6	Cysts 108				
8.7	Eversion / inversion of the nictitating membrane 108		10.6.1.2	Eosinophilic keratitis 136	
8.8	Hyperplasia / hypertrophy of the gland of the nictitating membrane ("cherry eye") 110		10.6.2	Deep or interstitial keratitis or keratitis profunda (without defects) 136	
			10.6.3	Ulcerative keratitis 137	
			10.6.3.1	Superficial ulcers 137	
8.9	Subconjunctival hemorrhages 113		10.6.3.2	Deep ulcers 140	
8.10	Injuries 113		10.6.3.3	Hernia of Descemet's membrane (descemetocele) 140	
8.11	Conjunctivitis 113				
8.11.1	Catarrhal (or serous) conjunctivitis 114		10.6.3.4	Corneal perforation (staphyloma) 142	
8.11.2	Purulent conjunctivitis 114		10.6.3.5	Nictitating membrane, conjunctival, and corneal oversuturing techniques 142	
8.11.3	Follicular conjunctivitis 116				
8.11.4	Plasmacellular conjunctivitis 116		10.6.4	Corneal sequestration / cornea nigrum / corneal necrosis / corneal mummification ... 147	
8.11.5	Papillary / nodular / granulomatous conjunctivitis 117				
			10.6.5	Keratitis punctata 149	
8.11.6	Conjunctivitis neonatorum 117		10.6.6.	Keratitis herpetica 150	
8.11.7	Infectious bovine / ovine keratoconjunctivitis (pinkeye) 118		10.6.7	Infectious bovine / ovine keratoconjunctivitis 150	
8.12	Eosinophilic granuloma 119		10.6.8	Corneal cysts 150	
8.13	Allergic conjunctivitis 119		10.6.9.	Corneal abscess 150	
8.14	Conjunctival adhesions 119		10.7	Dystrophic / degenerative deposits in the cornea 151	
8.14.1	Symblepharon 119				
8.14.2	Conjunctival stricture in the rabbit 120		10.7.1	Corneal dystrophies 151	
8.15	Neoplasia of the conjunctiva 122		10.7.1.1	Epithelial / stromal dystrophy 151	
			10.7.1.2	Endothelial dystrophy or senile endothelial degeneration 152	
9	**Globe**				
9.1	Introduction 125		10.7.2	Local degenerative crystal deposits 153	
9.2	Exophthalmos, enophthalmos 125		10.7.3	Deposits resulting from systemic diseases ... 153	
9.3	Pseudo-exophthalmos / pseudo-enophthalmos 125		10.7.4	Corneal edema in the Manx cat 153	
			10.7.5	Mucopolysaccharidosis 154	
9.4	Setting sun phenomenon 126		10.7.6.	GM1 and GM2 gangliosidosis 154	
9.5	Strabismus 126		10.8	(Epi)scleritis 154	
9.6	Nystagmus 126		10.9	Neoplasms 155	
9.7	Anophthalmia, cyclopia, microphthalmia 127				
			11	**Intraocular Pressure and Glaucoma**	
9.8	Phthisis bulbi 127		11.1	Introduction 157	
9.9	Macrophthalmia 128		11.2	Glaucoma 159	
9.10	Buphthalmos / hydrophthalmia 128		11.2.1	Etiology 159	
9.11	Endophthalmitis, panophthalmitis 128		11.2.1.1	Primary glaucoma 159	
			11.2.1.2	Secondary glaucoma 160	
10	**Cornea and Sclera**		11.2.1.3	Absolute glaucoma 160	
10.1	Introduction 129		11.2.2	Irido-corneal angle abnormalities 161	
10.1.1	Symptoms of corneal disease 129		11.2.2.1	Open irido-corneal angle glaucoma 161	
10.1.2	Localization and causes of corneal abnormalities 132		11.2.2.2	Narrowed or closed irido-corneal angle glaucoma 161	
10.1.3	Corneal regeneration 132		11.2.3	Conditions of the drainage angle 161	
10.1.4	Retardation of healing 133		11.2.3.1	Open pectinate ligament glaucoma 161	
10.2	Microcornea 133		11.2.3.2	Primary morphologically abnormal pectinate ligament 161	
10.3	Persistent pupillary membrane (PPM) . 133				
10.4	Dermoid 133		11.2.4	Length of time of development and progression of glaucoma 161	
10.5	Trauma 134				
10.6	Keratitis 134		11.2.4.1	Acute glaucoma 161	
10.6.1	Superficial keratitis (without ulceration) 134		11.2.4.2	Chronic glaucoma 162	

11.2.4.3	Hydrophthalmia or buphthalmos	162
11.3	**Clinical aspects of glaucoma**	**162**
11.3.1	Acute glaucoma	162
11.3.2	Chronic glaucoma	164
11.3.3	Therapeutic possibilities in glaucoma	165
11.4	**Secondary glaucoma**	**168**
11.4.1	Secondary glaucoma associated with the lens or vitreous	168
11.4.1.1	Dislocation of the lens	168
11.4.1.2	Lens proteins	168
11.4.1.3	Cataract	168
11.4.2	Secondary glaucoma associated with uveal changes	168
11.4.2.1	Uveitis	168
11.4.2.2	Iris atrophy / iridoschisis	168
11.4.3	Secondary glaucoma associated with trauma	169
11.4.4	Secondary glaucoma associated with intraocular neoplasia	169
11.4.5	Secondary glaucoma associated with medication	169
11.4.6	Secondary glaucoma associated with ocular surgery	169
11.4.6.1	Extracapsular lens extraction	169
11.4.6.2	Intracapsular lens extraction	169
11.5	**Phthisis bulbi**	**169**

12	**Uvea**	
12.1	**Introduction**	**171**
12.1.1	Iris	171
12.1.2	Ciliary body	172
12.1.3	Choroid	173
12.2	**Persistent (epi)pupillary membrane**	**173**
12.3	**Coloboma**	**174**
12.4	**Acorea / aniridia**	**175**
12.5	**Heterochromia of the iris**	**175**
12.6	**Blue iris / white coat**	**175**
12.6.1	Oculocutaneous albinism and deafness	175
12.6.2	Partial oculocutaneous albinism	175
12.7	**Acquired color differences in the iris**	**175**
12.8	**Iris cysts**	**176**
12.9	**Hyphema**	**176**
12.9.1	Dysplastic abnormalities	176
12.9.2	Trauma	176
12.9.3	Leaking of vessels	176
12.9.4	Coagulation disorders	176
12.9.5	Uveitis	177
12.9.6	Neoplasms	177
12.10	**Uveitis (anterior)**	**177**
12.10.1	Traumatic uveitis	179
12.10.2	Metabolic uveitis	179
12.10.3	Infections	179
12.10.3.1	Viral	179
12.10.3.2	Rickettsia	180
12.10.3.3	Bacterial	180
12.10.3.4	Mycotic	180
12.10.3.5	Algae	180

12.10.3.6	Protozoa	180
12.10.3.7	Parasites	180
12.10.4	Immune reactions	180
12.10.4.1	Uveo-dermatologic syndrome (UDS)	181
12.10.4.2	Lupus erythematosus (LE)	181
12.10.5	Idiopathic uveitis	181
12.10.6	Pseudo-uveitis caused by neoplasia	181
12.10.7	Equine recurrent (chronic) uveitis (ERU)	182
12.10.8	Anterior uveitis in the rabbit	183
12.11	**Iris atrophy**	**183**
12.12	**Dysautonomia or pupil dilatation syndrome (Key-Gaskell Syndrome)**	**184**
12.13	**Horner's syndrome**	**184**
12.14	**Other pupillary abnormalities**	**184**
12.15	**Neoplasia**	**184**
12.16	**Posterior Uvea**	**186**

13	**Lens and Vitreous**	
13.1	**Introduction**	**189**
13.1.1	Ontogenesis	189
13.1.2	Anatomy and physiology	190
13.1.3	Vitreous	191
13.2	**Developmental disorders of the lens**	**192**
13.2.1	Aphakia / coloboma / spherophakia / microphakia / lenticonus / lentiglobus	192
13.2.2	Persistent hyaloid artery (PHA)	192
13.2.3	Persistent hyperplastic tunica vasculosa lentis / persistent hyperplastic primary vitreous (PHTVL / PHPV)	193
13.3	**Cataract**	**193**
13.3.1	Types of cataract	196
13.3.2	Secondary cataract	197
13.3.2.1	Diabetic cataract	197
13.3.3	Therapeutic possibilities	197
13.3.4	Prevention of cataract	201
13.4	**Lens luxation or ectopic lens**	**201**
13.5	**Vitreous floaters, asteroid hyalosis, and synchysis scintillans**	**206**
13.5.1	Vitreous floaters	206
13.5.2	Asteroid hyalosis	206
13.5.3	Synchysis scintillans	206
13.6	**Hemorrhages and / or exudates in the vitreous**	**206**
13.6.1	Blood	206
13.6.2	Hemorrhagic or other exudate in the vitreous	207
13.7	**Retinal detachment and intraocular neoplasms**	**207**

14	**Fundus and Optic nerve**	
14.1	**Introduction**	**209**
14.1.1	Ontogenesis	209
14.1.2	Retina	209
14.1.3	Optic nerve or tract	211
14.1.4	Vascular supply	213

14.1.5	Choroid (vascular membranes) 214
14.2	**Symptoms, pathologic changes, and reaction patterns of the fundus** 214
14.3	**Aplasia** 218
14.4	**Micropapilla and hypoplastic papilla** . . . 218
14.5	**Coloboma** 218
14.6	**Retinal dysplasia (RD)** 219
14.7	**Collie eye anomaly (CEA)** 219
14.8	**Inherited enzyme deficiencies** 221
14.9	**Hereditary (progressive) retinal dysplasias / atrophy / degeneration (PRA)** 221
14.9.1	Hereditary progressive retinal degeneration / progressive retinal atrophy 222
14.9.2	Hereditary (stationary) night blindness 224
14.9.3	Hereditary day blindness 224
14.9.4	Pigment epithelial dystrophy (PED) 224
14.10	**Hemorrhages and other vascular abnormalities** 224
14.10.1	Vascular occlusion 225
14.10.2	Hyperlipoproteinemia 225
14.11	**Trauma** 225
14.12	**Intoxications** 225
14.12.1	Iatrogenic intoxications 225
14.13	**Abnormalities of nutritional origin** 225
14.13.1	Vitamin A and vitamin E deficiencies 225
14.13.2	Thiamine (aneurine) or vitamin B_1 deficiency 227
14.13.3	Taurine deficiency 227
14.14	**Posterior uveitis / chorioretinitis / retinitis** 227
14.15	**Retinal detachment** 228
14.16	**Hypertensive Retinopathy** 229
14.17	**Non-hereditary degenerative abnormalities** 230
14.17.1	Feline central retinal degeneration (FCRD) . 230
14.18	**Papilledema** 230
14.19	**Papillitis, optic neuritis** 231
14.20	**Neoplasia** 231
14.21	**Amblyopia / amaurosis** 232
14.21.1	Sudden acquired retinal degeneration (SARD) 232

15	**Breed Predispositions and Hereditary Eye Diseases**
15.1	**Introduction** 237
15.2	**Modes of inheritance** 237
15.2.1	Simple inheritance 237
15.2.1.1	Autosomal dominant (not sex-linked) 237
15.2.1.2	Autosomal recessive (not sex-linked) 237
15.2.1.3	Sex-linked inheritance 237
15.2.1.4	Incomplete recessive or dominant, or incomplete penetrance 238
15.2.2	Multiple (polygenic) transmission 238
15.3	**Is the abnormality inherited?** 238
15.4	**Breed predispositions and inherited eye abnormalities** 240

16	**Glossary of Terms Relating to the Eye** 247

Index 251

Authors

Frans C. Stades, DVM, PhD, Dip. ECVO
Associate Professor of Veterinary Ophthalmology
Department of Clinical Sciences of Companion
   Animals
Faculty of Veterinary Medicine
Utrecht University, The Netherlands

Milton Wyman, DVM, MS, Dip. ACVO
Professor of Veterinary Clinical Sciences
Ohio State University College of Veterinary
   Medicine
Professor of Ophthalmology
Ohio State University College of Medicine
Columbus, Ohio, USA

Michael H. Boevé, DVM, PhD, Dip. ECVO
Associate Professor of Veterinary Ophthalmology
Department of Clinical Sciences of Companion Animals
Faculty of Veterinary Medicine, Utrecht University,
   The Netherlands
Honorary Professor of Veterinary Ophthalmology, Stiftung
   Tierärztliche Hochschule Hannover, Germany

Willy Neumann, DVM, Dip. ECVO
Specialist for Veterinary Surgery, Veterinary Ophthalmology
Am Drosselschlag 25
Giessen-Heuchelheim, Germany

Bernhard Spiess, DVM, PhD, Dip. ACVO/ECVO
Department for Small Animals, Ophthalmology Unit
Vetsuisse Faculty
University of Zurich, Switzerland

Abbreviations

a.	artery	long.	longus
ACE	angiotensin converting enzyme	m.	muscle
ant.	anterior	med.	medial
BAB	blood–aqueous barrier	MRI	magnetic resonance imaging
BCE	before the Common Era	OD	oculus dexter (right eye)
brev.	brevis	OS	oculus sinister (left eye)
BSS	balanced salt solution	OU	oculus uterque (both eyes)
CE	Common Era	PDT	parotid duct transposition
CEA	Collie eye anomaly	PHA	persistent hyaloid artery
CH	choriodal hypoplasia	PHTVL/PHPV	persistent hyperplastic tunica vasculosa lentis/ persistent hyperplastic primary vitreous
CRD	chorioretinal dysplasia		
CSNB	congenital stationary night blindness		
CT	computed tomography	PM	pupillary membrane
dv	dorsoventral	PMMA	polymethylmetacrylate
ERG	electroretinogram	post.	posterior
ERU	equine recurrent uveitis	PRA	progressive retinal atrophy
ext.	external	PU/PD	polyuria/polydipsia
FCRD	feline central retinal degeneration	RD	retinal dysplasia
FHV-1	feline herpes virus type 1	RPE	retinal pigment epithelium
HA	hyaloid artery	SARD	sudden acquired retinal degeneration
IOL	intra-ocular lens	STT	Schirmer tear test
IOP	intraocular pressure	TVL	tunica vasculosa lentis
KCS	keratoconjunctivitis sicca	UDS	Uveo-dermatologic syndrome
lat.	lateral	v.	vein
LE	lupus erythematosus	VEP	visual evoked potential

Origin of Plates and Figures

Plates:

7.16, 7.17: G. Kása; Kleintierklinik, Lörrach, Germany.

7.33, 7.34, 8.19, 10.34: W. Klein, Department of Equine Sciences, Faculty of Veterinary Medicine, University of Utrecht, The Netherlands.

3.4, 3.5, 4.10, 6.11, 6.12, 7.8, 7.9, 7.26, 7.27, 10.15, 10.16, 10.17, 10.18, 12.11, 14.6, 14.9, 14.26, 14.27: W. Neumann, Am Drosselschlag 25, Giessen-Heuchelheim, Germany.

10.30, 14.2: B. Spiess, Department for Small Animals, Ophthalmology Unit, Vetsuisse Faculty, University of Zurich, Switzerland.

13.3: Th. M. van Balen, University Medical Center, Amsterdam, The Netherlands.

14.25: A. Heijn, Veterinaire Specialisten Oisterwijk, The Netherlands.

Remaining plates: F. C. Stades and M. H. Boevé, Department of Clinical Sciences of Companion Animals, Faculty of Veterinary Medicine, University of Utrecht, The Netherlands.

Figures:

2.2, 7.2, 7.6, 7.16, 13.2 and **13.9** are, with permission of the publisher, taken from: F. C. Stades/M. H. Boevé, Ogen, in: Anamnese en lichamelijk onderzoek bij gezelschapsdieren, A. Rijnberk & H. W. de Vries, Editors, Bohn, Scheltema & Holkema, 1990.

2.2, 4.5, 6.1, 6.2, 6.5, 7.2, 7.4, 7.6, 7.16, 7.23, 10.3, 12.3, 13.2, 13.9: B. Jansen, Department of Clinical Sciences of Companion Animals, Faculty of Veterinary Medicine, University of Utrecht, The Netherlands.

Remaining figures: F. C. Stades.

1 Introduction

The previous editions of this book have clearly proved their value. After the Dutch, German and English first editions in 1996, the second and third editions in German, Spanish, Portuguese, Italian and Japanese versions of the book have been published.

Over the past 10 years, continued progress has been made in the knowledge and medications associated with veterinary medicine, and in veterinary ophthalmology, in particular. Of direct interest to the practitioner are not only those drugs that are not available anymore, but also and more importantly, the new drugs and medications that have become available in the recent years. All together, these are good reasons for a thoroughly revised, new edition of this book.

We are very happy about the willingness of Prof. Dr. B. Spiess, Dip. ACVO/ECVO to join the team as coauthor. All the coauthors have each screened a part of the chapters and the editor has screened all and has tried to bring any differences in opinion, if necessary and possible, to a consensus.

The morphologic and physiologic features of the eye and the characteristics of ocular diseases are similar among domestic animals. Nevertheless, there are species differences in structure, in reactions of the eye, and in diagnostic procedures. There are also specific diseases and treatments in the different species.

Ophthalmologic diseases comprise a large proportion of the patients seen by the small animal practitioner. Eye problems are especially frequent in dog breeds with redundant nasal and forehead skin folds, misdirected hairs, or poorly apposed lids, and they cause discomfort to the animal. The large animal practitioner will see eye problems in horses similar to those in small animals, but usually less frequently, and some conditions are specific to the horse. In cattle, sheep, goats, swine, small mammals, and birds, eye diseases are also generally less frequent than in pet animals, but they may cause considerable problems when larger groups of animals are affected. Breed predisposition and hereditary ophthalmic disorders are frequent in all species, but are mainly recognized in the dog. A knowledge of breeds predisposed to eye anomalies and hereditary eye diseases is of major importance. In addition, the authors have tried to pay special attention to the recognition of eye abnormalities such as trichiasis, glaucoma, lens luxation, and progressive retinal atrophy, all of which are difficult to diagnose without specialized ophthalmic equipment.

Much has been published on the subject of veterinary ophthalmology and there are many excellent and detailed books on ophthalmology as well as beautiful atlases. The majority of ophthalmic disorders can be diagnosed using relatively simple equipment and without the need for additional or specialized procedures. However, there is little practical information available for the veterinary student or the non-specialist practitioner.

This book is written primarily to provide the veterinary student and the general practitioner with the necessary information for the recognition and basic treatment of ophthalmic disorders. Over 180 photographs illustrate the abnormalities and more than 200 schematic drawings are included to clarify the text and the different approaches to treatment.

A fully problem-oriented approach appears to be less suitable in the work up of eye diseases. The chapter sequence in this book follows, as closely as possible, the recommended order of the ophthalmic examination, with the exception of the chapters on ocular diagnostics and therapy, surgical procedures, and breed predisposition and hereditary eye diseases. There is a separate chapter on primary ocular emergencies as this should be readily available in hectic practical situations.

Each chapter begins with a very brief introduction to the morphology and physiology of the specific structure; this helps in understanding the etiology, clinical behavior, and therapy of the associated diseases. The eye abnormalities are then presented in the same sequence in each chapter according to pathogenesis, with congenital anomalies being dealt with first. These are followed by diseases caused by environmental influences such as trauma, intoxications, and deficiencies. Inflammatory processes, including infections, are presented next. The final parts of each chapter deal with degenerative, autoimmune, and neoplastic diseases.

The most commonly encountered ocular problems receive the most detailed attention. Priority is given to the way the authors recognize and work up ophthalmologic emergencies and how they are treated. For other ophthalmic problems, the authors have tried to provide adequate information to aid in their recognition and to give general rules for treatment, with special emphasis on preventing mistakes. Details about the specific species are preceded by the species icons.

All of this has been done with an understanding of the limitations in equipment and training of the non-specialist practitioner. Therefore, the authors have also indicated which patients should be referred and when, and how the eye should be protected during transport. The authors have tried to inform practitioners about what the referred owner might expect, which different treatments are possible, and the necessary after-care referring veterinarians must provide when the animal returns to them. At the end of the description of each disease, brief information is given about the prognosis, the genetic aspects, and the consequences for breeding.

The authors are very grateful to the students, interns, and residents who have played a part in making this book possible. Their critiques of the diagnostic and therapeutic keys were

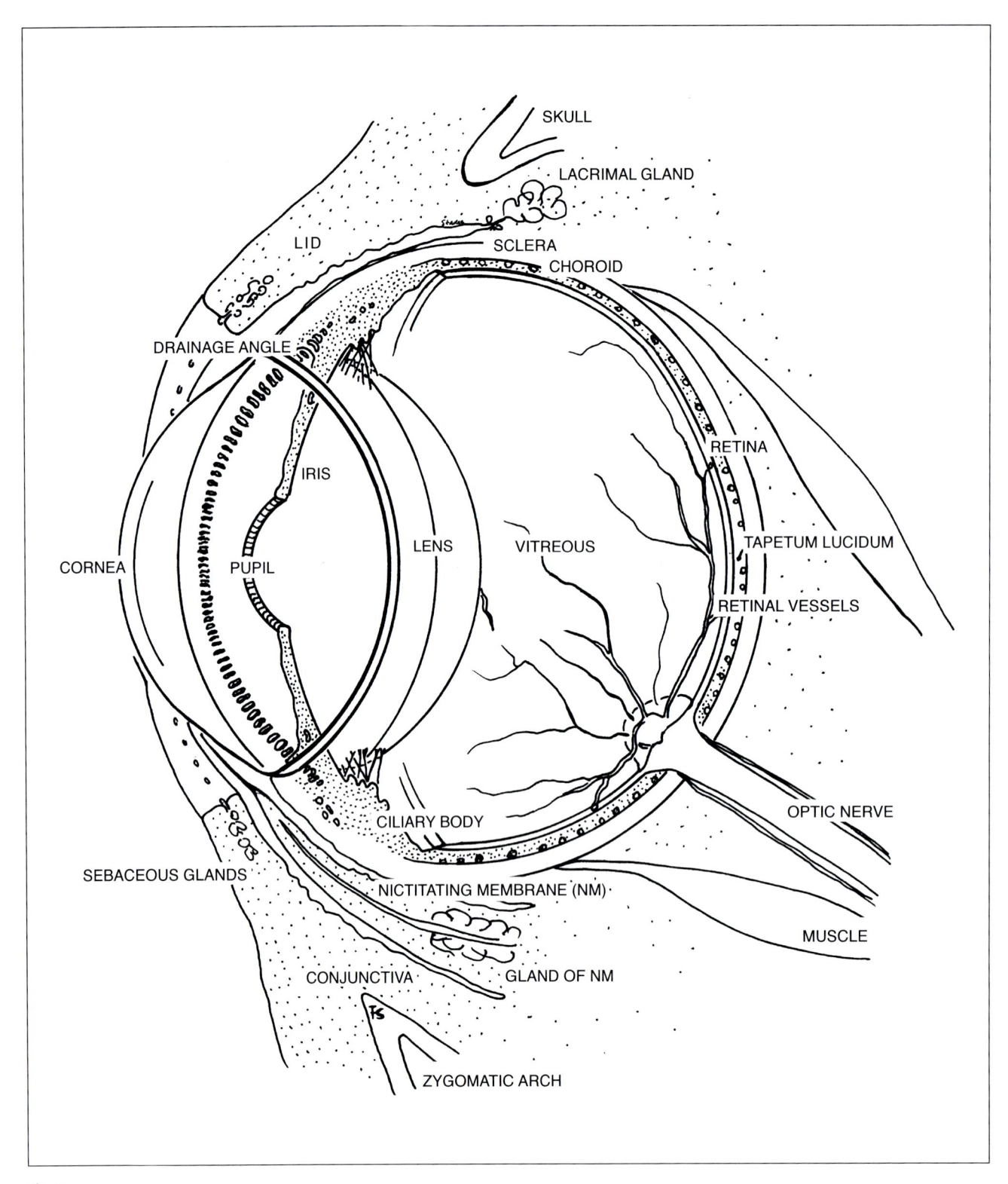

Fig. 1:
Partly opened section of the eye and the nomenclature.

most helpful. We are also most grateful for the helpful criticism of Prof. Dr. J. Fink-Gremmels and Dr. C. Görig. The many hours spent by Dr. Bruce Belshaw in editing the original manuscript were vital for the book. His devotion to this task is gratefully acknowledged. We are also greatly indebted to Dr. Peter Beyon for his thorough, final correction of the manuscript

The authors are especially grateful for the encouragement, understanding, and active help of their families during the preparation of this book.

2 Clinical and Differential Diagnostic Procedures

Emphasis should be placed at the start on both the patient's history and those diagnostic procedures that are specific to the eye and adnexa when presented with an animal with an ocular problem. The general history and examination should be dealt with only briefly. If there are indications that another system is involved or that there is a systemic disease (e.g. sneezing, hemorrhage, loss of weight, neoplasia), then a general physical examination must also be performed.

It is important to follow a routine examination protocol as a checklist (Fig. 2.1) in order to provide a complete evaluation of the eye and adnexa. The recommended ophthalmic examination is described briefly; for further details of ophthalmic examination procedures, the reader is referred to specialized literature on the subject.[1,2,3]

2.1 Description of the patient

In addition to the age and sex of the patient, the species, breed and origin are of special importance. Many disorders of the eye have a predisposition in certain breeds or are inherited in specific breeds, and specific breed characteristics such as brachycephaly and/or redundant skin folding have to be considered.

2.2 Patient history

The following questions are important when taking the history:
- Was the onset of the problem acute or gradual, or was it present when the dog was obtained? Does it affect one or both eyes and if the latter, which eye is worse? Is the problem improving, static, or becoming worse?
- Have there been signs of general illness as well? Has the patient been vaccinated recently? Are there signs such as rubbing or scratching at the eyes, excessive blinking, blepharospasm, photophobia, or pain during barking, yawning, chewing, or biting?
- Is there a discharge from the eye (watery, mucoid, purulent)? Does it result in periocular soiling and to what degree? Is the surface of the eye dry and encrusted?
- Is there deterioration of vision, disorientation, or a change in the patient's behavior, and if there are such changes, are they more pronounced in bright or dim light?
- If the owner describes the eye as bulging, is it protruding from the orbit (exophthalmic) or is the globe itself enlarged (microphthalmos/buphthalmos)? Or, in contrast, is the eye too small (microphthalmos/phthisis bulbi) or lying too deep in the orbit (enophthalmos)?

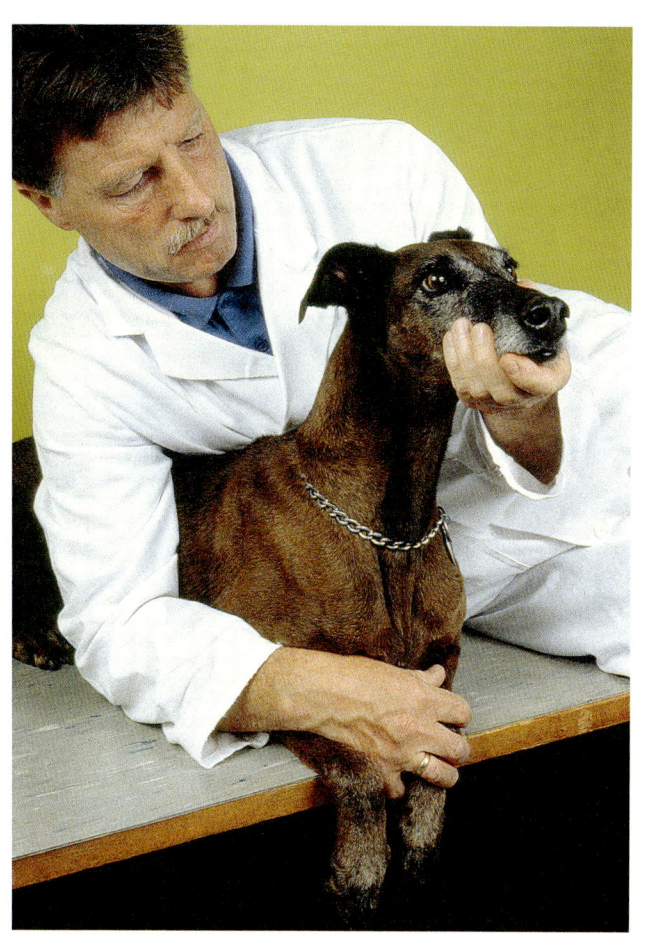

Plate 2.1:
A dog in the "Sphinx" position for eye examination (see also Plate 2.6).

- Are there changes in the color, position, or form of the globe?
- What are the normal living conditions of the animal: does it have to climb stairs, is it on a leash outdoors, is it restricted to its own terrain or free to roam, or has the animal a specific function (e.g. hunting, watchdog, jumping horse)?
- What is the composition of the family: are there children, are there other animals?
- What previous illnesses has the patient had, and what eye diseases? What information is available about illnesses of other animals in the same household or of parents or siblings of the patient?
- Are there any abnormalities in eating, volume of water drunk, urination, or defecation?
- Has the patient received eye washes or topical and/or systemic medication for the present ophthalmic problem?

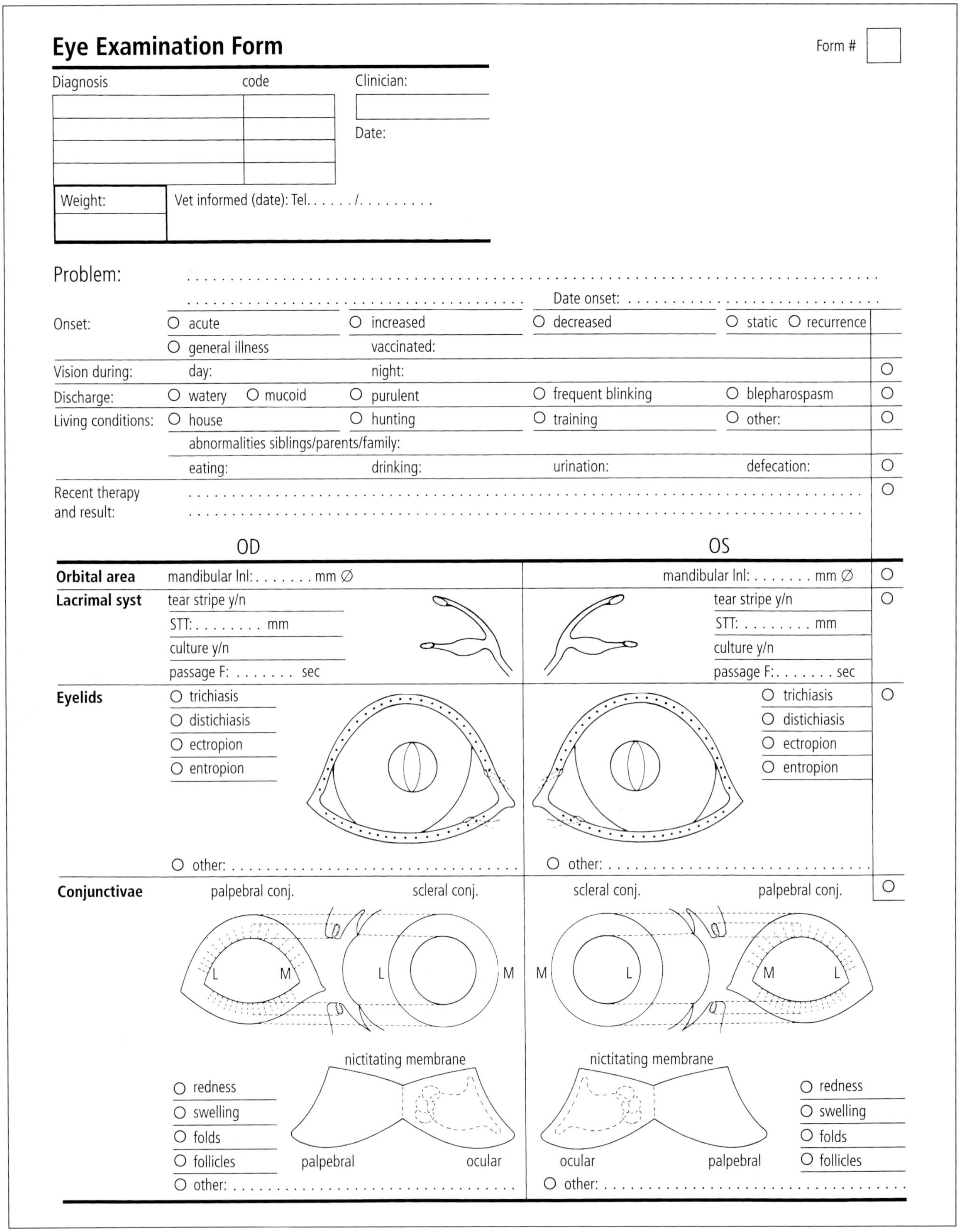

Eye Examination Form

Form #

Diagnosis	code

Clinician:

Date:

Weight:

Vet informed (date): Tel. . . . . . /. . . . .

Problem: . . . .

Date onset: . . . .

Onset: O acute O increased O decreased O static O recurrence

O general illness vaccinated:

Vision during: day: night: O

Discharge: O watery O mucoid O purulent O frequent blinking O blepharospasm O

Living conditions: O house O hunting O training O other: O

abnormalities siblings/parents/family:

eating: drinking: urination: defecation: O

Recent therapy and result: . . . . O

OD / OS

Orbital area mandibular lnl: . . . . mm ∅ | mandibular lnl: . . . . mm ∅ O

Lacrimal syst tear stripe y/n; STT: . . . . mm; culture y/n; passage F: . . . . sec | tear stripe y/n; STT: . . . . mm; culture y/n; passage F: . . . . sec O

Eyelids O trichiasis O distichiasis O ectropion O entropion O other: . . . . | O trichiasis O distichiasis O ectropion O entropion O other: . . . . O

Conjunctivae palpebral conj. L M; scleral conj. L M | scleral conj. M L; palpebral conj. M L O

nictitating membrane: palpebral, ocular | nictitating membrane: ocular, palpebral

O redness O swelling O folds O follicles O other: . . . . | O redness O swelling O folds O follicles O other: . . . .

Clinic for Companion Animals, University of Utrecht

Fig. 2.1:
Example of an eye examination protocol.

	OD	OS	
Bulbus	○ exophthalmus ○ enophthalmus ▼▲ I.O.press: .... mmHg ▼▲ retrobulb. p. ○ buphth. ○ norm. ○ microphth. ○ phthisis	○ exophthalmus ○ enophthalmus ▼▲ I.O.press: .... mmHg ▼▲ retrobulb. p. ○ buphth. ○ norm. ○ microphth. ○ phthisis	○
Cornea **Sclera** **Ant chamber**	○ fluoresc. pos goniosc.:	goniosc.: .... ○ fluoresc. pos.	○
Iris P.reflex ○ direct: ○ consens.:	○ < 2 sec ○ slow ○ none OD → OS: ○ < 2 sec ○ slow ○ none pupil: .... mm dark .... mm light ○ PPM ○ other: .... ○ mydriaticum ○ iridodonesis	○ < 2 sec ○ slow ○ none OD ← OS: ○ < 2 sec ○ slow ○ none pupil: .... mm dark .... mm light ○ PPM ○ other: .... ○ mydriaticum ○ iridodonesis	○ ○ ○
Lens **Vitreous**	ant. post. ○ cataract ○ lux ○ other:	ant. post. ○ cataract ○ lux ○ other:	○
Fundus	vision light: .... dark: .... obstacle test: .... lat.	vision light: .... dark: .... obstacle test: .... lat.	○

pigment (black)   edema (blue)   infiltrate   scar   dystrophy   synechia   defect (green)
                  cataract (lens), atrophy (ret)   granulation (red)   F = positive

Therapy
....
....
....
....

○ **Radiology**
○ **Cytology**   **Follow-up:**
○ **Histology**
○ **Haematology**

© Department of Clinical Sciences of Companion Animals – Utrecht University

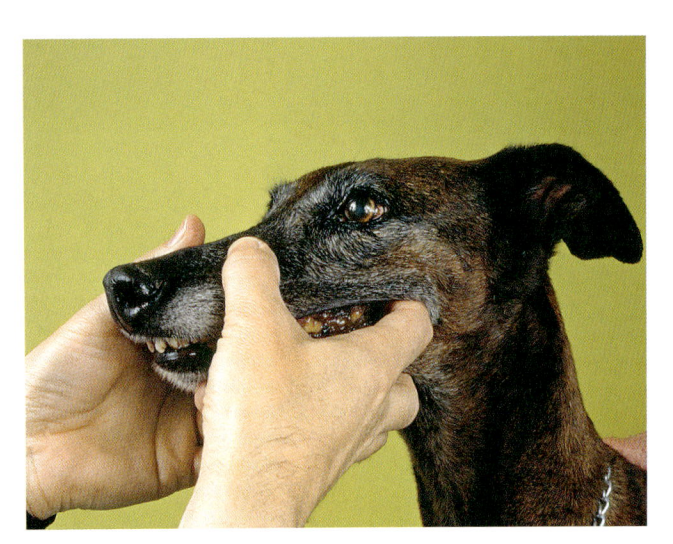

Plate 2.2:
Palpation of the weak bottom of the orbit in the mouth (with a closed mouth) behind the last upper molar (M 2).

2.3 Animal handling, equipment, and instruments

The examination should be performed in a room that can be dimmed and completely darkened, with a strong spotlight available above the patient. The examiner should be seated during the examination. Dogs and cats are held in a "Sphinx" position (Plate 2.1) at the edge of the examination table. All four feet of cats should be fixed to prevent injury. Materials for culturing like moist sterile swabs and cytobrushes are important aids in ophthalmologic diagnostics.

2.3.1 Restraint and sedation

Dogs should be muzzled if they are nervous, unreliable, or unfriendly. In dogs and cats, tranquilizers usually cause enophthalmos, inwards rotation of the globe, and protrusion of the nictitating membrane. For these reasons, they should only be used in low doses. In cats, a low dose of ketamine-xylazine results in excellent positioning of the globe for ophthalmic examination. More convenient is a very low dose of medetomidine (0.01 mg/kg; for which an antagonist is available). It can be used in cats and dogs without significantly interfering with the ophthalmic examination, although some miosis may be caused.

In horses a very low dose of detomidine (1–1.5 mg/100 kg) results in excellent positioning of the globe for ophthalmic examination. Blocking or infiltration anesthesia (supraorbital and/or auriculopalpebral) is also possible. However, general anesthesia is preferred for more extensive surgery, because of the lack of swelling and the better positioning for the surgeon.[4]

2.3.2 Materials and instruments

The instruments that should be available include a penlight, a direct ophthalmoscope with a slit beam and a blue filter, Von Graefe or other suitable forceps, a curette, and a spatula. Disposable materials include the Schirmer tear test, fluorescein test strips (or single dose drops), rose bengal strips or single dose vials, and tubes containing transport medium for microbiological culturing. For ocular irrigation, 0.9% NaCl solution in a soft plastic infusion bottle with a 2-mm cannula can be used. Proparacaine, lidocaine, or tetracaine, which can cause irritation during induction, can be used for topical anesthesia. Tropicamide can be used as a short-acting mydriatic. In puppies and kittens, and in adult animals or patients with apparent congenital intraocular abnormalities, 0.5–1% atropine can be used.

2.4 Examination of the eye and its adnexa

General examination of the eye should start with a gross observation of the position and symmetry of the eyes and adnexa. In principle the specific examination begins with the adnexa and progresses inwards into the globe. However, the lacrimal tear film should be examined before it is influenced by other procedures, and thus before inspection of the lids. The globe as a whole can be examined either after the examination of the lids or after examination of the conjunctiva, but this important step should not be forgotten. The presence or absence of periocular swelling and the gross appearance of the cornea and conjunctiva should be determined. Observe the animal's ability to move freely in a room with obstructions and its ability to follow moving objects such as cotton balls.

For purposes of recording findings, the points of reference are anterior or posterior, nasal/medial or temporal/lateral, dorsal/superior or ventral/inferior, and positions corresponding to the numbers on a clock.

2.4.1 Head, skull, and orbital area

The position of the head and its relationship to the body (e.g. tilted left or right) and the muscle tone are noted while the animal walks into the examination room, when it is at rest, and when it is placed on the examination table. The patient is stroked on the head not only as an introduction, but also for the inspection of its chewing muscles for pain, warmth, swelling or atrophy, and asymmetry. The mandibular lymph nodes are palpated. If abnormalities are found, all nodes are examined. The sinuses and the bony and soft tissue parts of the orbits are examined by percussion and are inspected for swelling, atrophy, abnormally hard or soft areas, pain, and asymmetry. If there are signs of a retrobulbar process, the mouth is opened to determine whether it can be fully opened and whether opening causes pain. The soft tissue area behind the upper last molars (Plate 2.2), forming the bottom of the orbit, is examined for abnormalities such as discoloration, abscesses, swelling, etc. With the dog's mouth closed, the same area can be palpated via the corners of the mouth with the tips of ones fingers. When pressure is applied, the globe will be displaced 1–2 mm or more anteriorly in the orbit. If there is a retrobulbar mass, this may be painful, the globe will move much more, and/or the area will be found to be hard and indurated.

The medial canthus area is inspected for the presence of tear-moistened hairs. In cats, these areas may contain particles of pigment. Hairs surrounding the eye can irritate the conjunctiva and/or eyeball (trichiasis, especially in the Bloodhound, Chow Chow, and short-nosed animals such as the Pekingese and the "Peke-faced" Persian cat), and will show wetness.

2.4.2 Tear film and tear production

The tear film and tear production are inspected before they can be influenced by further examinations. The tear film is examined at the junction of the cornea and the lid margin or at the edge of the nictitating membrane (Plate 2.3). The cornea and the image it reflects are inspected to see whether the image is intact, not distorted, and has regular margins. If there is doubt about the integrity of the tear film or there is a mucopurulent exudate, the Schirmer tear test (STT) is performed (Plate 2.4). The test strip is grasped with a dry forceps and the round sterile end is placed in the ventral conjunctival sac about one-third of the distance from the lateral canthus. After 60 seconds, the strip is removed and the length of strip that has become moistened, from the notch, is measured in millimeters. The reference values are 13–23 mm in dogs, 10–20 mm in cats, 20–30 mm in horses, and 15–20 mm in rabbits (Table 2.1). Values of 9 mm or less in dogs and 6 mm or less in cats indicate keratoconjunctivitis sicca (KCS).[5,6,7] If the value is between 10 and 13 mm in dogs or cats, rose bengal stain can be performed after fluorescein staining has been completed.[8] Rose bengal staining reveals intact but devitalized epithelial cells in areas where the tear film has broken down. However, this examination requires magnification, preferably a slit lamp (biomicro-

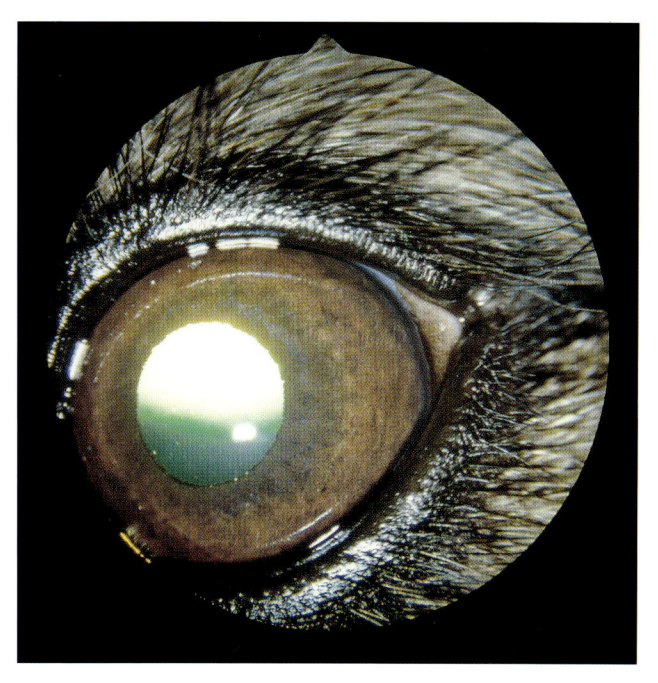

Plate 2.3:
Eye with an intact precorneal tear film showing a clear and transparent adhesion line of tears between the cornea and free lid margin in the 12- and 1-o'clock positions (OS, dog). The central reflection on the precorneal tear film is disturbed by the fundus reflection. NB: The borderline of the eyelash hairs and the hairs on the upper and lower lids in dogs and cats, are placed more outside the free lid margin than eyelashes in man.

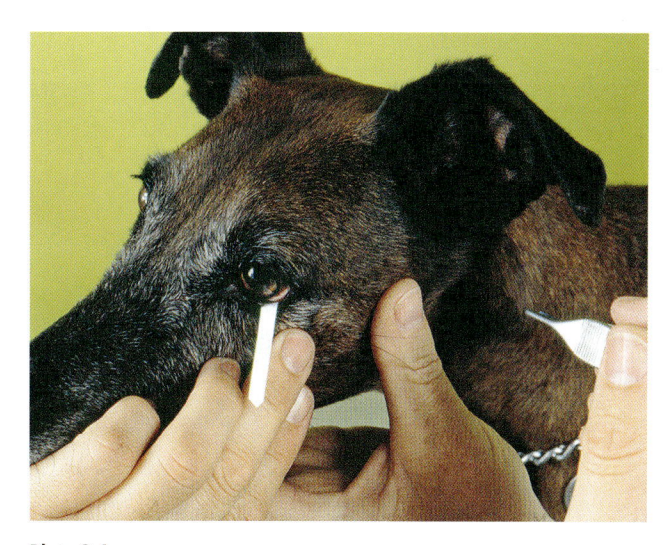

Plate 2.4:
The Schirmer tear test. The rounded end of the strip is placed in the ventral conjunctival sac about one-third of the distance from the lateral canthus. After 60 seconds, the length of the strip that has become moistened from the notch is measured in millimeters.

scope), which is not usually available in general practice. It should be noted that rose bengal will stain devitalized epithelial cells that are infected with the rhinotracheitis virus (herpes virus) in cats. The resulting stained areas with a dendritic appearance are pathognomonic for this disease.

Table 2.1: Reference values for tear production (Schirmer tear test [type 1])

	µl	SD	Author
Dog	20.2	3.0	Hamor[9]
	18.8	2.6	Saito[10]
Cat	16.2	3.8	McLaughlin[11]
Horse	22/26 (summer/winter)	6.0	Beech[12]
Rabbit*	4.85	2.90	Biricik[13]
	5.30	2.96	Abrams[14]

* There are significant breed differences in rabbits (Abrams[14])

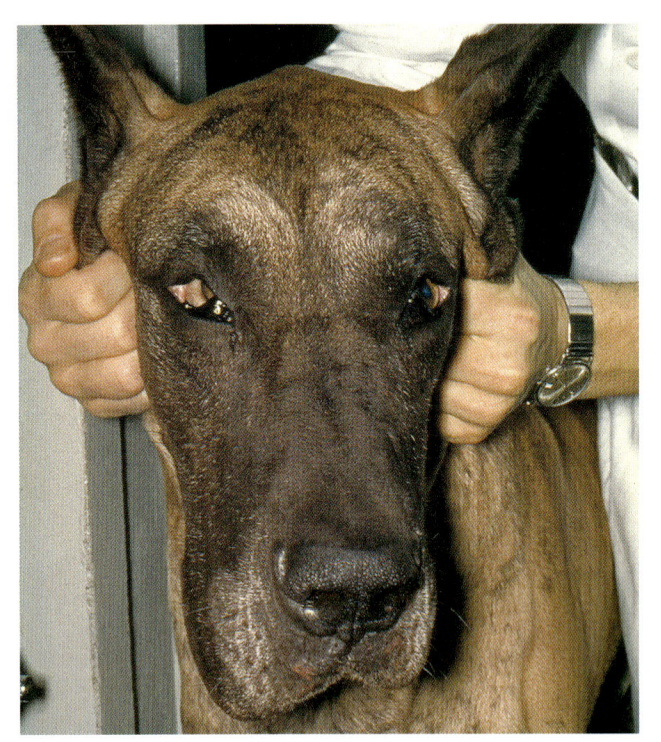

Plate 2.5:
Incorrect fixation of the head of an eye patient. By traction on the skin, the eye fissure is under tension and thus possible faults in the lid positioning are masked. Compare with the fixation shown in Plate 2.1.

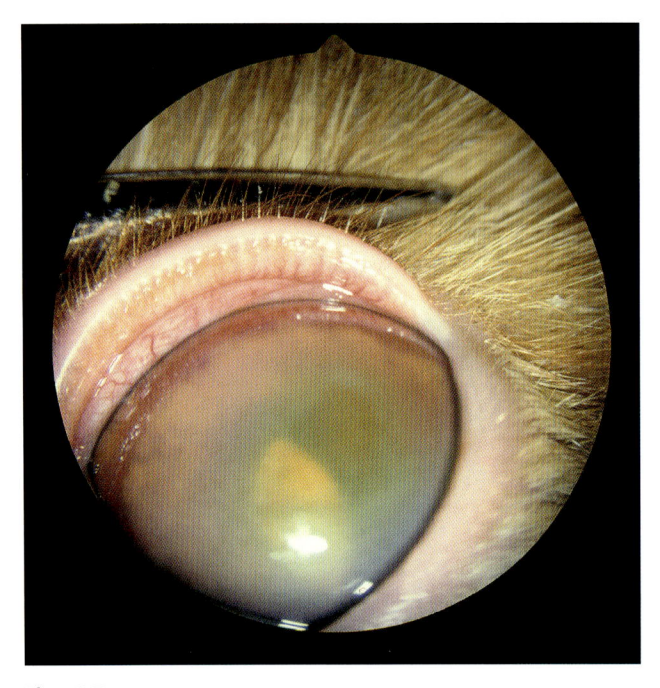

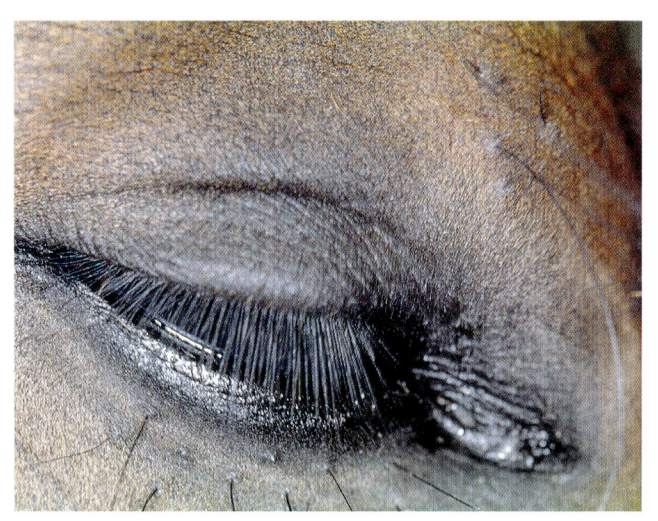

Plate 2.6:
Lid margin in a horse. On the upper lid there are lashes as in humans.

2.4.3 Ocular discharge

Discharge, in spite of normal tear production, can have an infectious cause and thus, a sample should be collected for microbiologic culture. If the transport time is likely to exceed one hour, the specimen should be placed in transport medium and kept refrigerated to prevent drying and thus the death of the organisms. After collection of the sample, the conjunctival sac is irrigated with 0.9% NaCl solution.

2.4.4 Eyelids (palpebrae)

During examination of the lids, ectropion or entropion may be artificially corrected if the patient is restrained in a way that places traction on the skin behind the lids (Plate 2.5). The lid reflex and the apposition of the lid margins to the globe are inspected. The lid edges should be in contact with and follow the curvature of the cornea. The margins should be hairless in cats, while some eyelash hair is to be expected in dogs, horses, and cattle. The lid margins should also be pigmented, smooth, glossy, and intact. Plate 2.6 shows the lid margins in a horse with lashes on the upper lid as in humans. The lid margins should be inspected for discoloration, swellings, alopecia, and moisture. Scrapings are made of suspicious areas for examination for parasites (demodex, sarcoptes). Defects in the lid margins or absence of meibomian glands (Plate 2.7) may be due to aplasia palpebrae or injury to the lid. Wet lid margins or lid hairs indicate a disturbance of the normal lid function due to abnormalities, such as distichiasis, chalazion, or hordeolum, or direct contact between the hairs on the outer surface of the lid

Plate 2.7:
Ectropionizing of the upper lid, showing the overfilled meibomian glands and their openings in the free lid margin. The center of the cornea of this Persian cat has a brownish pigmentation, the beginning of a corneal sequester (OS). At the limbus, a ring of vessels is growing into the cornea.

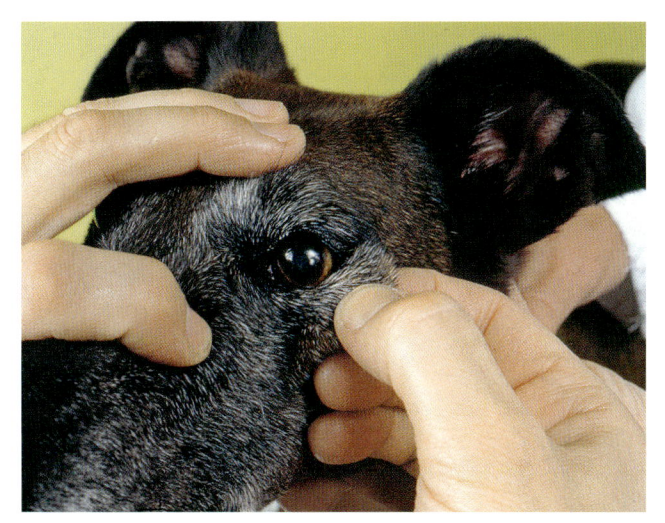

Plate 2.8:
Entropion test. A small skin fold, about 15 mm below the lid margin, is retracted so that the lid margin entropionizes. This should be immediately corrected by blinking and its persistence indicates entropion.

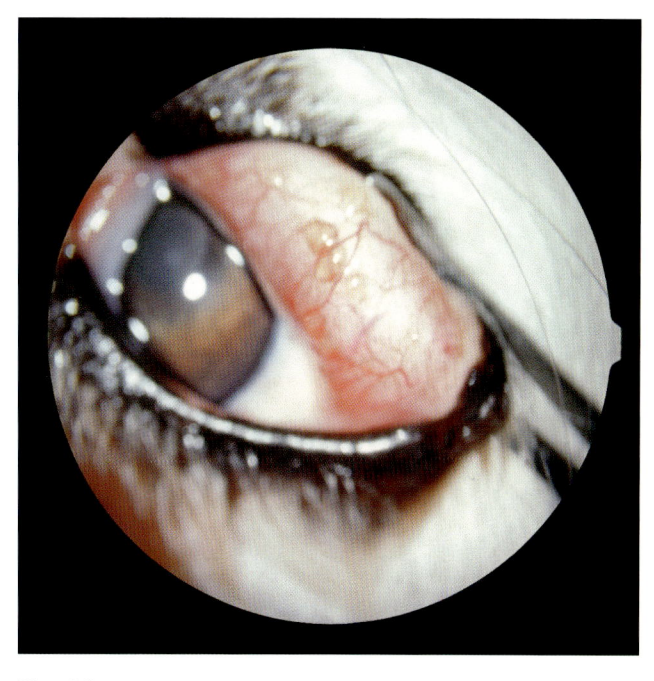

Plate 2.9:
Inspection of the lid edge and the palpebral conjunctiva of the upper lid. The lid margin is everted and the conjunctiva stretched with a Von Graefe's forceps. A group of follicles centrally located in the conjunctiva is now shown (OS, dog).

and the conjunctiva and/or cornea (entropion, trichiasis, exophthalmos). Wet, hairless, discolored areas may be due to chronic blepharospasm. Suspected entropion can be confirmed by the entropion test. For this purpose, a small skin fold, approximately 10–15 mm below the lower lid margin, is retracted slightly so that the lid margin turns inwards and the outer edge lies against the cornea (Plate 2.8). This should be corrected by a single blink, and its persistence indicates (habitual) entropion.

2.4.5 Conjunctiva

The conjunctiva is a thin, transparent membrane, through which the sclera and subconjunctival tissues should be clearly recognizable. The bulbar conjunctiva is usually very pale, especially in the cat. The palpebral conjunctiva is much redder in appearance because of the arborization of its vessels. Because of anastomoses between the uveal and bulbar conjunctival vascular systems, inflammation in the globe (uveitis) or increased intraocular pressure (IOP) will result in an engorgement of the conjunctival vessels at the limbus. These vessels are located more or less perpendicular to the limbus and they will be seen to move with the conjunctiva when it is moved. Chronic irritation by dust or bacteria causes a diffuse inflammatory redness, primarily in the lower conjunctival sac. The conjunctiva is examined for abnormalities such as discoloration, wetness, smoothness, or the presence of follicles (Plate 2.9). Follicles are small, glassy eruptions on the surface, especially on the inner surface of the nictitating membrane near its margin.

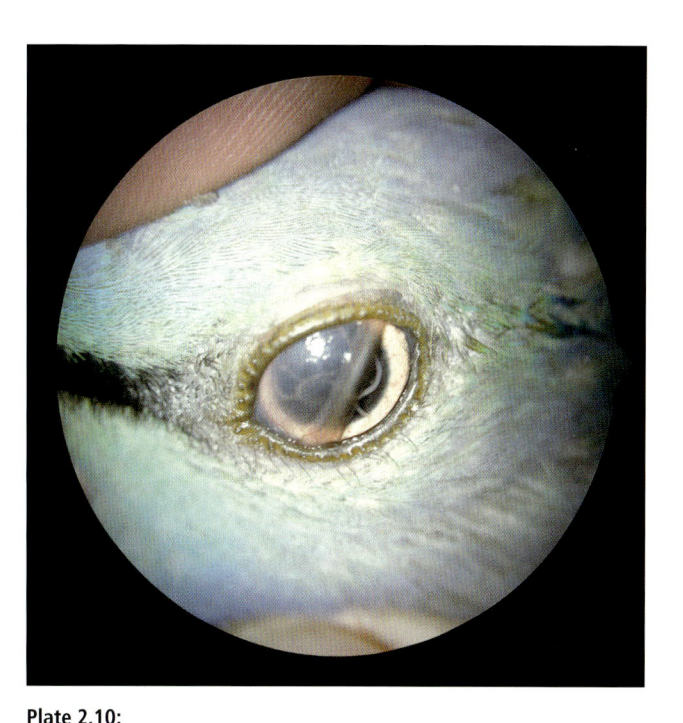

Plate 2.10:
The "blinking" of the nictitating membrane (NM) of birds comes from the dorsomedial (OD). The NM in birds is almost transparent, blinks frequently and makes the precorneal tear film. In the anterior chamber in this eye is a worm, which is also visible through the NM, demonstrating its transparency.

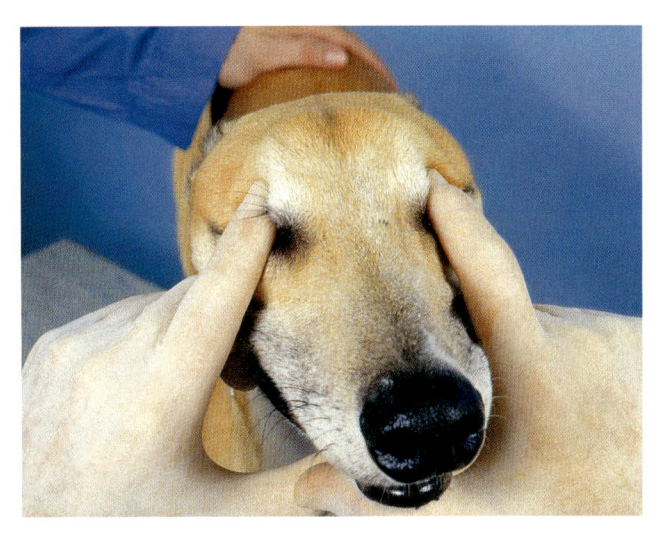

Plate 2.11:
Palpation of the retrobulbar pressure. The tips of the forefingers are placed on the closed upper lids covering the globes, gently pressing the globes backwards into the orbit.

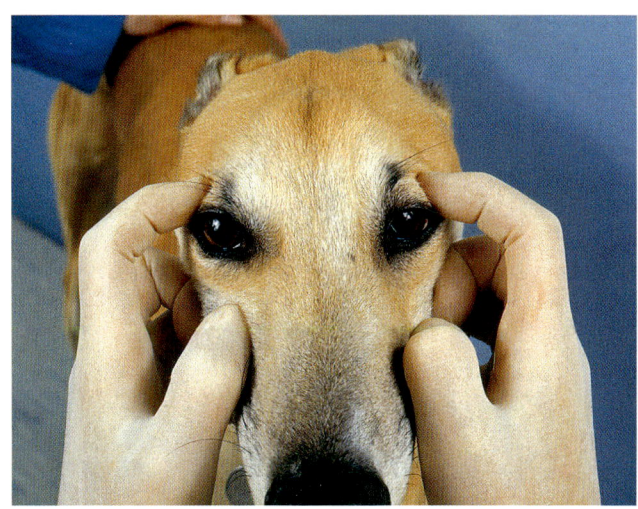

Plate 2.12:
Bilateral palpation of the ocular tension by placing the tips of the slightly curved forefingers over the closed lids on the globes, pressing them medially against the orbital wall.

Protrusion of the nictitating membrane may be the result of enophthalmos or a swelling at the base of the membrane. The combination of protrusion and exophthalmos indicates increased retrobulbar pressure, e.g. as a result of retrobulbar swelling. If there is swelling or discoloration of the conjunctiva, a swab, smear, or scraping should be taken for cytologic examination.[15]

2.4.6 Globe (bulbus)

The symmetrical movement of the eyes, both horizontally and vertically, and the ability to fix both eyes on a distant point (as far as possible for the species) are evaluated. Abnormalities of gaze such as strabismus (Siamese; Plate 9.1) or rapid oscillations of the globe (nystagmus) should be assessed. The position of the globe in the orbit is examined for enophthalmos or exophthalmos. Enophthalmos may be a response to pain, but it can also be secondary to loss of retrobulbar pressure or support, neurological (e.g. loss of sympathetic tone, Horner's syndrome), or loss of condition, or a lack of well-being (especially in the cat); thus symmetry is an important consideration. The retrobulbar pressure (or retropulsion) is evaluated by placing the tips of the two forefingers on the closed upper lids covering the globes, and gently pressing the globes into the orbits (Plate 2.11). Space-occupying lesions within the orbit behind the eye will prevent its displacement into the orbit and/or make this painful.

Both globes should be of the same diameter (approximately 22–24 mm in the dog and cat) and in proportion to the orbit and the head of the patient. It is usually easy to recognize if one globe is too large (buphthalmos or macrophthalmia) or too small (microphthalmia or phthisical). The diagnosis of bilateral microphthalmia is more difficult. In cases of doubt, ultrasonography (or MRI) measurements have to be performed. A difference in color between the eyes, especially involving the cornea, may give the impression that the globes are of different sizes. An edematous, white, cloudy cornea will suggest enlargement of the globe. A microphthalmic eye may suggest enophthalmos or, vice versa, enophthalmos may suggest microphthalmos. When this is in doubt, measurement of the horizontal corneal diameter may be helpful (normally about 17 mm in the adult dog, 18 mm in the cat).

Measurement of IOP is still a major problem for the practitioner (Table 2.2). Manual tonometry is a crude method of determining very hard and very soft eyes (Plate 2.12). It is performed by placing the tips of the slightly curved forefingers over the closed eyelids of the globes, and pressing them medi-

Table 2.2: Intraocular pressure reference values

	mmHg	SD	Author
Dog	18.7	5.5	Gelatt[20]
Cat	19,7	5.6	Miller[21]
Horse	23.3	6.89	Miller[22]
Rabbit	24.4	1.3	Poyer[23]
Guinea pig	5–20 (Variationsbreite)	–	Wagner[24]
Rat	17.30	5.25	Mermoud[25]
Pigeon	13.4	1.4	Korbel[26]

ally against the orbital wall (not posteriorly toward the apex of the orbit; this is retropulsion and does not measure indentation of the globe). When the spherical curvature of the globes is felt, the globes are indented slightly so that the pressure is perceived. This perception of the pressure can be compared with that of a dog without ocular problems, or with that of the examiner. If manual tonometry is the only method available to the practitioner, and glaucoma is suspected, the patient should be referred immediately. Indentation (Schiötz) tonometry is influenced by the different radius of the cornea in different species and in different individuals, and of the globe during the progress of glaucoma. However, it can be performed with reasonable reliability when performed frequently and with carefully cleaned equipment. Then it is more applicable to the management of this devastating disease than gross observation. In addition, the Tonopen® (applanation tonometer) is available; this can be used very effectively with practice, but is expensive. Recently, a new rebound tonometer, TonoVet®, has become available. The apparatus is easy to handle and can be used without topical anesthesia. These tonometers are most accurate at the ranges of IOP of direct interest in glaucoma, but are less reliable with low or very high pressures.[16,17,18,19]

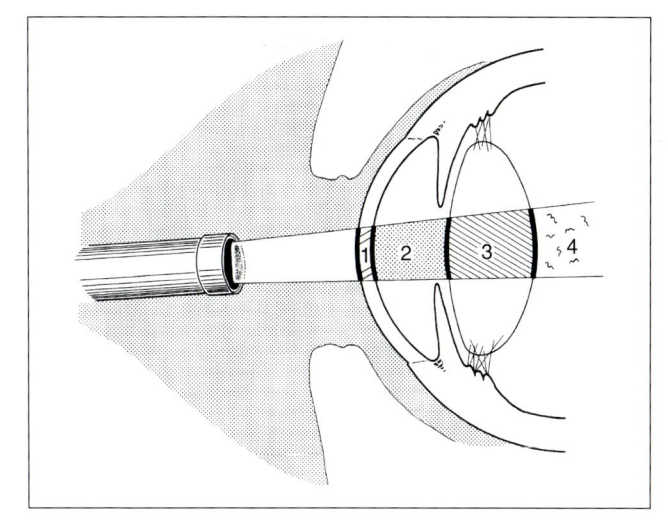

Fig. 2.2:
Slit-lamp section through the anterior media of the eye: (1) Reflection of the slit light on the surface of the cornea and the corneal section; (2) anterior chamber; (3) reflection on the convex anterior capsule of the lens, the section, and the reflection on the concave posterior capsule of the lens; (4) vitreous.

2.4.7 Sclera

The sclera is inspected for defects, discoloration, swelling, as well as injected and/or congested vessels. The scleral vessels run more or less parallel to the limbus and they are darker than the overlying conjunctival vessels.

2.4.8 Cornea

The normal cornea has an intact lacrimal tear film, is without defects, and is smooth, spherical, reflective, transparent, and highly sensitive. The corneal surface is inspected in a darkened room, preferably with a loupe (as in the direct ophthalmoscope: +20 to +40 and its slit beam; Fig. 2.2.). This inspection should be done by looking from all sides, and also with the light source coming from all sides. Corneal edema (island pattern, bluish-white, irregular) must be differentiated from scar tissue (dense, white, sclera-like tissue) and corneal lipidosis or dystrophy (glittering, white, resembling sugar, or glass fiber crystals). Pigmentation of the cornea resulting from chronic irritation is found especially in the dog as a reaction to chronic irritation. Corneal pigmentation is rare in the cat; however, a darkly pigmented deposit (corneal sequestration; Plate 2.7, 10.23) can occur in the central or pericentral cornea. If there are irregularities of the corneal surface, the cornea is stained by fluorescein dye to search for epithelial defects. Strips impregnated with the dye are held either in the ventral conjunctival sac or adjacent to the dorsal bulbar conjunctiva for 1–2 seconds. If the lacrimal passage to the nose is also being tested (passage time 30–60 seconds in the dog and cat), the strips are held in place longer, and the conjunctival sac and the cornea must be irrigated and the nose lowered. Defects in the cornea will be seen as intense yellow-green fluorescent irregularities. To potentiate the florescence, the blue filter of an ophthalmoscope or a Wood's lamp may be used.

2.4.9 Anterior and posterior chambers

The anterior chamber is examined for transparency, flare, contour, and depth. The inferior inner surface of the cornea is checked for precipitates adhering to the endothelium, and the anterior chamber is examined for free precipitates (hypopyon), flare, clots, or blood (hyphema; signs of uveitis). Transparent, variably pigmented and sized spheres that are free-floating in the anterior chamber or fixed at the edge of the pupil are usually harmless iris or ciliary body cysts. Pigmented or discolored bulging areas on the iris surface may indicate neoplasms of the anterior uvea. A large, transparent or white disc in the anterior chamber may indicate a luxated lens. If the lens is luxated posteriorly, the anterior chamber will be deep, the iris hangs straight down and it will "flutter" after an eye movement (iridodonesis). If the lens is dislocated to one side, an aphakic, luminescent crescent may be seen between the contour of the lens and the pupil. The posterior chamber cannot normally be inspected. If a mass between the anterior surface of the lens and the back of the iris presses the iris forward, the lesion can be seen in the posterior chamber.

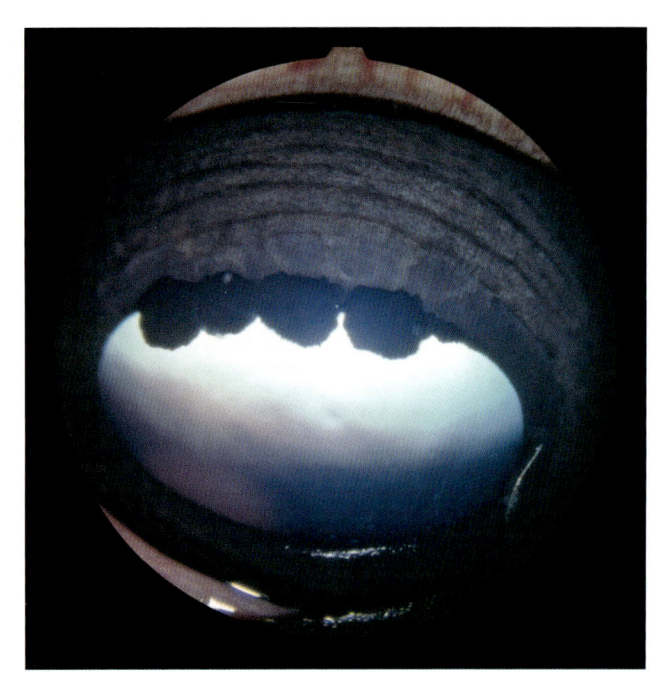

Plate 2.13:
Iridal granulae on the edge of the iris in a horse eye.

2.4.10 Pupil and iris

The normal iris is generally pigmented, but it may be blue in the Siamese (in the Siamese the anterior layers of the iris are unpigmented, the pigment of the pigmented epithelium on the posterior surface of the iris causes the blue aspect) or white, as in blue merle dogs. In miosis, the pupil of the cat has a vertical slit form, while that in horses, sheep, goats, and cattle is horizontally oval. In mydriasis, the pupils in all species are more or less round. The edge of the pupil bears iridic granules, varying from microscopically small ones in small animals to large ones in horses and ruminants (Plate 2.13). They are most prominent in the dorsal pupillary margin and are referred to as "corpora nigra". The absence of these in horses indicates previous inflammatory disease.

The margin of the iris (pupil) is inspected for adhesions to the surface of the lens (posterior synechia) or adhesions to the cornea (anterior synechia). The pupil should react in 2–3 seconds when a pen-light is shone into the visual axis of the eye. The contralateral eye should also respond within a few seconds. Unilateral miosis can be a sign of uveitis or Horner's syndrome (other signs of Horner's syndrome are enophthalmos, ptosis, and protrusion of the nictitating membrane). Unilateral or bilateral mydriasis can be due to dysfunction of the afferent part of the reflex arc, the retina, the optic nerve, or the brain and the oculomotor nerve, but it can also be due to glaucoma. In nervous, frightened, or angry animals, the release of epinephrine may block the pupillary response.

The iris is examined for discoloration, smoothness of its surface, bulging areas, remains of the embryological vascular systems (persistent pupillary membrane or vascular tunic of the lens), defects (coloboma), or synechia from the iris to the lens or to the cornea.

2.4.11 Lens

During examination in the dark with the slit beam (Plate 13.3), special attention is paid to the transparency, diameter, and form of the lens. This examination should also be performed after inducing total mydriasis (15–20 minutes after one drop of 0.5% tropicamide; in young animals 20–45 minutes after 1% atropine).

In birds, a topical mydriatic does not induce mydriasis. Mydriasis can be induced by injecting d-tubocurarine into the anterior chamber[27], but because of the risks associated with this, it is almost exclusively used as a last resort. Alternatively, topical or intra-ocular tubocurarine, vecuronium, can be used.[28]

If there are signs of luxation of the lens (clouds over the pupil edge, aphakic crescent, "disc" in the anterior chamber, or a deeper anterior chamber) or of glaucoma (mydriasis and complete diffuse corneal edema), the use of a mydriatic is contraindicated. The lens can be displaced anteriorly or posteriorly. If there is no associated cataract, the luxation may go unnoticed by the owner for some time. In the cat, secondary glaucoma usually occurs less acutely and rapidly than in the dog.

2.4.12 Vitreous

The vitreous is inspected by slit beam for white strings (persistent hyaloid artery from the center of the posterior pole of the lens), glittering (cholesterol) crystals, or larger clumps. Flares of exudate, blood, membranes, vessels, or tissue may be signs of posterior uveitis, retinal detachment, or intraocular neoplasia.

2.4.13 Fundus

In animals, the fundus can usually be examined quite satisfactorily with a direct ophthalmoscope. Dogs and cats must be positioned symmetrically on the table, like a sphinx. If the animal is uncooperative, the inexperienced clinician should consider sedation, unless the condition of the animal prevents this. If there are signs of defective vision, mydriasis should be induced after carrying out vision tests.

Vision is ideally tested, especially in the horse, when the animal is allowed to move around freely in an unfamiliar area containing obstacles. Testing vision in cats is not simple, because of their independent behavior; it is also difficult in puppies. Alternatives are:
- Observing the animal moving freely and almost falling from the examination table may be informative, but is more time-consuming.
- Observing how the eyes follow a small piece of cotton (distance about 20 cm).
- Optical placing reflex. Although less dependable, this test is useful in light-weight animals such as puppies, kittens, cats, and small dogs.
- The menace reaction, pointing at the eye with a finger, must be done without eliciting air currents, otherwise it is very unreliable.

The optic disc or papilla is located slightly ventral and nasal to the posterior pole of the fundus (Plate 2.14). The optic disc in dogs is more or less rounded and, in some animals, surrounded by a small edge of white glial tissue. The retinal arterioles are thinner and bright red; the venules thicker and dark red. In dogs, the venules may anastomose in the disc. In cats, the optic disc is small (about 1 mm) and pale pink. The retinal vessels disappear into the disc just inside the edge of the disc. In ruminants and pigs, there is a central vein within the confines of the disc. In horses, the small retinal vessels course to and from the disc like the rays of the sun, while in other species they follow a more or less inverted T-pattern. The area of the retina located temporal to the optic disc, referred to as the area centralis, has the highest concentration of cones but is not usually grossly visible. In humans, this area is referred to as the macula; it contains the fovea, a region which is composed entirely of cones.

A tapetum lucidum is found in most animals (tapetum; Gr.: carpet or covering structure; lucidum: L.: clear; tapetal fundus in Anglo-American literature) in approximately the upper half circle of the posterior part of the globe, which reflects the incoming light as orange-yellow to green-blue. The remaining surface of the posterior part of the globe is generally heavily pigmented because of the pigment in the interstices of the choroid and in the pigmented epithelium of the retina. This area is referred to as the tapetum nigrum (nigrum: L.: black) or non-tapetal fundus in Anglo-American literature. In very young animals, before the tapetal areas have matured, the whole fundus appears dark purple-blue. In white, blue merle, and albino animals, both parts of the tapetum may be partially or completely absent; in which case, ophthalmoscopy reveals the large choroidal vessels. These vessels have a more or less sun-ray pattern and in between these vessels, a sun-ray, striped pattern of white sclera may be distinguishable. The optic disc is usually located on, or just below, the junction of the tapetum lucidum and tapetum nigrum.

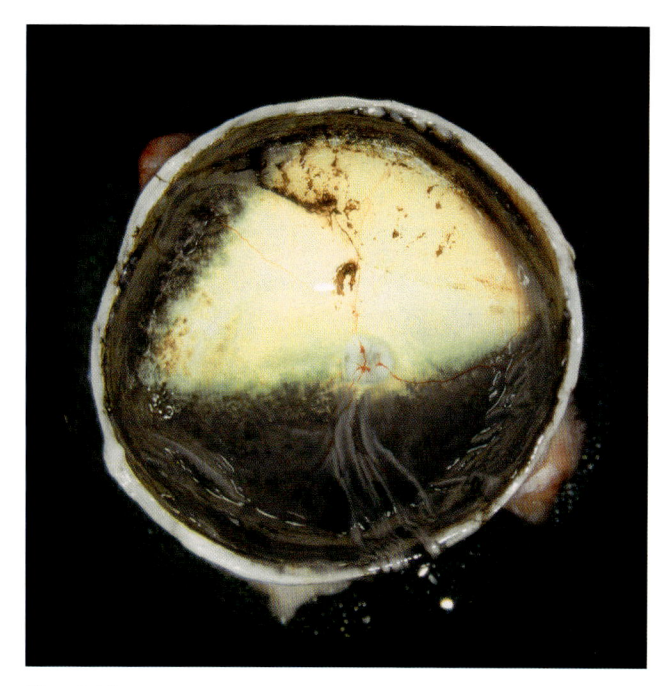

Plate 2.14:
The posterior calotte of the globe of a dog (OD). The outer white ring is the sclera. The darkly pigmented inside part is the tapetum nigrum of the choroid and the pigment epithelium of the retina. The yellow-green area in the posterior pole is the tapetum lucidum. Centrally, the optic disc or papilla is located at the junction of the lucidum and the nigrum. The folded inner membrane is the neural retina with the retinal veins.

Distinct, local or total, hyperreflectivity of the retina may indicate neuroretinal loss of function, e.g. degeneration, whilst blood or cloudy, bullous, membranous, or elevated areas may indicate inflammation, and/or retinal detachment, or neoplasia.

The individual variation in the normal fundus pattern is enormous. For this reason, patients should be referred for ophthalmoscopy when interpretation of findings is uncertain.

2.4.14 Additional and specific examinations

Additional examinations that may be indicated include biopsy, binocular indirect ophthalmoscopy, slit-lamp biomicroscopy, tonometry, gonioscopy, electroretinography, visual evoked responses, fundus angiography, endothelial microscopy, ultrasonography, computed tomography (CT), magnetic resonance imaging (MRI), and other radiologic techniques.[29,30,31,32,33] If the equipment or assessment is not available, the patient should be referred.

2.5 Differential diagnosis

2.5.1 Introduction

A fully problem-oriented clinical work up of the general ophthalmologic patient is not useful, because many eye diseases can be localized and diagnosed by the description of the patient, a good case history, and the results of a thorough clinical examination. However, in some problems it can be useful to have lists of groups of abnormalities or individual abnormalities that differentially may be the cause of the problem. The lists below are reminders and do not pretend to be complete.

The differential diagnoses are presented when possible in order of the etiology of the disease (congenital/acquired) and furthermore, in order of external influences (trauma, intoxications, deficiencies), inflammatory processes (including infection), degenerative processes, autoimmune diseases, and neoplasia. In some cases, more specific details are presented or differentially important diagnostic steps are given.

2.5.2 The "red" eye

Local with increase of tissue:
- hypertrophy of the nictitans gland
- episcleritis (nodular/diffuse)
- granulation into an ulcer/around a foreign body
- eosinophilic granuloma/pannus
- neoplasia

Diffuse:
- results from severe excitement
- keratoconjunctivitis sicca (Schirmer tear test)
- conjunctivitis/dacryocystitis (foreign body/infectious disease)
- keratitis (fluorescein: negative/positive)/(epi)scleritis
- hyphema (traumatic/coagulation/vascular disorder/hypertension/neoplasia)
- glaucoma (lens luxation)
- uveitis (rubeosis iridis)

2.5.3 Epiphora without distinct blepharospasm

- results from blockage of the tear drainage system:
  - atresia: punctum/canaliculus/sacculus/nasolacrimal duct/ostium
  - blockage: foreign body/dacryocystitis/symblepharon (upper respiratory disease)
- distichiasis
- conjunctivitis (follicular/plasmacellular, allergic/atopic)

2.5.4 Blepharospastic/painful eye (Schirmer tear test not decreased)

- results from trauma (contusion of the globe/foreign body/burns/perforation)
- results from irritation by hairs (ectopic cilia/entropion/trichiasis/distichiasis)
- blepharitis
- corneal defect/ulcer
- infectious keratoconjunctivitis:
  - distemper/upper respiratory disease/symblepharon
  - bovine/ovine infectious keratoconjunctivitis
- anterior uveitis
- glaucoma

2.5.5 Protrusion of the nictitating membrane with enophthalmos

- results from blepharospastic/painful eye: see 2.5.4
- results from discomfort/general malaise/sedation/general illness
- Horner's syndrome
- results from loss of retrobulbar support (fat/dehydration/muscle atrophy)
- results from pressure from rostral to bulbus (manual/fracture/tumor, including neoplasia)
- tetanus
- results from local disease of the nictitating membrane:
  - foreign body/hyperplasia or hypertrophy of the nictitans gland/eversion/scars
  - follicular/plasmacellular conjunctivitis/symblepharon

2.5.6 Exophthalmos

- results from trauma
- mucocele/aneurism
- orbital fracture
- myositis
- results from endocrine disease: Cushing's syndrome, acromegaly
- retrobulbar inflammation (cellulitis/abscess)
- retrobulbar neoplasia

2.5.7 The "blue-white" cornea

- blue-white irregular (overstretching/edema):
  - local (superficial/deep corneal disease/Descemet tear)
  - diffuse (endothelial dystrophy/glaucoma/uveitis)
- white as sclera:
  - scar tissue
- crystalline/angel's hair aspect:
  - dystrophic process: precipitates (lipidosis)
  - arcus lipoides (hypothyroidism)

2.5.8 The "pigmented" eye

- granula iridis/iris cyst
- foreign body
- results from chronic corneal irritation (keratoconjunctivitis sicca/lagophthalmos/hairs)
- chronic keratitis (general, pannus, sequestrum)
- staphyloma
- melanoma

2.5.9 The "blind" eye

- results from congenital disease (hypo-/dysplasia, e.g. hypoplastic papilla/retinal dysplasia/Collie eye anomaly/brain disease [portocaval shunt])
- results from trauma
- results from intoxication (plants/organophosphates/lead/quinolone/antibiotics in the cat)
- results from deficiency disease (taurine/vitamin A/vitamin E)
- glaucoma, excavation papilla
- anterior and/or posterior uveitis
- cataract/lens luxation
- retinal degeneration/atrophy
- chorioretinitis (high blood pressure/infection/immune disease/etc.)
- retinal detachment
- sudden acquired retinal degeneration
- results from acquired optic disc/nerve/brain abnormality (inflammation/neoplasia)

Literature

1. STADES, F.C. & BOEVÉ, M.H.: Ogen. In: Anamnese en lichamelijk onderzoek bij gezelschapsdieren. Ed.: A. Rijnberk & H.W. de Vries, Stuttgart, G. Fischer, pp. 243, 1993.

2. BOEVÉ, M.H., STADES, F.C. & DJAJADININGRAT-LAANEN, S.C.: Ogen. In: Anamnese en lichamelijk onderzoek bij gezelschapsdieren. Ed.: A. Rijnberk & F.J. van Sluijs, Bohn Stafleu van Lochem, Houten, pp. 211–240, 2005.

3. GELATT, K.N.: Examination of the eye. JAAHA. Proc. **37**: 326, 1970.

4. RUBIN, L.F.: Auriculopalpebral nerve blocks as an adjunct to the diagnosis and treatment of ocular inflammation in the horse. JAVMA **144**: 1387, 1964.

5. VEITH, L.A., CURE, T.H. & GELATT, K.N.: The Schirmer tear test in cats. Mod. Vet. Pract. **51**: 48, 1970.

6. STADES, F.C, BEIJER, E.G.M. & HARTMANN, E.G.: Use of lysozyme test in the diagnosis of keratoconjunctivitis sicca in dogs and cats. Tijdschr. Diergeneesk. **101**: 1141, 1976.

7. WILLIAMS, R.D., MANNING, J.P. & PEIFFER, R.L.: The Schirmer tear test in the equine: Normal values and the contribution of the gland of the nictitating membrane. J. Equine Med. Surg. **3**: 117, 1979.

8. GELATT, K.N.: Vital staining of the canine cornea and conjunctiva with rose bengal. JAAHA **8**: 17, 1972.

9. HAMOR, R.E., ROBERTS, S.M., SEVERIN, G.A. et al.: Evaluation of results for Schirmer tear tests conducted with and without application of a topical anesthetic in clinically normal dogs of 5 breeds. Am. J. Vet. Res. **61**: 1422, 2000.

10. SAITO, A., IZUMISAWA, Y., YAMASHITA K. & KOTANI, T.: The effect of third eyelid gland removal on the ocular surface of dogs. Vet. Ophthalmol. **4**: 13, 2001.

11. MCLAUGHLIN, S.A., BRIGHTMAN, A.H., HELPER, L.C., PRIMM, N.D., BROWN, M.G. & GREELEY S.: Effect of removal of lacrimal and third eyelid glands on Schirmer tear test results in cats. Am. J. Vet. Res. **193**: 820, 1988.

12. BEECH, J., ZAPPALA, R.A., SMITH, G. & LINDBORG, S.: Schirmer tear test results in normal horses and ponies: effect of age, season, environment, sex, time of day and placement of strips. Vet. Ophthalmol. **6**: 251, 2003.

13. BIRICIK, H.S., OGUZ, H., SINDAK, N., GÜRKAN, T. & HAYAT, A.: Evaluation of the Schirmer and phenol red test for measuring tear secretion in rabbits. Vet. Rec. **156**: 485, 2005.

14. ABRAMS, K.L., BROOKS, D.E., FUNK, R.S. & THERAN, P.: Evaluation of the Schirmer tear test in clinically normal rabbits. Am. J. Vet. Res. **51**: 1912, 1990.

15. CELLO, R.M.: The use of conjunctival scrapings in the diagnosis and treatment of external diseases of the eye. 6th Gaines Vet. Symp. **6**: 22, 1956.

16. MILLICHAMP, N.J. & DZIEZYC, J.: Evaluation of the Tonopen applanation tonometer in dogs and horses. Trans. Am. coll. Vet. Ophthalmol. **19**: 39, 1988.

17. MILLER, P.E., PICKETT, J.P. & MAJORS, L.J.: In vivo and in vitro comparison of Mackay-Marg and Tonopen applanation tonometers in the dog and cat. **19**: 53, 1988.

18. GÖRIG, C., COENEN, R.T.I., STADES, F.C., DJAJADININ-GRAT-LAANEN, S.C. & BOEVÉ, M.H.: Comparison of the use of new handheld tonometers and established applanation tonometers in dogs. Am. J. Vet. Res. **67**: 1, 2006.

19. GÖRIG, C., SCHOENMAKER N.J., STADES F.C. & BOEVÉ M.H.: Evaluation of different tonometers in exotic animals. Vet. Ophthalmol. **8**(6): 430, 2005.

20. GELATT, K.N. & MACKAY, E.O.: Distribution of intraocular pressure in dogs. Trans Am. Coll. Vet. Ophthalmol. **28**: 13, 1997.

21. MILLER, P.E., PICKETT, J.P., MAJORS, L.J. & KURZMAN, I.D.: Evaluation of two applanation tonometers in cats. Am. J. Vet. Res. **52**: 1917, 1991.

22. MILLER, P.E., PICKETT, J.P. & MAJORS L.J.: Evaluation of two applanation tonometers in horses. Am. J. Vet. Res. **51**: 935, 1990.

23. POYER, J.F., GABELT, B. & KAUFMAN, P.L.: The effect of topical PGF2 alpha on uveoscleral outflow and outflow facility in the rabbit eye. Exp. Exe. Res. **54**: 277, 1992.

24. WAGNER, F., GÖRIG, C., HEIDER, H-J., *et al.*: Augenerkrankungen beim Meerschweinchen (*Cavia porcellus*). Teil 1: Anatomische und physiologische Besonderheiten, Untersuchungsgang, extraokuläre Erkrankungen. Tierärztliche Praxis **28**: 247, 2000.

25. MERMOUD, A., BAERVELDT, G., MINCKLER, D.S., LEE, M.B. & RAO, N.A.: Intraocular pressure in Lewis rats. Invest. Ophthalmol. Vis. Sci. **35**: 2455, 1994.

26. KORBEL, R. & BRAUN, J.: Tonometrie beim Vogel mit dem Tonopen XL. Tierärztliche Praxis **27**: 208, 1999.

27. MURPHY, C.J.: Raptor Ophthalmology. Compend. Contin, Educ. Pract. Vet. **9**: 241, 1987.

28. MIKAELIAN, I., PAILLET, I. & WILLIAMS, D.: Comparative use of various mydriatic drugs in kestrels (*Falco tinnunculus*). Am. J. Vet. Res. **55**: 270, 1994.

29. DONOVAN, E. F. & WYMAN, M.: Fundus photography of the dog and cat by means of the Noyori hand fundus camera. JAVMA **25**: 865, 1964.

30. GELATT, K. N., HENDERSON, J.D., JR. & STEFFEN, G.R.: Fluorescein angiography of the normal and diseased ocular fundi of the laboratory dog. JAVMA **169**: 980, 1976.

31. GELATT, K.N. & LADDS, P.W.: Gonioscopy in dogs and cats with glaucoma and ocular tumors. J. Small Anim. Pract. **12**: 105, 1971.

32. CARTER, J. D.: Orbital venography, J. Am. Vet. Radiol. Soc. **13**: 43, 1972.

33. LECOUTEUR, R. A. *et al.*: Indirect imaging of the canine optic nerve, using metrizamide (optic thecography). Am J. Vet. Res. **43**: 1424, 1982.

3 Diagnostics and Therapeutics for Eye Diseases

3.1 Introduction

The majority of ophthalmological drugs are administered topically. This route guarantees the highest levels of drug for the conjunctiva, cornea, and the anterior chamber. The use of the systemic route may be beneficial for the deeper parts of the eye. Parenteral or oral administration of drugs is used only in special cases, e.g. to treat infections (antibiotics), glaucoma (dichlorphenamide, glycerin, mannitol), inflammation (corticosteroids), hypertension (amlodipine, enalpril) or KCS (pilocarpine). Only biphasic agents with a good distribution coefficient can penetrate into the globe when administered topically, with only the non-ionized fraction being able to penetrate.[1,2,3,4] Penetration is generally better when the globe is affected by inflammatory processes. Other essential properties of a topical medication are a smooth consistency (artificial tears, gel, oil, or highly liquid ointment), isotonicity, a pH similar to tears, and sterility. If an adjuvant is necessary, its penetrance must be high and it should not cause allergies or other types of irritation.

When drugs are administered topically, local resorption will take place, thus systemic side effects may also occur.[5] Drugs are drained to the nose via the lacrimal drainage system (especially eye drops), pass through the naso- and oropharynx, and are finally swallowed.

Note: the possible toxic side effects in very small animals caused by the swallowing and licking, mainly of eye drops.

Ophthalmic drugs may also either diffuse directly into the vascular system of the conjunctiva or reach the circulatory system via the cornea or sclera, and thus the aqueous humor.

Local administration of drugs can be performed as follows:

3.1.1 Into the conjunctival sac

Before the drug is given, any mucus or purulent exudate should be removed from the conjunctival sac. The exudate can first be dissolved with 10% acetylcysteine. The conjunctival sac is then irrigated from the lateral side (Plate 3.1) with 0.9% NaCl solution at body temperature. Pekingese dogs and cats usually detest such irrigations and they should not be used in these animals unless the exudate is abundant. After irrigation, the drug is administered in the following manner: the tube(s) and/or dropper bottle(s) are opened and put aside ready for use. The patient is placed in a corner of the room. The head is held with one hand, the thumb being placed under the lower jaw and pressing the head upwards in such a way that the gaze is directed towards the ceiling; this results in a doll's eye reaction, rolling the eye downwards and exposing the dorsal bulbar conjunctiva. The upper lid is raised with the middle and/or index finger of the same hand. Afterwards a drop of liquid or ointment is dropped onto the eyeball from a height of 2–3 centimeters above the eye (Plate 3.2). Eye ointment should melt at body heat and not be spread over the cornea by hand.

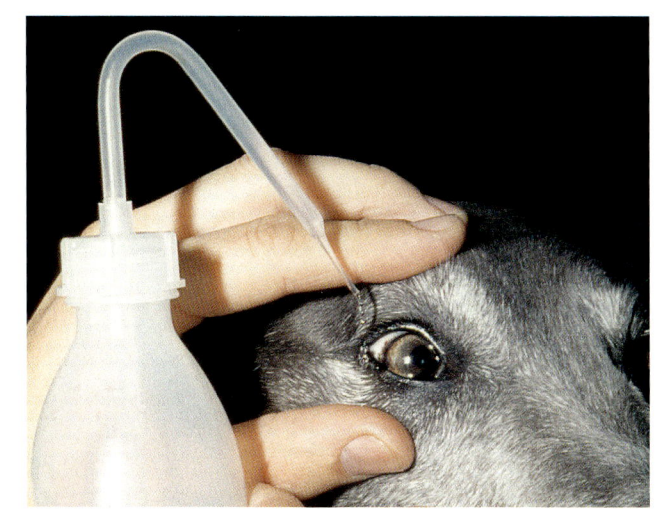

Plate 3.1:
Conjunctival flush with 0.9% hand-warm saline. The stream is directed on the globe from the dorsolateral. Under no circumstances should the opening of the flushing bottle be contaminated by the hairs around the eye.

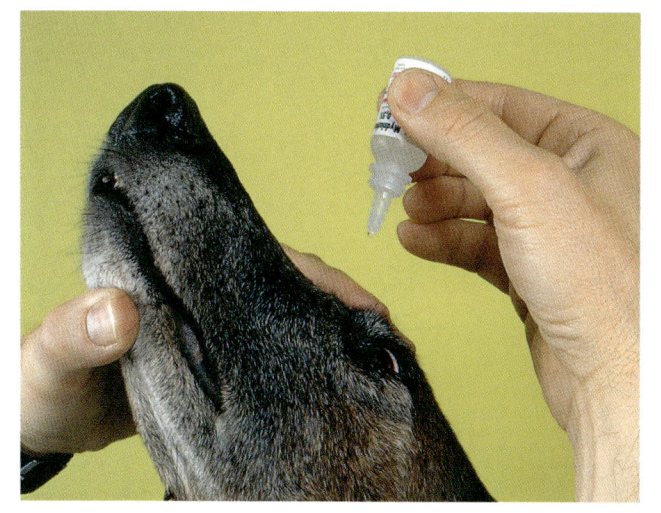

Plate 3.2:
The application of eye drops in a dog's eye. The head is lifted upwards in such a way that the gaze is directed to the ceiling. The upper lid is raised and the drop of liquid or ointment is dropped onto the eyeball. Care should be taken to avoid touching the hairs around the eye, because dirt and/or bacteria can be aspirated into the bottle.

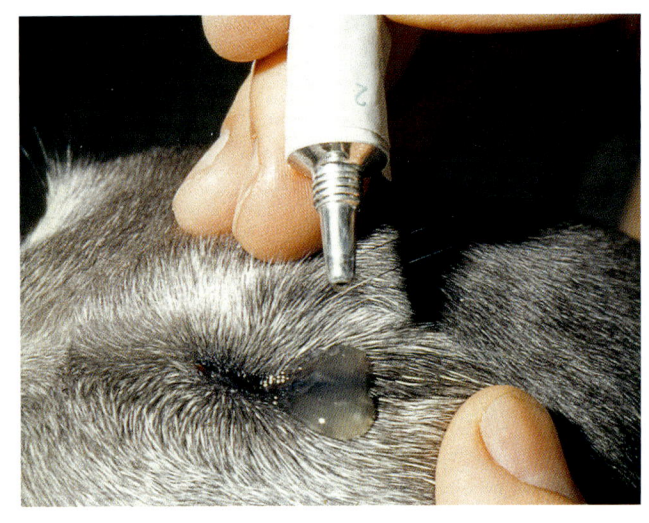

Plate 3.3:
Incorrect way of applying eye drops or ointment. Also, if too much of the drug is applied, the surplus will end up on the lid margins.

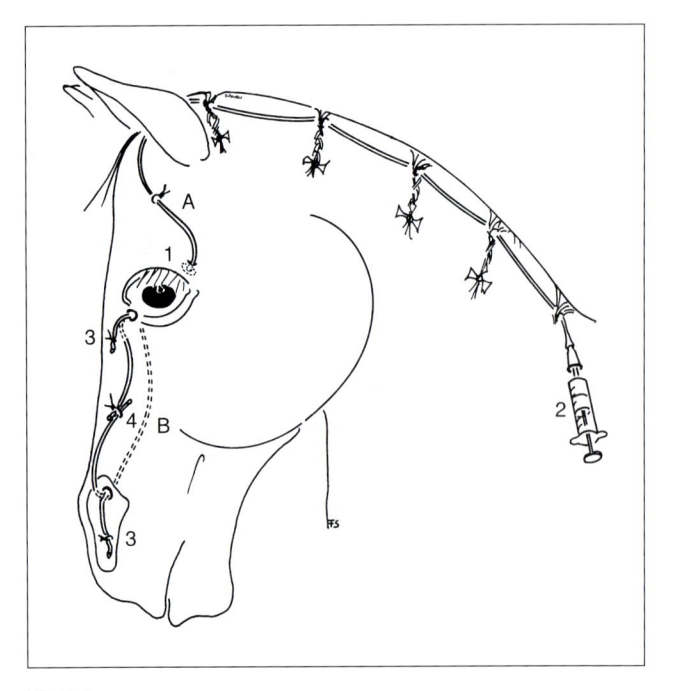

Fig. 3.1:
A. subpalpebral medication tube placement for the horse for the topical application of eye drops or ointments into the dorsal fornix (1). The medication is introduced through a syringe (2). The alternative nasal technique, via the nasolacrimal duct (3).
B. Catheterization of the nasolacrimal system in the horse. Silicon tubing can be sutured in place in the medial canthus and in the opening of the nose (3) or the two ends can be sutured together, halfway between these points (4).

Care should always be taken to avoid touching the hairs around the eye with the tip of the irrigation or dropper bottle, because hair and dirt can be aspirated into the tip, thus contaminating the contents (Plate 3.3). Ophthalmic drugs usually contain a preservative; however they should not be used any later than 1 month after opening.

The ventral cul-de-sac is used in large animals. Three millimeters of eye ointment may be applied directly to the bulbar conjunctiva and allowed to melt due to the warmth of the eye. The patient should be allowed to blink, but the eye should not be rubbed. Large animals do not always allow topical application of drugs. In such cases, a syringe with a thin, broken, blunt cannula can be used to squirt the eye drops into the conjunctival sac. Also, a tubing system can be introduced via a sufficiently large, sharp cannula through the lid skin above the eye (Fig. 3.1 A; Plate 3.4). Before introducing the tubing, small holes are cut in the tube, in the part that will be positioned in the fornix, thus enabling the drug to reach the conjunctival sac. The tubing is attached along the mane crest to the shoulder area by suturing or using the mane itself. From there, the drug can be applied by the use of a syringe or infusion pump.[6] Nowadays, commercial subpalpebral lavage systems are available with a special footplate. They can be placed either in the dorsolateral conjunctival sac or in the medioventral conjunctival sac where the nictitating membrane will protect the cornea (Fig. 3.1 A, Plate 3.4).

An alternative route is via a urine catheter (diameter 3–5 mm), which is introduced into the ostium of the nasolacrimal duct in the nose and fixed onto the ridge of the nose (Fig. 3.1 B).

Either eye ointments or eye drops may be used. Drops are simpler to administer and have less influence on vision. Their duration of action, however, is very brief (about 5 minutes). Two drops have the same duration of action as a single drop and they are more likely to flow over the lid edge onto the skin, so there is no advantage to the use of more than one drop. Drops should be clear solutions; suspensions are less suitable. Drops have a more lubricating and soothing effect and a longer contact time (7–10 minutes) when they are viscous, i.e. based on artificial tears or gel or oil.

Eye ointments are active for a longer time than drops (about 15 minutes, e.g. useful during the night) and are transported less easily to the nose. The ointment's greasy/viscous vehicle has a better soothing and lubricating effect, which is an advantage in such disorders as entropion or distichiasis. More of the vehicle will remain in the conjunctival sac, resulting in a discharge; thus a yellow ointment will produce a yellow discharge (the owner has to be informed!). When ointments and drops are used in combination, both should have an

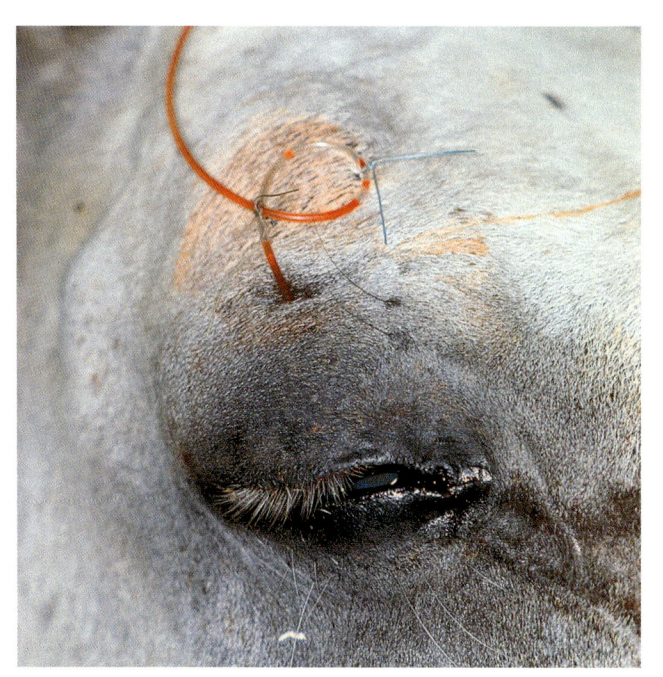

Plate 3.4:
Horse with a subpalpebral lavage and medication application system. The silicon tubing device ends in the upper fornix. The other end is fixed in the crest. Drugs can be administered from that entrance to the conjunctival sac (see Fig. 3.1 and Plate 6.12).

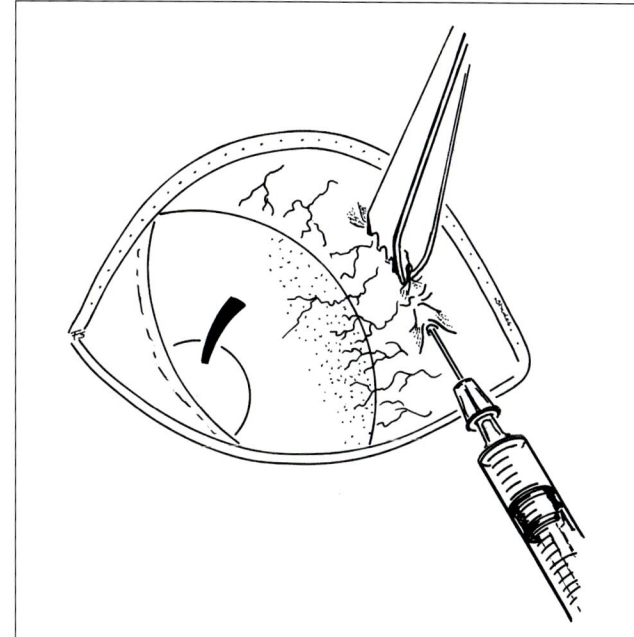

Fig. 3.2:
Subconjunctival injection. The bulbar conjunctiva may be lifted by Graefe's forceps. The cannula is injected from ventral.

oily base. If this is not possible, aqueous drops should be administered before an oil or an ointment. A minimum of five minutes should then elapse between medications.

3.1.2 Subconjunctival

Subconjunctival injections (Fig. 3.2) are generally tolerated quite well as long as no more than 1 ml of liquid is used. Absorption into the globe via the sclera is good and of relatively long duration. However, subconjunctival injections should only be used when there is absolute certainty regarding the diagnosis and treatment, as they cannot be reversed. Before an injection is made, the eye is anesthetized locally. Patients are sedated before the injection if they are uncooperative or if the eye is painful (e.g. uveitis). The best procedure is to use a short cannula of 3- to 4.5-mm diameter on a short syringe. The syringe is evacuated with the palm of the hand. The cannula is inserted through the lateral conjunctiva from the ventral side (if the patient retracts, it will be upwards), with the hands relaxed and in contact with the patient's head. If necessary, a small fold of conjunctiva is lifted up first with a forceps. Indications include keratitis pannosa, granulomas of the cornea and sclera, (e.g. episcleritis), uveitis, and treatment following intraocular surgery.

3.1.3 Retrobulbar

Retrobulbar injections are used rarely. They can, for example, be used for retrobulbar anesthesia.

3.1.4 Intraocular

Injection into the anterior chamber or into the vitreous is used almost exclusively as a last resort. It should only be performed by veterinarians specializing in ophthalmology. A possible indication is panophthalmia. Intraocular gentamycin injections directly in the vitreous will result in a vast iridocyclitis, thus lowering the IOP. These injections are very painful and not in the direct interest of the patient, which is ethically not outweighed by the cosmetic appeal to the owner in that the globe is retained, unless all other treatments fail and the animal's systemic health does not allow enucleation.

3.1.5 General rules

The following are general rules for the use of ocular medications:
1. There should be a thorough clinical examination to identify and remove any irritating factors and provide a basis for the choice of medication.
2. Exudates and other residues (e.g. ointment) should be dissolved with acetylcysteine and/or removed with 0.9% NaCl solution prior to medication, thus preventing dilution, inactivation, or antagonism of the selected agent.[7]
3. The nutritional condition of both the patient and the local tissue should be optimal and must be corrected if necessary. Vitamins such as A and C are important for the cement substance of the cornea.[8] Vitamin A deficiency may cause xerophthalmia and night blindness. In cats, taurine is an essential amino acid, functioning as a neurotransmitter. Vitamin E (α-tocopherol) deficiency may cause retinopathies in the dog.
4. Irritation of the eye by hairs should be reduced by application of a neutral oil or ointment (e.g. vitamin A oil or ointment).
5. Infections should either be prevented or treated initially with antimicrobials, hereafter referred to as "initial choice" antimicrobials (e.g. chloramphenicol, fusidic acid, chlorhexidine). A change to a specific antibiotic may be indicated when there is clear evidence of a specific infectious agent (e.g. gram-stained smear or a melting corneal ulcer) or as a result of culture and sensitivity testing. These antimicrobials are referred hereafter as "specific choice" antimicrobials
6. Signs of pain are often due to ciliary muscle spasm and are best counteracted by atropine, which suppresses the ciliary spasm (cycloplegia). Atropine or other mydriatics are contraindicated if there are any signs of glaucoma. Local anesthetics inhibit corneal re-epithelization; therefore, their use as painkillers must be considered as being a professional mistake. They are only used as an aid to diagnosis.

If there is little or no response to treatment, the cause may be due to factors related to:

1. The patient: such as impairment of the immune system, the patient's environment, poor compliance, side effects, or a wrong diagnosis.
2. The veterinarian and the owner: because of an incorrect diagnosis, alarming side effects, or the unwillingness or incapability of the owner to administer the drugs correctly (non-compliance).
3. The drug itself: because it is the wrong drug, is given too early or too late, or at the wrong intervals, or in a dosage that is too high or too low, or because the etiologic agent is resistant, the tissue accessibility is poor, a combination of drugs prevents penetration of one of the drugs (watery eye drops instilled after an ointment), antagonisms (sulfa-pH), or failing penetration of the drug (sulfa on purulent discharge).

3.2 Ocular therapeutic agents

For the veterinarian, the most important ocular therapeutic agents are the following:

3.2.1 Vasoconstrictors

1. Epinephrine (=adrenaline) 0.1–1% drops or injection: (mostly α-adrenergic) to stop minor hemorrhages. Epinephrine 1%, buffered. May also be used as a diagnostic and palliative agent in Horner's syndrome. Also used as an intraocular mydriatic.
2. Phenylephrine 2.5–15% drops: (α-adrenergic), to stop hemorrhages. Phenylephrine 10%: moderately powerful mydriatic. May also be used as a diagnostic and palliative agent in Horner's syndrome.

3.2.2 Antihistamines (nowadays mostly replaced by corticosteroids)

1. Antazoline 0.5% drops: vasoconstrictor in conjunctivitis.
2. Naphazoline 0.1% drops: as 1.
3. Cromoglicic acid drops: 2–4 times daily. Stabilizes mast cells, prevents release of histamine, etc. Allergic conjunctivitis. Effectiveness in dog and cat not clear.

3.2.3 Antiglaucoma agents

3.2.3.1 Miotics. Facilitating drainage of aqueous

a) Short-acting miotics (parasympathomimetics, direct acting)

1. Pilocarpine 1–4% drops: 4 times daily. Side effects: irritation of the conjunctiva, exception: 0.5–2%, orally starting with one drop. Animals of 1–10 kg: 0.5%; 10–20 kg: 1%; above 20 kg: 2%. In KCS, stimulation of the lacrimal glands. May be increased from one drop up to a maximum of 3–4 drops, 3–4 times daily, provided that the patient eats properly and does not vomit.
2. Acetylcholine 1% injection: potent miotic, for intraocular surgery, induces instant miosis.

b) Long-acting miotics (parasympathomimetics, indirect acting)
Irreversible cholinesterase inhibitors.
1. Ecothiophate iodine 0.06–0.2% drops: 1–2 times daily. Very potent miotic, in cases of acute glaucoma. Side effects: vomiting, diarrhea, panting. Especially in low-body-weight patients resorbed via nasopharynx. Not available in the EU; in future possibly as gel.
2. Fluostigmine 0.01% (oil base): alternative to pilocarpine.
3. Demecarium bromide 0.25–0.5%: alternative to 1. Not available in the EU; in future possibly as gel.

3.2.3.2 Moderating production of aqueous: carbonic anhydrase inhibitors

1. Dichlorphenamide tablets: 0.5–2.5 mg/kg, 4 times daily. Starting with a maximum of 2.5 mg/kg, reducing to 0.5–2 mg/kg after a few days. Side effects: diuretic effect with increased excretion of Na^+, K^+ and HCO_3^-, causing drowsiness, vomiting, and diarrhea. The potassium can be substituted using powder or effervescent tablets (resorption from bananas is too low).
2. Acetazolamide tablets and I.V.: 0.5–2.5 mg/kg, 3 times daily. Side effects: as 1, but more pronounced. I.V. for direct lowering of the IOP.
3. Ethoxyzolamide tablets: 1.0–2.5 mg/kg, 4 times daily. Side effects as 1.
4. Methazolamide tablets: 1.0–2.0 mg/kg, 3 times daily. Side effects as 1.
5. Dorzolamide[9] 2% drops: 3 times daily, pH 5.6. Side effects: conjunctival hyperemia, blepharitis.
6. Brinzolamide[10] 1% drops: 2–3 times daily; pH 7.5, because of this less irritating to the cornea than dorzolamide. No proven effect in glaucoma in the cat.

3.2.3.3 Osmotic agents[11]

1. Mannitol 20% solution: 1–5 ml/kg/24 hours, strictly I.V. Do not give water to the patient for 1 hour after administration.
2. Isosorbide 50% solution: 1–1.5 g/kg/24. For direct lowering of the IOP. Not registered in the EU.
3. Glycerol (glycerine) P.O.: 0.1–0.6 ml/kg, 4–6 times daily, in acute attacks of glaucoma and not for long term antiglaucoma therapy. Do not give water to the patient for 1 hour after administration.

3.2.3.4 Other agents used to reduce ocular pressure

1. Epinephrine (= adrenaline) 1% (buffered): reduces IOP by both alpha- and beta-adrenergic effects, and may cause mydriasis at the same time. Indications: occult glaucoma and combinations of uveitis and glaucoma. Side effects: slight reddening of tears may occur immediately after administration.
2. Dipivalyl epinephrine (propine) 0.1%: a pro-drug which converts to epinephrine when it passes through the cornea. Provides the same mechanism for reduction of IOP as epinephrine. Is more stable and more slowly resorbed than epinephrine, therefore longer acting.
3. Timolol[12] 0.25–6%: beta-blocking action, reduces IOP with only a minor effect on pupil size (slight miosis).
4. Other beta-blockers: other beta-blockers such as: levobunolol, optipropanol, metipranolol, betaxolol and arteolol, are alternatives to 3.
5. Latanoprost 0.0025–0.005% drops: 1–2 times daily (at least in the evening). Very powerful miotic in acute glaucoma (use in cats less well known). Prostaglandin analogue, which can be used alone or in combination of other antiglaucoma agents. Side effects: punctate keratitis, iris pigmentation.
6. Bimatoprost[13,14] 0.03% drops: potent miotic in acute glaucoma (use in cats less well known).
7. Travoprost 0.004% drops: potent miotic in acute glaucoma (use in cats less well known).
8. Apraclonidine[15] 0.5% drops: 3 times daily. Inhibits the aqueous production, selective alpha-2-adrenergic agonist, lowers blood pressure and IOP. Can be administered as prophylactic for postoperative increase of the IOP (e.g. after lens extraction). Side effects: conjunctival hyperemia, miosis, bradycardia; vomiting in cat.
9. Brimonidine 0.2% drops: 2 times daily. As apraclonidine.
10. Combinations: e.g. of timolol and dorzolamide, or pilocarpine (2%) und epinephrine.

3.2.4. Mydriatics

Side effects: profuse salivation, foaming, particularly eye drops in cats and brachycephalic dogs. The owner should be warned so that they continue to medicate.

1. Atropine 0.5–1% drops or ointment: 1–4 times daily, duration of action 3–10 days, therapeutic. When the signs of uveitis decline: 1–2 times daily. If salivation is expected, the use of ointment is preferred; exception: drops used as diagnostic agent in puppies and kittens and animals with such disorders as congenital cataract and persistent pupillary membrane. Before lens extraction, topically if pre-operative mydriasis is indicated. Ocular pain is caused in many causes by spasm of the ciliary muscle, even in conditions affecting the cornea. It can best be treated with atropine, which suppresses the ciliary spasm (cycloplegia).

Note: Contraindicated if sings of glaucoma or KCS are present. Exception: in normotensive horse eyes atropine does not influence the IOP, it may even lower the IOP in glaucomatous horse eyes. But only to be used when strictly monitored.

Indications: uveitis, corneal ulcers, with or without risk of perforation of the cornea and associated uveitis. If there is no evidence of anterior uveitis, atropine is not indicated because it does not reduce corneal pain itself and it reduces lacrimation with time.

Note: In low body weight animals toxic side effects possible!

Some rabbits produce atropinesterase, able to inactivate atropine; phenylephrine can be used as an alternative.

Ineffective in birds.

2. Tropicamide 0.5%: weak, short-acting mydriatic; used mostly as diagnostic agent, 15–20 minutes prior to examination.
3. Phenylephrine 10%: 60 and 15 minutes before lens extraction. Also used as diagnostic and palliative agent in Horner's syndrome.
4. Epinephrine 0.01–1% (= adrenaline; see 3.2.1 and 3.2.3.4): moderately powerful mydriatic. Used during lens extraction as an intraocular instant mydriatic (0.01–1.00%)

3.2.5 Antimicrobial agents

Topical agents. **Minimum 4 times daily**, sometimes more often, especially in the first three days of use.

3.2.5.1 "Initial choice" antibacterials
"Initial choice" antibacterials defined as antibiotics initially used without clear evidence of a specific agent, a stained smear or culture and sensitivity testing.
1. Chlorhexidine 0.1% drops: 4–6 times daily, broad spectrum, also as antimycotic; *Proteus* spp. and *Pseudomonas* spp. may be resistant. Indication: preoperative and in conjunctivitis. Side effect: local irritation.

2. Chloramphenicol 0.4–1% drops or ointment: 4–6 times daily. Bacteriostatic, broad spectrum, small molecule, penetrates easily into the globe. Also effective against common, low pathogenic eye infections. Indications: conjunctivitis, keratitis, uveitis. Side effect: hypersensitivity (very rare). Following extremely prolonged use in humans: irreversible aplastic anemia; not known to occur in animals, but reversible changes in the blood are possible. After use careful hand washing.
Note. Not to be used in production animals.
3. Fusidic acid 1% gel: Broad spectrum, against common gram-positive and gram-negative bacteria, not effective against *Pseudomonas* spp.
4. Bacitracin / gramicidin: against gram-positive bacteria, fewer problems with resistance.
5. Neomycin 0.5% drops: for gram-negative and some gram-positive bacteria, less effective against some *Pseudomonas* spp.
6. Polymyxin B 0.1–1% ointment / drops: bactericidal, specifically against gram-negative bacteria such as *Pseudomonas* spp. Plasmid inhibiter, thus resistance inhibiter. Does not penetrate the intact globe.
7. Combined preparations of 4–6: do not penetrate the intact globe; e.g. bacitracin / gramicidin-polymyxin-B; neomycin-polymyxin-B.

If there is evidence of a specific infectious agent (i.e. from the symptoms or after a gram-stained smear, culturing, or sensitivity tests), the following "specific choice" antimicrobial agents or combinations thereof may be used:
1. Povidone-iodine 0.1% drops: 4–6 times daily. Broad spectrum; *Proteus* spp. and *Pseudomonas* spp. may be resistant. Indication: conjunctivitis. Disadvantage: unstable, should be freshly prepared. Side effects: histamine-induced local irritation. 5% solution: very effective for preoperative use. Local lid skin disinfectant. One or two drops in the conjunctival sack, directly followed by removal with 0.9% NaCl solution.
2. Framycetin 0.5% drops: as for neomycin. Moderately effective against *Pseudomonas* spp.
3. Gentamycin 0.3% drops or ointment: as neomycin. Effective against *Pseudomonas* spp.
4. Chlortetracycline 1% and oxytetracycline 0.5% ointment or drops: broad spectrum and effective against Mycoplasma spp. and Chlamydia spp. (Chlamydophilae)
5. Cloxacillin: semi-synthetic penicillin.
6. Tobramycin 0.3%, drops or ointment: against gram-negative bacteria, including *Pseudomonas* spp., but less effective against Streptococci.
7. Norfloxacin / ciprofloxacin / ofloxacin 0.3% drops or ointment: last-effort broad spectrum antibiotic; e.g. in lytic corneal ulcers.
8. Combined preparations of 2–7.

Note: **Sulfonamides**. Systemic sulfonamides in dogs may result, within some weeks, in KCS. Alternatively, **olsalasine**, 20 mg/kg/day orally can be used as an alternative.

3.2.5.2 Antimycotics
1. *Natamycin* 5% suspension: effective against mycoses and saccharomycoses.
2. *Amphotericin B* 0.1–1% solution: topical, but only with an intact cornea.
3. *Miconazole and other imidazoles:* effective against mycoses and saccharomycoses.
4. *Chlorhexidine* 0.1% drops: 4–6 times daily. Broad spectrum disinfectant, also against mycoses und yeasts.
5. *Povidone-iodine* AT 0.1% drops: 4–6 times daily. Broad spectrum disinfectant against mycoses und yeasts.

3.2.5.3 Antiviral drugs: DNA-synthesis inhibitors[16,17]
1. *Trifluorothymidine* (TFT) 1–2% ointment: against DNA viruses like *Herpes* spp. First day every hour, there after 5 times daily.
2. *Idoxuridine* 0.1–0.2% ointment: against DNA viruses like *Herpes* spp. Effectiveness not well known.
3. *Adenine arabinoside* 3% ointment: against DNA viruses like *Herpes* spp. Effectiveness not well known.
4. *Acyclovir* (AS; vidarabine) 3%: against *Herpes spp*. Effectiveness not well known.
5. *Gamma-interferon* 4.000 iu/ml: 4 times daily; 1 drop, will inhibit intracellular virus synthesis.
6. *Alpha-lysine:*[18,19] 500 mg orally, 2 times daily. Competitive inhibition of arginine (essential for virus replication).
7. *Famcyclovir* 30 mg tablets: 2 times daily P.O. Possibly effective in chronic herpetic keratitis in cat.

Note: Veterinary antibiotic eye ointments and drops often come combined with corticosteroids. This fact, however, is often indicated on the packing in only very small print and without a clear warning. See corticosteroids (3.2.6).

3.2.6 Corticosteroids

Corticosteroids have a membrane-stabilizing effect, but also an inhibiting effect both with regard to inflammatory reactions and epithelialization of the cornea, and they potentiate proteolytic activity. Vitamin A oil may be administered at the same time for its epithelialtrophic effect.

Indications for the use of corticosteroids are:
- Inflammatory reactions such as allergy, chronic conjunctivitis, keratitis, uveitis, undesirable granulation.
- Postoperatively against corneal vascularization and edema, and fibrin formation in the anterior chamber.

Contraindications for the use of corticosteroids are:
- Epithelial lesions of the cornea; therefore, fluorescein staining should always be performed before use.
- Viral / mycotic / bacterial infections.
- Glaucoma.[20,21]
- Absence of a valid indication.

Administration
3.2.6.1 Topical, into the conjunctival sac
(listed in order of increasing anti-inflammatory action)
1. *Methylprednisolone,* 0.5%–1% drops (phosphate solution or acetate suspension): possibly irritating; ointment (acetate).
2. *Dexamethasone,* 0.1% drops: dexamethasone phosphate: superficial penetration; dexamethasone alcohol: deep penetration.
3. *Fluorometholone,* 0.1% drops (suspension).
4. *Betamethasone,* drops: very effective, but only superficial penetration. Indications: blepharitis, conjunctivitis, episcleritis and keratitis.

3.2.6.2 Subconjunctival
1. *Methylprednisolone:*[22] side effects – when in suspension the vehicle itself may cause inflammatory reactions.
2. *Flumethasone.*
3. *Dexamethasone.*

3.2.6.3 Oral
1. *Prednisolone:* 1–3 mg/kg, P.O., once daily, in the morning for 4–5 days, then every other day for 8–10 days; thereafter decreasing to half the dosage every other day, and so on until the prednisolone is stopped.
2. *Dexamethasone:* alternative to 1.

3.2.7 Non-steroidal anti-inflammatory drugs (NSAIDs)
3.2.7.1 Prostaglandin synthesis inhibitors[23,24,25]
1. *Carprofen* 20/50 mg tablets: dog 2 mg/kg, 2 times daily, for 3–5 days.
2. *Ketoprofen* 5/10/20 mg tablets: dog, 1 mg/kg/day; cat, ¼–½ mg/kg/day; for 3–5 days
3. *Meloxicam* 1.5 mg/ml oral suspension: dog, 0.1 mg/kg/day, for 3–5 days.
4. *Flunixin meglumine:* horse, 1 mg/kg/day, for 3–5 days. Against post-traumatic or non-traumatic uveitis.[26] Side effects: gastrointestinal ulceration and renal failure.
5. *Indomethacin* 1%: before/after lens extraction surgery, 4 times daily, topical. Side effects: corneal irritation.
6. *Flurbiprofen* 0.03%: 2–4 times daily, topical. Against uveitis.
7. *Ketorolac* 0.5%: 2–4 times daily, topical. Against uveitis.
8. *Diclofenac* 0.1% drops: 1–4 times daily, topical. Against (post-traumatic) uveitis.

3.2.8 Local anesthetics

Note: Diagnostic agents. Not to be administered by the patient's owner.

Local anesthetics reduce blinking activity, influence corneal nutrition, inhibit corneal epithelialization, and have an addictive effect (anesthesia dolorosa). Indications: diagnostic agent, minor surgical interventions of the conjunctiva and cornea (e.g. removal of foreign bodies), as a less deep level of general anesthesia is necessary. Allergic reactions are more likely with the ester group. Such allergic reactions also can easily be caused by the frequently used preservative benzalconium chloride.

1. ***Proparacaine*** (ester) 0.5% drops: low epitheliotoxicity, but also less anesthesia. Less stable after opening.
2. ***Oxybuprocaine*** 0.4% drops: shorter working than proparacaine or tetracaine.
3. ***Benoxinate hydrochloride*** (ester) 0.4% drops: identical to oxybuprocaine.
4. ***Tetracaine*** 0.5–2% drops.
5. ***Lidocaine*** (amide) 4% drops: initial burning sensation directly after use. Strong anesthesia, but also more epitheliotoxic. Not registered by the FDA in the USA yet.
6. ***Cocaine*** 0.5–4% drops: most toxic to the epithelium, but also the strongest anesthesia. Causes also vasoconstriction. Controlled drug!

Note: Ocular pain is caused in many cases by spasm of the ciliary muscle, even in conditions affecting the cornea. It can best be treated with atropine, which suppresses the ciliary spasm (cycloplegia).

3.2.9 Vitamins, epithelializing agents, and neutral agents

1. ***Vitamin A*** 15,000–60,000 IU, in drops, ointment, gel: 1–4 times daily. Supports epithelialization; the vehicle smoothes, lubricates, and shields. In pannus, an UV-light protection is suspected. Also used in KCS and retinal rod degeneration caused by vitamin A deficiency.
2. ***Vitamin C*** tablets: 50 mg once daily, orally. Important for the corneal cement substance.
3. ***Vitamin B_1*** tablets: 50 mg/kg once daily, P.O. In cats whose diet contains a large amount of fish; bilateral protrusion of the nictitating membrane could be a consequence of deficiency of this vitamin. Possibly also useful in Horner's syndrome
4. ***Vitamin E*** tablets: 5–10 mg/day orally. Deficiency can cause retinopathies.
5. ***Artificial tears*** drops, ointment: in general based on hydroxypropyl methylcellulose 1–2% or similar preparations. Treatment of KCS. These are also a good vehicle to increase the duration of action of other pharmaceuticals on the eyeball.
6. ***Hyprolose:*** 3.5 × 1.3 mm rods that are introduced into the ventral conjunctival sac where they slowly dissolve, thereby suppressing irritation. Treatment of KCS.

7. ***Viscoelastics:*** high viscosity "gel" for topical lubrication and moistening, and intraocular surgery. Protects corneal epithelium and endothelium, separates tissues, contains hemorrhage, lubricates, and keeps the anterior chamber in form. Contains hyaluronic acid or hydroxypropylmethylcellulose. For topical use e.g.: i-drop®: preservative free, long lasting lubricant and moistening agent in e.g. KCS.

3.2.10 Collyria

Always administer hand warm (approx. 37 °C). Irrigate from the lateral to the medial side, e.g. using a laboratory irrigator bottle (Plate 3.1). Remove excess moisture with paper tissue.
1. ***NaCl*** solution 0.9%: isotonic, neutral, irrigation solution.
2. ***$ZnSO_4$*** 0.1%: mildly astringent. Against chronic conjunctivitis.
3. ***Povidone iodine*** 2–5% buffered: for the conjunctival sac followed by irrigation with 0.9% NaCl.[27] Given pre-operatively to counteract contamination of the conjunctival sac and the lid skin. Use in a 1:20 dilution as irrigation solution against purulent conjunctivitis. Side effects: in some animals swelling of the skin and/or of the conjunctiva as sign of irritation directly after application or some minutes later.
4. ***EDTA*** 1–2% solution: against salivary crystals on the cornea after parotid duct transposition.

3.2.11 Other "drugs" for ocular use

3.2.11.1 Diagnostic agents

1. ***Fluorescein sodium*** 2% (strips or drops in single-dose package): for the diagnosis of corneal (only epithelial and stromal) lesions. *Pseudomonas* spp. and mycotic agents may grow in the drops.
2. ***Rose bengal:*** stains intact but non-vital epithelial cells in areas where the tear film has broken down. To be used only if the cornea does not show any lesions (fluorescein negative).
3. ***Tropicamide*** 0.5%: mydriasis after 15–20 minutes, active for 4–6 hours.
4. ***Homatropine*** 2–5%: mydriasis after 15–20 minutes, as tropicamide, but less active.
5. ***Atropine*** 0.5–1%: duration of action in animals over 6 months of age – up to 10 days. Drops or ointment: mydriasis after about 20 minutes. Only as a diagnostic agent in puppies, kittens, and animals with disorders such as congenital cataract and persistent pupillary membrane.
6. ***Cyclopentolate*** 0.5–1% drops: as tropicamide but less active. Side effects: conjunctival irritation.
7. ***Schirmer tear test (STT):*** sterile, standardized filter strips for measuring tear production.

3.2.11.2 Chemical cauterizing agents
1. Phenol, saturated solution: to activate indolent ulcers. The cauterized ulcer will whiten immediately upon application. Irrigate thoroughly after use.
2. Iodine tincture 2–4%: like phenol, but does not aid visualization (brown) of the cauterized area.

3.2.11.3 (Discharge-)dissolving agents
1. Acetylcysteine 5–10%; in ampoule as 10–20% solution: aspirate into syringe (and dilute 1:1 with NaCl 0.9%), close syringe air-tightly (anti-oxidation).[28] Instruct owner to give drops directly from that syringe and to close it again after use. Good purulent discharge-dissolving agent, e.g. in KCS and mucopurulent conjunctivitis. Proteolytic, against bacterial enzymes in aggressively deepening ulcers, especially when there is a softening or dissolution of the edges due to collagenase activity.
2. Tissue plasminogen activator 250 μg/ml: 0.2–0.3 ml in the anterior chamber for dissolving fibrin, hypopyon, and hyphema. Not to be used during or directly after hemorrhage.

3.2.11.4 Anti-hypertensive agents (in secondary retinopathy)
Against hypertension (most likely after renal, adrenal or thyroid disease):
1. Amlodipine: calcium antagonist; 0.625–1.25 mg/cat/day; dog: 0.1–0.2 mg/kg/day.
2. Atenolol: 0.5–0.65 mg/cat/day.
3. Enalapril: ACE inhibitor, less effective than amlodipine; 0.5 mg/kg/day. Alternatives: **Benazepril, Captopril.**

3.2.11.5 Other drugs used on the eye
1. Cyclosporine A 0.2% (ointment) to 2% (oil): 1–2 times daily, locally. T-cell inhibitor,[29] epithelialtrophic mechanism is not yet fully understood.[30]
Side effects: with topical use – irritation, conjunctival redness. Indicated in KCS, and as extra therapy in pannus and other granulomatous changes. Systemic side effects: nephrotoxic.
2. Tacrolimus 0.02% drops, suspension:[31] likely to be 10 × stronger than cyclosporine 2%. Alternative in cyclosporine-resistant KCS patients; as extra therapy in pannus and other granulomatous changes. Topical side effects not yet well known.
Note: Not yet registered for the use on the eye.
3. Pimecrolimus 1% drops: identical to tacrolimus.[32]
Note: Not yet registered for the use on the eye.
4. Butylcyanoacrylate: tissue glue, to cover and protect deep corneal ulcers. Apply in a very thin layer over the dried defect.

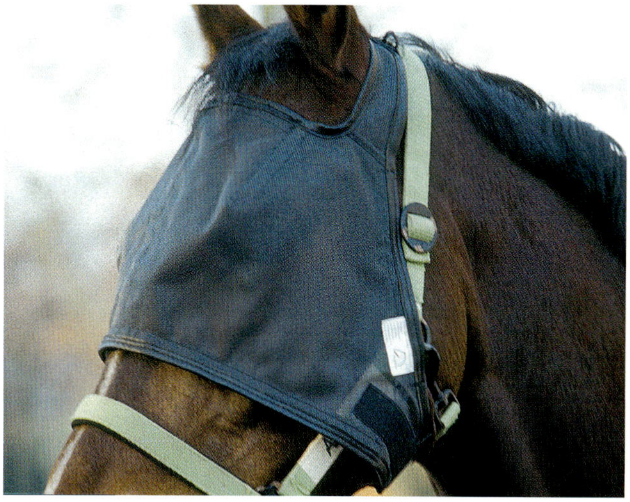

Plate 3.5:
Protecting fly net in a horse.

3.2.12 Radiation

Beta radiation, 500–1000 rads: penetrates about 2 mm into the tissue. For treatment of excessive granulation, keratitis pannosa, and neoplasia.

3.2.13 Protective devices

1. Elizabethan collars, goggles, protective hoods: to prevent self-mutilation or trauma caused by bumping against objects.
2. Fly net: to protect against insects (Plate 3.5).

3.3 Surgical possibilities

3.3.1 Anesthesia

If sedation and local anesthesia are insufficient or inadequate, general anesthesia is performed.

As premedication in dog and cat use e.g. medetomidine (0.01–0.05 μg/kg I.V.) in combination with propofol (10 mg/ml bolus, I.V. to effect). General anesthesia can be continued thereafter with inhalation anesthesia.

However, this type of anesthesia induces a distinct rotation of the globe and enophthalmos, which makes it less desirable for ocular or intraocular surgery. An advantage is the quiet and quick recovery (antidote: atipamezole).

In dogs, premedication is also possible after sedation with acepromazine (0.03–0.1 mg/kg) and methadone (0.5–1 mg/kg) (S.C., I.M., or I.V.).

Inhalation anesthesia in combination with a muscle relaxant (e.g. (cis)atracurium or norcuronium) is necessary to prevent rotation and enophthalmos, but this also necessitates artificial respiration.

Detomidine is very useful for examination or as premeditation in the horse.

3.3.2 Preparation of the operative field

The lid skin is usually shaved. The smaller "mini shave" is very suitable. The last row of eyelash-like hairs is cut using scissors with some ointment on the blades, so that the cut hairs will stick to the ointment. Afterwards, the conjunctival sac and the skin are washed copiously with hand-warm saline. The skin is then dried with gauze sponges. If intraocular surgery is to be performed and/or a contaminated conjunctival sac is expected, buffered povidone iodine solution 2–5% can be instilled and the washing repeated. Starting at the margins, the lids are penciled with povidone iodine solution. Care should be taken not to allow any iodine to reach the (other) eye. The globes should not be covered with neutral ointment, as practiced by anesthetists to prevent drying of the cornea during surgery. The greasing effect may make handling of the lids or globe almost impossible. Drying out of the eye surface may be prevented by the use of artificial tears.

3.3.3 Positioning on the operating table

The patient is positioned on the operating table with the head higher than the rest of the body. For lid surgery, the lid fissure has to be positioned more or less horizontally. For ocular or intraocular surgery, the limbal plane has to be positioned more or less horizontally. The positioning of the head is best carried out by using a vacuum pillow (be careful of sharp claws). The surgeon always works in a sitting position, with his/her hands resting on the animal's head, thus preventing the risk of uncontrolled movements and minimizing tremor. For surgery of the adnexa, the surgeon sits at the ventral side of the head. For ocular or intraocular surgery, the surgeon is generally positioned dorsolateral to the head.

Powerful, well-focused operating lights, a head-mounted light, or operating microscope lights are essential during ocular surgery.

3.3.4 Draping

Special soft, non slippery ocular drapes with an opening for the eye, or disposable drapes with a hole cut during surgery, can be used for eye surgery. The drapes may be fixed by towel clamps (Jones or Scheadel). During surgery, the drapes are fixed below the head, otherwise they may be pulled downwards by the surgeon's knees, thus influencing the shape of the lid fissure or position of the eye. The nictitating membrane and/or the globe may be fixed by stay sutures. The lid hairs and margins may also be covered by surgical plastic or the back part of a surgical glove. An eye speculum will fix the plastic or rubber to the lid opening. The rubber and also the gloves must be cleaned of powder to prevent inflammatory reactions, especially after intraocular surgery.

3.3.5 Magnification equipment

One of the most important factors for eye surgery is good magnification. For eyelid surgery x3–5 magnification is sufficient in most cases. For more subtle surgery of the lids or globe, or for intraocular surgery, a high quality (x5–6 magnification) operating loupe or an operating microscope (x5–27) is necessary.

3.3.6 Surgical equipment

Depending on the type of operation, a basic eye set and special sets for surgery of the lacrimal system, eyelids, and globe, and for intraocular surgery should be available.

3.3.7 Suture material

Atraumatic suture material is always used for eye surgery. For lid skin, which may be extremely leathery, especially in cats, 10- to 20-mm, ⅜–½ circle, extra-sharp-pointed round, or micro-pointed, or extra-fine cutting needles are used. For the cornea, very sharp spatula or taper needles are necessary.

If there is any likelihood of post-surgical irritation of the cornea by the suture material (e.g. recurrence of entropion), soft material such as silk should be used. If strength is important, 5-0 or 6-0 mono- or polyfilament nylon (temporary tarsorrhaphy, nictitating membrane flap, etc.) is needed, while for corneal suturing 8-0 or 9-0 monofilament can be used. For absorbable material, polyglactin 910 or polyglycol acid can be used (enucleation 4-0, conjunctiva 7-0, 8-0, cornea, monofilament, 8-0 to 10-0, etc.). If there is a high risk of infection, monofilament nylon is used (blepharoplasties 6-0), or in extreme cases 6-0, 7-0, or 8-0 steel can be used.

3.3.8 Hemostasis

Hemorrhage may be stopped by suturing or (bipolar) electrocoagulation. Topical application of 0.1–1% epinephrine eye drops may stop bleeding, too. For hemorrhages of very fine vessels, special ophthalmic (battery) microcautery units are available. Cautery will cause a local area of necrosis and for this reason one should not cauterize too quickly or too much. Diffuse hemorrhages will usually stop spontaneously. To avoid delay caused by waiting for the hemorrhage to stop spontaneously, cutting should be done from the lowest to the highest point.

3.3.9 Cryosurgery

In cryosurgery, use is made of the destructive effect of freezing the intracellular water, which results in rupture of the cell membranes in unwanted tissues. In general, two cycles of rapid freezing and slow, spontaneous thawing are used. The tissues are frozen to at least −25 °C by the use of carbon dioxide or nitrous oxide.

Cryosurgery may be of use for the destruction of reactive granulation tissue, hair follicles, parts of the ciliary body in case of glaucoma, or the destruction of several types of neoplasia.

Cryosurgery is also used in retinal detachment surgery to induce local inflammation, thus causing scar tissue bridges between the loose retina and the uvea.

Furthermore, the cryotechnique is used for the removal of the lens in intracapsular lens extraction (lens luxation). The tip of the extractor is frozen to the capsule and the contents of the lens, thus enabling the extraction of the lens *in toto*, without breaking its capsule; otherwise, the lens proteins could be released into the anterior chamber and induce anterior uveitis.

3.3.10 Laser techniques

Laser techniques can be used for destroying tissues such as posterior capsular after-cataract, ciliary body tissue in glaucoma, or neoplasia. The laser is also used in retinal detachment surgery, inducing local inflammation with secondary scar formation, thus causing bridges between the retina and the choroid.

Literature

1. BURSTEIN, N. L. & ANDERSON, J.A.: Review: Corneal penetration and ocular bioavailability of drugs. J. Ocular Pharmacol. **1**: 309, 1985.
2. SHELL, J.W.: Pharmacokinetics of topically applied ophthalmic drugs. Surv. Ophthalmol. **26**: 207, 1982.
3. BENSON, H.: Permeability of the cornea to topically applied drugs. Arch. Ophthalmol. **91**: 313, 1974.
4. ROWLEY, R.A. & RUBIN, L.F: Aqueous humor penetration of several antibiotics in the dog. Am. J.Vet. Res. **3**: 43, 1970.
5. POLAK, B.C.P.: Drugs used in ocular treatment. In: Meylers' Side Effects of Drugs, 10th edition. Ed.: M.N.G. Dukes, Amsterdam, Elsevier, pp 875–886, 1984.
6. LAVACH, J.D.: Large animal ophthalmology. St. Louis, Mosby, pp 25–26, 1990.
7. BERMAN, M. & DOHLMANN, C.: Collagenase inhibitors. Arch. Ophthalmol. **35**: 95, 1975.
8. TEI, M., SPURR-MICHAUD, S.J. *et al.*: Vitamin A deficiency alters the expression of mucin genes by the rat ocular surface epithelium. Invest. Ophthalmol.Vis. Sci. **41**: 82, 2000.
9. GELATT, K.N. & MACKAY, E.O.: Changes in intraocular pressure associated with topical dorsolamide and oral methazolamide in glaucomatous dogs.Vet. Ophthalmol. **4**: 61, 2001.
10. GRAY, H.E., WILLIS, A.M. & MORGAN, R.V.: Effects of topical administration of 1% brinzolamide on normal cat eyes. Vet. Ophthalmol. **4**: 185, 2003.
11. LORIMER, D.W., *et al.*: The effect of intravenous mannitol or oral glycerol on intraocular pressure in dogs. Cornell.Vet. **79**: 249, 1989.
12. WILKIE, D.A. & TATICUMSON, C.A.: Effects of topical administration of timolol maleate on intraocular pressure and pupil size in dogs. Am. J.Vet. Res. **52**: 432, 1991.
13. GELATT, K.N. & MACKAY, E.O.: Effect of different dose schedules of bimatoprost on intraocular pressure and pupil size in the glaucomatous beagle. Ocul. Pharmacol. Ther. **18**: 525, 2002.
14. BARTOE, J.T., DAVIDSON, H.J. *et al*: Effect of topical bimatoprost and unoprostone isopropyl on the intravascular pressure of normal cats. Trans. Am. Coll.Vet. Ophthalmol. **35**: 9, 2004.
15. MILLER, P.E. & RHOSIA, S.L.: Effects of topical administration of 0.5% apraclonidine on intraocular pressure, pupil size and heart rate in clinically normal cats. Am. J.Vet. Res. **57**: 83, 1996.
16. NASISSE, M.P., *et al.*: In vitro susceptibility of feline herpesvirus-1 to vidarabine, idoxuridine, trifluridine, acyclovir, or bromovinyl-deoxyuridine. Am. J.Vet. Res. **50**: 1672, 1989.
17. WEISS, R.C.: Synergistic antiviral activities of acyclovir and recombinant human leukocyte (alpha) interferon on feline herpesvirus replication. Am. J.Vet. Res. **50**: 1672, 1989.
18. MAGGS, D.J., NACISSE, M.P. & KASS, P.U.: Efficacy of oral supplimentation with L-lysine in cats latently infected with feline herpes virus. Am. J.Vet. Res. **64**: 37, 2003.
19. STILES, J. *et al.*: The effect of oral L-lysine on the course of feline herpes virus conjunctivitis. Trans. ACVO 2000, p. 30.

20. CHEN, C.L., GELATT, K.N. & GUM, G.G.: Serum hydrocortisone (cortisol) values in glaucomatous and normotensive Beagles. Am. J. Vet. Res. **41**: 1561, 1980.

21. GELATT, K.N. & MACKAY, E.O.: The ocular hypertensive effects of topical 0.1% dexamethasone in beagles with inherited glaucoma. J. Ocul. Pharmacol. Ther. **14**: 57, 1998

22. FISCHER, G.A.: Granuloma formation associated with subconjunctival of a corticosteroid in dogs. JAVMA **174**: 1086, 1979.

23. BRIGHTMAN, A.H., HELPER, L.C. & HOFFMANN, W.E.: Effect of aspirin on aqueous protein values in the dog. JAVMA **178**: 572, 1981.

24. YOSHITOMI, T. & YUSHI, I.: Effects of indomethacin and prostaglandins on the dog's iris sphincter and dilator muscles. Invest. Ophthalmol. Vis. Sci. **29**: 127, 1988.

25. KROHNE, S. & VESTRE, W.A.: Effects of flunixin meglumine and dexamethasone on aqueous protein values after intraocular surgery in the dog. Am. J. Vet. Res. **48**: 420, 1987.

26. REGNIER, A. *et al.*: Effect on flunixin meglumine on the breakdown of the blood-aqueous barrier following paracentesis in the canine eye. J. Ocul. Pharmacol. **2**: 165, 1986.

27. ROBERTS, S.M., SEVERIN, G.A. & LAVACH, J.D.: Antibacterial activity of dilute povidone-iodine solutions used for ocular surface disinfection in dogs. Am. J. Vet. Res. **47**: 1207, 1986.

28. COSTA, N.D. & SLATTER, D.H.: Potency of N-acetylcysteine as a collagenase inhibitor in pharmaceutical preparations. Effects of temperature and storage. Aust. Vet. J. **60**: 195, 1983.

29. KASWAN, R.L., SALISBURY, M.A. & WARD, D.A.: Spontaneous canine keratoconjunctivitis sicca: A useful model for human keratoconjunctivitis sicca. Treatment with cyclosporine eye drops. Arch. Ophthalmol. **107**: 1210, 1989.

30. YOSHIDA, A., FUJIHARA, T. & NAKATA, K.: Cyclosporin A increases tear fluid secretion via release of sensory neurotransmitters and muscarinic pathway in mice. Exp. Eye Res. **68**: 541, 1999.

31. BERDOULAY, A., ENGLISH, R.V. *et al.*: The effect of topical 0.02% Tacrolimus aqueous suspension on tear production in dogs with KCS. Trans. Am. Coll. Vet. Ophthalmol. **34**: 33, 2003.

32. OFRI, R., ALLGOEWER, I. *et al.*: Successful treatment of keratoconjunctivitis sicca (KCS) in dogs with pimecrolimus drops: a comparison with cyclosporin A (CyA) ointment. Trans. Am. Coll. Vet. Ophthalmol. **35**: 24, 2004.

4 Ocular Emergencies

4.1 Introduction

Ophthalmologic emergency patients can be divided into two main groups:
a) Trauma caused by direct or indirect injuries. Examples within this group include luxation of the globe as well as burns, or blunt, superficial or perforating trauma to the lids, conjunctiva, cornea, or the entire globe.
b) Ocular diseases which, because of their aggressiveness or rapid development (1–2 days), can lead to severe pain, loss of sight, or loss of the entire globe, and thus require direct treatment. Examples of these include retrobulbar processes;[1] aggressive ulcers with melting edges (see 10.6.3.2), which may perforate; anterior uveitis; glaucoma; lens luxation; and acute blindness due to such causes as posterior uveitis, retinal detachment, and involvement of the optic papilla and nerve by hemorrhage, inflammation, or neoplasia. These diseases are discussed in the subsequent relevant sections of this book, organized on a morphologic and pathogenetic basis.

Trauma to the bony orbit, globe, and/or adnexa can be caused by foreign bodies or by direct or indirect injuries in the form of moderate or severe blows (automobile accidents or even punishing blows from the owner), or from being stabbed, shot, bitten, or scratched.

4.2 Luxation and proptosis of the globe

Luxation of the globe refers to a dislocation of the globe through lid fissures, as proptosis can be defined as frontal dis-

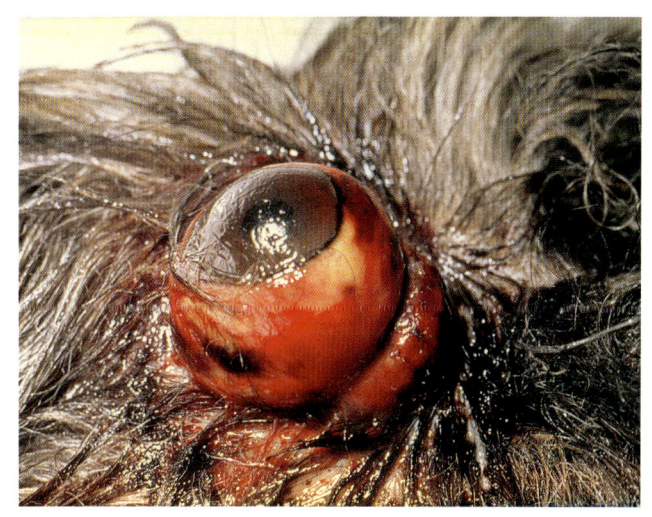

Plate 4.2:
Luxation or proptosis of the globe approximately 20 minutes after a car accident (OD, dog).

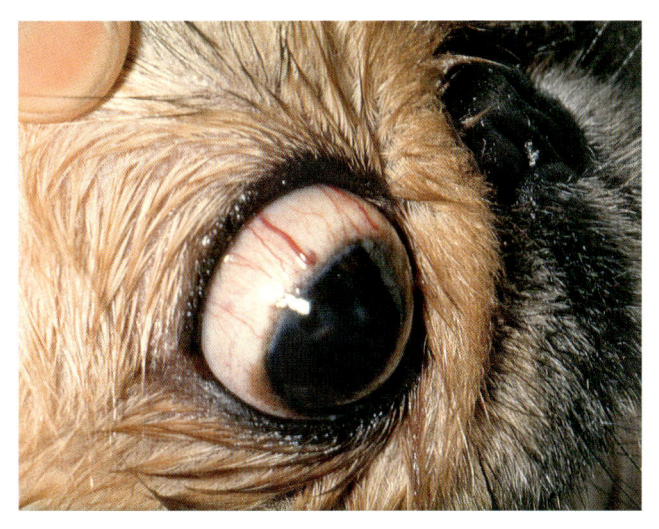

Plate 4.1:
Provoked luxation (proptosis) of the globe in a Pekingese. Pekingese and Shih Tzu should be restrained by the owner, taking care that no undue pressure is exerted on the head, resulting in forced propulsion of the globe. The length of the fissure (usually 30–34 mm) and the tension of the orbicular muscle prevent spontaneous replacement. The scleral, conjunctival, and venous drainage is blocked, which causes additional swelling.

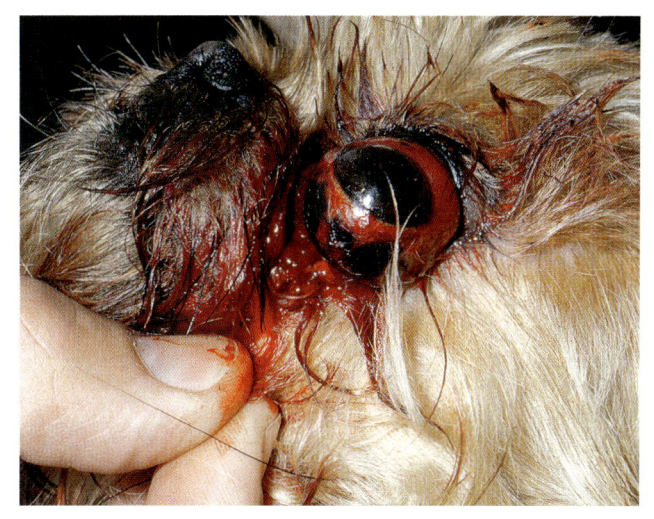

Plate 4.3:
Luxation or proptosis of the globe approximately 40 minutes after a car accident. Note: ventrally to the globe is free blood, indicating tissue rupture. In this patient, almost all of the eye stalk had been torn away, making reposition senseless.

placement of the globe in general. Luxation of the globe (Plate 4.1–4.3) is one of the ophthalmologic and veterinary emergencies. The luxation is usually caused by an automobile accident or injury from another animal such as bites from another dog or kicks from a horse. The direct contact with the automobile bumper and/or compression of the zygomatic arch can force the globe forward so that it is luxated out of the orbit and rostral to the palpebral fissure. If the eye is bitten, it may be pulled outwards by a canine tooth. The arterial supply remains intact but the venous drainage is blocked. If the lid fissure is of normal length (in dogs with macroblepharon there may be proptosis but rarely luxation), the globe will be blocked outside the lid fissure, the lid margins will entropionize, and will stick with their dry, hairy outer surface behind the globe. The conjunctiva becomes congested and thus quickly swells and goes intensively red. The cornea is severely damaged and the optic nerve irreversibly damaged either immediately or within a few hours. Brachycephalic breeds such as the Pekingese and the Shih Tzu deserve separate attention here. In these breeds the globe lies in such a shallow orbit and the opening between the eyelids is so large that the globe can luxate through the opening with ease (Plate 4.1). Hyperactivity or a tantrum of the dog can be enough to cause luxation. The globe can also luxate easily if the animal requires excessive restraint on the examination table. Such dogs should be restrained by the owner with the hand around the animal's neck, taking care that undue pressure is not exerted to the head resulting in a forced propulsion of the globe. These dogs should never be held by the skin of the neck.

Therapy: As a first step, the eyelids must be immediately pulled back over the globe. Unfortunately, an owner seldom succeeds in doing this. If immediate replacement of the eye in the orbit is impossible, the globe should be protected against further damage and drying by applying, for example, salad oil. The patient should then be brought as soon as possible to the veterinarian. During transport, self-mutilation must be prevented by fixation.

The veterinarian should first inspect the eye for total rupture of the muscles or the optic nerve, especially when free blood is present (Plate 4.3). Thereafter, the eye is protected with "initial choice" antibiotic and lacrilube ointments. If the patient is still somewhat dazed by the accident, a lateral canthotomy (incision with a pointed scalpel) can be performed immediately (Fig. 4.1). Otherwise, the patient is anesthetized (if its condition allows it) and then the canthotomy is performed. If minimal inflammatory sequelae are present and no traumatic myotomies are manifest, canthotomy is sometimes not necessary. The eyelids are then pulled over the globe by the use of two Allis forceps or two strabismus hooks. Sometimes, gentle pressure must be applied to the globe via a moistened cotton bud.

A temporary tarsorrhaphy is performed by placing two or three horizontal mattress sutures (4-0 or 5-0, cutting, micropoint or round body needle), using infusion set tubing or sterile wide rubber bands to prevent the suture from cutting into the tissues. The mattress sutures are placed by inserting the needle 5–7 mm from the edge of the lid and exiting through the edge itself, in or just outside the orifices of the meibomian glands and inside the cilia (Fig. 4.1, 4.2). Sutures placed too far outside can cause entropion. Sutures placed through the conjunctiva may result in an egg slicing effect to the cornea. The needle is introduced at the corresponding location in the edge of the opposite lid. The canthotomy incision is closed very

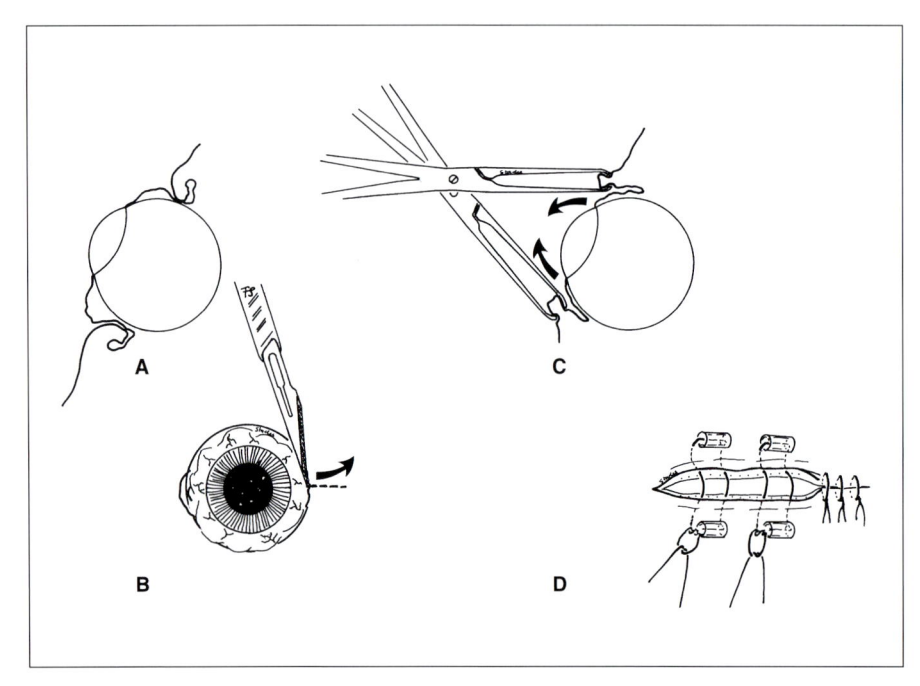

Fig. 4.1:
Luxation of the globe (A). Canthotomy (B), reposition (C), suturing method (D).

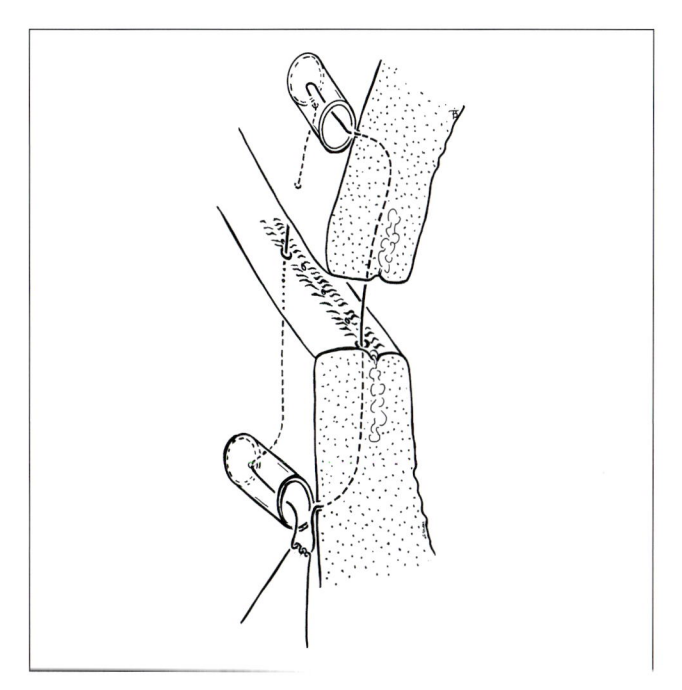

Fig. 4.2:
Temporary tarsorrhaphy. Method of suturing in section.

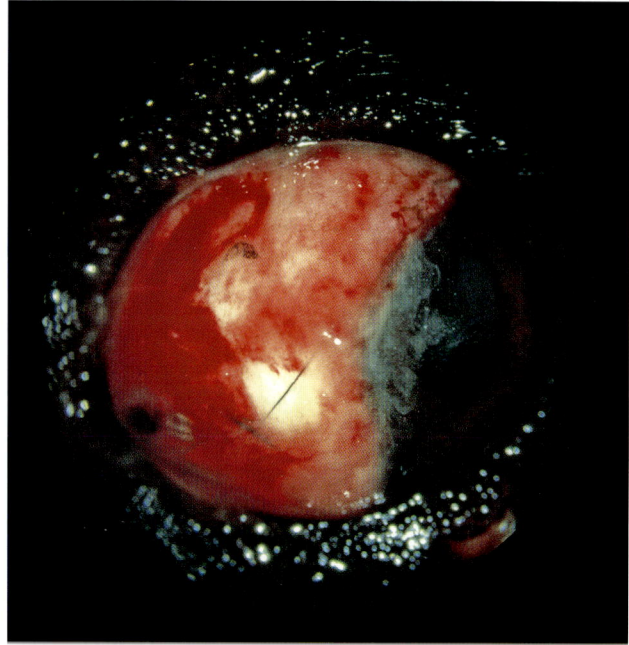

Plate 4.4:
Luxation or proptosis of the globe after repositioning (OS). The medial rectus muscle is ruptured, causing a divergent strabismus.

precisely, starting with a figure-of-eight suture. Prophylactic "initial choice" antibiotic and atropine ointments are applied behind the nictitating membrane before the sutures are knotted. After-care consists of applying the same medication in the lateral canthus, between the eyelids, and anti-inflammatory drugs are prescribed (e.g. carprofen). After 3–5 days the medial suture is removed. If there is still an apparent tendency to luxation, the remaining suture is left in place for a few more days.

A complicating tearing of the medial rectus and medial retractor oculi muscles often results in a diverging strabismus after the luxation (Plate 4.4). Not much can be done about this in the field; even veterinary ophthalmologists can rarely perform this type of muscle surgery for the re-establishment of a normal position. Searching for the torn muscle ends will cause severe surgical trauma unless the surgeon is experienced in this procedure. In an attempt to correct the strabismus as much as possible, the leading margin of the nictitating membrane can be attached to the lateral scleral conjunctiva by the use of 1 or 2 mattress sutures (see 10.6.3). This method does not prevent a recurrence of globe luxation, but may assist in repositioning the globe. The divergent strabismus may disappear or improve spontaneously within 6–8 weeks.

After the tarsorrhaphy sutures are removed, appropriate antibiotic ointment is administered. Atropine ointment is further used if anterior uveitis is present. In addition, anti-inflammatory agents may be indicated as frequently as 4 times daily, for about 10 days. The canthotomy sutures are removed 10–12 days after the accident.

Prognosis: Usually, the prognosis for preservation of the globe and restoration of vision is reasonably favorable, provided that the luxation has not been present for longer than 1–2 hours (<15 minutes in Pekingese). However, the prognosis for vision is dependent on the severity of the injury. If there has been severe trauma to the globe resulting in avulsion of the medial extrinsic muscles or the optic nerve, retinal detachment, hyphema, or contusion of the globe (see 4.4.2), blindness or phthisis bulbi is inevitable. In the case of very severe damage to the muscles and the optic nerve, direct enucleation is usually the best solution.

Complications: If there seems to be a tendency for the luxation to recur after the first suture has been cut, the second suture should remain in place for a few more days. If exophthalmos is still present, a permanent tarsorrhaphy can be performed. For this purpose, a strip of skin 10–15 mm long and 1 mm wide is removed just outside the upper and lower lid margins. The proximal edges of the upper and lower wounds are then sutured together over the lid edges (5-0 silk or nylon). The result is a tissue bridge over the rims of the lids that holds the globe in place. After-care consists of administration of "initial choice" antibiotic ointment for 10 days, followed by an indifferent, protective ointment (e.g. vitamin A ointment). After a few months the tissue bridge can be transected. The wounds close spontaneously. In cases of very severe damage, especially after rupture of multiple muscles or the optic nerve, enucleation of the eye may be unavoidable.

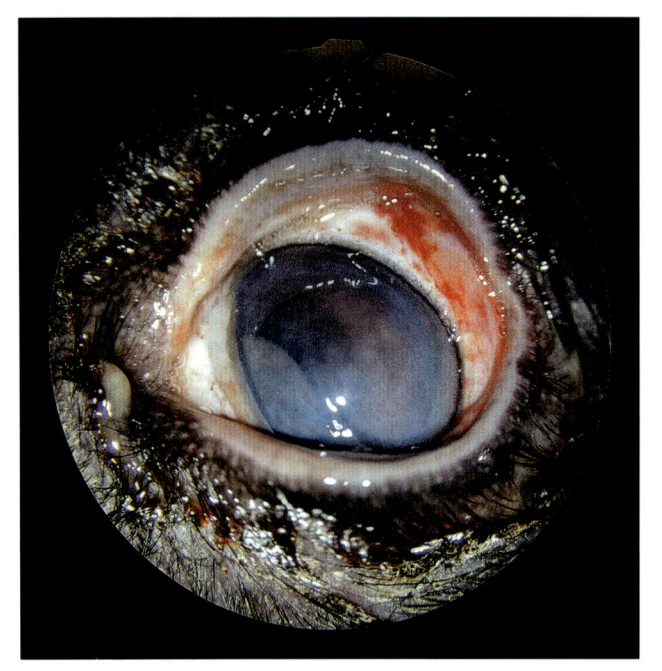

Plate 4.5:
Chemical burn (quick lime) of the eye (OS, dog). The lid margins are depigmented and swollen. The scleral conjunctiva shows defects and hemorrhages. The cornea is very edematous.

Prevention: In the brachycephalic breeds (e.g. Pekingese, Shih Tzu), a medial canthoplasty can be considered as a preventive measure, in which the palpebral fissure is shortened (see 7.8.1).

Note: not in the lateral canthus; a medial canthoplasty also prevents nasal fold, caruncle trichiasis and medial canthus entropion irritation. If necessary, the animal should be referred to someone experienced in this surgery. The buyers as well as the breeders of dogs of predisposed breeds need to be reminded emphatically that the eye should be able to function freely and requires a real orbit for protection.

4.3 Chemical burns

Acids and alkalis, such as battery acid, detergents, and quicklime, can cause very severe corneal burns (Plate 4.5). Acids are slightly less dangerous because they cause precipitation of protein which hinders a deeper penetration into the cornea. Alkalis penetrate quickly and cause severe damage to the cornea and the deeper structures. This results in irreversible damage to those structures involved, leading to complete scarring of the cornea and irreparable damage to the anterior uvea.

There is profuse, diffuse edema of the cornea. The conjunctiva is edematous and has hemorrhagic defects. The owner must irrigate the eye immediately, preferably with liberal amounts of lukewarm tap water, or any other water available. The first seconds / minutes are, by far, the most important. In the case of a distinct alkali burn, vinegar or boric acid solutions may be useful. After local anesthesia, the veterinarian can then irrigate the eye for 5–10 minutes with lukewarm 0.9 % NaCl solution (1–2 l) or with an EDTA solution. The conjunctival sac should be examined for possible residues of the injurious material.

After-care consists of "initial choice" antibiotic and 1 % atropine eye drops and, for a few days, if fluorescein staining is negative, topical anti-inflammatory agents. Parenteral antiprostaglandins and corticosteroids may be necessary. If the endothelium has been destroyed, only a corneal transplant offers a solution, but even this is unlikely to be successful if the peripheral endothelium or anterior uvea has also been damaged.

4.4 Blunt trauma

Blunt trauma can be recognized by the tearing of the tissues of the orbit, the adnexa, the globe, and its contents, and all the consequences of this. Hemorrhages and post-traumatic inflammation can cause severe swelling, especially in the cat. Tearing of the zonular fibers of the lens can induce lens luxation and subsequent glaucoma. There may also be orbital fractures. Appropriate therapy requires an accurate diagnosis, in which radiographic and ultrasound examination are of great importance.

4.4.1 Orbital fractures

Closed orbital fractures which result in little displacement require no special treatment except rest and the provision of soft food. Fractures of the zygomatic arch, in which the globe is either pressed anteriorly or, less often, posteriorly, should be repositioned and fixation should be by osteosynthesis. Fracture of the symphysis of the mandible, with secondary rotation of one-half of the mandible, can result in dislocation of the coronoid process and thus exophthalmos.

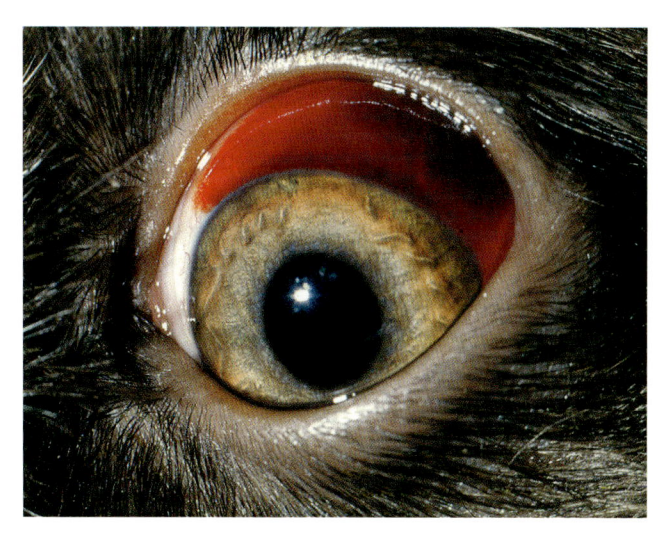

Plate 4.6:
Suffusion between the scleral conjunctiva and the sclera after a corrective blow with the leash (OS, dog).

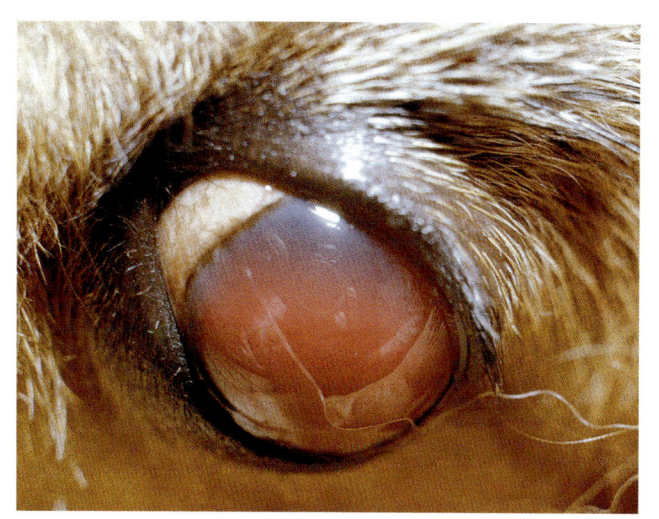

Plate 4.7:
Diffuse hyphema after a car accident (OS, dog).

4.4.2 Contusion of the globe

Contusion of the globe can have very different effects. Although the trauma is most often rostrolateral, the pressure wave can be transmitted deep into and behind the eye, so that retinal and retrobulbar damage are among the possible sequelae. Thus, a complete examination of the eye, possibly including additional examinations (e.g. indirect ophthalmoscopy, slit-lamp biomicroscopy, tonometry, ultra-sonography, MRI), is essential.

4.4.2.1 Suffusion (hyposphagma)
Suffusion or (subconjunctival) hemorrhages usually result from rupture of the subconjunctival vessels above the relatively stiff sclera, and hence the blood spreads out in the space between the sclera and the conjunctiva (Plate 4.6). Severe swelling results, which may prevent closure of the lid fissure. Often the trauma is caused by a blow with the hand or some object, or by strangulation. Hemorrhages can, however, be caused by diseases such as coagulation disorders or malignant lymphoma. Acute hemorrhages can sometimes be stopped by application of 0.1–1.0 % epinephrine drops. Therapy consists of a prophylactic "initial choice" antibiotic ointment for 5–8 days. If there much swelling, preventing lid closure, additional indifferent ointment or artificial tears should be administered every hour. Suffusion hemorrhages are normally absorbed within 5–10 days if the cause is removed.

4.4.2.2 Traumatic corneal edema
Traumatic corneal edema usually progresses into the stroma. This cloudiness is usually reversible. The administration of steroidal anti-inflammatory drops, 2–4 times daily, for a few days, can be considered after the cornea has been found to be negative on fluorescein staining.

In birds, keratitis is often caused by handling or by cage trauma.

4.4.2.3 Hyphema
Hyphema or hemorrhage in the anterior chamber is a frequent complication after trauma (Plate 4.7). There is little evidence that any therapy is of much benefit. However, keeping the animal quiet with cage rest is beneficial. Some ophthalmologists advocate the administration of 0.1 % epinephrine and/or 1 % atropine drops in the acute stage to stop the hemorrhage, but it has almost always stopped spontaneously before the drops take effect. Atropine may prevent posterior synechiae. Prescription of "initial choice" antibiotics and dexamethasone eye drops must be considered if synechia formation is expected, especially in horses. Within 1–2 days, the erythrocytes in the anterior chamber will settle to the bottom, resulting in a dense red horizontal line with a cleared area lying above it (Plate 4.8). Removal of the blood via a ventral paracentesis (small opening in the limbus) is seldom indicated

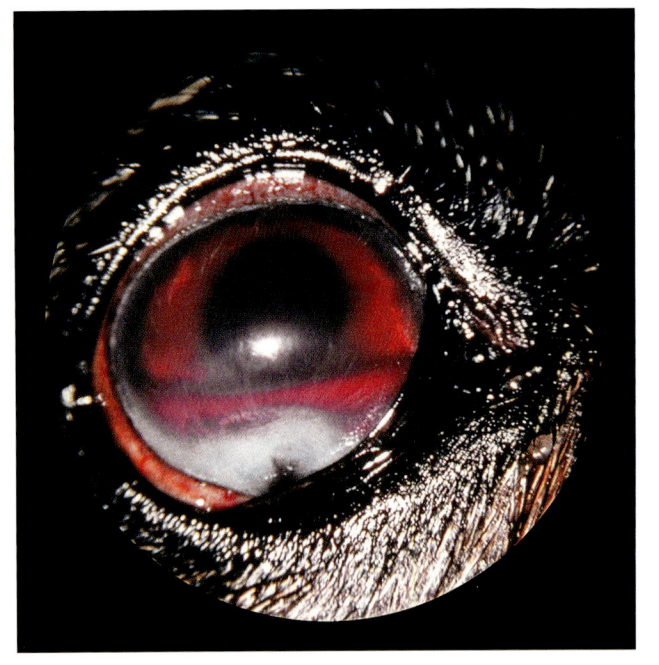

Plate 4.8:
Horizontal line of erythrocytes in the anterior chamber, 36 hours after a car accident (OD, dog). In the part undergoing clearing above the line, the pupil is just visible again.

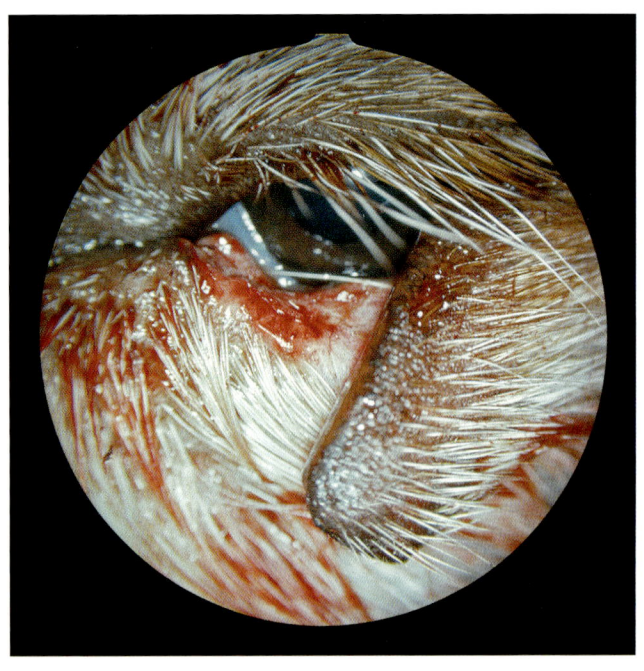

Plate 4.9:
Laceration of the lower lid after a dog bite (OS). Lid wounds should be almost without exception sutured immediately (see also Plate 4.10).

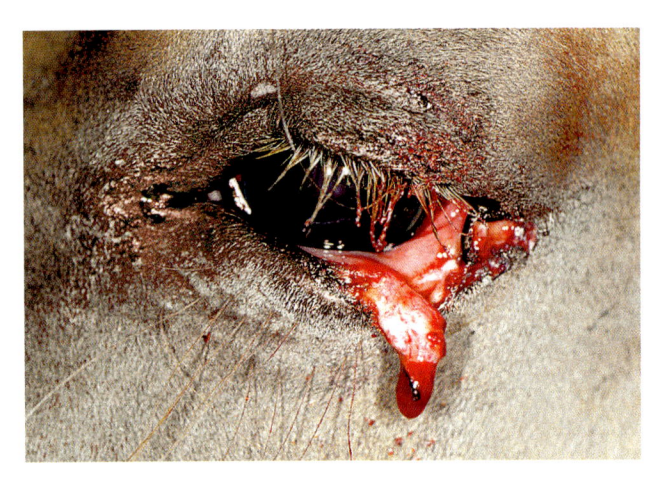

Plate 4.10:
Lid laceration caused by barbed wire in a horse (OS). Lid lacerations should be surgically treated immediately (see also Plate 4.11).

in animals. In addition, the alternating administration of atropine and pilocarpine or the use of heparin ointment does not really hasten absorption. A hyphema that does not clear, or bilateral hyphema, is usually not the result of trauma but more likely a sign of hemorrhagic diathesis, e.g. in malignant lymphoma (see 12.9) and further examination should be carried out in that direction.

4.4.2.4 Trauma with deeper penetration

Trauma with deeper penetration can have extremely variable consequences. Hence in addition to hyphema, there can be tearing of the iris, tearing of the zonular fibers with subsequent lens luxation, hemorrhage in the vitreous or the fundus, and retinal edema or retinal ablation. Treatment thus depends upon the findings. Hemorrhages can sometimes be stopped with topical epinephrine, though direct surgical intervention may be indicated in some cases. If lens luxation is found, treatment for glaucoma is started as an emergency measure (see 11.3.3). Inflammatory processes can be suppressed with steroidal anti-inflammatory drops or parenteral steroidal or NSAIDs; though with the latter one must be aware of their anti-thromboxane effect and hence the increased bleeding tendency with NSAIDs. Often it is advisable to refer patients with signs of deep trauma to the skull also to an eye specialist.

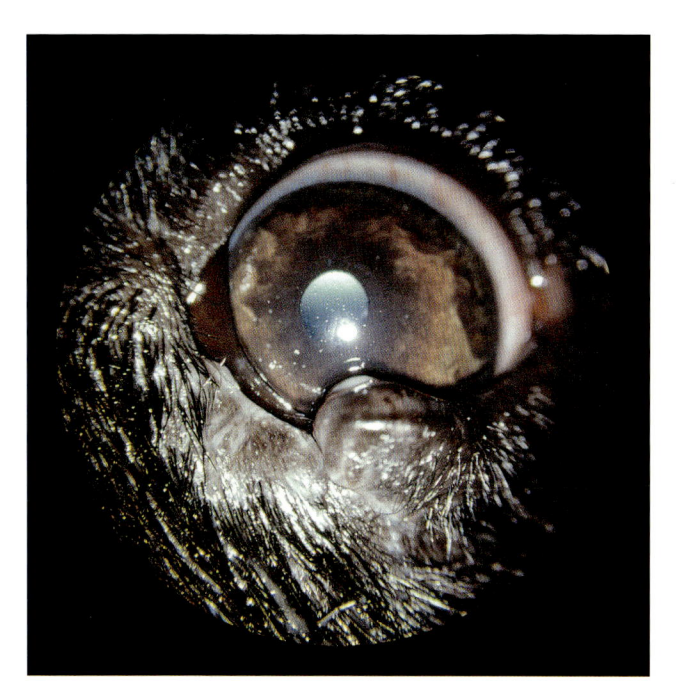

Plate 4.11:
Scar of a lid laceration almost identical to the one shown in Plate 4.9, but after spontaneous healing (OS, dog). The retraction of the orbicularis muscle and scar retraction have resulted in a nodule of scar tissue and ventral traction of the lid edge. Because of the "lucky" location of the wound, the nictitating membrane has partly taken over the lid function and protects the cornea.

4.5 Penetrating or perforating trauma

Perforating trauma and tissue separation are usually caused by thorns, splinters, claws, or teeth. In horses, training whips and nails in the stalls are often incriminated. In the case of periocular soft tissue swelling, the use of corticosteroids or NSAIDs has to be considered.

Because the skin around the eye is almost directly over the bony skull, the skin is frequently torn away or complicating fractures are present with this type of trauma. Therapy is as given below. Adequate tetanus prevention is essential.

4.5.1 Lid lacerations and conjunctival sac wounds

Eyelids and conjunctival sac wounds are often right-angled and bleed heavily (Plate 4.9–4.11). If the lid edge has been cut through, the defect will enlarge spontaneously in the lid via contraction of the orbicularis oculi muscle. Wounds in the eyelid should therefore always be sutured immediately, even if they are more than 8 hours old. The use of topical anesthesia and/or sedation for the necessary surgical correction is generally not adequate, especially in the horse. The correction has to be performed under general anesthesia, using a high-quality magnification operation loupe. Hair along the wound edges can be clipped away if it does not lead to unnecessary damage. Both the wound in the lid and the conjunctival sac must be very thoroughly irrigated. Mechanical wound debridement should be kept to a minimum. A water-pick is an excellent method of providing irrigation and wound debridement.

The wound in the edge of the lid must be closed very precisely with a figure-of-eight or mattress suture (5-0 or 6-0 monofilament nylon, [cutting] round body needle; absorbable only for aggressive or difficult to handle, high anesthesia-risk patients). The suture is started 1–2 mm from the margin, where hair growth starts (Fig. 4.3). The meibomian gland openings

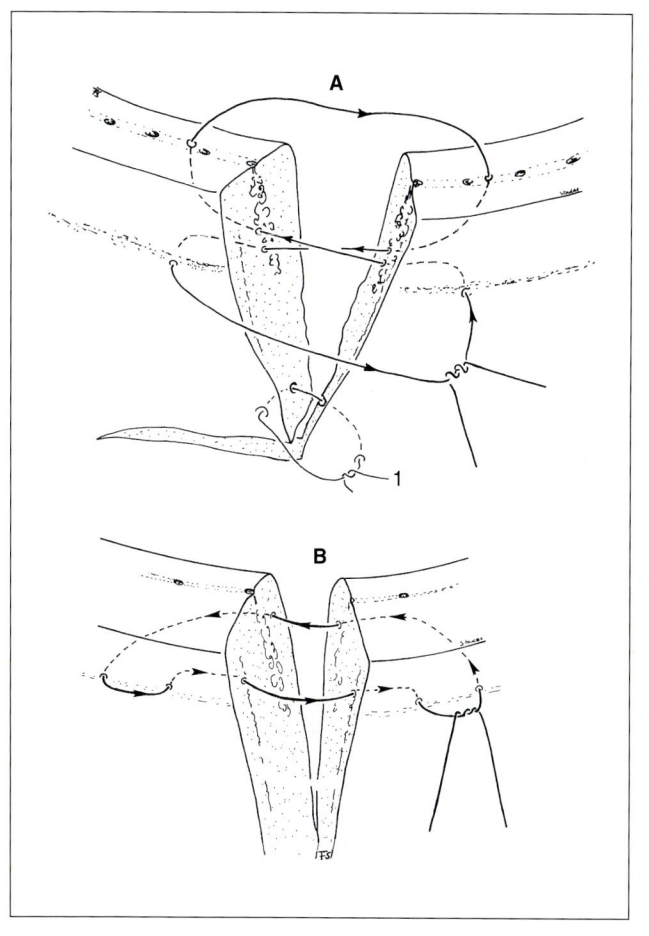

Fig. 4.3:
Laceration of the lid margin. Methods of suturing using a figure-of-eight (A) or a U-form (B) suture. Thereafter, the conspicuous points of the wound are sutured (1).

38 Ocular Emergencies

are used as a guide line for precise realignment. Horizontal or vertical mismatching (Fig. 4.4 and Plates 4.11, 4.12) of the two parts of the lid edge are unacceptable. Small defects in the conjunctiva rarely have to be sutured. Sometimes, non-perforating U-sutures can be used (see also 4.5.2). After the lid edge has been closed, the most conspicuous points of the wound (e.g. angles) are brought together with simple interrupted sutures. The remaining parts of the wound are then closed by placing additional sutures halfway between the previous sutures until the wound edges are adequately closed. This method prevents unequal traction upon the wound edges. The maximal distance between sutures should not be more than 2 mm. After-care consists of applying topical antibiotic ointment to the eye and the wound. Other clinicians avoid topical therapy and administer antibiotics parenterally. If contamination is evident and concern about bacterial infection is present, culture and sensitivity tests are indicated. The veterinarian should evaluate the progression of healing and modify the treatment as necessary.

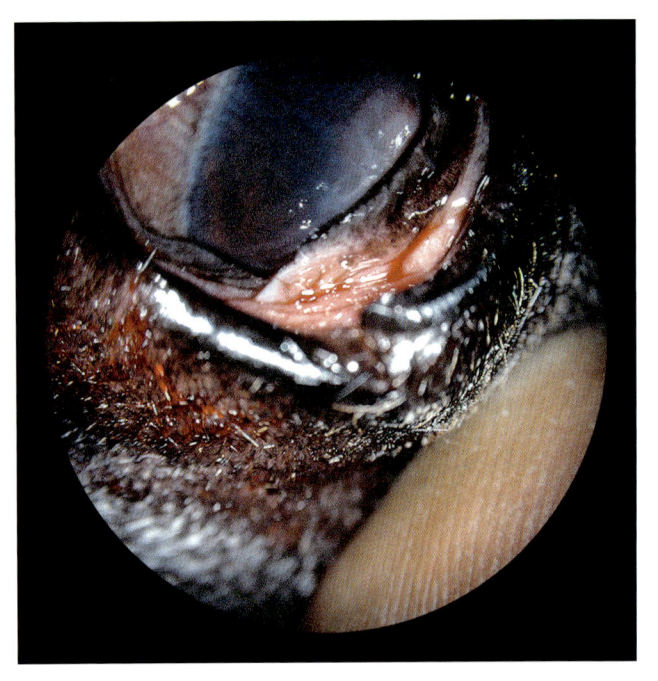

Plate 4.12:
Scar of a not "lege artis" sutured lid laceration (OD, dog), as shown in Figs. 4.4 E and F.

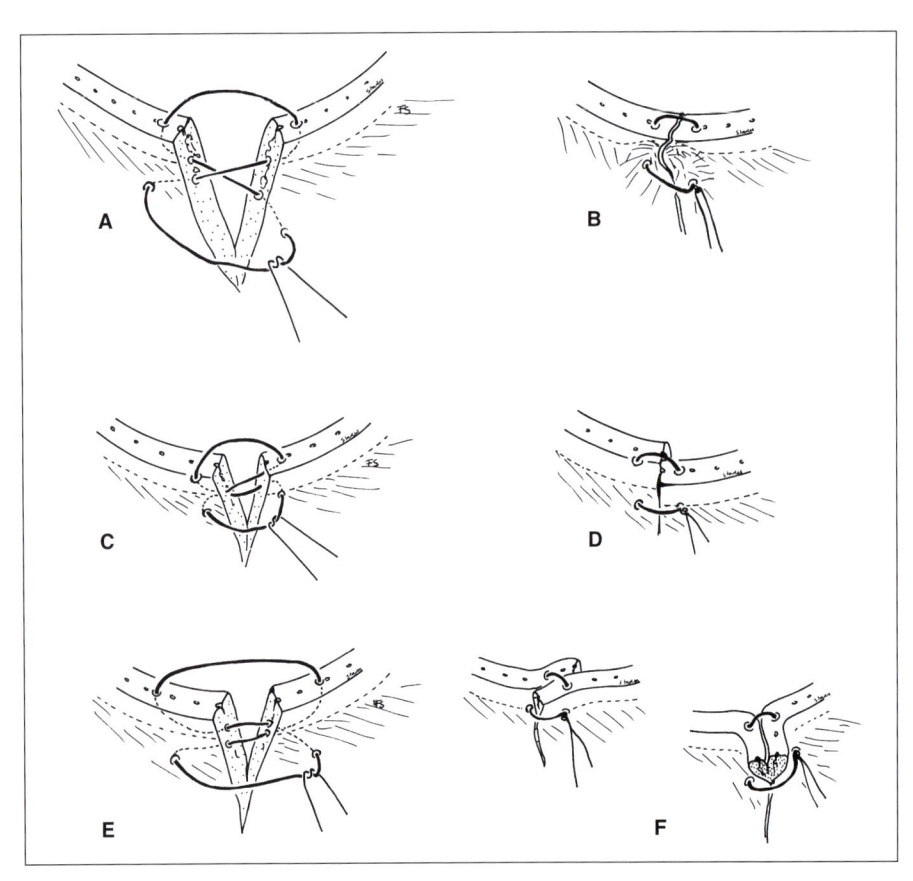

Fig. 4.4:
Suturing of a laceration of the lid margin as it should not be done. The figure-of-eight-suture has been started at an unequal distance and too far away from the margin (A), with the result (B). Incongruous suture: at the left side 1 mm outside of the margin and at the right side in the line of the meibomian gland openings (C) and its result (D). Suture located too far away from the margin (E) and its result (F).

4.5.1.1 Lacerations of the lid edge including the lacrimal canaliculus

Lacerations of the medial canthus are rare, though when they occur they are usually in the lower lid and accompanied by laceration of the lacrimal ducts. The canaliculi are located in the swollen wound by intubation. An S-shaped 000 probe or Worst pigtail probe (preferably with an eye in the tip) is introduced via the upper punctum into the wound (Fig. 4.5). A 0.7- to 1.3-mm diameter silicone tube is either placed over the tip of the probe or cut on a slant and inserted into the eye in the tip of the probe. The tube is pulled through the upper punctum via the entrance in the wound and the sacculus. The probe is then introduced through the lower punctum to the wound and the other end of the silicone tube is pulled through the rest of the lower canaliculus to the lower punctum. The ends are tied together by a 5-0 silk suture. This way of tying is quick, but both ends may irritate the cornea. Irritation from the ends can be avoided by making a circular tubing (Fig. 4.5, 6.8) or if the ends are fixed to the medial canthal skin using a simple interrupted suture. A strand of 6-0 monofilament nylon is passed through the tube, the length of the tube is adjusted and the strand is knotted, leaving the tube in a ring through the canaliculi and sacculus (see 6.4.2). The wound in the lid margin is closed with a figure-of-eight suture and the rest of the wound by single interrupted sutures. The tubing is left in place for 2–3 weeks.

4.5.1.2 Lacerations with loss of tissue

When there is loss of tissue at the margin of the lid, retraction will enlarge the defect even more. If reconstructive blepharoplasty cannot be done directly, 1–2 tension sutures should be inserted (Fig. 7.26). Cutting into the tissue by the sutures should be prevented by the use of pieces of silicone or infusion tube. If possible a blepharoplasty should be performed immediately. The reverse triangle method (Fig. 7.23) is appropriate for closure of a small, deeper defect. Broad, shallow defects should be corrected by an H-plasty (Fig. 7.25). Even larger defects can be closed by a rotating (Fig. 7.3) or sliding flap, or a Z-plasty.

4.5.2 Conjunctival lacerations

Larger defects of the conjunctiva or nictitating membrane are closed with continuous sutures (6-0 to 8-0 absorbable material, [cutting] round body or spatula needle), preferably free of knots. The animal should be referred if necessary. The suturing

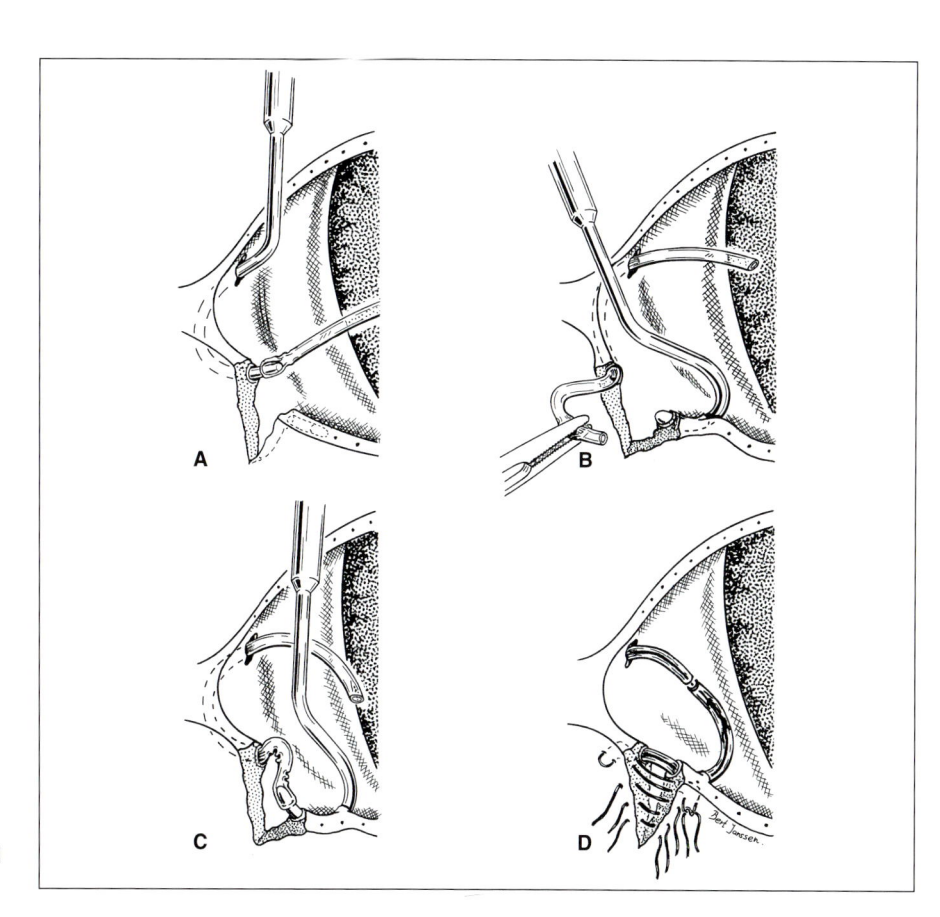

Fig. 4.5:
Lid-edge laceration through the inferior canaliculus. Connection is guaranteed by the introduction of a silicone tube. After that the wound is sutured (alternative suturing, see Fig. 4.3).

Fig. 4.6:
Defect in the nictitating membrane. Method of suturing with as few knots as possible.

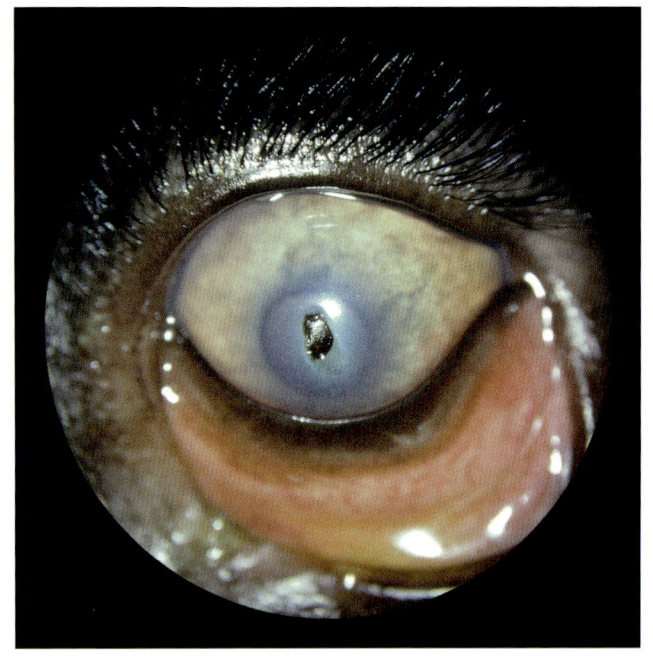

Plate 4.13:
Foreign body centrally on / in the cornea (OS, dog), one day after contact. It is the covering layer of a plant bud. It has been sucked with its concave side into the tear film and subsequently into the cornea (see also Plate 4.14).

must never result in traction scars, as these lead to irritation. If traction cannot be avoided it is better to leave the conjunctival wound open. Knots should be avoided or placed beneath the conjunctiva. The defect in the conjunctiva accompanying a wound in the lid edge rarely needs to be sutured.

4.5.3 Corneal lacerations

Corneal wounds can occur with or without a foreign body and can be superficial, deep, or perforating. The patient has severe blepharospasm, profuse tear production, corneal edema, and possibly a prolapse of coagulated material, even iris, into the wound.

4.5.3.1 General rules of treatment
Veterinarians who do not have all the necessary materials or who lack the experience or confidence to undertake procedures involving the cornea should refer patients with foreign bodies or severe corneal defects. When there are very deep defects in the cornea that reach Descemet's membrane (which does not stain with fluorescein) or penetrate into the anterior chamber, oversuturing of the nictitating membrane can be considered (see 10.6.3), but this requires considerable time, is not the method of initial choice and will require an extra anesthesia.

Before referral, severely contaminated wounds should be cultured and sensitivity tests run to select the best antibiotic. Further treatment will dictate the type of "specific choice" antibiotic to be used afterwards. Exudate may be dissolved by a collagenase inhibitor such as acetylcysteine, and the contamination removed by saline lavage. Bacterial invasion is stopped by effective, penetrating "initial choice", broad-spectrum antibiotic drops. Pain caused by ciliary muscle spasm is relieved (cycloplegia) with 1 % atropine, also in eye drops. "Treatment" with topical anesthetics will delay epithelial healing, mask further damage, and therefore must be seen as a professional mistake. The release of prostaglandins is decreased by anti-prostaglandins. For transport and during the healing period, the patient can be fitted with a protective collar or hood.

4.5.3.2 Non-perforating corneal wounds
Non-perforating corneal wounds can be shown by fluorescein staining. Foreign bodies such as plant material (Plates 4.13, 4.14) and particles of food which have been thrown to the dog to catch (e.g. potato chips, dried shrimp) can be irrigated or removed under local anesthesia using foreign body forceps. Thorns that have penetrated into the corneal stroma (Plates 4.15–4.17) and lie completely within it, but have not

Penetrating or perforating trauma **41**

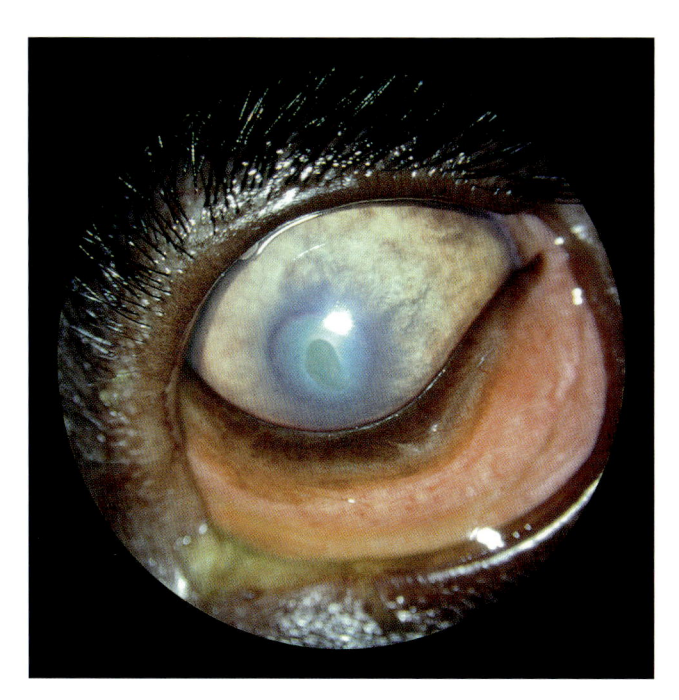

Plate 4.14:
Defect after the removal of the foreign body shown in Plate 4.13 (OS, dog).

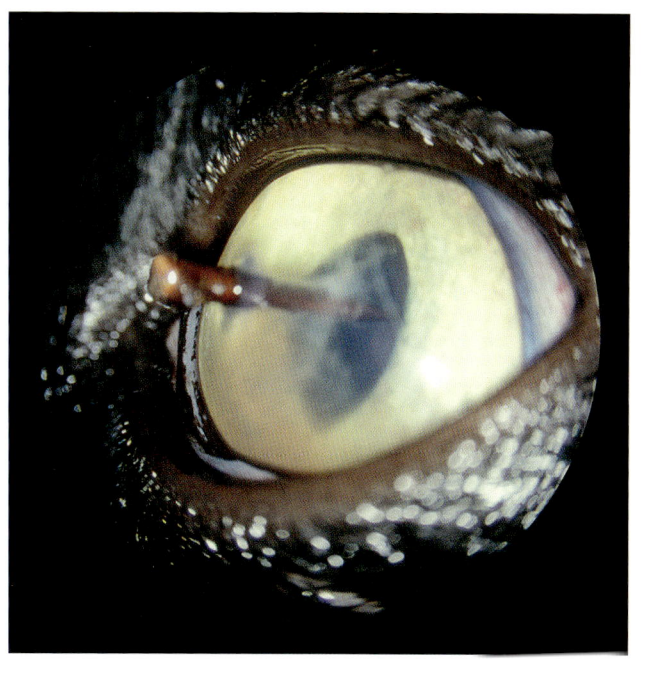

Plate 4.15:
Corneal perforation of a thorn into the lens in the eye of a cat (OS; see also Plate 4.16).

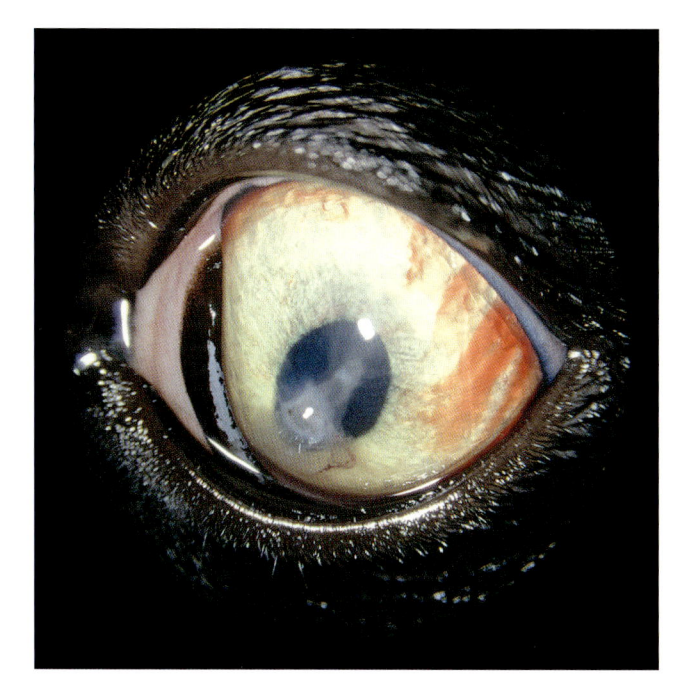

Plate 4.16:
Corneal defect directly after the removal of a thorn: a covering "tube" around the channel of introduction of the thorn and flares of free blood in the anterior chamber. (OS; same eye as shown in Plate 4.15).

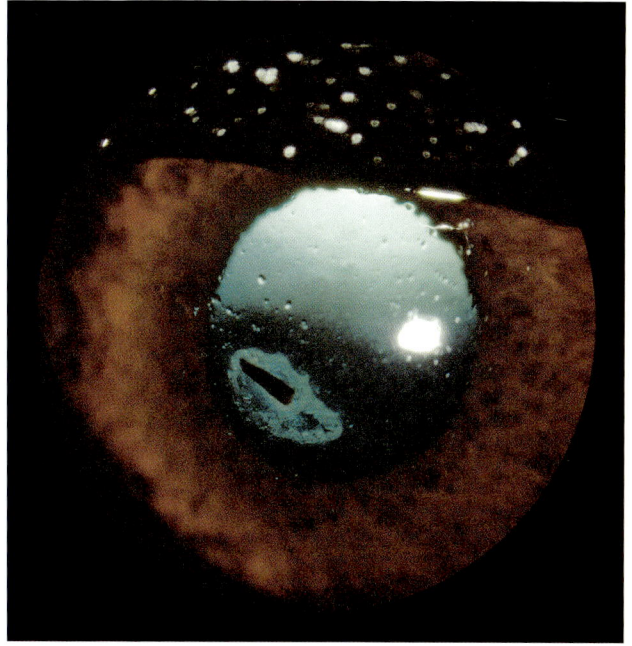

Plate 4.17:
Thorn in the corneal stroma with a ring of edema around it (OS, dog). The darker spot ventral to the back of the thorn is the port of entry.

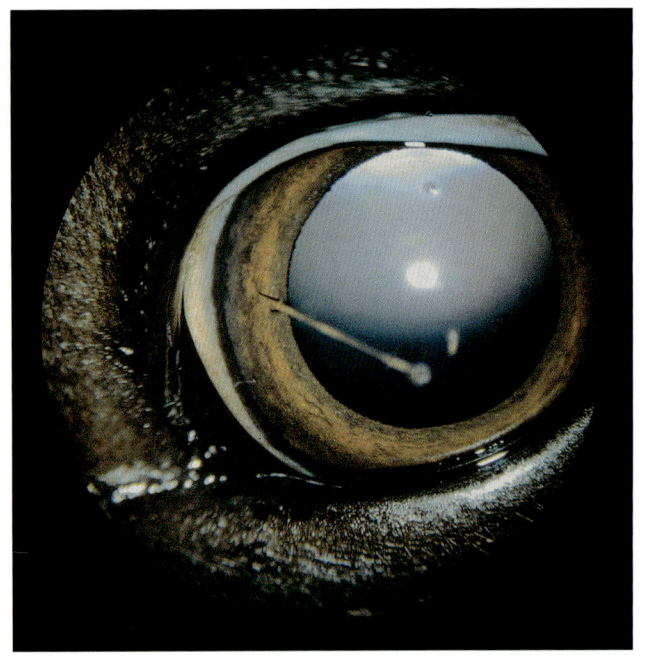

Plate 4.18:
Eye of a dog with the history: "for some days there has been a thorn or a worm in the anterior chamber" (OS). The strand from the cornea to the collarette on the surface of the iris at 9 o'clock is a persistent pupillary membrane.

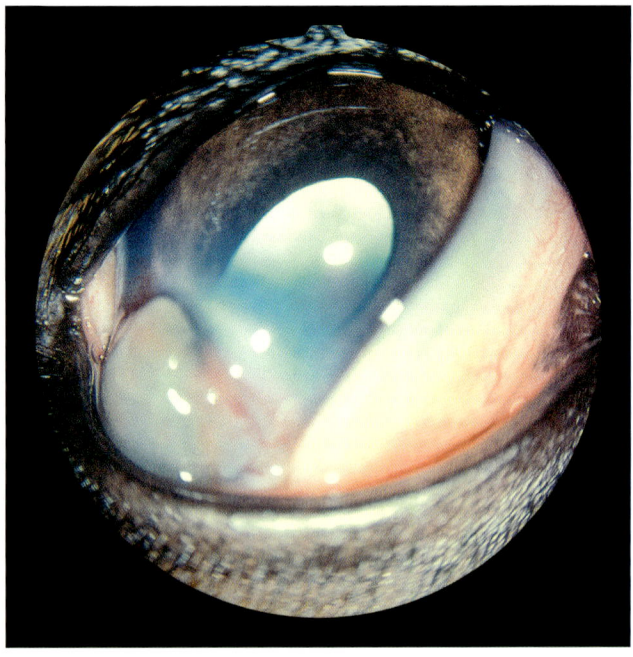

Plate 4.19:
Staphyloma near the limbus at 7 o'clock, after a traumatic corneal perforation, one day after the accident (OD, dog). The anterior chamber is clear, the edge of the pupil is sharp, and the surface of the iris does not show distinct signs of uveitis.

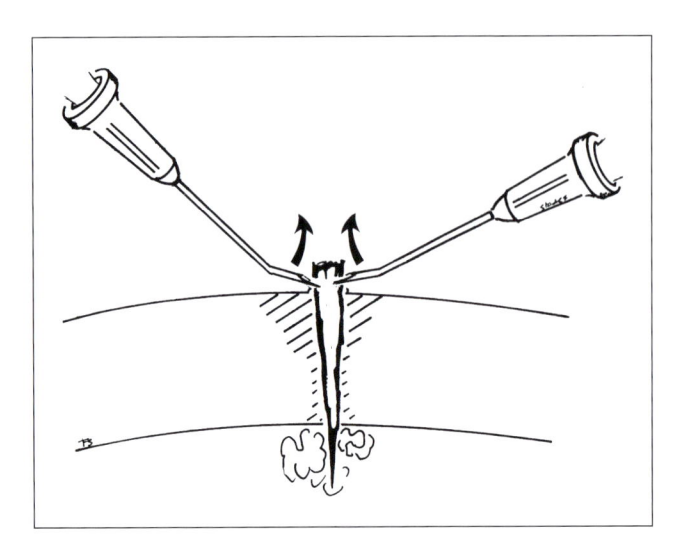

Fig. 4.7:
Removal of a thorn out of the cornea by the use of two fine cannulas. At the tip of the thorn is a lump of exudate.

penetrated into the anterior chamber, should be removed by incising the overlying cornea with a corneal scalpel. If the animal is quiet, a local anesthetic is sufficient. If insufficient help is available, or the animal is difficult to restrain, the patient is sedated or anesthetized. Eye trauma located medially usually requires inhalation anesthesia with muscle relaxation (and so artificial respiration), especially in large animals, and the use of stay sutures. After thorough irrigation of the conjunctival sac and further inspection of the eye, treatment following removal of such a foreign body consists of topical "initial choice" antibiotics 4 times daily. If anterior segment involvement is manifest, 1 % atropine to effect is also indicated. Also the use of special contact lenses may be indicated. The defect should heal within a few days.

Defects that are deeper than one third of the thickness of the cornea require a longer time to heal. There is usually also a temporary ingrowth of vessels and granulation tissue, leading to formation of a scar. Once epithelialization has occurred, some clinicians prescribe steroidal anti-inflammatory agents to control or reduce the development of granulation tissue and vascularization. However, this is only safe if the healing process can be evaluated by slit-lamp biomicroscope, and the results should not be overestimated.

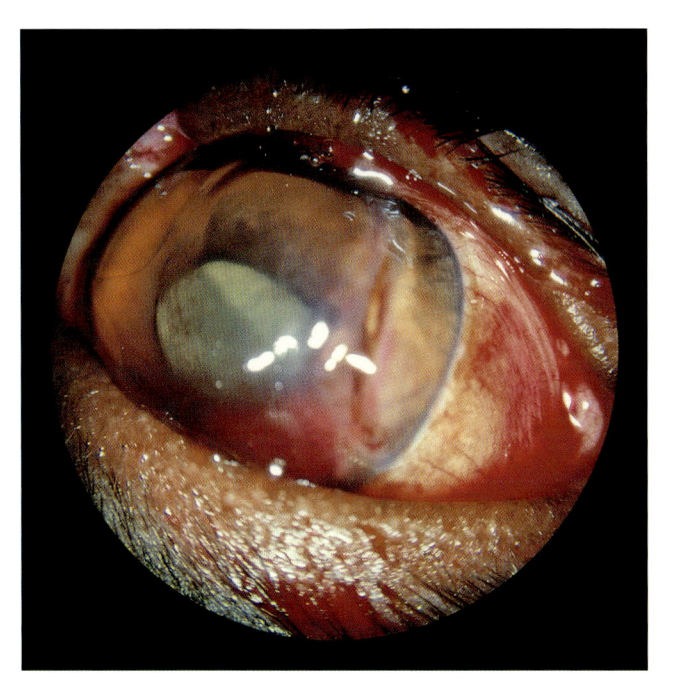

Penetrating or perforating trauma **43**

Plate 4.20:
Corneal laceration of a dog's eye, some hours after a cat scratch (OS). There is an aqueous flare and the iris shows signs of post-traumatic uveitis. The wound was closed with seven interrupted sutures (monofilament nylon, 9-0; see also Plate 4.21).

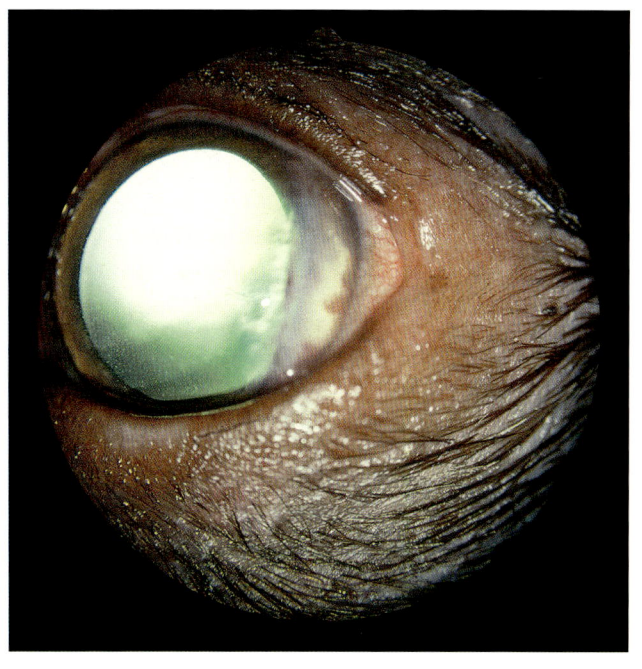

Plate 4.21:
Corneal scar of a cat scratch, after the removal of the stitches, 18 days after the accident (OS, dog; same eye as shown in Plate 4.20). The aqueous flare has resorbed and the pupil is round and in mydriasis (induced by atropine).

4.5.3.3 Perforating corneal defects

Perforating corneal defects are usually caused by objects that strike the cornea at great speed, such as cat claws, thorns, or airgun/shotgun pellets. The associated trauma to the iris can cause hemorrhage into the anterior chamber as well as outside the eye, via prolapse of the iris through the corneal wound. This will be accompanied by a severe inflammatory reaction in the uvea. When there is deeper penetrating trauma, cataract or hemorrhage into the vitreous or retina can occur. The eye should not be irrigated, and any substances prolapsing through the wound should be left undisturbed until just before suturing. If the animal is tractable and further examination to determine course of action is necessary, a topical anesthetic should be administered. In addition, topical "specific choice" broad-spectrum antibiotic and atropine eye drops should be given.

Thorns which are in part still clearly visible above the corneal surface can be extracted with a foreign body forceps (Plate 4.15, 4.16). If the thorn is deeper, attempts to remove it with forceps only cause corneal edema and there is a great risk that the thorn may be propelled by the forceps into the anterior chamber or, worse, into the iris and/or lens. An attempt can be made to remove a thorn lying deep in the cornea by lifting it out with two bent 0.45-mm (26 gauge) hypodermic needles (Fig. 4.7). In the case of a penetrating foreign body, one should be sure that the resulting defect can be sutured immediately after removal; otherwise the patient should be referred immediately.

Perforating wounds in the cornea (Plates 4.19–4.21) should be sutured under general anesthesia with muscle relaxation, using e.g. 8-0 or 9-0 monofilament nylon or absorbable material with a spatula-shaped needle. Muscle relaxation is preferred so that the eye will rotate in a standard gaze position; this results in less traction during surgery to the compromised eye. Corneal tissue is scarce and thus the laceration is not debrided. Small, clean iris prolapses can be replaced through the cornea with a spatula. A large or contaminated iris prolapse (Plate 4.19) should be excised by electrocautery. The corneal sutures should be placed into about two thirds of the depth of the stroma (Fig. 4.8). Caution should be exercised not to penetrate the full thickness of the cornea. An air bubble or a viscoelastic is introduced to move the iris away from the cornea, and then the pressure in the anterior chamber is reformed by introducing a special aqueous fluid replacement solution, such as balanced salt solution (BSS).

When a larger part of the cornea is missing, a conjunctival oversuturing method (see 10.6.3.5) or a free transplant can be used for closure.

After-care consists of "specific choice" antibiotics, atropine, and steroidal anti-inflammatory drops to treat the anterior uveitis that is present in every patient that suffers this type of injury. These agents should be used 6 times daily for the first few days and the frequency modified as the situation dictates. The use of steroidal anti-inflammatory drops is only safe if the healing process can be evaluated frequently by a slit-lamp biomicroscope. In many patients, parenteral steroidal or NSAIDs are given. After 1–2 days, the eye should be examined and evaluated for severity of post-traumatic uveitis (see 12.10) and secondary glaucoma (see 11.2). The sutures are removed after 14–16 days.

Shotgun and airgun (Plates 4.22–4.24) pellets can produce disastrous destruction in the eye. Cats, in particular, which come home with a damaged eye after a few days absence (Plate 4.22), should be examined radiographically for the possible presence of a pellet. Usually, such a damaged eye can only be treated for post-traumatic uveitis (see 12.10.1). Pellets can seldom be removed without causing even more severe operative trauma. However, they usually become encapsulated and then seldom cause problems. Lead intoxication is only a consideration if there are many (>50) lead pellets present.[2]

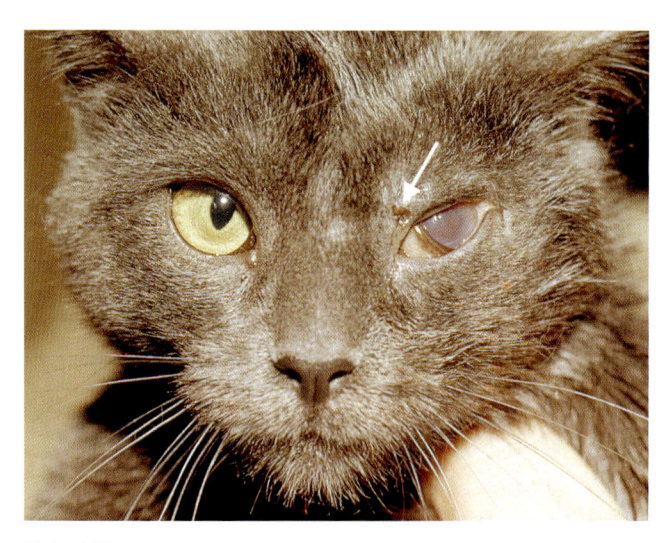

Plate 4.22:
Lid (see arrow) and corneal laceration caused by an air rifle bullet (24 hours after the shooting; OS).

Literature

1. BISTNER, S.I. & AGUIRRE, G.D.: Management of ocular emergencies. Vet. Clin. North Am. **2**: 359, 1972.

2. SCHMIDT, G.M., DICE, P.F. & KOCH, S.A.: Intraocular lead foreign bodies in four canine eyes. J. Small Anim. Pract. **16**: 33, 1975.

Penetrating or perforating trauma **45**

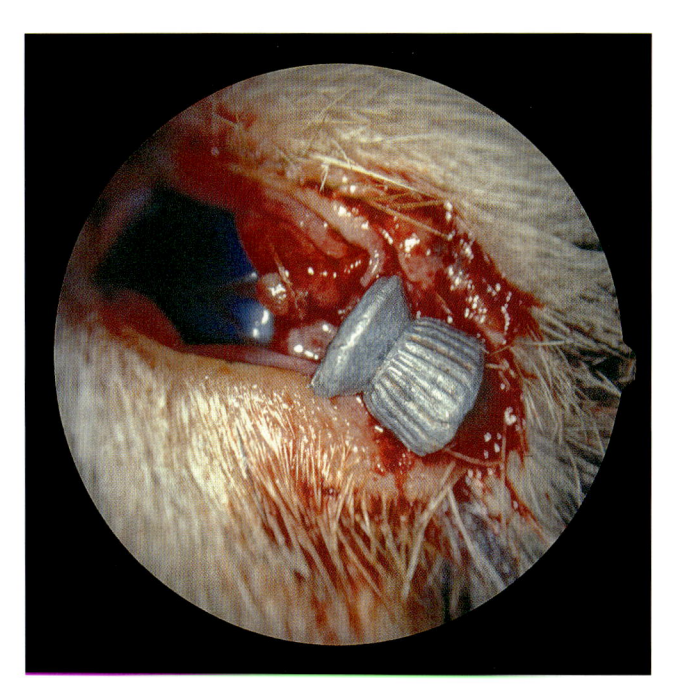

Plate 4.23:
Air rifle bullet, directly after removal from the retrobulbar tissues behind the right eye of a cat.

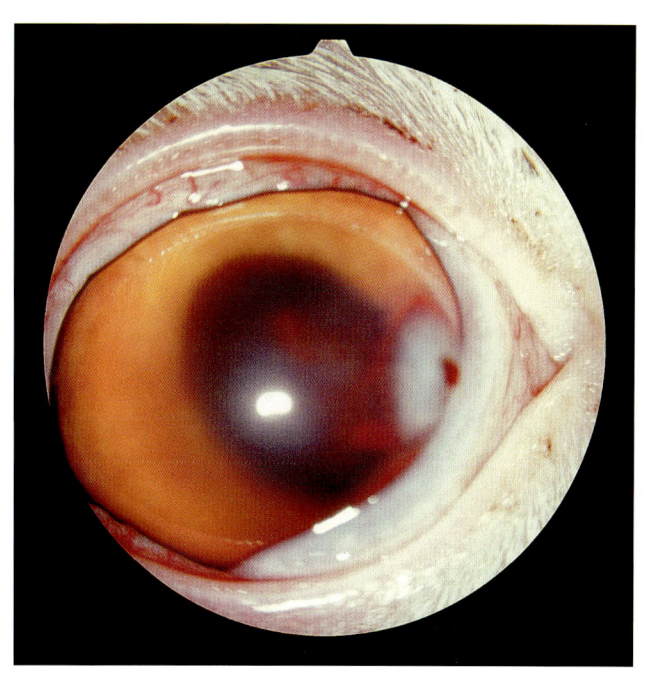

Plate 4.24:
Corneal defect with a ring of edema and blood in the anterior chamber, after the penetration of a shotgun pellet (OD, cat).

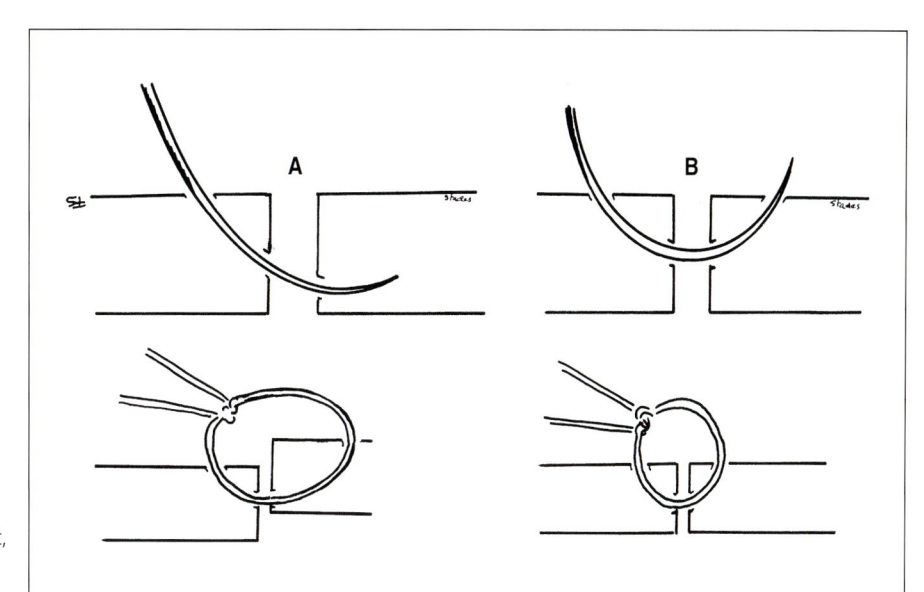

Fig. 4.8:
Suturing of tissue layers has to be done at the same level and the same distances (left incorrect, asymmetrical; right correct, symmetrical). In this way the layers will fit together correctly.

5 Orbital and Periorbital Structures

5.1 Introduction

A large number of different causes of diseases affecting the orbit and periorbital structures (Fig. 5.1) are possible, including congenital, traumatic, inflammatory, degenerative, and neoplastic disorders. The disease process can originate from (1) tissues outside the orbit, such as the nose, the sinuses, or the oral cavity posterior to the last molar; (2) from tissues of the orbit itself, including bone, muscles, nerves, fat, and blood vessels; and (3) tissues of the globe itself.

Abnormalities within the orbit and/or orbital tissues are often characterized by exophthalmos and/or protrusion of the nictitating membrane (Fig. 5.2). There are exceptions, however, depending on the localization of the space-occupy-

Fig. 5.1:
Positioning of the globe in the orbit (side view). Lacrimal gland (gl), zygomatic gland (gz), zygomatic arch (z), frontal bone (f), coronoid process (pc) of the mandible.

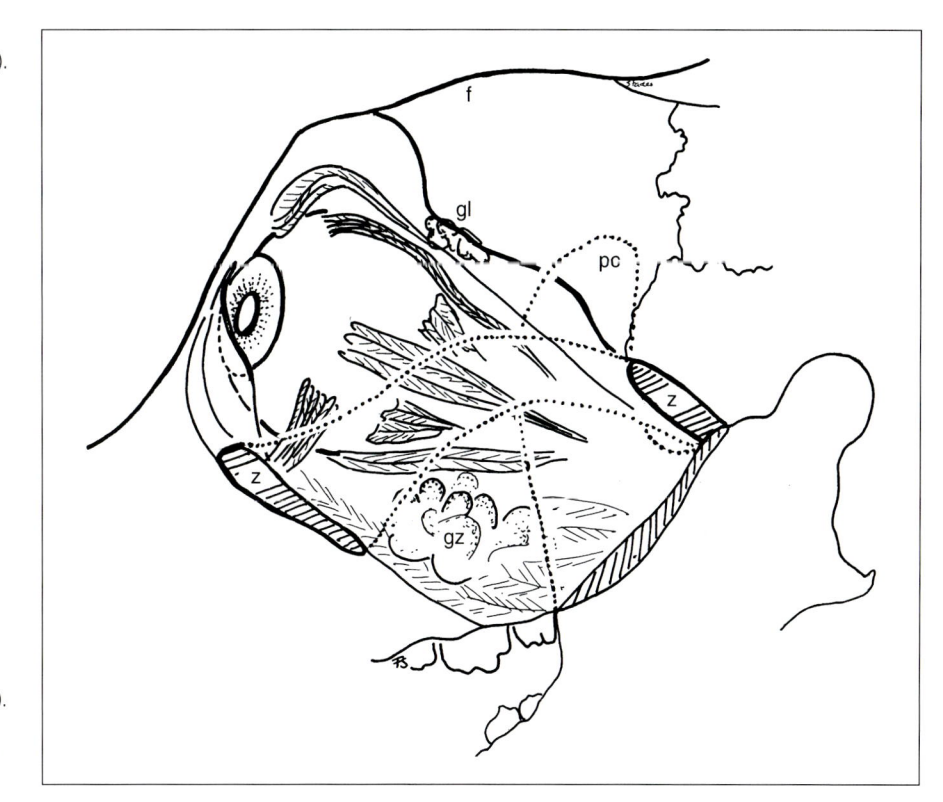

Fig. 5.2:
Exophthalmos due to a retrobulbar process (A). Enophthalmos due to a process positioned anterior to the globe (B; this position will only rarely be encountered).

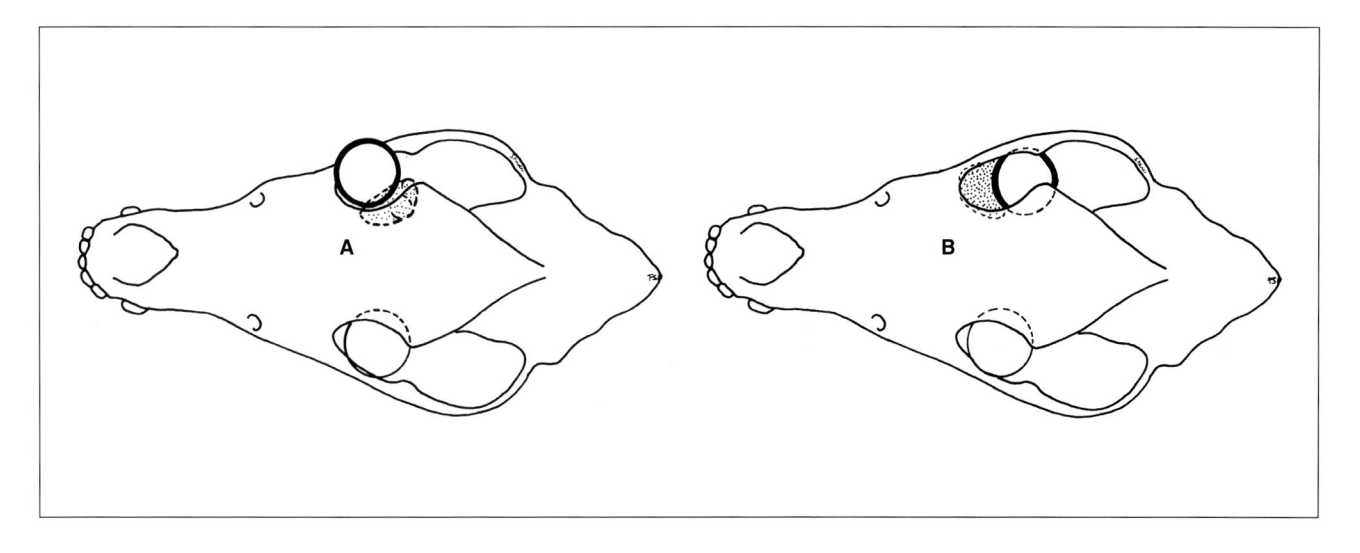

ing process (Fig. 5.3) or, indeed, processes causing loss of tissue. If a space-occupying lesion or a fragment of a fractured bone compromises the orbit caudal to the eyeball, exophthalmos will be more prominent and the retrobulbar pressure will be increased. If the process lies more to the nasal side of the orbit (e.g., a neoplasm arising from the base of the nictitating membrane or from the nasal cavity), or if the support behind the eye is reduced (by dehydration, resorption of retrobulbar fat, or muscle atrophy), enophthalmos will occur instead, with a normal or lowered retrobulbar pressure. The enophthalmos will be associated with protrusion of the nictitating membrane. For further diagnostic procedures, such as biopsy, specialized radiographic[1,2] and angiographic studies, ultrasonography, CT, MRI, and orbital angiography, the patient must usually be referred.[3,4]

With the exception of luxation of the eyeball, orbital or periorbital diseases occur infrequently.

5.2 Congenital abnormalities

Among the congenital abnormalities that must be considered are anophthalmia, hydrocephalus (sometimes associated with a "setting sun" position of the globes), orbital dysplasias, and cysts. In view of the rarity of these disorders and the variation in the forms in which they occur, they will not be considered further.

5.3 Trauma

(See 4, Ocular Emergencies)

5.4 Enophthalmos

Enophthalmos may be a response to pain but it can also be secondary to a loss of retrobulbar pressure or support, general malaise, a loss of condition, or sympathetic denervation (Horner's syndrome).

5.4.1 Enophthalmos due to loss of support

Enophthalmos due to general malaise or a loss of condition is usually a transient condition in which both eyes lie deep in the orbits and there is a secondary protrusion of the nictitating membranes. The primary cause must be found and treated.

If the enophthalmos is caused by a rupture of the periorbital muscles (horse) or severe atrophy of the temporal muscles due to a myositis (usually in German Shepherd Dogs, eosinophilic myositis), the eyes lie very deep in the orbits and there is severe protrusion of the nictitating membranes and, possibly, secondary entropion of the lower lids. In cases of atrophy, the skin loses all its supportive tissues and will lie almost directly over the skull and the zygomatic arch.

The eye may appear blind, because it is unable to look over the edge of the nictitating membrane and the zygomatic arch. Irritation of the eye results in lacrimation and a mucus discharge.

Therapy: Treatment consists of correction of the secondary entropion, frequent eye washes, and protection of the globe by, for example, vitamin A oil or ointment. In some cases a retrobulbar silicone implant of 5–15 ml can be considered. The implants can be introduced from behind the orbital ligament

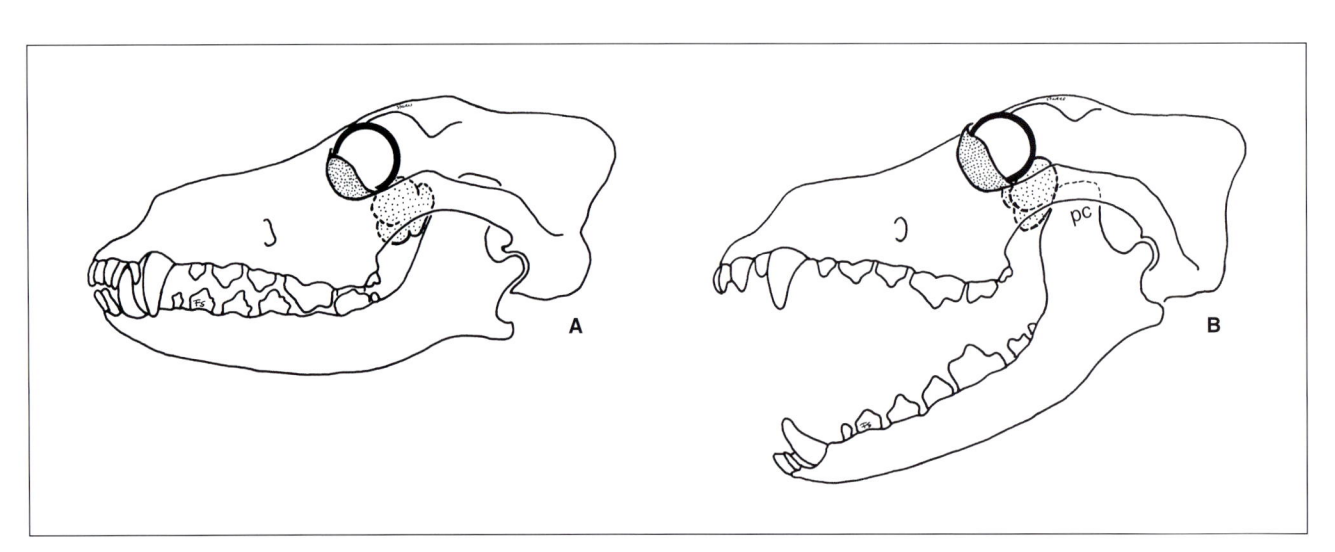

Fig. 5.3:
Retrobulbar process with a closed (A) and opened mouth (B). The coronoid process (pc) produces pressure on the process.

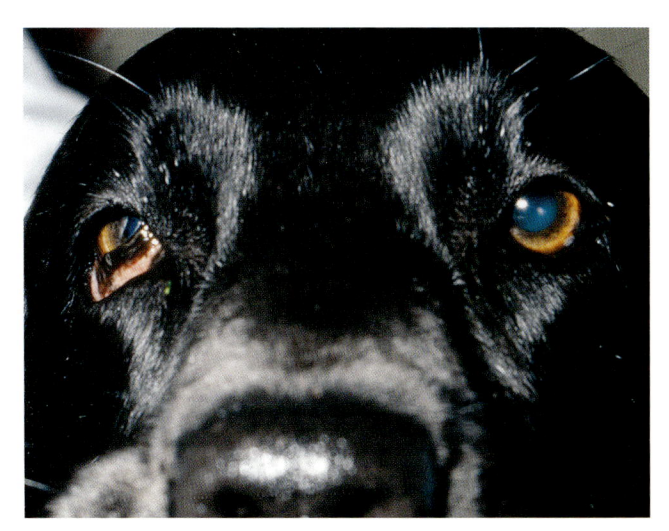

Plate 5.1:
Horner's syndrome (OD) in a Labrador Retriever, after peripheral trauma to the sympathetic fibers. There is enophthalmos, protrusion of the nictitating membrane, miosis, and ptosis (see also Plate 5.2).

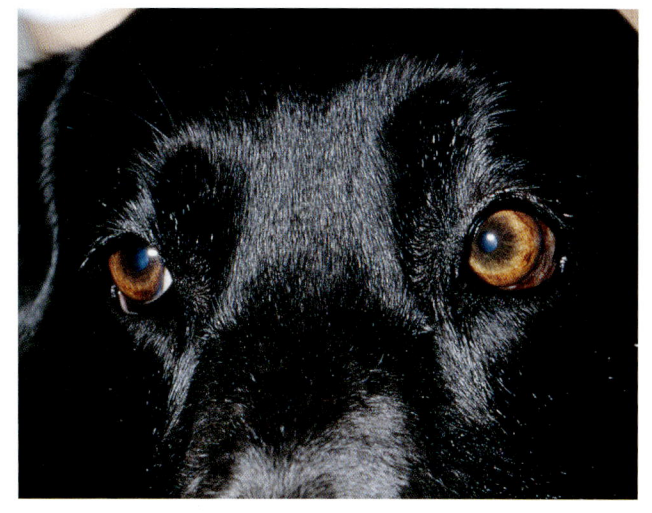

Plate 5.2:
Horner's syndrome (OD) of a Labrador Retriever after peripheral trauma, 15 minutes after one drop of topical 10% phenylephrine. The signs of the syndrome, except for the miosis, have almost disappeared (same eye as shown in Plate 5.1).

or through the conjunctival sac. Because absolute sterility is almost impossible to maintain in these cases, complications such as retrobulbar infection are likely.

5.4.2 Enophthalmos due to Horner's syndrome

Horner's syndrome (Plate 5.1) is caused by lesions of the sympathetic nerve fibers in the brain stem, the cranial plexus, or the pre- and postganglionic peripheral sympathetic fibers. Possible causes to be considered include congenital abnormalities, trauma, inflammation, infection, or neoplasia. In dogs, the causes are frequently idiopathic or unrecognized traumatic injuries (e.g. lunging on a chain) and are postganglionic. Lesions in the chest such as neoplasia or inflammatory disease can result in the clinical signs observed and these are also classified as Horner's syndrome. In cats, lymphosarcoma may cause lesions in the thoracic inlet and mediastinum (thoracic x-ray), again causing Horner's syndrome.[5]

Symptoms: Horner's syndrome is characterized by unilateral enophthalmos, protrusion of the nictitating membrane, miosis, and a variable degree of ptosis (slight drooping of the upper eyelid).

> Warmness and sweating of the ipsilateral part of the neck, ear, and face occurs in horses, which can only be detected during careful examination.[6,7]

Diagnosis: For diagnosis, as well as for prognosis and therapeutic purposes, one drop of 10% phenylephrine or 1% epinephrine is applied to both the affected and the unaffected eye (Plate 5.2). Also an extended neurological case history and a full neurological examination are indicated. If mydriasis occurs within 15–30 minutes, it is more likely that there is a postganglionic peripheral nerve lesion. In that case, the medication can be continued 2–3 times daily, as a palliative treatment.

Prognosis: The prognosis is favorable, as the signs often disappear within 1–6 months. If mydriasis does not occur, or is very slow, the lesion is probably more central and the prognosis is reserved.

5.5 Exophthalmos

Exophthalmos may be a response to space-occupying processes behind the eye, preventing its normal position in the orbit as previously discussed. Exophthalmos may be due to enlargement of the temporal muscles; extension of processes from the nasal or oral cavity, sinuses, and teeth; Cushing's syndrome and acromegaly; zygomatic mucocele; vessel anomalies behind the globe[8]; or edema, inflammation, abscesses, or neoplasia of the orbit.[9]

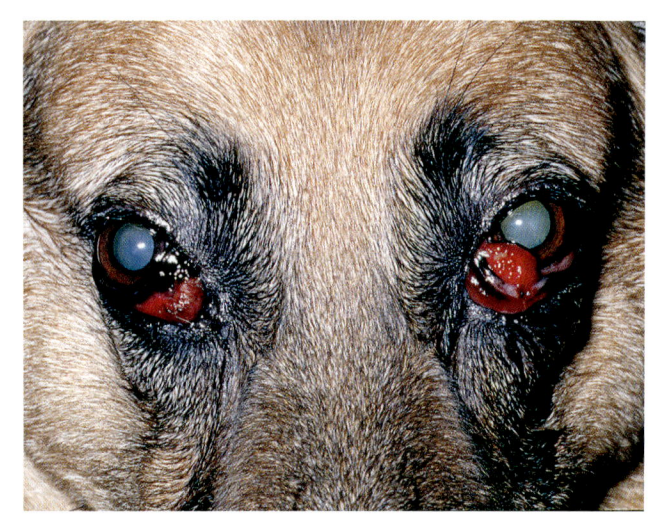

Plate 5.3:
Severe bilateral exophthalmos, protrusion of the nictitating membrane and swelling of the muscles of the cheeks in a German Shepherd, due to myositis (eosinophilic).

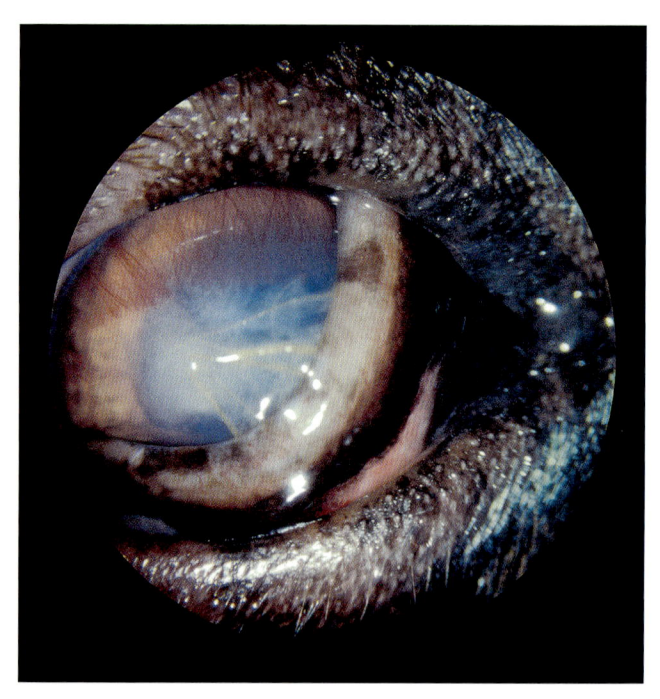

Plate 5.4:
Eye trauma due to a foreign body (OD, dog). The yellow spurs of a grain of wheat, covered with slimy exudate, peek from behind the nictitating membrane. The dog had had a severe blepharospasm for five days.

5.5.1 Exophthalmos due to swelling of the temporal muscles[10]

Inflammatory, degenerative, or autoimmune disorders involving the masseter, temporal, or pterygoid muscles are often associated with pain, exophthalmos, and protrusion (medial) of the nictitating membrane, although the signs are easily missed by the owner. Usually, the disorder results in subacute or chronic atrophy of these muscles, with subsequent protrusion of the nictitating membrane and enophthalmos. It is mainly found in larger dog breeds, especially the German Shepherd (eosinophilic myositis; Plate 5.3).

Diagnosis: Diagnosis "myositis" is made on the results of hematologic examination (increased lymphocytes, neutrophils, and eosinophils), muscle biopsy (most sensitive test), and electromyography.

Therapy: Therapy consists of prednisolone, 1–2 mg/kg, orally, once daily in the morning for one week and then on alternate days in decreasing dosage. For the treatment of chronic enophthalmos, see 5.4.

5.5.2 Exophthalmos due to retrobulbar processes (Plate 5.6–5.8)

There are numerous causes of swelling behind the eye, including the rare mucoceles of the lacrimal gland or the zygomatic glands, or arising from retained glandular tissue.[11] Usually, there will be an associated inflammation. In the dog, the most important causes of retrobulbar inflammation are penetrating foreign bodies, such as grass awns (Plates 5.4, 5.5, 5.7), which can work through the conjunctiva within a few hours, or slivers of wood which enter via the conjunctiva or from the mouth via the bottom of the orbit. The inflammation can spread diffusely (cellulitis) or can form an abscess (Plate 5.6). In the cat, retrobulbar inflammations are less frequent. This is probably because cats are more on their guard when playing, moving, and eating than dogs are.

In rabbits and rodents, inflammatory orbital ingrowth of molars (caused by e.g. hypocalcaemia) or fat retention may produce retrobulbar processes.

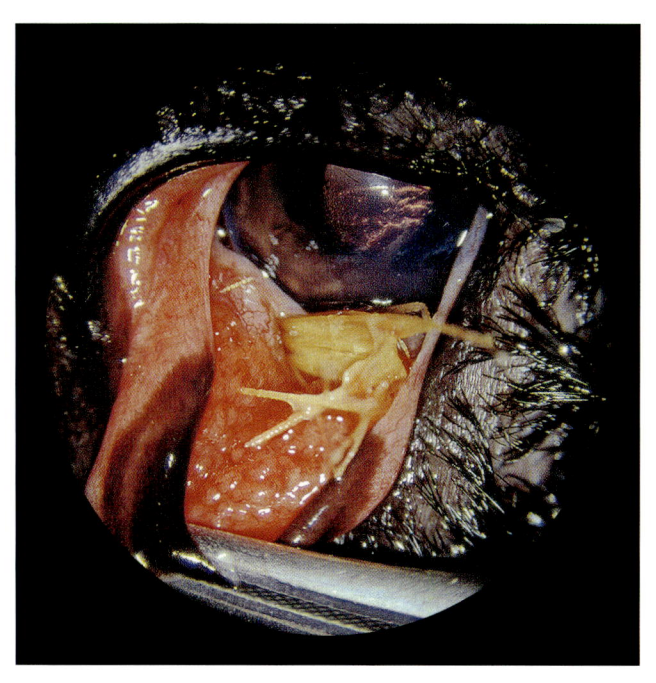

Exophthalmos 51

Plate 5.5:
Eye trauma due to a foreign body, about 5 hours after the start of the blepharospasm (OS, dog). The grain of wheat has already penetrated the conjunctiva for several millimeters. Such foreign bodies can penetrate the conjunctiva fully in less than one day and can be the cause of a retrobulbar abscess developing afterwards.

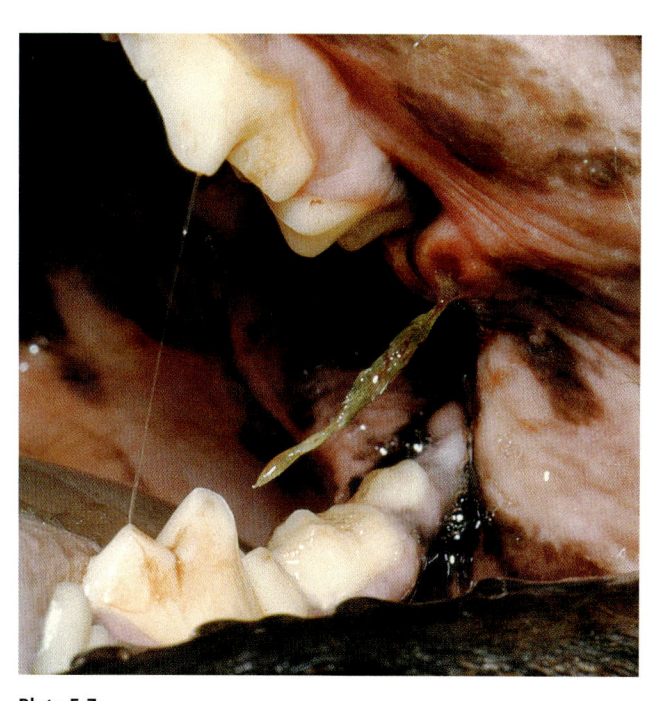

Plate 5.7:
Grass seed bulging out of a just-opened retrobulbar abscess (behind M 2; left side, dog).

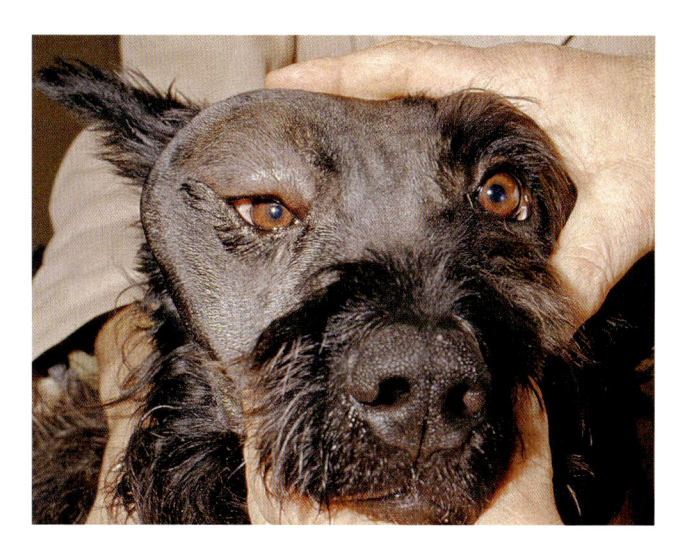

Plate 5.6:
Retrobulbar abscess (right side) in a Bouvier des Flanders. After shaving, the swelling is obvious. Note that there is no distinct protrusion of the nictitating membrane because of the dorsolateral location of the abscess. The miosis is due to mild uveitis.

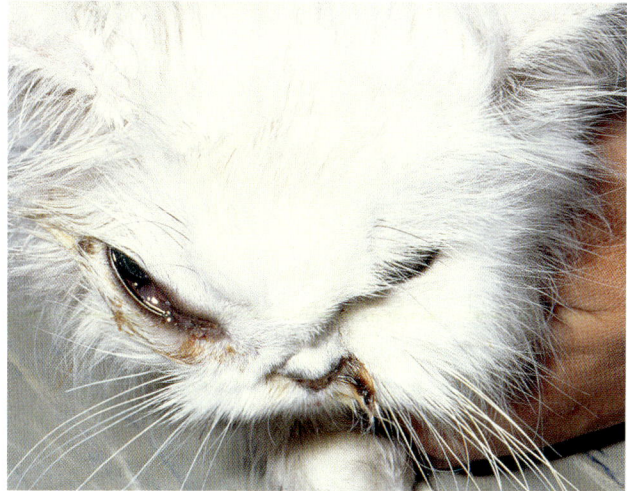

Plate 5.8:
Retrobulbar neoplasia (right side) in a 12-year-old Persian cat, seen from above. Due to the neoplasm, the globe is dislocated laterally and rostrally. Furthermore, there is a severe deformation of the head.

Proliferative inflammatory disease (e.g. of the deep gland [Hardens] of the nictitating membrane), abscesses or neoplasia may cause exophthalmos in birds.

Primary orbital neoplasms (Plate 5.8) can develop from each type of orbital and periorbital tissue.[12,13] Secondary neoplasms can arise from adjacent tissues (e.g. the mouth, nasal cavity, and sinuses)[14] or they can be metastases from neoplasms elsewhere in the body. Both primary and secondary forms are rare.

Usually, it is not easy to determine whether a retrobulbar process is cystic, inflammatory, or neoplastic. For this reason, it is best to start by considering a patient with a retrobulbar process in general.

In the history, it is usually noted that the animal has had difficulty eating for some time and that the eyeball has been very gradually protruding (exophthalmos) or that its position has otherwise changed. Questions must then be asked to determine whether the patient can still bark, chew, pick up its bone or ball, or yawn, and whether in doing so it shows pain.

Symptoms: The most noticeable sign is unilateral exophthalmos or, in exceptional cases, lateral displacement of the eyeball. In bilateral exophthalmos, processes by the optic chiasm must be considered or diseases such as myositis (swelling of the chewing muscles; most often in the German Shepherd Dog [eosinophilic]), Cushing's disease or acromegaly, or malignant lymphoma. Usually, there is also protrusion of the nictitating membrane, but this may not occur if the process is located more laterally. The eyeball itself is not enlarged but it can show the effects of the pressure or damage, which frequently leads to the referral of such patients because of a suspicion of glaucoma. The retrobulbar pressure is increased. Opening of the mouth is limited and, especially when the process is inflammatory, it can be extremely painful. It is advisable to ask the owner to open the animal's mouth for examination, but very carefully. Palpation of the soft floor of the orbit, behind the last molar, sometimes reveals thickening and/or sensitivity to pressure. Swelling of the optic disc can be expected if there is pressure or inflammation around the optic nerve, but this is difficult to confirm using monocular direct ophthalmoscopy.

Diagnosis: The differential diagnoses include all lesions arising from the orbit and the immediately adjacent tissues. The diagnosis can only be confirmed satisfactorily by additional examinations and/or biopsy and drainage. Simple diagnostic procedures can include blood examinations (which may reveal very high or low numbers of leukocytes, or eosinophilia) and aspiration biopsy of the mandibular lymph node or, rarely, of a peripherally located, fluctuating swelling. Only if the cytology of the biopsy reveals evidence of metastasis is the diagnosis thereby completed. However, more complex procedures are usually necessary to arrive at a definitive diagnosis, so the patient must be referred. These procedures must be carried out under general anesthesia and can include radiography in several projections (also with contrast media to detect bone destruction, cysts, or proliferation), ultrasonography (masses and especially fluid accumulation), CT, MRI, cytologic or histologic examination of biopsies of thickened tissue and/or exudates, and culture and antibiotic sensitivity testing.

Therapy: If there is no direct evidence of malignancy, drainage of the retrobulbar process should be carried out. The patient is anesthetized with the endotracheal tube sealed to prevent insufflation of blood or purulent material into the trachea. For this purpose, a short probe (with an eye) or a mosquito forceps is introduced from the oral cavity, behind the last molar, in the direction of the orbit (Fig. 5.4). If clear, viscid fluid without direct signs of inflammation is aspirated, a cystic lesion of the zygomatic gland is likely.[15,16] Complete surgical removal of the mucocele via orbitotomy is usually the only possible therapy.

If purulent material is aspirated, it is used for culture and antibiotic sensitivity testing. If foreign bodies such as grass awns are found (Plate 5.7), they are removed. Usually, however, it is necessary to insert a Penrose drain starting behind the M2, following the sondage route as shown in Figure 5.4. The drain is fixed to the skin dorsolateral to the eye. This is fixed to the skin. The drain serves to maintain an open channel through which any foreign material will exit and/or the abscess can be drained (Plate 5.7).

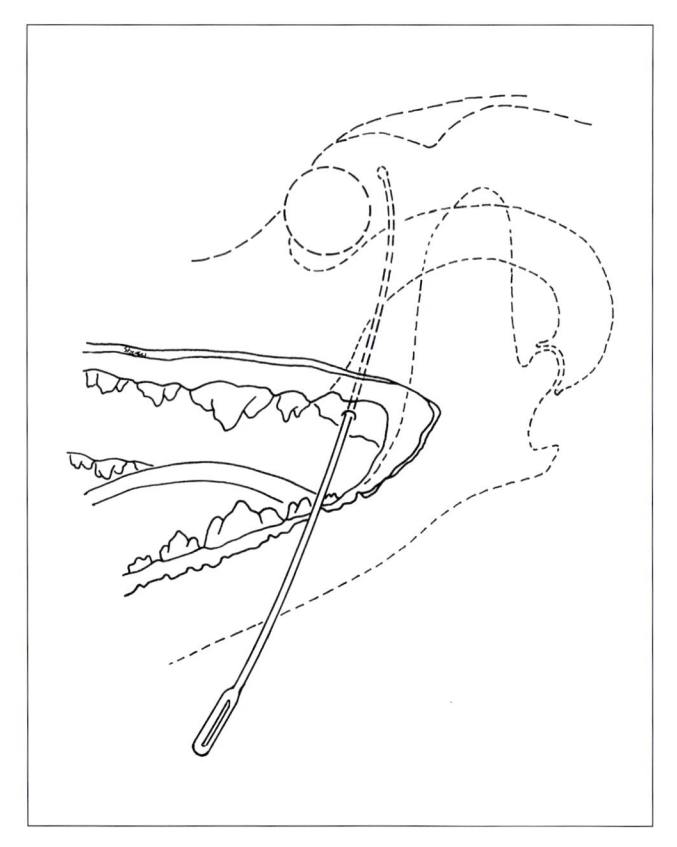

Fig. 5.4:
Retrobulbar process. Sondage inserted dorsally behind the last molar.

After drainage, the patient receives an broad-spectrum antibiotic (e.g. amoxicillin with clavulanic acid) or an appropriate antibiotic according to the sensitivity test, for 10 days, eventually together with corticosteroids. Some ophthalmologists also insert an antibiotic-corticosteroid ointment along the drain, into the orbit. The eyeball is protected with an "initial choice" antibiotic ointment. In exceptional cases (e.g. when the patient is very young or in very poor condition), a decision may be made to avoid anesthesia, start with medical therapy, and evaluate its results first.

Therapeutic possibilities in retrobulbar abscesses in the rabbit are limited. Frequently, they contain very thick, granular purulent material, which is very difficult to drain. With molar abscesses, it is generally better to extract the affected molar.

The treatment possibilities for retrobulbar neoplasms are limited. Sometimes, the disease can be slowed, but in almost all cases the well-being of the animal can be improved by the use of high doses of corticosteroids. This can be continued until the owner agrees to the usually unavoidable euthanasia.

For the purpose of diagnosis, when a retrobulbar process is resistant to the initial therapy, or for orbitotomy if a well-circumscribed neoplasm (e.g., of the zygomatic salivary gland) is suspected, referral of the patient can be considered. In an orbitotomy, a part of the zygomatic arch is lifted to allow inspection of the orbit (see 5.10). If the tumor is inoperable, specific cytostatics or corticosteroids may stop the process. High doses of corticosteroids, at least, may improve the general well-being of the patient before the often unavoidable euthanasia.

5.6 Enucleation of the globe including the conjunctiva

(Fig. 5.5)

Indications for enucleation of the globe include a painful eye with irreversible blindness or damage as a result of severe trauma, panophthalmitis, glaucoma, or an intraocular neoplasm that cannot be treated locally.

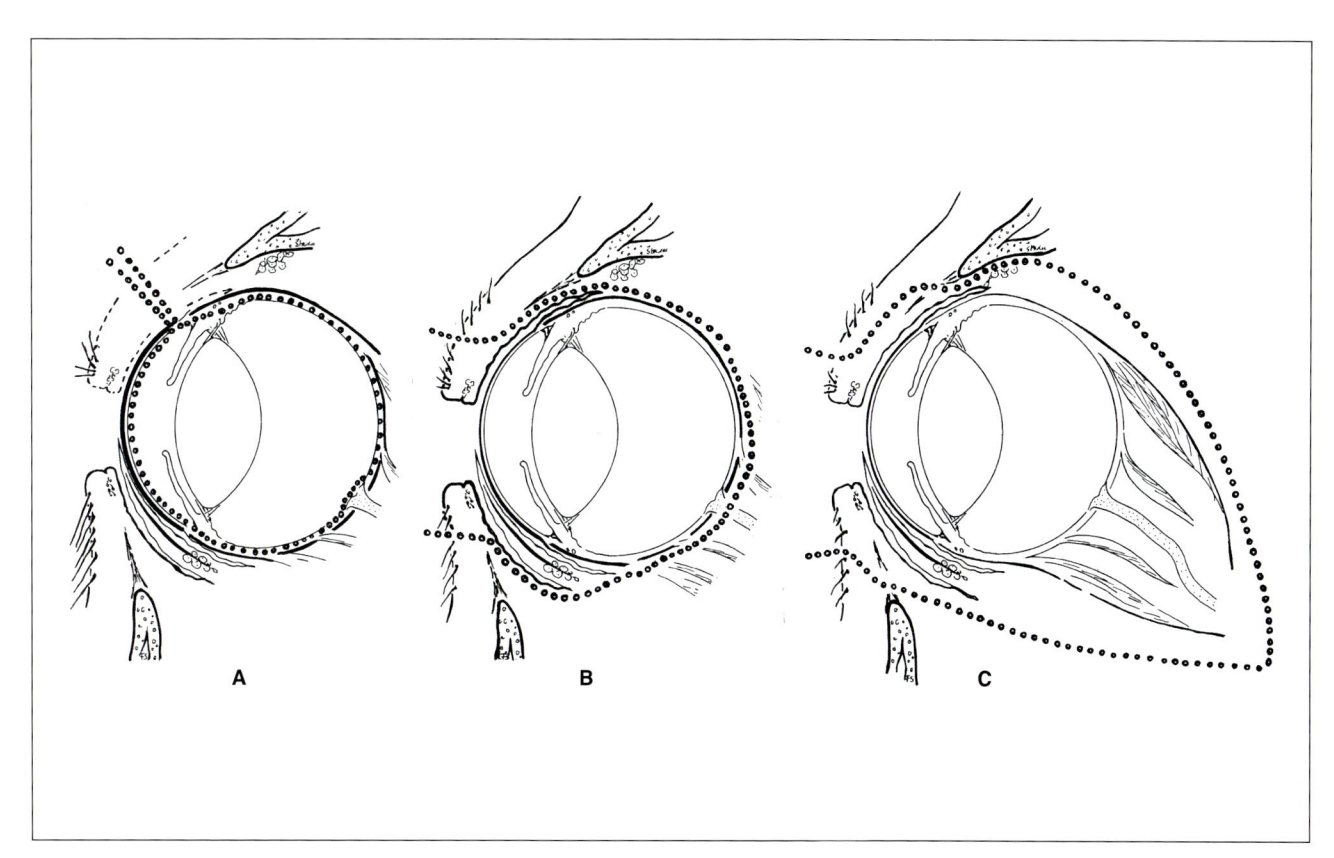

Fig. 5.5:
Evisceration of the globe (A); enucleation of the globe including the conjunctiva (B); exenteration of the orbit (C).

54 Orbital and Periorbital Structures

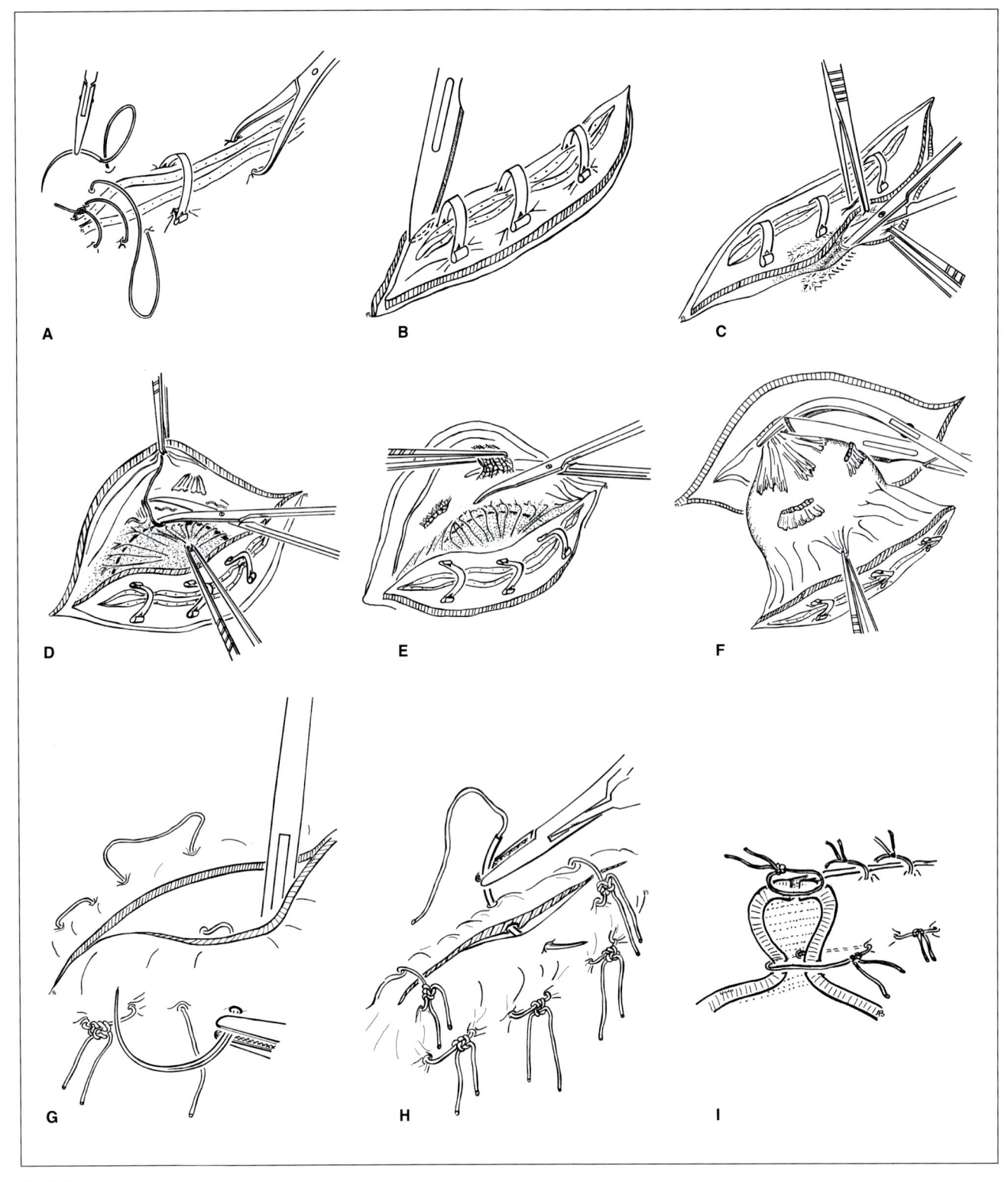

Fig. 5.6:
Enucleation of the globe and conjunctiva. Closure of the lid margin by sutures, clamps or staples (A); incision (B); dissection of the conjunctiva (C, D); cutting of the straight muscles (E); clamping and cutting of the optic stalk (F); suturing in two layers (G-I).

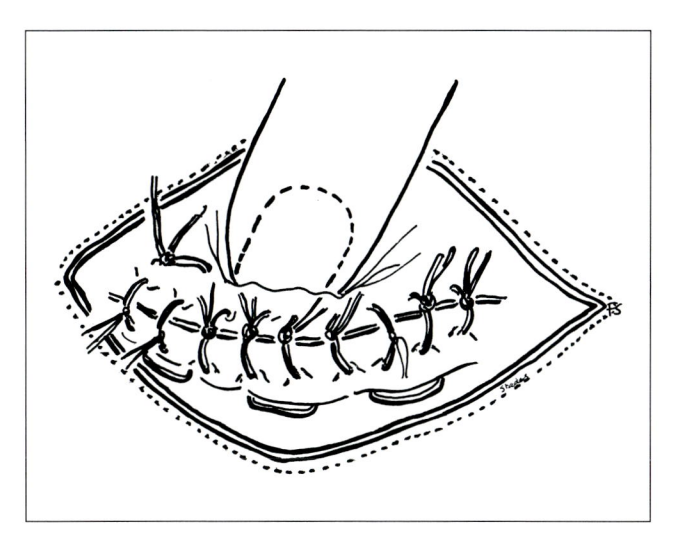

Fig. 5.7:
Postoperative check for "blood-tight" closure of the wound.

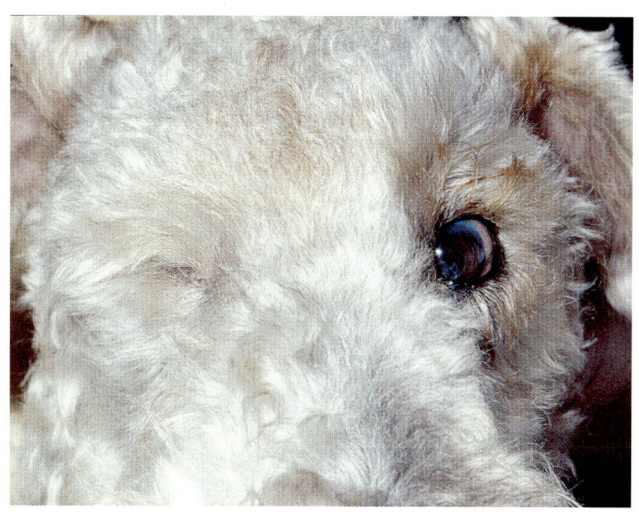

Plate 5.9:
Postoperative result 2 months after an enucleation in a Wire-haired Fox Terrier.

The objective is to remove the eye completely, so that an intraocular neoplasm (possibly not yet diagnosed) cannot metastasize, without complicating hemorrhage or infection, and while still achieving a reasonable cosmetic effect (Fig. 5.5, 5.6 and Plate 5.9).

Prior to surgery, the animal should be given "initial choice" antibiotics orally or parenterally (e.g. amoxicillin with clavulanic acid) and examined again to confirm that the eye to be enucleated is indeed the diseased one. Under general anesthesia, the operative field is prepared, with disinfection (povidone iodine) of the conjunctiva and cornea as well as the skin. The lid fissure can either be left open or closed with clips or sutures, or with Allis or towel forceps. An elliptical incision is made around the eye opening, 3–5 mm from the lid edges, and including the tarsal glands. The upper and lower eyelid skin is then freed from the subconjunctival tissue. During this dissection no pressure should be placed on the eyeball. The orbital septum is perforated and the opening is enlarged first medially and then laterally, and around the lateral canthus. The sclera is dissected bluntly and dissection is continued over the sclera along the limbus and around the eye, except for the medial canthus. If the preparatory dissection has been close enough to the sclera, there is usually no problem with hemorrhage. The medial canthus skin is cut free to the septum and the medial septum is also perforated. Dissection is extended over the medial part of the sclera, parallel to the limbus. The four straight eye muscles are freed and cleaved over the sclera. It should now be possible to rotate the eye (no traction!) through 180 degrees. The stalk of the eye is clamped with a strong curved clamp (e.g. Mixter-Baby) after which the stalk can be cut off over the clamp.

The wound is closed with 3 or 4 flat mattress sutures of 3-0 to 4-0 absorbable material such as polyglactin. These sutures are placed 10–15 mm from the edges of the wound. Just before the last suture is tied, the clamp is carefully removed from the stalk, which does not have to be ligated. The placement of these sutures results in a large ridge of skin, preventing post operative retraction of the skin into the orbit. The wound edges are now carefully closed with simple interrupted sutures, approximately 5 mm apart, using the same suture material. Pressure is applied to the skin over the orbit to be certain that the wound does not leak (Fig. 5.7). The wound can be covered with spray bandage and a ball of cotton wool. The owner should be warned of the possibility of a loss of a few drops of blood from the nostril on the same side (via the nasolacrimal duct).

Postoperative treatment consists of continuing the antibiotics for 4 days. The sutures are removed after 10–12 days. The ridge flattens out and an eyebrow-like edge remains. The eyeball is submitted to an ophthalmic pathologist for pathologic examination, especially to determine whether there is an intraocular malignancy.

In birds, one has to be aware that the globes are enormous compared to the size of the head, that the retractor muscle does not exist, and that the distance to the chiasm is extremely short. Moreover, there is a bony plate system in the sclera which does not allow any changes in the form of the globe, and the space between the globe and the bony orbit is very limited. Centrally, the globes are only separated by a very thin bony septum. For enucleation, a highly curved pair of scissors is required. More space is available when the operation wound is enlarged by including the opening of the ear. During enucleation any traction on the optic nerve has to be avoided, to prevent damage to the optic chiasm.[17]

5.7 Evisceration of the globe

(Fig. 5.5 A)

In this procedure, the contents of the eye are removed but the sclera and cornea are left intact and an artificial ball is inserted to prevent collapse. If there are no complications, a good cosmetic effect is achieved. This is, however, not in the interest of the animal. In 10–20% of cases there may be short-term complications.[18] In particular, the fact that intraocular neoplasms often cannot always be recognized during the presurgical examination (even when ultra-sonography is used; about 8–13% of buphthalmic eyes) is a risk for the patient that is ethically not outweighed by the cosmetic appeal to the owner. A proper explanation to the owner is thus essential.

5.8 Enucleation of the globe

(Fig. 5.5 B)

In this procedure only the globe is removed. Some surgeons preserve the conjunctiva, to prevent traction of the skin into the orbit. The lid margins are removed and the wound is closed over the conjunctival tissues. This can lead to a continued activity of the remaining glandular tissues, resulting in a fluctuating orbital cavity. For these reasons, the removal of the globe including the conjunctiva is preferred (see 5.6).

Enucleation of the globe can be done in order to facilitate the subsequent introduction of an artificial eye. Artificial eyes (in the form of a shell, with painted iris and conjunctival vessels) must be removed regularly from the conjunctival sac for cleaning of both the prosthetic contact lens and the sac. This procedure preserves the adnexa of the eye. The globe is isolated by an incision at the limbus, dissecting through Tenon's capsule, and identifying the extrinsic muscles including the recti, obliques, and the retractor oculi cone. These muscles should be incised as close to the sclera as possible. A prosthetic sphere is placed in the orbital cone and the muscles are either attached to them or the muscles are sewn over the sphere to allow later movement of the prosthesis. The conjunctiva is then oversewn and a plastic conformer is placed in the cul-de-sac to prevent contraction and provide a support for the prosthetic contact lens. This procedure requires the skill of an ophthalmic surgeon. Few people perform this procedure because of the expense and the laxity of the lids in dogs, which may result in loss of the expensive contact lens. The method is more frequently used in horses, particularly those that are shown. Because of the cost and the difficulty in achieving a successful outcome, enucleation with direct removal of the total conjunctiva is preferred.

5.9 Exenteration of the orbit

(Fig. 5.5 C)

In this procedure, the entire orbital contents are removed. Exenteration of the orbit is indicated if a neoplasm has extended outside the eyeball and is the treatment of last resort.

5.10 Orbitotomy

In this procedure, the orbit is opened via the zygomatic arch. The arch is cut with a saw medially and laterally. Holes are first drilled on each side of the line of cutting, so that the piece of bone can later be replaced and held by steel cerclages.[19,20] About 3–5 cm of the arch can be lifted out. This method can be used by the specialist for diagnosis of orbital processes or for the removal of a well-circumscribed neoplasm in the orbit.

Literature

1. GELATT, K.N., GUFFY, M.M. & BOGGESS, T.S.: Radiographic contrast techniques for detecting orbital and nasolacrimal tumors in dogs. JAVMA **156**: 741, 1970.

2. LECOUTEUR, R.A. et al.: Indirect imaging of the canine optic nerve, using metrizamide (optic thecography). Am. J. Vet. Res. **43**: 1424, 1982.

3. MILLER, W.W. & CARTREE, R.E.: B-scan ultrasonography for the detection of space-occupying ocular masses. JAVMA **187**: 66, 1985.

4. EISENBERG, H.M.: Ultrasonography of the eye and orbit. Vet. Clin. North. A, **15**: 1263, 1985.

5. MORGAN, R.V. & ZANOTTI, S.W.: Horner's syndrome in dogs and cats: 49 cases (1980–1986). JAVMA **194**: 1096, 1989.

6. JONES, B.R. & STUDDERT, V.P.: Horner's syndrome in the dog and cat as an aid to diagnosis. Aust. Vet. J. **51**: 329, 1975.

7. SWEENEY, R.W. & SWEENEY, C.R.: Transient Horner's syndrome following routine intravenous injections in two horses. JAVMA **185**: 802, 1984.

8. RUBIN, L.F. & PATTESON, D.F.: Arteriovenous fistula of the orbit in a dog. Cornell Vet. **55** (3): 471, 1965.

9. MCCALLA, T.L. & MOORE, C.P.: Exophthalmos in dogs and cats. Part 1. Anatomic and diagnostic considerations. Comp. Cont. Ed. Vet. Med. **11**: 784, 1989.

10. GLAUBERG, A. & BEAUMONT, P.R.: Sudden blindness as the presenting sign of eosinophilic myositis: A case report. JAAHA **15**: 609, 1979.

11. KNECHT, C.D.: Treatment of disease of the zygomatic salivary gland. JAAHA **6**: 13, 1970.

12. CARLTON, W.W.: Orbital neoplasms. In: Comparative Ophthalmic Pathology. Ed.: R. L. Pfeiffer. Springfield, Charles C. Thomas, pp 47–63, 1983.

13. GROSS, S., AGUIRRE, G. & HARVEY, C.: Tumors involving the orbit of the dog. Trans. Am Coll. Vet. Ophthalmol. **10**: 229, 1979.

14. GELATT, K.N., LADDS, P.W. & GUFFY, M.M.: Nasal adenocarcinoma with orbital extension and ocular metastasis in a dog. JAAHA **6**: 132, 1970.

15. HOFFER, R.E.: Surgical treatment of salivary mucocele. Vet. Clin. North Am **5**: 333, 1975.

16. SCHMIDT, G.M. & BETTS, C.W.: Zygomatic salivary mucoceles in the dog. JAVMA **172**: 883, 1983.

17. MURPHY, C.K.J., BROOKS, D.E., KERN, T.J. *et al.*: Enucleation in birds of prey. JAVMA **183**: 1235, 1983.

18. KOCH, S.A.: Intraocular prosthesis in the dog and cat: The failures. JAVMA **179**: 883, 1981.

19. BISTNER, S.I., AGUIRRE, G. & BATIK, G.: Atlas of Veterinary Ophthalmic Surgery, Philadelphia, W. B. Saunders, 1977.

20. SLATTER, D. H. & ABDELBAKI, Y.: Lateral orbitotomy by zygomatic arch resection in the dog. JAVMA **175**: 1179, 1979.

6 Lacrimal Apparatus

6.1 Introduction

The tear film actively and passively protects the cornea and conjunctiva (it contains e.g. lysozyme, lactoferrin, IgA, IgM and IgE),[1,2,3] keeps them clean, moist and lubricated, supplied with nutrients, and transports white blood cells. The eyelids spread the tear film over the surface of the eyeball and maintain its thickness within very narrow limits.[4] The upper eyelid, in particular, has a very important function in this regard. In birds, the thickness of the tear film is mainly maintained by the nictitating membrane (Plate 2.10). Some cats have a relatively low frequency of blinking and often a markedly lower tear production than dogs. This may be one of the causes of the frequent occurrence of central corneal sequester formation in the cat, especially the Persian, Himalayan and Burmese which have very large, protruding eyes.

The tear film (Fig. 6.1) is approximately 0.04–0.07 mm thick and consists of three layers.[5,6] The outer layer is the lipid layer, which is produced by the sebaceous glands in the margins of the lids, and reduces evaporation, lubricates and prevents adhesion of debris. The middle layer is formed by the aqueous fraction of the tears. It washes away foreign bodies and contains, for example, antimicrobial agents, soluble mucins, immunoglobulins, enzymes and cellular debris. This layer blends gradually into the inner, mucous layer of the tear film, which is mainly produced by the intra-epithelial goblet cells of the conjunctiva. This hydrophilic layer attaches to the glycocalyx,[7] which serves as an adhesive between the hydrophobic microvilli of the corneal epithelium and the mucous layer of the tear film, thus lubricating and protecting the cornea. The mucous layer also entraps debris and microbes in a mucous thread, which moves continuously, via the lower cul-de-sac, to the medial canthus. There it dries and is rubbed away.

About 60% of the aqueous portion of the precorneal tear film is produced by the lacrimal gland, which is located dorsolateral to the globe, under the zygomatic process of the frontal bone (Fig. 6.2). The remaining 40% of the tears is produced by the gland (or glands in some species) of the nictitating membrane (main producer of tears in birds) and by the accessory tear glands.[8]

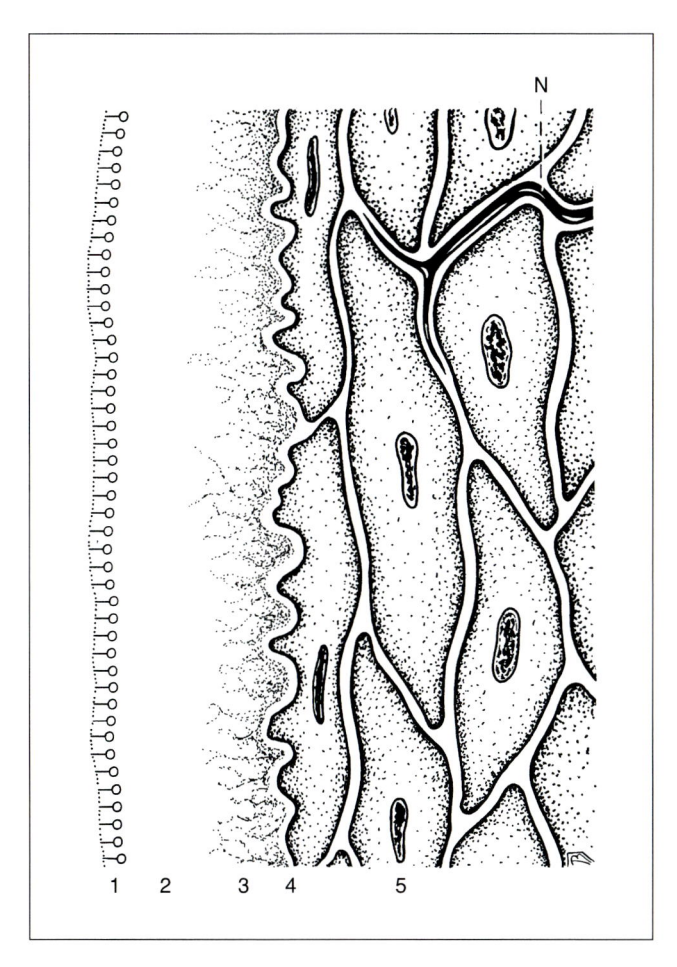

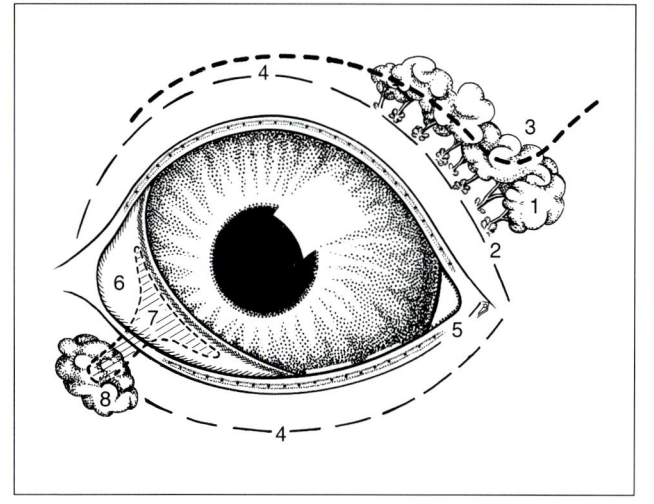

Fig. 6.2:
Tear production apparatus. (1) Lacrimal gland, (2) accessory lacrimal glands, (3) zygomatic process of the frontal bone, (4) fornix, (5) tarsal glands (meibomian), (6) nictitating membrane (NM), (7) NM cartilage, (8) superficial gland of the NM.

Fig. 6.1:
Tear film and the superficial corneal epithelium. (1) Lipid layer, (2) watery fraction, (3) mucous layer, (4) microvilli, (5) epithelial cell; N: nerve fiber.

60 Lacrimal Apparatus

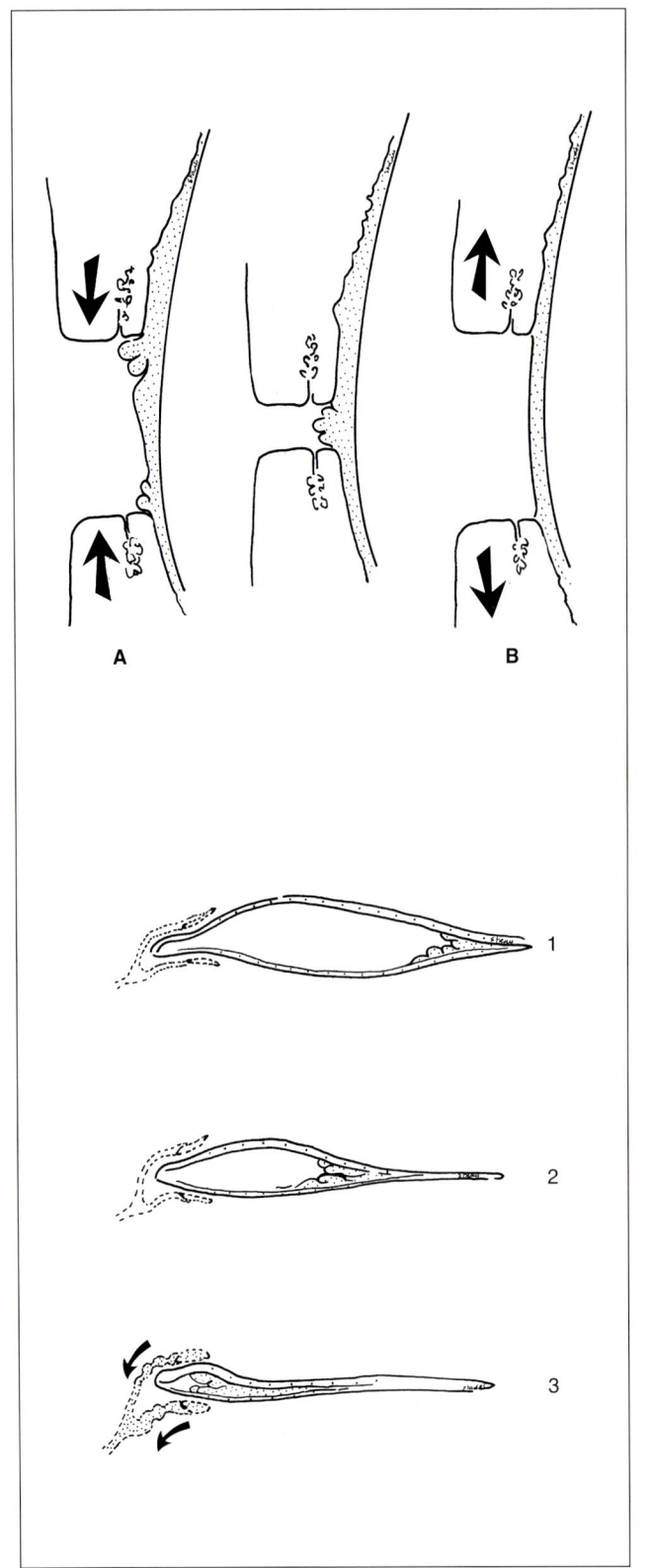

Fig. 6.3:
The push-up of the tears (A) during the closure phase of blinking; "drawing" of the tear film (B) during opening of the lids. The drainage of the used tear fluid by the "zipper" mechanism of blinking (1, 2, 3).

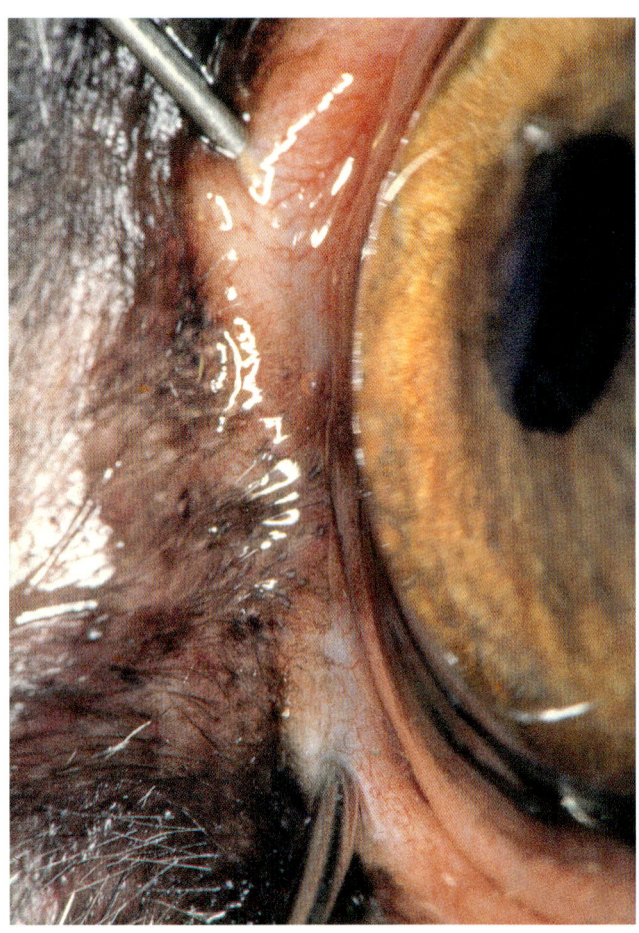

Plate 6.1:
Superior and inferior lacrimal punctum in a dog, probed by a tear duct cannula (OS). The first 3–4 mm of the canaliculus is parallel to the lid edge and just covered with a conjunctival sheet. The (normal) caruncle hairs are easily recognizable.

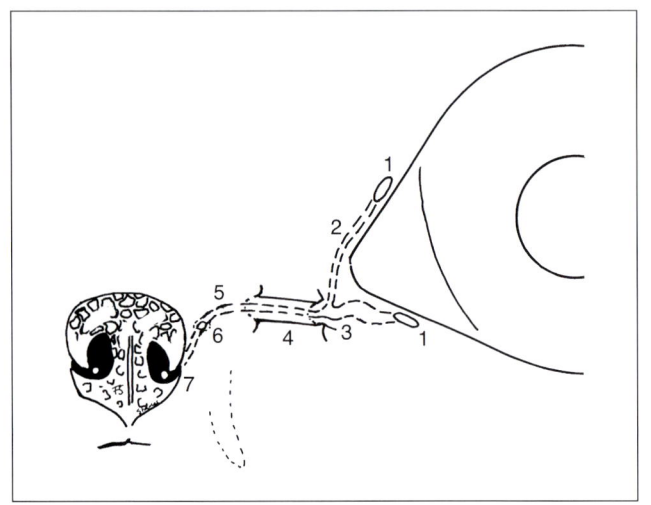

Fig. 6.4:
Tear drainage. (1) Lacrimal punctum, (2) lacrimal canaliculus, (3) lacrimal saccus, (4) nasolacrimal duct (NLD) in the bony tunnel, (5) NLD in the nasal mucosa, (6) opening of the duct at the level of canine tooth, (7) ostium in the nasal opening.

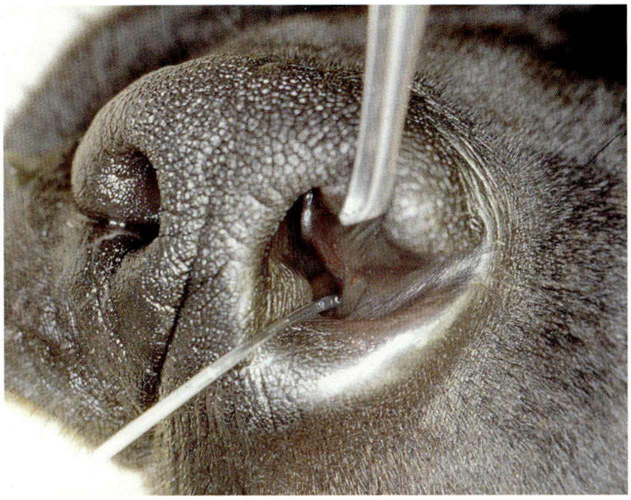

Plate 6.2:
Location of the ostium of the nasolacrimal duct in the lateral nares of a dog. The silicon tube peeks out of the ostium, which is positioned one mm more laterally, inside of the nose.

Stimuli that are painful or irritating to the cornea and conjunctiva or to the adnexa can increase tear production, while anesthesia, atropine, and drugs such as some sulfonamide derivatives and etodolac can reduce it.

Part of the tear film evaporates. The remainder drains away via the lacrimal punctae (oval, 2–3 mm diameter; Figs. 6.3, 6.4 and Plate 6.1), which are located 6–10 mm from the medial canthus in the conjunctiva at the mucocutaneous junctions of the lower and upper lids. From there, the tear fluid drains via the lacrimal canaliculi (Fig. 6.4), the saccus, and nasolacrimal duct to the external nares (Plate 6.2). In some animals, the nasolacrimal duct does not extend all the way to the nose but empties into the nasopharynx at the level of the canine tooth. Obstruction or compression along the path of drainage and/or overproduction of tear fluid quickly leads to epiphora and tear stripe formation (tear staining syndrome; Plate 6.7).

In the cat, this epiphora is often accompanied by pigmented detritus, possibly resulting from oxidized catecholamines in the tears that can accumulate as small pigmented stripes on the margins of the lids and in the tear stripe, and which can infiltrate the corneal surface resulting in sequestra.[9]

In rabbits and swine only a lower punctum exists.

6.2 Keratoconjunctivitis sicca (KCS)

KCS (Plates 6.3–6.6) can be defined as a tear film deficiency of the cornea and conjunctiva, and hence it is not a primary keratitis. KCS is usually caused by an inadequate production of tears by the lacrimal glands, thus of the watery fraction, and therefore the STT values are low and the tear film break-up time is less than 20 sec. This deficiency can also occur because the tear film breaks up due to an abnormal composition (e.g. of the mucous layer). In these cases, there are often low-normal STT values in addition to minor sicca signs.

There are many known causes of KCS:
1. KCS can be congenital and possibly inherited.
2. Traumatic injuries to the lacrimal glands or in the area of its innervation near the base of the ear can result in inflammation and/or atrophy of the glands themselves or in a disturbance to their innervation.
3. Surgical trauma to the nerve supply or the tear glands or their ducts can cause KCS. Also, the removal of the nictitans gland may result in KCS.[10] KCS, after hypophysectomy has been ascribed to traumatic or ischemic neuropraxia of the major petrosal nerves.[11] In rats, hypophysectomy-induced regression of the lacrimal gland was partially restored by the administration of androgens and prolactin, suggesting trophic action of these hormones on the gland.[12]
4. Nutritional deficiencies such as hypovitaminosis A.
5. Intoxications such as locoweed,[13] belladonna, and botulism can cause KCS.
6. Medications such as phenazopyridine,[14] etodolac and sulpha derivatives (*note: sometimes used in geriatrics or for chronic kidney/bladder disease*) can cause permanent KCS in less than 14 days. Atropine can cause temporary KCS.[15,16] Tear production ceases during general anesthesia.[17,18] An unprotected cornea will dry out very quickly, especially under anesthesia during which the eyelids remain open (e.g. anesthesia with ketamine in the cat), and certainly if the eye also lies directly under the heat of the surgical lights. During anesthesia the eyes should be protected by application of a neutral eye ointment.
7. Inflammation, especially due to infection of the tear glands, is an important cause of KCS. Infections of the conjunctival sac presumably provide an important port of entry for infection of the tear glands, but can also result in blockage of the drainage system. In addition, inflammation in the middle ear can cause a disturbance to the parasympathetic innervation of the tear glands.
8. Autoimmune diseases resulting in a plasmacytic, lymphocytic adenitis, can cause KCS.[19] This is a T-cell reaction and justifies using T-cell inhibitors for treatment. This is the most frequent cause of KCS in the dog. Autoimmune and degenerative diseases such as Sjögren's syndrome and the dysautonomia syndrome have been reported to cause KCS. Sjögren's syndrome, in which all mucous membranes are excessively dry, is the most important cause of KCS in humans. Sjögren's syndrome has also been described as a

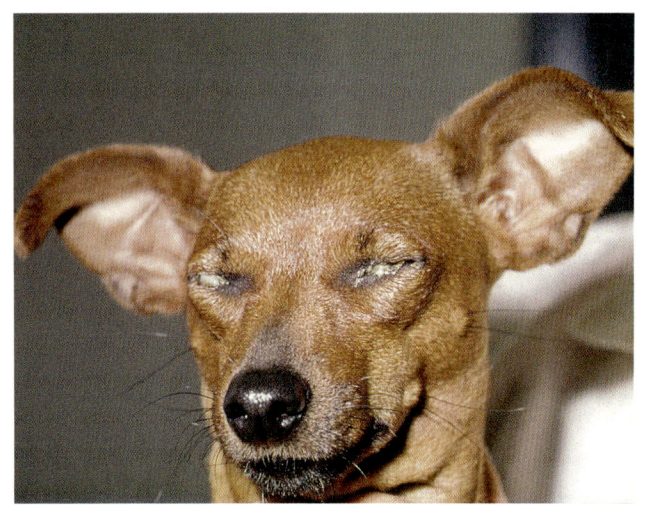

Plate 6.3:
Severe bilateral blepharospasm with mucopurulent discharge, without signs of epiphora. Conclusion: keratoconjunctivitis sicca. The nasal plane is wet, thus making Sjögren's syndrome a less plausible cause.

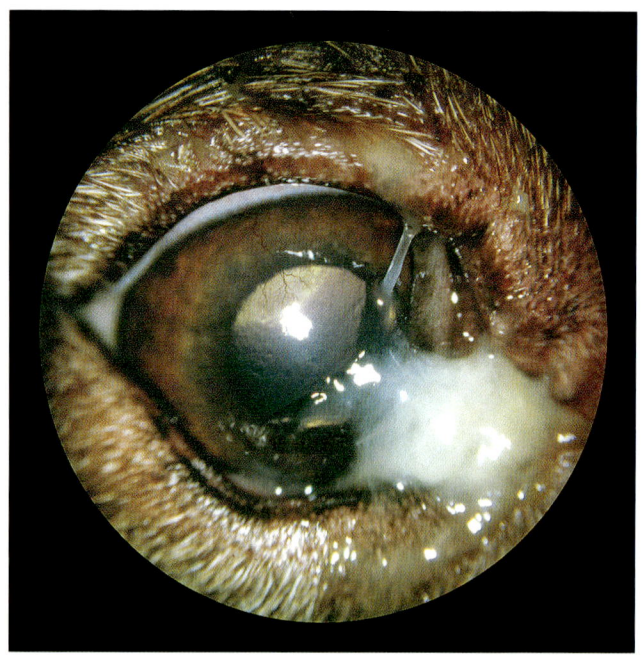

Plate 6.4:
Keratoconjunctivitis sicca (OD, dog). Mucopurulent discharge with crusts. There is pus instead of clear tears. The corneal reflex is malformed. The Schirmer value was 0 mm/minute.

cause of KCS in dogs[20], but not as yet in cats. In dysautonomia syndrome in cats and dogs (see 12.12), the sympathetic and parasympathetic neurons of the autonomic ganglia are degenerate. Mydriasis is found in approximately 90% of these cats, and in 80% there is a distinct KCS.

9. Neoplasia can directly or indirectly destroy the lacrimal glands.
10. Idiopathic causes. In many patients with KCS, the primary cause cannot be determined. The glands atrophy or no longer function because of denervation, for example.
11. Secondary to lid defects, exophthalmos, proptosis, luxation of the globe, lagophthalmos etc., a local KCS or KCS over the whole conjunctiva and cornea may develop.

In the dog, KCS occurs regularly and since only a small proportion of these patients recover completely, they will continue to require regular follow-up examinations and attention. In the cat, KCS is seen much less frequently. However, tear film that breaks up too quickly in the central area of the cornea could easily be the initiating factor in the development of mummification or sequestration of the cornea in large-eyed and often short-nosed cats (see 10.6.4). KCS is usually bilateral (about 60%) and occurs more often in female animals (about 65%). Breed predisposition includes small dogs in general, with a high prevalence in the Long-haired Dachshund, Cavalier King Charles Spaniel, and West Highland White Terrier.

Symptoms: The cornea and conjunctiva lose their normal luster and have a dull matted appearance. The reflected image can no longer be seen sharply on the "cornea". There are variable signs of mucopurulent conjunctivitis, such as redness, swelling, slight blepharospasm, and mucopurulent discharge (Plates 6.3–6.6), although without the expected overproduction of tears and/or wet hair around the eye (Plate 6.3). If KCS has existed for some time, signs of a chronic superficial keratitis are to be expected, often beginning in the centrolateral part of the cornea, which is the part most exposed to drying. These signs include edema, injection of vessels, epithelial defects, fibrosis and pigmentation. Usually there is no edema, but epithelial keratinization and fibrosis cause the grayish-white corneal cloudiness. In the cat, there may be sequestration of the cornea. In addition, the ipsilateral half of the nasal plane (Plate 6.6) and the oral cavity can have a dry appearance. Sometimes, the dry nasal plane is the only sign of KCS that has come to the attention of the owner.

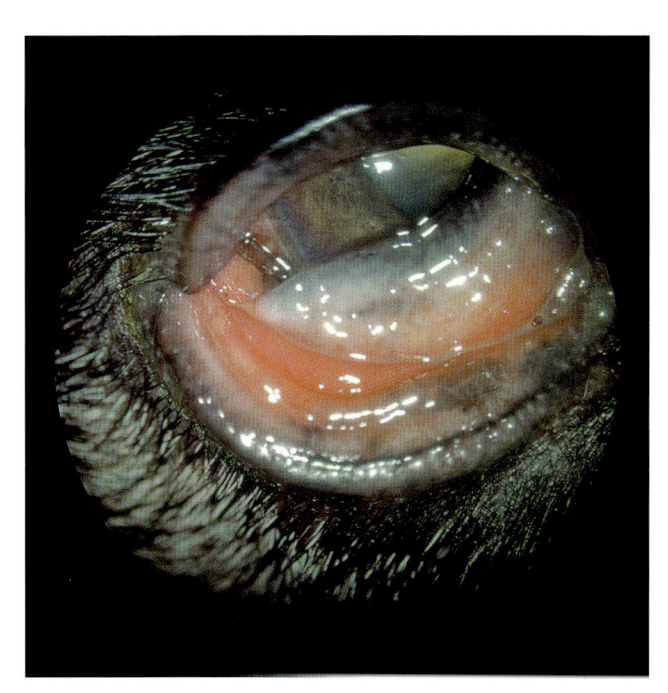

Plate 6.5:
Keratoconjunctivitis sicca (OD, dog). The mucopurulent discharge has been dissolved and washed out. The conjunctiva is red, swollen, folded, and dull. The cornea shows superficial vessels, and is not nicely reflective.

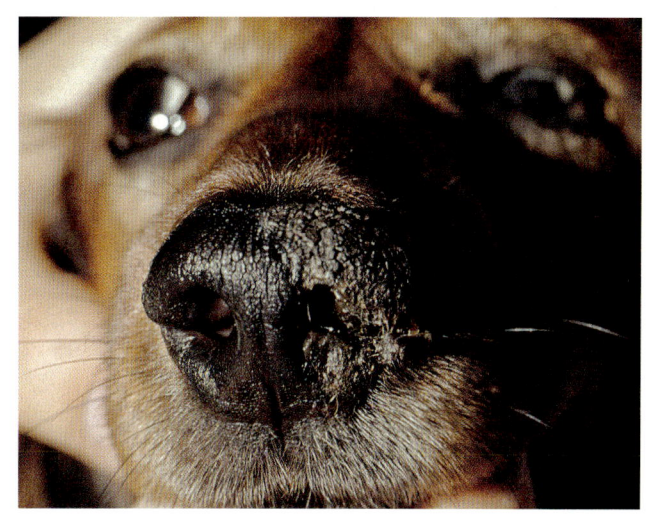

Plate 6.6:
Mucopurulent, crustose nasal discharge (left side) and an ipsilateral keratoconjunctivitis sicca. The abnormal eye had not been recognized by the owner.

Diagnosis: The diagnosis is based on the lowered STT value and the clinical signs. If the STT value is normal or low-normal, but there are still clinical signs consistent with KCS, referral for rose bengal staining of the cornea and tear film break-up time measurement, both with the aid of a slit-lamp biomicroscope, can be of additional diagnostic value.

Many forms of conjunctivitis and keratitis come into consideration in the differential diagnosis, but in these disorders, normal or even elevated tear production is to be expected.

Therapy: Treatment of mild KCS is medical. Severe chronic forms are treated medically or in specific cases surgically. If there are only minor signs of KCS, together with a low-normal STT and a positive rose bengal staining, then initially it will be sufficient to wash the eyes and apply e.g. cromoglycate and vitamin A oil, or dexamethasone, both 4 times daily, or 0.2% cyclosporine 2 times daily.

In severe, distinct acute KCS, antibiotics and corticosteroids are given orally for 7–10 days.[21] The client is educated to understand the nursing care necessary to provide comfort and function for the patient. Further treatment consists of dissolving the mucopurulent discharge with 10% acetylcysteine, washing the eye, and then applying 0.2% cyclosporine 2 times daily.[22] Cyclosporine can also be applied to both eyes even though the condition may only be unilateral. It takes at least 3 weeks before the drug reaches an effective level, and therefore ancillary therapy must be provided until the drug becomes effective. In a number of patients, an increased tear production does not occur, but the subjective signs of the disease are markedly reduced and the patient is much more comfortable. As more potent alternatives cyclosporine 2% can be used or the stronger 0.02–0.03% tacrolimus[23] or pimecrolimus (all T-cell inhibitors, see 3.2.11.5) *Note: the latter three are not registered for the use on the eye.*

Fifteen minutes after the cyclosporin ointment, a topical, "initial choice" antibiotic and if there is no overt ulceration, a corticosteroid or an "initial choice" antibiotic-corticosteroid combination are used. This procedure is repeated 4 times daily for 4–6 weeks. Artificial tears should be used as necessary at times other than those described. Additional pilocarpine can be administered orally[24] (see 3.2.3.1).

On the day of the follow-up examination (after 3–4 weeks), the topical medications are not given but, if prescribed, the pilocarpine should be given orally as usual. If the signs of KCS have disappeared and the STT value has become normal, the antibiotic-corticosteroid combination is adjusted to fit the patient's needs. Often one can discontinue them and maintain the patient on the T-cell inhibitor and the artificial tears or other mucocinomimetics (e.g. *i-drops*®). If the STT value is still low or has declined, the more potent T-cell inhibitors can be tried. Thereafter, a maintenance level is determined and the patient is kept on that level and monitored as needed. At the last resort, if the STT remains 0 and the owner is not able to continue the treatment, referral for a parotid duct transposition (PDT) can be considered. There must, however, be a normal production of saliva.

In the PDT operation[25,26] (difficult in the cat), the terminal portion of the parotid duct is freed in the mouth and is brought to the conjunctival sac either via a tunnel running totally under the skin of the cheek[27] or from an incision in the skin of the cheek, (Fig. 6.5). The opening of the duct is implanted in the ventrolateral fornix, between the nictitating membrane and the palpebral conjunctiva. The disadvantages of PDT are that calcium deposition can occur on the cornea and an excess of saliva/mucus can lead to inflammation of the skin of the cheek.

Prognosis: The prognosis for healing of distinct, acute KCS is relatively good, however, the prognosis for chronic KCS is less favorable. The prognosis for KCS is often somewhat better in cats than in dogs. Because only the smaller proportion of this group will heal completely, the majority of patients will need continuous veterinary care and thus, the owner must be motivated to do so.

6.3 (Sialo)dacryoadenitis

Dacryoadenitis of the deep gland of the nictitating membrane in rats and mice may cause porphyrine-containing tears and result in a redness of the skin around the eyes (chromodacryorrhea).

The sialodacryoadenitis virus in the rat is a highly infectious corona virus of the respiration apparatus of the rat. It causes rhinotracheitis, bronchitis and alveolitis. It may also cause an inflammation of the salivary glands and a necrotizing inflammation of the deep (Hardens) gland of the nictitating membrane and/or the other lacrimal glands

Symptoms: There may be exophthalmos, epiphora and keratoconjunctivitis. The symptoms will generally disappear spontaneously within a week, but may be complicated by uveitis and multifocal retinal degeneration.

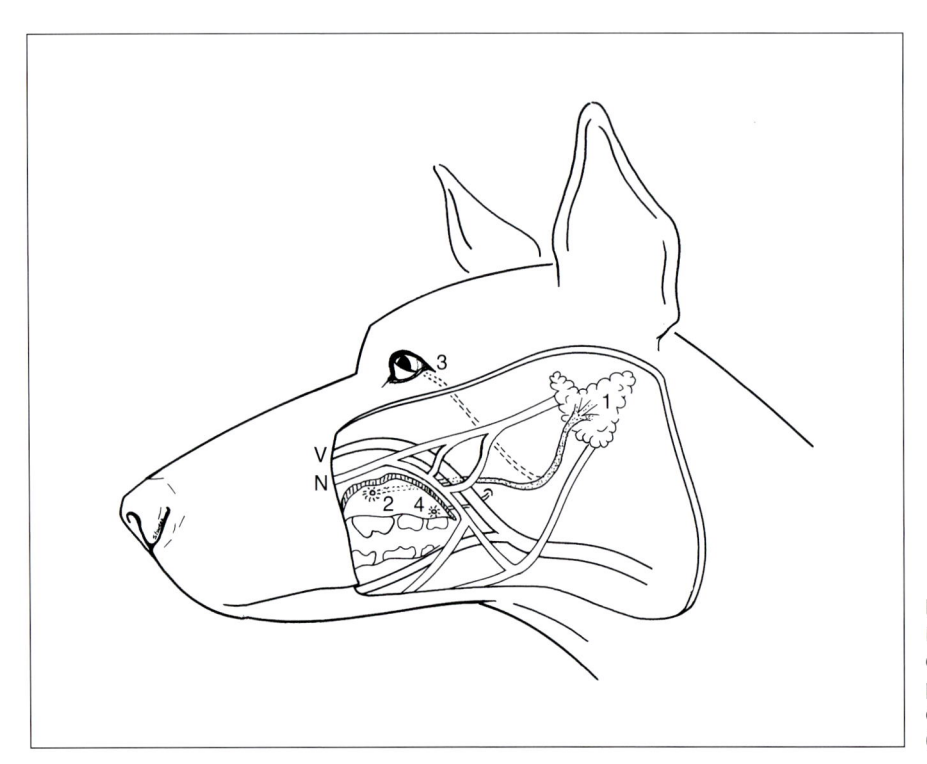

Fig. 6.5:
Location of the parotid gland (1), the opening of the duct (2), and the situation after transpositioning of the duct (3). The opening of the duct of the zygomatic gland near the last molar (4); V: facial vein, N: facial nerve branches.

6.4 Tear stripe formation

By means of the "zip-closure action" of the blinking of the lids (Fig. 6.3), tear fluid is moved towards the medial canthus, where, if there is any functional obstruction to its drainage or simply excessive production, it flows over the edge of the eyelid. If this situation persists, a tear stripe will form under the medial canthus; this being a brown-colored, moist stripe (tear staining syndrome; Plate 6.7). In cats, small aggregates of pigmented material can be found between and on the hairs. Tear stripe formation can, therefore, be caused by a problem in the drainage of tear fluid or by overproduction of tears, or a combination of the two. During the diagnosis, possible causes of overproduction should be excluded first, such as medial entropion (short-nosed Persian cat), distichiasis, trichiasis, conjunctivitis, or keratitis. Causes of a disturbance to the drainage should then be considered. These include:

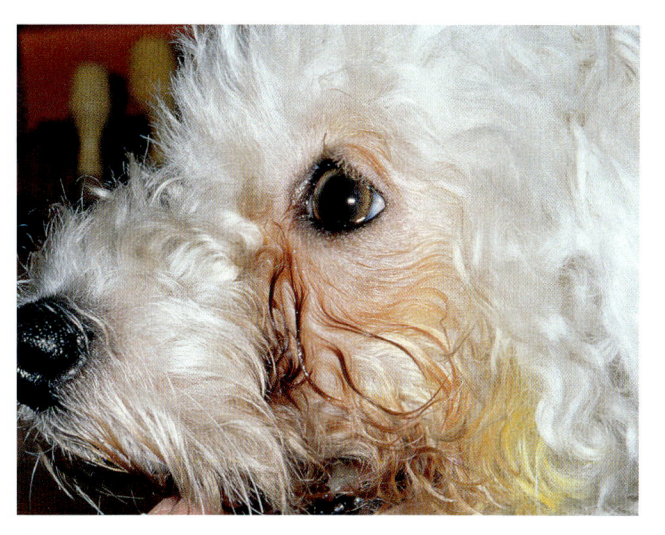

Plate 6.7:
Tear stripe (left side) due to obstructed tear ducts or over-production of tears, or both.

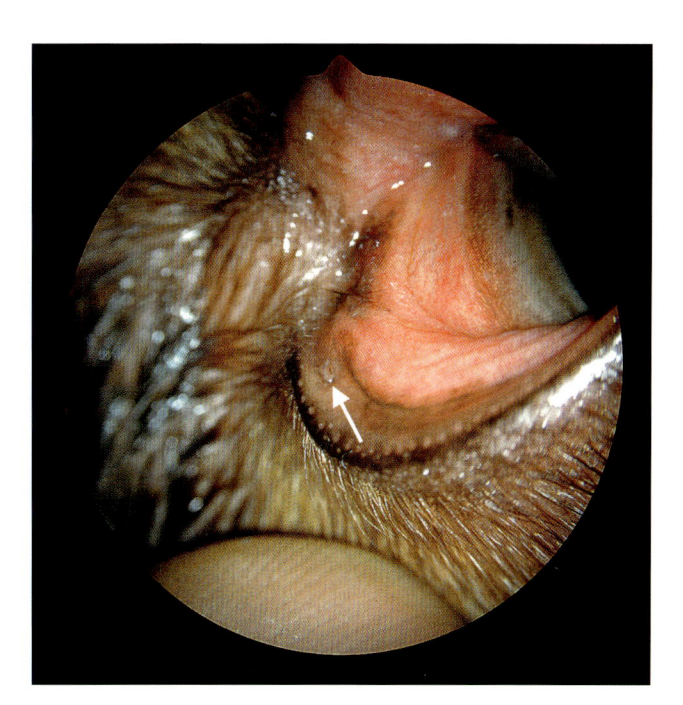

6.4.1 Micropunctum or stenosis of the lacrimal punctum

Narrowing of a punctum only causes a problem in drainage if it involves the inferior punctum (Plate 6.8). It can be a congenital defect.

In the cat, it is usually a residual complication of upper respiratory disease e.g. feline herpes virus type 1 (FHV-1), calici virus, or chlamydia infections.[28,29]

The most important sign is chronic tear stripe formation. The passage of fluorescein is retarded or absent. A lacrimal tear duct cannula can only be introduced with difficulty or not at all, but the passage is otherwise good (Fig. 6.6; Plate 6.8).

Therapy: Treatment consists of stretching the punctae with a lacrimal dilator and irrigating the drainage apparatus with a collyrium. In easily handled patients, this can be done under local anesthesia, but in most cats it is necessary to carry out the stretching and flushing under general anesthesia.

Plate 6.8:
Micropunctum (inferior, OS; see arrow) in a dog. Note the meibomian gland openings and just outside of them, some openings of the Zeis and Moll glands.

6.4.2 Atresia and secondary closure of the punctum

One or both punctae and/or canaliculi may have failed to open or have become closed. In the dog, this abnormality is often congenital (inheritance unknown), while in the cat the cause is usually adhesions after damage to the epithelial lining of the drainage system in the course of upper respiratory disease, e.g. FHV-1 and calici virus and/or chlamydia infection. Examination will reveal either no recognizable punctum, or that the lacrimal cannula almost immediately encounters an obstruction preventing the outflow of tears.

Therapy: The treatment, carried out under anesthesia, consists of opening the relevant punctum. This requires somewhat specialized instruments and skill, without which the patient should be referred. If the opposite punctum is open, this can be used for insertion of a round-tipped, hooked probe with a slit-hole in the tip (e.g. a modified Worst "pigtail" probe). The epithelium at the level of the punctum is raised and snipped off. In order to prevent the punctum from closing again, a silicone tube with a diameter of 0.7–1.5 mm can be introduced (Figs. 6.7, 6.8.). After-care consists of a "specific choice" antibiotic and corticosteroid in artificial tear drops (4 times daily), and a protective collar. The tube is left in place for about 3–6 weeks. It is then cut and both parts removed.

If both punctae are closed, the dorsal one is opened with a pointed blade and the above procedure is carried out. If one or both canaliculi are found to be closed over a greater distance, opening in the above manner will not usually be possible. If the abnormality is not too severe a hindrance for the patient, further attempts at opening should be avoided. In exceptional cases, conjunctivo-rhinostomy can be considered.

Atresia of the lacrimal drainage apparatus[30] (and dacryocystitis) in horses is characterized by copious mucous or mucopurulent exudate from the involved eye. This is usually seen in young horses. The tear ducts can be irrigated (cat catheter) via the tear ducts; nevertheless, to start with, it is simpler to try to irrigate from the ostium in the nose (urinary catheter, diameter 3–6 mm; Plate 6.12). However, the obstruction is most frequently at the distal opening and can easily be corrected by antegrade irrigation with a collyrium and observing the "bulging" at the distal end in the nose. Under local anesthesia, this bulge can be incised, either with a pointed scalpel or by electrocautery. After opening the distal end, the duct is irrigated thoroughly with a collyrium and an antibiotic (some clinicians include corticosteroids). Cannulation is possible, but is usually not necessary for maintaining a patent duct.

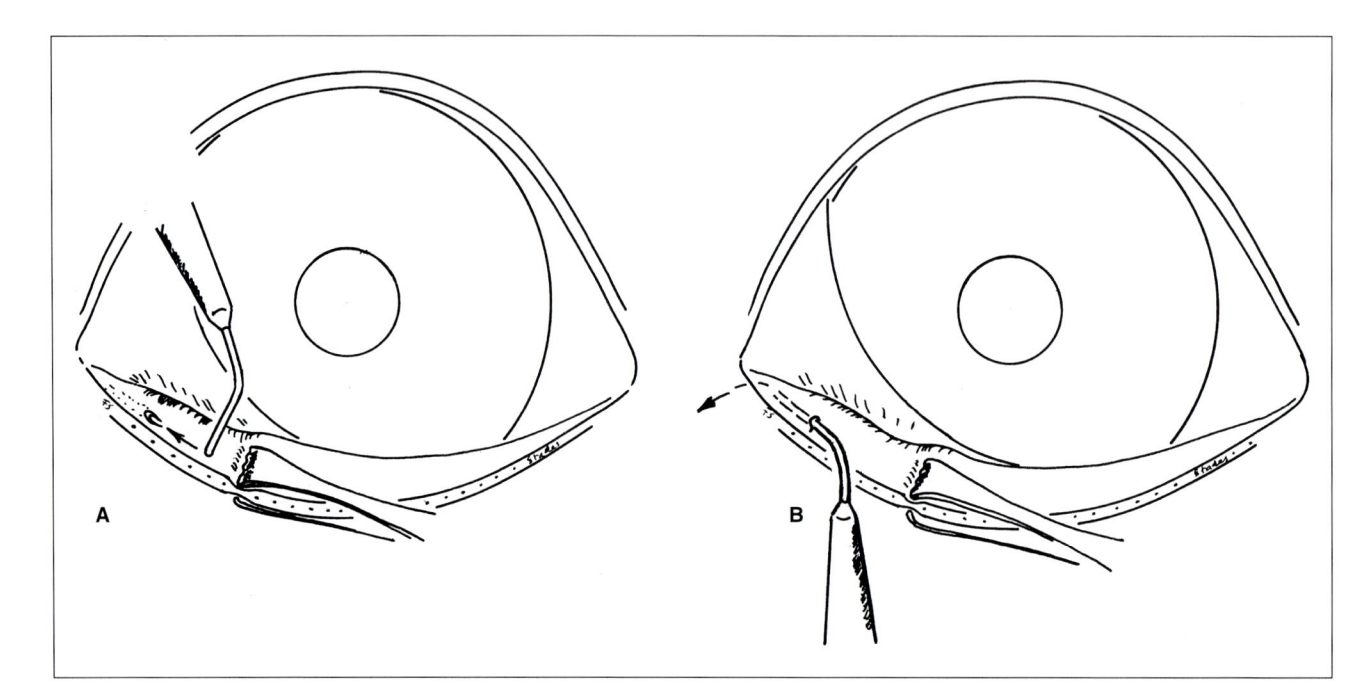

Fig. 6.6:
Check for patency of the tear ducts. The cannula, perpendicular on the palpebral conjunctiva and starting 8 mm away from the medial canthus, is moved medially approximately 1 mm away from the lid edge, until it sticks (A) in the punctum. Afterwards it is introduced in the canaliculus (B), parallel to the lid margin.

6.5 Dacryocystitis

Dacryocystitis (Plates 6.9–6.11) is an infrequent disorder and consists of inflammation of the lacrimal sac, canaliculi, and nasolacrimal duct. It often follows a viral, bacterial, or mycotic infection, and/or a foreign body. Additionally, trauma to the nose or neoplasms can predispose to obstruction of the drainage apparatus. In horses, it can also be caused by a *Thelazia* spp. infection (see 8.11.5).[31] The secondary inflammation causes swelling, by which the drainage system is compromised and the passage further reduced. The problems especially occur in the upper part of the duct, where the duct is surrounded by a bony canal. Swelling in this part can only press inwards, so obstruction develops rapidly. The purulent exudate that is formed seeks an exit and it usually takes the path of least resistance, which is upwards towards the conjunctival sac, or it eventually forms a fistula to the lower lid skin, a few millimeters under the medial canthus. The purulent exudate often causes and sustains a chronic conjunctivitis.

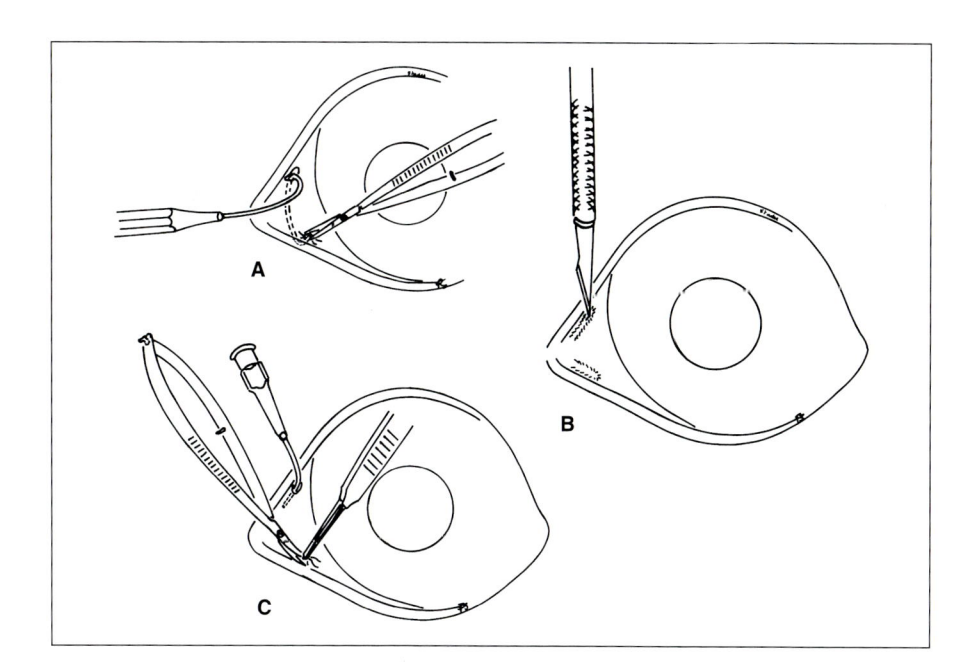

Fig. 6.7:
Opening of the lower punctum via the upper one using probing (A), and flushing (C), and opening if both punctae are closed using a pointed blade (B).

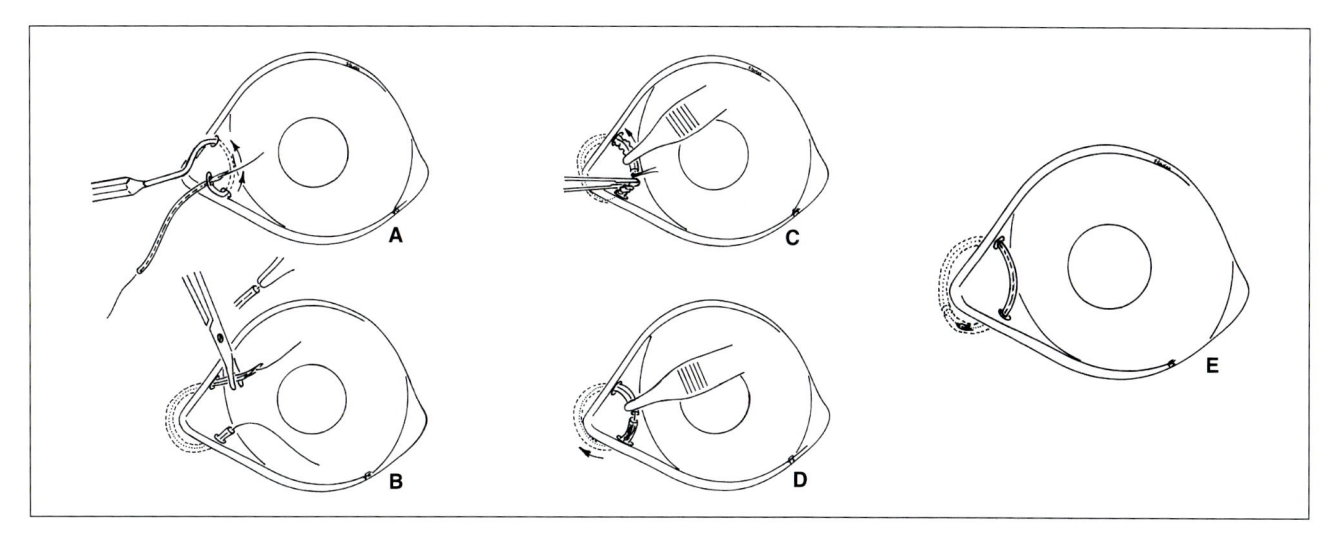

Fig. 6.8:
The introduction of a silicone tube through the lower punctum in the case of atresia of the punctum/canaliculus lacrimalis.

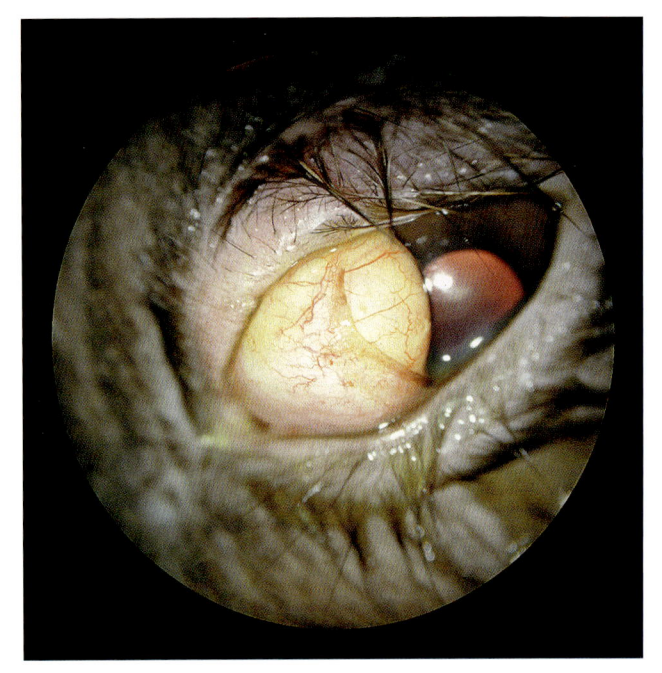

Plate 6.9:
Dacryocystitis in a rabbit (OS). The lacrimal saccus and inferior canaliculus (in the rabbit the superior is absent) is bulging with cheese-like pus.

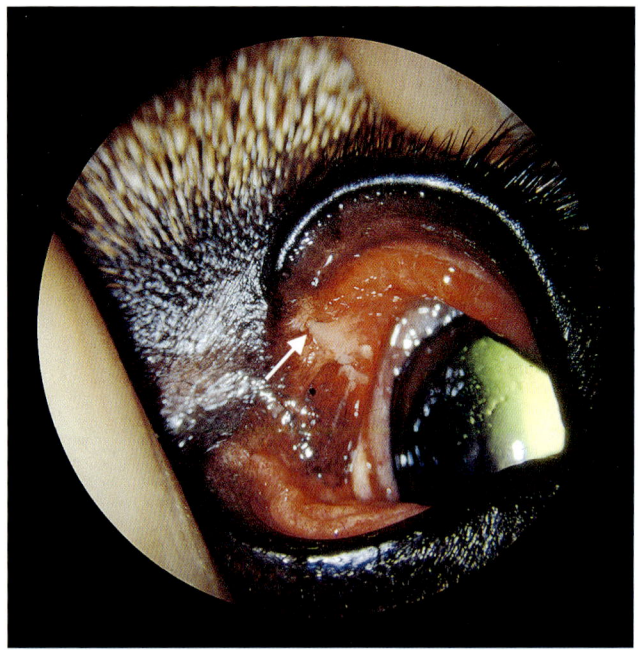

Plate 6.10:
Dacryocystitis in a dog (OS). The purulent discharge has been washed out. When pressure is applied at the medial canthus, pus emerges from the dorsal punctum (see arrow).

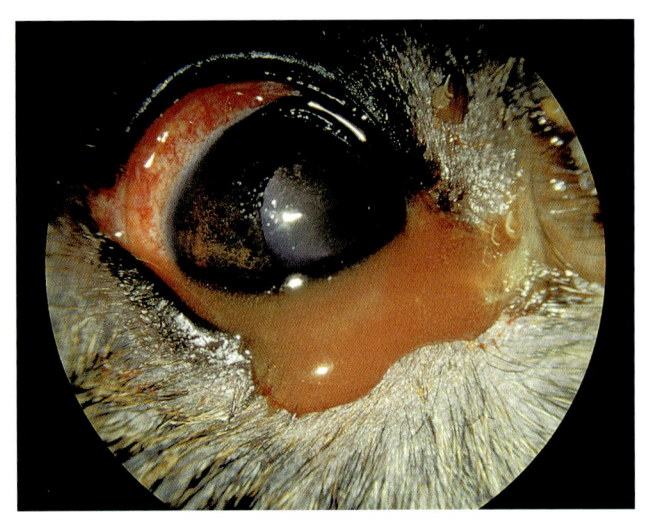

Plate 6.11:
Severe, hemorrhagic discharge from a dacryocystitis in a dog with a foreign body in the nasolacrimal duct (OD).

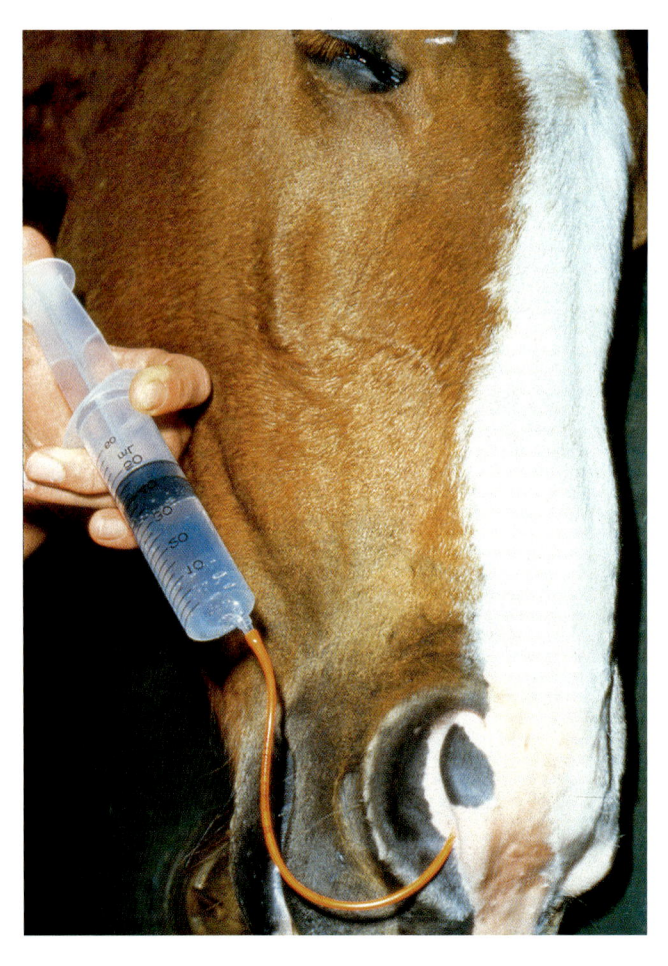

Plate 6.12:
Nasolacrimal flush in a horse, using a urinary catheter (diameter 5 mm), via the ostium in the nares. If the animal objects to the local application of drugs, they can be injected into the conjunctival sac in this way (alternative possibility: see Fig. 3.1 and Plate 3.4).

Diagnosis: Dacryocystitis has the appearance of a chronic purulent conjunctivitis, with a normal or elevated STT value. After the conjunctival sac has been irrigated, pressure on the medial canthus produces a purulent exudate from the punctae (Plate 6.10, 6.11). Dacryocystorhinography and/or CT scanning can be used for diagnosis and also to determine the most effective method of correcting the lesion.

Therapy: For purposes of both diagnosis and therapy, the tear drainage system is irrigated (10% acetylcysteine can be added to the irrigation fluid) to remove the exudate. If the passage is thereby opened, a viscous antibiotic-corticosteroid combination solution (preferably after sensitivity testing) is introduced into the lacrimal sac. This treatment is repeated 2–4 times daily for at least 1 week. If the animal resists or is too difficult to handle, the procedure must be carried out under anesthesia, but since repeated anesthesia is impossible, referral for catheterization should be arranged instead.[32]

The first step in catheterization is the introduction of a 0-0 to 3-0 monofilament nylon suture (its tip rounded by heating), preferably via the dorsal punctum and then through the nasolacrimal duct to the nose (Figs. 6.7–6.9). Retrograde irrigation and catheterisation of the nasolacrimal drainage apparatus can be performed, but is less easy. A silicone tube (0.7–1.3 mm) is passed over this suture and pulled through to the nose (Plate 6.2). After removal of the nylon thread, the end of the tube is fixed to the skin with sutures near the medical canthus and lateral to the angle of the nose. After-care consists of administering the same antibiotic-corticosteroid preparation 4 times daily. The tube is left in place for at least 3 weeks and the administration of the medication is continued for an additional 10 days. A protective collar is placed on the animal to prevent removal of the tube.

If the passage cannot be opened up by irrigation and/or if catheterization is not possible, the only solution is to perform a dacryorhinostomy, for which the patient has to be referred.

The simplest but also the most traumatic and least controlled method is a conjunctivorhinostomy. By using a Kirschner wire, a canal is drilled into the nose. As the wire breaks through into the nasal cavity, difficult controllable hemorrhage can occur. A silicone or polyethylene tube can be passed over the wire to keep the canal open.

A better method is a **conjunctivomaxillorhinostomy**[33] in which a hole about 7 mm in diameter is made rostral to the medial canthus, passing into the maxillary sinus in dogs and into the nasal passage in cats. The hole is then enlarged in the direction of the medial canthus until it reaches the edge of the orbit, so that the nasolacrimal duct is laid open to its orbital entrance. The two ends of a silicone tube are introduced through the existing puncta (or newly created if necessary) to the maxillary sinus (dog) or nasal passage (cat). Both tubes are encircled together by a separate "fixation suture" through the skin, to fix the tubing on its place. After-care consists of the previously described topical treatment and a protective collar. The tube should be left in place for at least 4–6 weeks. After cutting the "fixation suture" both tube ends can be removed from the puncta.

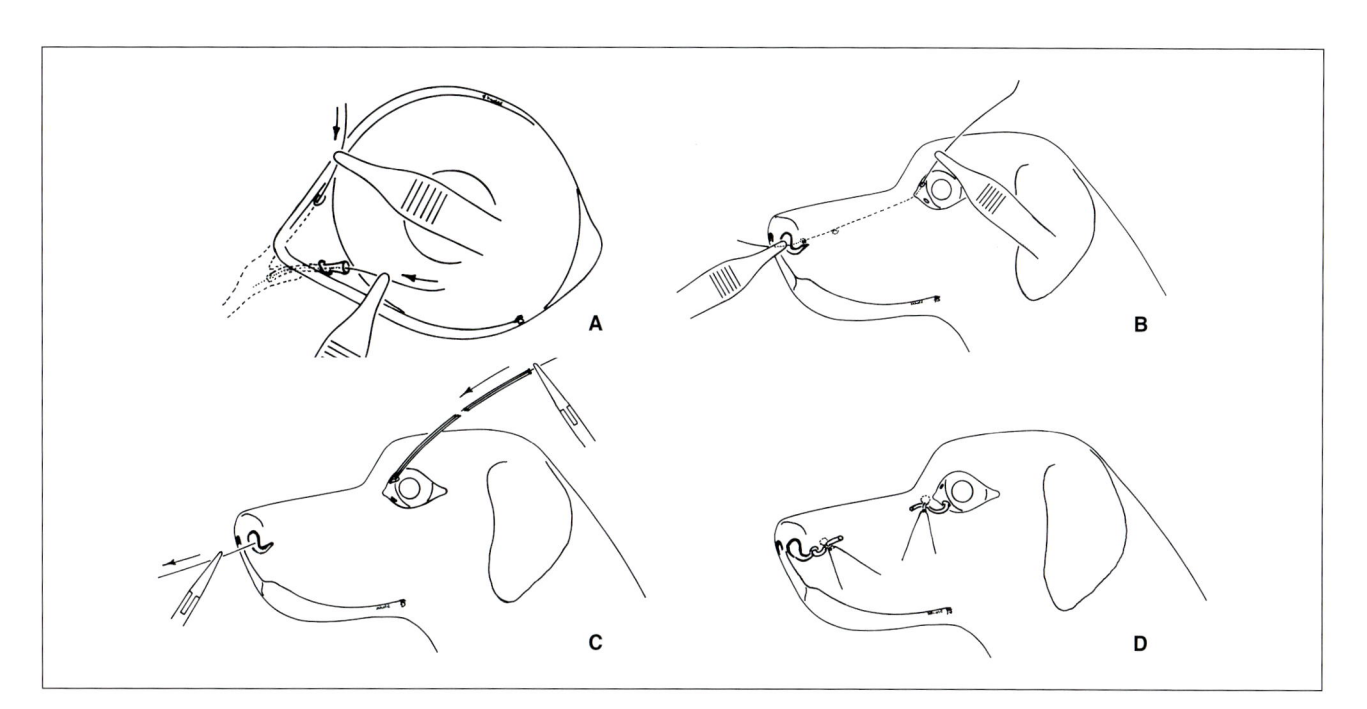

Fig. 6.9:
Probing of the nasolacrimal duct in dacryocystitis. A monofilament suture (prolene) is passed into the nose. A silicone tube is then passed over the suture into the nose. After removal of the thread, one end of the tube is sutured to the skin in the medial canthus and the other to the skin lateral to the angle of the nose.

In a recent described **conjunctivomaxillorhinostomy** method, via the surgically opened punctae and saccus, a fistula is broken through the lacrimal bone to the lacrimal sinus (dog) or the nose (cat) by opening a Mosquito artery clamp. Secondary closure of the fistula was prevented using Mitomycine-C®, as an anti-fibroblastic agent.[34]

Prognosis: Prognosis for healing is relatively good.

6.6 Lacerations

Eyelid wounds, in which the tear drainage apparatus is involved, should be sutured with extra care to avoid secondary obstruction of the tear duct by traction or adhesions. In order to prevent this, a silicone tube is inserted before the sutures are placed. The tube should be left in place for at least 3 weeks, as for atresia (Fig. 4.5; see 6.4.2). For further details, see 4.5.1.1.

Elongated roots of the upper teeth of the rabbit and other small mammals may cause obstruction of the nasolacrimal duct and result in tear stripes, but without signs of conjunctivitis or other ocular disease.

6.7 Cysts and neoplasia

The occurrence of congenital cysts or the development of neoplasms of the tear glands or of the lacrimal drainage system are rare. When such abnormalities are suspected, the patient should be referred for diagnosis and eventual treatment.

Literature

1. GINEL, P.J., NOVALES, M., GARCIA, M., et al.: Immunoglobulins in stimulated tears of dogs. Am. J. Vet. Res. **54**: 1060, 1993.
2. GERMAN, A.J., HALL, E.J. & DAY, M.J.: Measurement of IgG, IgM, and IgA concentrations in canine serum, saliva, tears and bile. Vet. Imm. Immunopath. **64**: 107, 1998.
3. DAVIDSON, H.J. & KUONEN, V.J.: The tear film and ocular mucins. Vet. Ophthalmol. **7**: 71, 2004.
4. CARRINGTON, S.D., et al.: Polarized light biomicroscopic observations on the pre-corneal tear film. I. The normal tear film of the dog. J. Small Anim. Pract. **28**: 605, 1987.
5. PRYDAL, J.I. & CAMPBELL, F.W.: Study of precorneal tear film thickness and structure by interferometry and confocal microscopy. Invest. Ophthalmol. Vis. Sci, **33**: 1996, 1992.
6. KING-SMITH, P.E., FINK, B.A., et al.: The thickness of the human precorneal tearfilm: evidence from reflection spectra. Invest. Ophthalmol. Vis. Sci. **41**: 3348, 2000.
7. GIPSON, I.K., YANKAUCKAS, M., SPURR-MICHAUD, S.J., et al.: Characteristics of a glycoprotein in the ocular surface glycocalyx. Invest. Ophthal. Vis. Sci. **33**: 218, 1992.
8. MCLAUGHLIN, S.A., et al.: Effect of removal of lacrimal and third eyelid glands on Schirmer tear test results in cats. JAVMA **193**: 820, 1988.
9. SAMS, R.: Ohio State University, personal communication. 2003.
10. PEIFFER R.L. & HARLING, D.E.: Third eyelid. In: Textbook of small animal surgery. Ed.: D. H. Slatter, Philadelphia, Lea & Febiger, 1501–1509, 1985.
11. MEIJ, B.P., VOORHOUT, G. et al.: Transsphenoidal hypophysectomy in beagle dogs: evaluation of a microsurgical technique. Vet. Surg. **26**: 295, 1997.
12. AZZAROLO, A.M., BJERRUM, K. et al.: Hypophysectomy induced regression of female rat lacrimal glands: partial restoration and maintenance by dihydrotestostrone and prolactin. Invest. Ophthalmol. Vis. Sci. **36**: 216, 1995.
13. SLATTER, D.: Fundamentals of veterinary ophthalmology. Philadelphia, W.B. Saunders, 249, 1990.
14. BRYAN, G.M. & SLATTER, D.H.: Keratoconjunctivitis sicca induced by phenazopyridine in dogs. Arch. Ophthalmol. **90**: 310, 1973.
15. LUDDERS, J.W. & HEAVNER, J.E.: Effect of atropine on tear formation in anesthetized dogs. JAVMA **175**: 585, 1979.
16. HOLLINGSWORTH, S.R., CANTON, D.D., BUYUKMIHICI, N.C. & FARVER, T.B.: Effect of topically administered atropine on tear production in dogs. JAVMA **200**: 1481–1484, 1992.
17. VESTRE, W.A. et al.: Decreased tear production associated with general anesthesia in the dog. JAVMA **174**: 1006, 1978.
18. ARNETT, B.D., BRIGHTMAN, A.H. & MUSSELMAN, E.E.: Effect of atropine sulfate on tear production in the cat when used with ketamine hydrochloride and acetylpromazine maleate. JAVMA **185**: 214, 1984.
19. KASWAN, R.L., MARTIN, C.L. & DAWE, D.L.: Keratoconjunctivitis sicca: immunological evaluation of 62 canine cases. Am. J. Vet. Res. **46**: 376, 1985.
20. STAMAN, J., GOUDSWAARD, J., STADES, F.C. & WOUDA, W.: Sjögrensyndrome (Keratoconjunctivitis in combination with xerostomy) in the dog. Proceedings Voorjaarsdagen, Neth. Sm. Anim. Vet. Assoc. 10–11 April, 1978.
21. LETTOW, E. & HILDEBRAND, B.: Keratoconjunctivitis sicca beim Hund. Tierärztliche Praxis **5**: 351, 1977.
22. KASWAN, R.L., SALISBURY, M.A. & WARD, D.A.: Spontaneous canine keratoconjunctivitis sicca: A useful model for human keratoconjunctivitis sicca. Treatment with cyclosporine eye drops. Arch. Ophthalmol. **107**: 1210, 1989.
23. BARDOULAY, A, ENGLISH, R.V. et al.: The effect of topical Tacrolimus aqueous suspension on tear film production in dogs with keratoconjunctivitis sicca. Trans. Am. Coll. Vet. Ophthalmologists **34**: 33, 2003.

24. RUBIN, L.F. & AGUIRRE, G.D.: Clinical use of pilocarpine for keratoconjunctivitis sicca in dogs and cats. JAVMA **151**: 313, 1969.

25. LAVIGNETTE, A.N.: Keratoconjunctivitis sicca in a dog treated by transposition of the parotid salivary duct. JAVMA **148**: 778, 1966.

26. WOLF, E.D. & MERIDETH, R.: Parotid duct transposition in the horse. J. Equine Vet. Sci. **1**: 143, 1981.

27. STADES, F.C.: Apparato Lacrimalia. *In:* Atlante di Oftalmologia veterinaria. Ed.: C. Perrucio, Torino, Edzione medico scientifico, 152–156, 1985.

28. HOOVER, E.A., ROHOVSKY, M.W. & GRIESEMER, R.A.: Experimental feline viral rhinotracheitis in the germ-free cat. Am. J. Pathol. **58**: 269, 1270.

29. NASISSE, M.P., GUY, J.S., DAVIDSON, M.G. *et al.*: Experimental ocular herpesvirus infection in the cat. Sites of virus replication, clinical features and effects of corticosteroid adminstration. Invest. Ophthalmol. Vis. Sci. **30**: 1758, 1989.

30. LUNDVALL, R.L. & CARTER, J.D.: Atresia of the nasolacrimal meatus in the horse. JAVMA **159**: 289, 1971.

31. LADOUCEUR, C.A. & KAZOCOS, K.R.: *Thelaxia lacrimalis* in horses in Indiana. JAVMA **178**: 301, 1981.

32. SEVERIN, G.A.: Nasolacrimal duct catheterization in the dog. JAAHA **8**: 13, 1972.

33. STADES, F.C.: Dacryozystomaxillorhinostomie. Eine neue chirurgische Therapie zur Dacryozystitis. Tierärztl. Prax. **6**: 243, 1978.

34. WÉVERBERG, F. & HONNEGER, N.: A new surgical approach to treat epiphora in dogs and cats: Dacryocystorhinostomy with topical applied Mitomycine-C® associated with eyelids correction. Proceeding Eur. Coll. Vet. Ophthalmologists, May 10–14, Brugge, pp. 81, 2006.

7 Eyelids

7.1 Introduction

In most animals, when the eye is open, the lids encircle the cornea, thus covering almost all the sclera. The average length of the palpebral fissure when stretched is approximately 28 mm in cats and 33 mm in dogs.[1] The circular muscle surrounding the palpebral fissure is the orbicularis oculi muscle (Fig. 7.1). The eye does not close by circular contraction, however, because of a ligament in the medial canthus and the retractor anguli lateralis muscle in the lateral canthus. The orbicularis oculi muscle/lateral ligament enables blinking, a movement in which the upper eyelid plays the most important part. In domestic animals, eyelid closure may be very firm, particularly when the animal is in pain (blepharospasm). Blepharospasm often occurs as a result of ocular pain, causing spasm of the orbicularis and enophthalmos, resulting in reduced support for the margin of the eyelid which allows the lid to turn in towards the globe (secondary entropion), and producing further pain and contraction of the orbicularis oculi, i.e. blepharospasm and associated enophthalmos. The levator muscles (innervated by the oculomotor nerve) open the upper eyelid and the malaris muscle opens the lower eyelid.

The free margins of the eyelids (Plates 2.3, 2.6; Fig. 7.2) are usually pigmented (but often non-pigmented if the skin around the eye is itself non-pigmented, e.g. in the area of a white spot around the eye), and they are hairless. In dogs and cats, the borderline of the eyelash-like hairs and the regular hairs in the upper lid begin about 1 mm away from the free lid margin (and not at the edge itself, as in humans). In the lower lid, hairs start about 2 mm away from the free margin. In the ungulate, more proximally placed, separate eyelash hairs can be found (in the same position as in humans). Furthermore, the margins are smooth, glossy and fatty, but dry. The 30–40 orifices of the meibomian glands are found in the free lid margin and open into a fine groove.[2] These openings and the groove are surgical landmarks used to re-appose lid margins in traumatic and surgical procedures discussed in this book. The meibomian glands are visible on the conjunctival surface, below

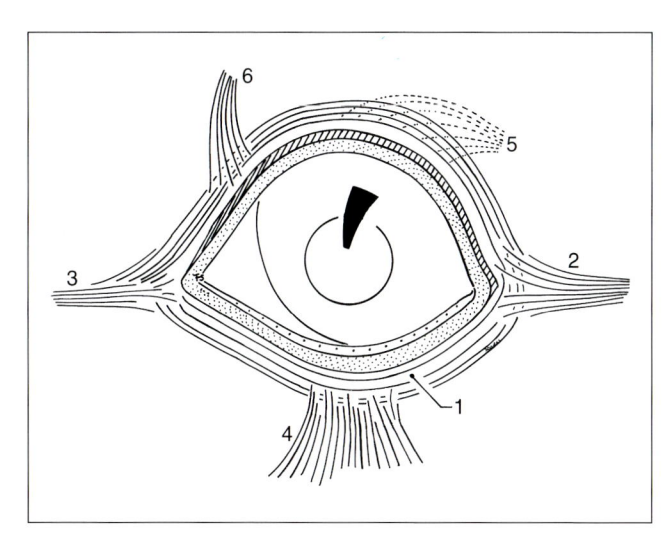

Fig. 7.1:
Muscles of the lids of the left eye: (1) orbicularis oculi m., (2) lat. palpebral ligament, (3) med. palpebral ligament; (4) malaris m., (5) levator palpebrae m., (6) levator anguli oculi med. m.

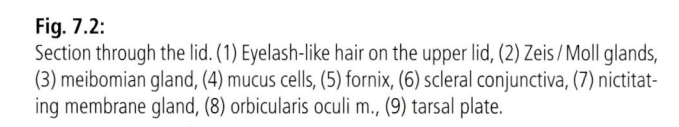

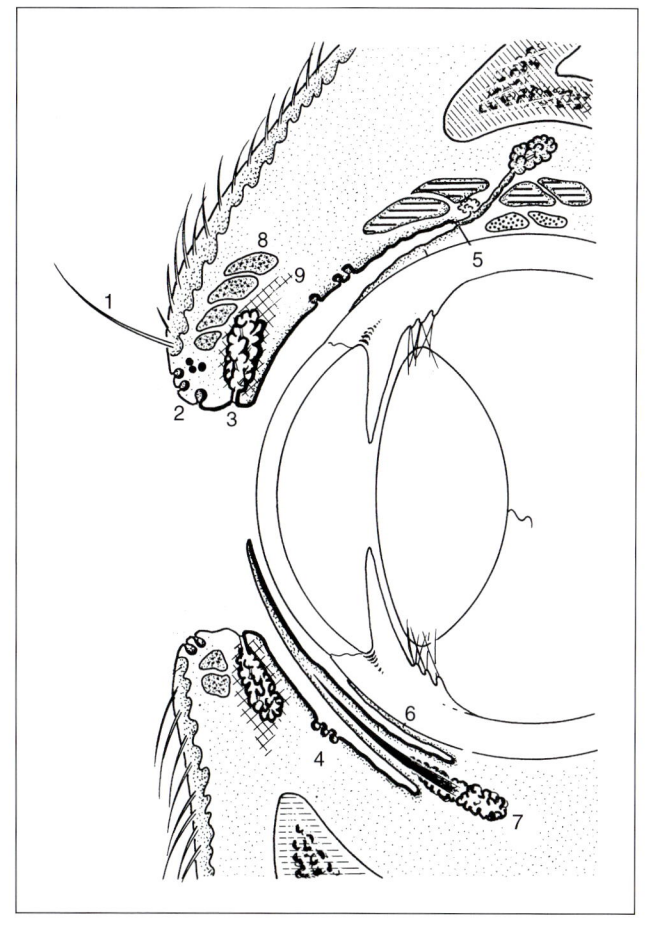

Fig. 7.2:
Section through the lid. (1) Eyelash-like hair on the upper lid, (2) Zeis / Moll glands, (3) meibomian gland, (4) mucus cells, (5) fornix, (6) scleral conjunctiva, (7) nictitating membrane gland, (8) orbicularis oculi m., (9) tarsal plate.

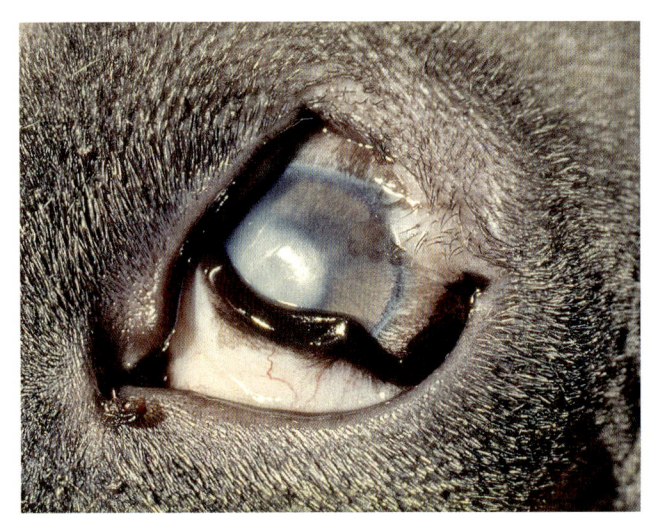

Plate 7.1:
Palpebral aplasia of the lateral part of the upper eyelid in a Persian cat (OS). The skin connects almost directly to the limbus. There is also a severe microphthalmia. A scar is located centrally in the cornea. From these strands of a persistent pupillary membrane connect to the iris collarette.

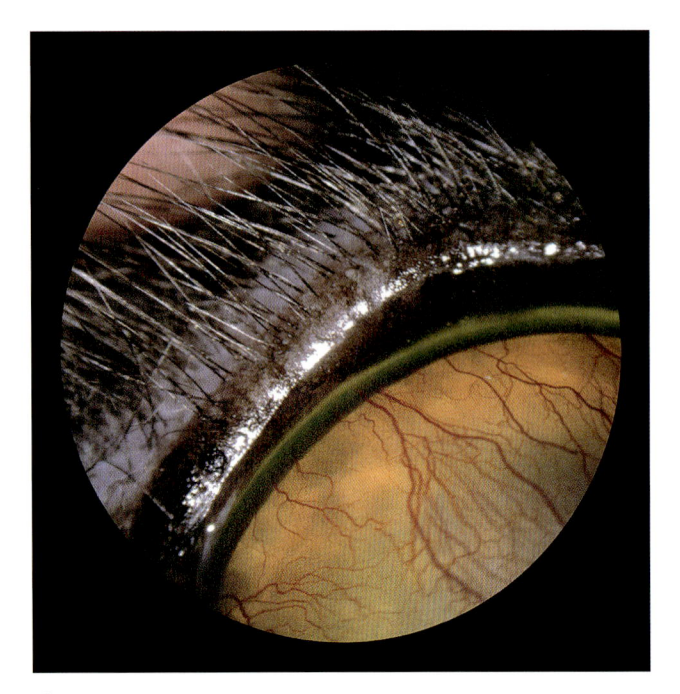

Plate 7.2:
Palpebral "aplasia" of the upper lid edge in a less distinct form (OD, cat). The lid edge is thin and no meibomian glands are presented in that area. Affected cats should be excluded from breeding.

the conjunctiva, as 2- to 4-mm long, whitish-yellow lines running perpendicular to the margin. Meibomian glands are not present in birds. Just outside the groove are the even smaller orifices of the glands of Zeis and Moll. The oily material secreted by these glands coats the margin of the lid with a lipid layer, preventing the tear fluid from flowing across it. This secretion also forms an extremely thin oily film on the watery tear fluid, thereby reducing evaporation, whilst providing lubrication and preventing adhesion of debris.

7.2 Ankyloblepharon

Ankyloblepharon is delayed or complete failure of opening of the palpebral fissure. The bridge of tissue in the palpebral fissure between the already developed margins of the eyelid normally atrophies 10–14 days post partum (dog, cat). Even though little is known about the cause of this regressive defect, some epidermal growth factor must be involved.

The anomaly is rare, and is usually bilateral. Conjunctivitis or ophthalmia neonatorum (see 8.11.6) must be considered in the differential diagnosis, but in these conditions the closed eyelids will bulge as a result of the exudate that accumulates in the closed pocket.

Therapy: Treatment consists of massaging the fissure cautiously until it opens. If this fails, mechanical spreading with mosquito forceps in the spontaneous first opening, or into the groove of the future fissure starting in the medial canthus, will open the fissure. Sometimes, a careful incision at the medial canthus with a pointed scalpel is necessary.

Postoperative treatment consists of topical "initial choice" antibiotic eye ointment, 4 times daily for 5 days.

Prognosis: The prognosis is favorable. There are no known means of preventing this condition.

7.3 Aplasia palpebrae

In aplasia palpebrae or lid colobomas (Plate 7.1), the margins of the eyelids are completely or partly undeveloped. This anomaly is congenital, most likely hereditary (recessive), and usually bilateral, affecting the lateral part of the upper eyelid. It occurs in many cat breeds and also in lions and tigers, but it is seen more frequently in Persian cats or their crossbreeds. Aplasia palpebrae is often associated with other congenital anomalies such as microphthalmia, absence of the lacrimal gland, KCS, or cataract.

The kittens are often born with their palpebral fissure partially or fully open. Sometimes, the margin of the eyelid is developed without meibomian glands (Plate 7.2). There are frequently ectopic hairs in such areas, directed towards the globe, which cause chronic irritation of the corresponding area of the cornea. When the defects are larger, a "deeper" part of the eyelid is usually also missing, in which case the skin directly joins the conjunctiva. The eyelids cannot be completely closed, if at all. As a result, parts of the cornea cannot be provided with the normal tear film and hairs come into direct contact with the cornea, leading to lesions of chronic irritation (edema, pannus, pigmentation, and sequestration). In the most severe cases, the problems are further complicated by the partial or complete absence of lacrimal secretion of the primary lacrimal glands.

Distichiasis and/or trichiasis must be considered in the differential diagnosis, but in these conditions the free lid margin and the meibomian gland openings can be easily recognized.

Therapy: If the margin of the eyelid is developed without meibomian glands, no therapy is necessary. If there are ectopic hairs in the area, these have to be removed (see 7.5). If the cornea is only slightly irritated, administration of topical fatty lubricants, to effect, on a daily basis will be sufficient. If the lesions are larger, a substitute eyelid should be created by blepharoplasty (usually arch- [Fig. 7.3] or pedicle-shaped).[3] The patient should be referred to a specialist with experience in these techniques. If lacrimation is also severely decreased, transposition of the parotid duct can be considered (see 6.2.1). However, this requires complex surgery and since the condition may be hereditary, some breeders or owners opt for enucleation or euthanasia.

Prognosis / prevention: In cases of a minor defect, the prognosis is favorable. In larger lesions, the substitute eyelid can function reasonably well. In some cases, lifelong administration of topical fatty lubricants will be necessary. In case of failing lacrimation, the prognosis is less favorable. If there are other congenital anomalies, these should be considered in the prognosis.

Owners should be instructed that these anomalies are most likely hereditary, and that the parents and littermates should be examined carefully for these and other anomalies (also for areas of lack of meibomian glands, most likely in the upper lateral part of the lid). Affected animals and, ideally, members of their immediate family should not be used for breeding (see 15).

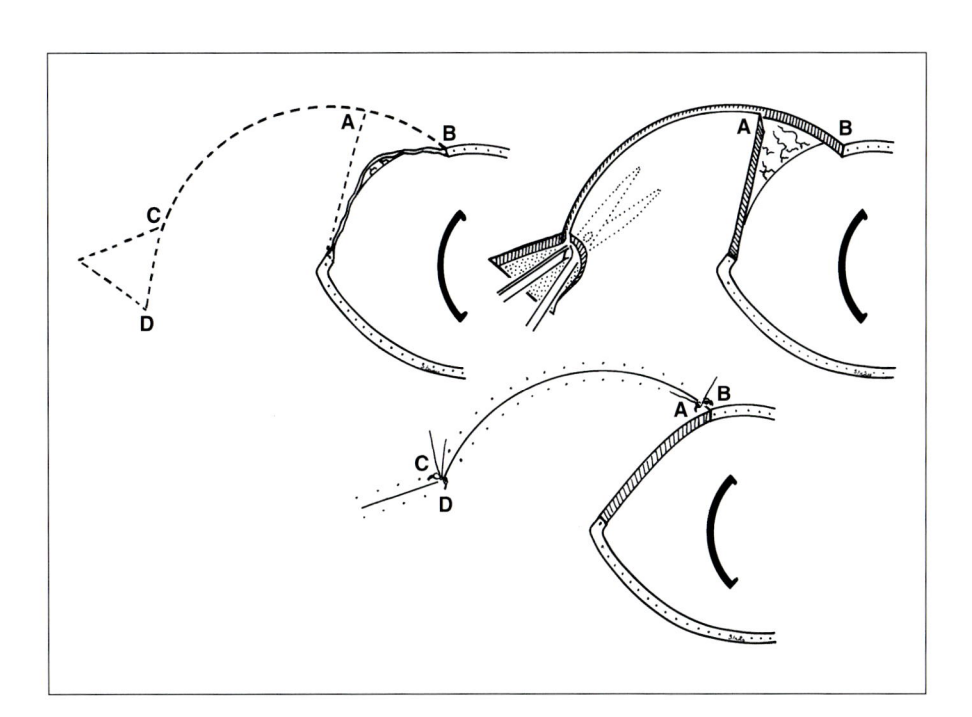

Fig. 7.3:
Rotation-flap correction method for large lid defects.

7.4 Dermoids / dysplasia of the lid

Dermoids and dysplasia of the lids are ectopic and abnormally developed islands of skin in or on the margin of the eyelid. They are rare, possibly hereditary, anomalies, usually of the lower lid near the lateral canthus. An island or fold of skin often disrupts the lid margin and is continuous with the conjunctiva (see also 10.4). Blinking is abnormal and hairs generally grow towards the cornea causing chronic irritation, and resulting in edema, vascularization, and pigmentation.

Therapy: Treatment consists of removal of the abnormal parts of the eyelid, after which the lid margin wound is closed with extreme care. Blepharoplasties are seldom necessary because the fissure length is sufficient in most cases. If the condition does not produce overt corneal disease, the operation may be delayed until 10–12 weeks of age, when the anesthesia risks are lower. For patients with severe defects it may be best to refer them to a specialist.

Postoperative treatment consists of topical "initial choice" antibiotic eye ointment or lubricating fatty solutions, 4 times daily for 10–14 days.

Prognosis / prevention: The prognosis is favorable. Parents and littermates should also be examined. Affected animals and, ideally, also members of their immediate family should not be used for breeding.

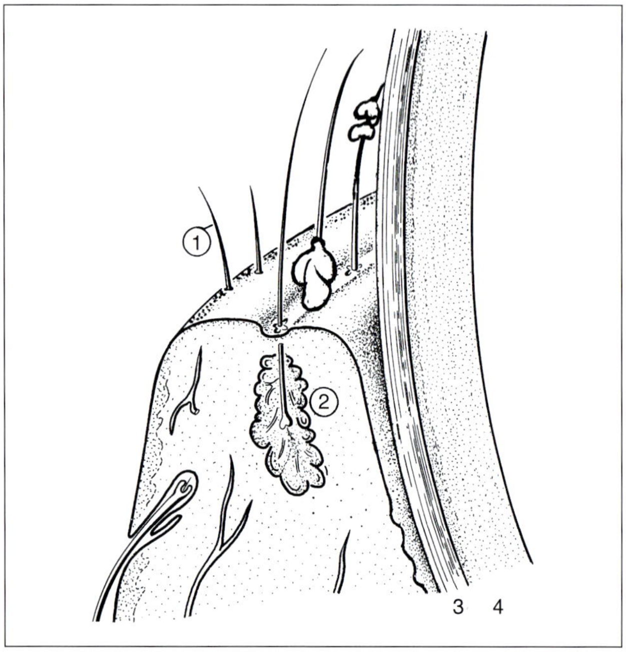

7.5 Distichiasis

Distichia are single or multiple hairs arising from the free lid margin (Fig. 7.4). They usually arise from the meibomian duct openings (Plate 7.3) and their hair follicles are located in the lid margin, in or near to the base of the meibomian glands. Stiff hairs that rub the cornea can irritate and injure it.[4] Irritation leads to increased lacrimation and slight blepharospasm, and thus epiphora. These abnormal hairs may act as a wick resulting in an overflow of tears over the lower lid margin, moistening the margin and the exterior skin of the eyelid. Although distichiasis is considered to be inherited, the mode of transmission is unknown.

It occurs frequently in dogs. Predisposed breeds are the American and English Cocker Spaniel, Boxer, English Bulldog, Eurasier, Flat-coated Retriever, Pekingese, Shetland Sheepdog, Shih Tzu, and Tibetan Terrier. It is rare in cats and horses, but does occur.

Irritation caused by distichia leads to variable degrees of epiphora, moisture on the margins of the lower eyelid, and corresponding corneal lesions such as edema, vascularization, ulceration, or in cats, sequestration. Distichia are hard to find without a magnifying glass, but a common sign of distichiasis is the mucus that adheres to the hairs, revealing their presence.

Trichiasis and entropion must be considered in the differential diagnosis, but in these conditions no hairs arise from the free lid margin.

Therapy: The simplest treatment is manual epilation by rounded tip epilation forceps at regular intervals; this can also be performed by some owners. The advantage of this method is that it allows detection of irritation caused by the hairs. More permanent treatment by electro-epilation requires general anesthesia and adequate magnification (x5–10) to detect the orifice of the hair follicle.[5] The hair follicle is destroyed by means of a very thin steel wire (Plate 7.4; e.g. Perma Tweez®), which is introduced into its root (Fig. 7.5).

Note: Excessive coagulation must be avoided, as it will cause formation of irritating scar tissue on the free lid margin (Plate 7.5).

Other methods of treatment which have been advocated include the use of electroscalpel, high frequency radio-hyperthermia or cryosurgery on the conjunctival surface adjacent to the follicle and destroying it.[6,7] The use of the PermaTweez causes very little trauma to the lid margin. Visualization of the removal of the hair follicle through the conjunctiva is possible using the electric scalpel. Cryodestruction is less selective and has the disadvantage of considerable postoperative swelling and long-term depigmentation. If a straight row of hairs exists, the base of the all meibomian glands can be excised (electric scalpel or pointed knife) from the conjunctival surface, but this may sometimes result in secondary entropion. Also, a wedge-shaped strip of cilia-bearing tissue can be excised from the free lid margin, but this requires a special lid clamp, the free lid margin is damaged and all the meibomian glands are lost.

Fig. 7.4:
Distichiasis (hairs in/on the lid margin) growing out of the meibomian (1), Zeis or Moll (2) gland openings; (3) tear film; (4) cornea.

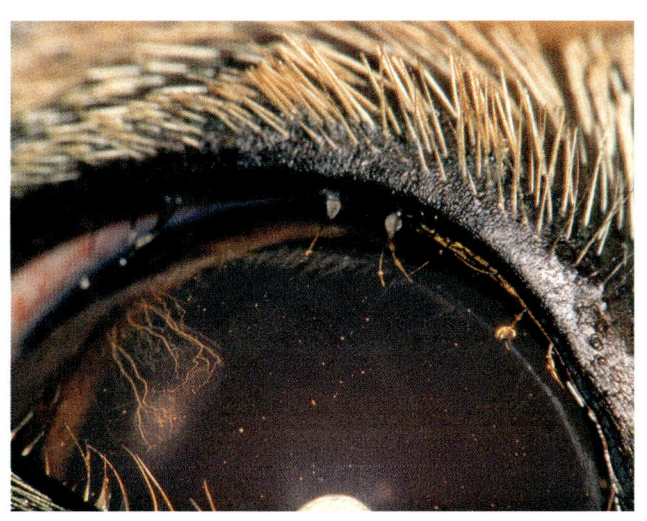

Plate 7.3:
Distichiasis of the upper lid in a dog (OS). Note the slime at the base of the cilia, produced as the result of direct corneal irritation, which gives away their position.

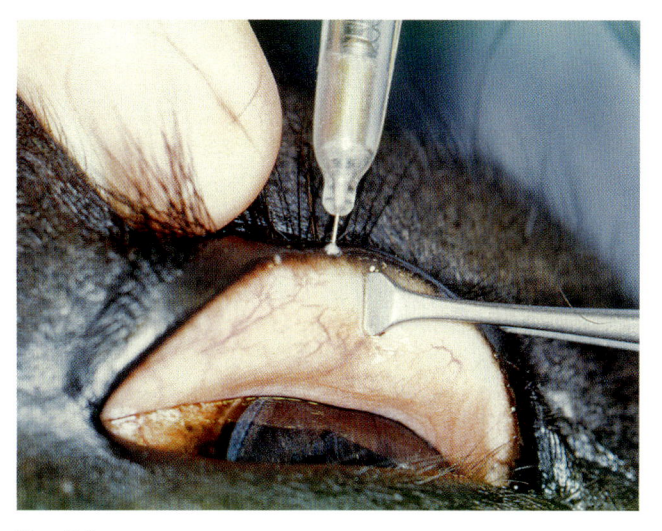

Plate 7.4:
Distichiasis in a horse (OD). The needle of the PermaTweez® coagulator (on a 9 Volt battery) is inserted into the hair follicle. The oily secretion of the gland "boils" out of the gland opening.

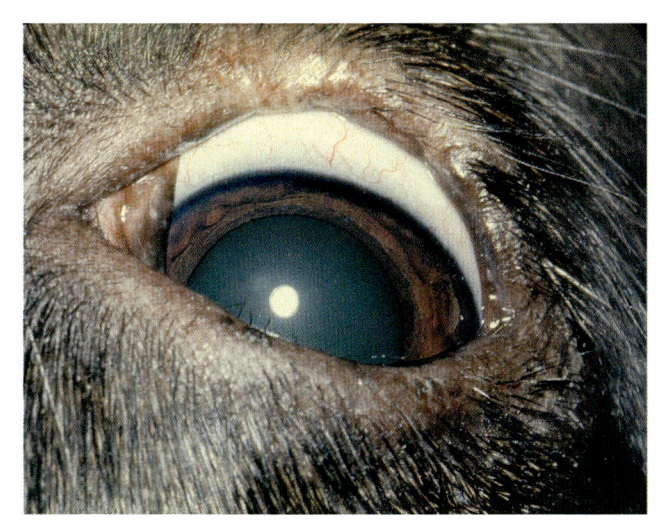

Plate 7.5:
Distichiasis of the upper and lower lid of a dog (OS). The scars in the lid edge of the upper eyelid are due to excessive coagulation. Not only the root of the distichia but the entire meibomian gland and the lid edge itself have been destroyed. In the lower lid "overseen" distichiasis is present.

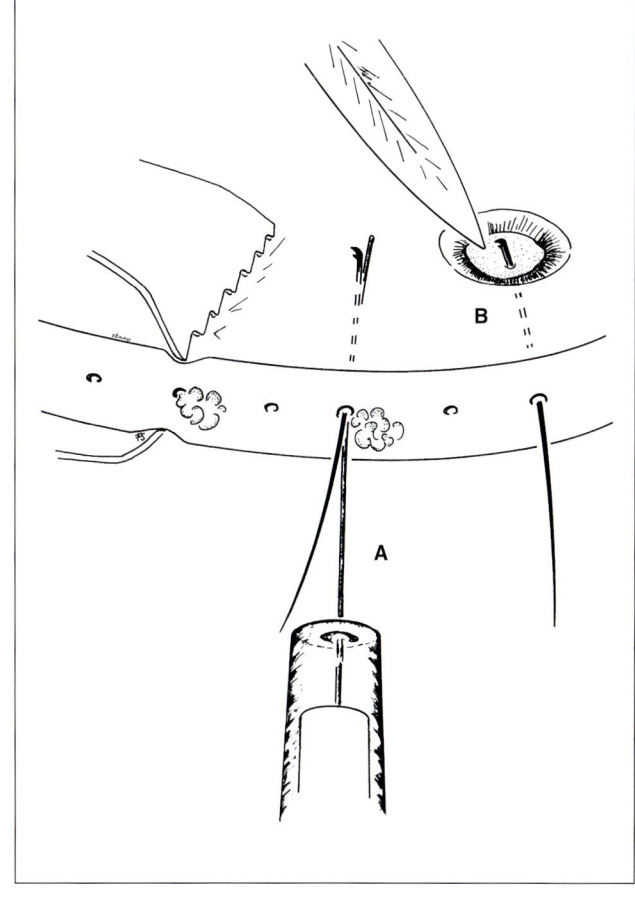

Fig. 7.5:
Distichiasis. Destruction of the hair follicle by needle coagulator via the opening of the gland (A), or via the conjunctiva (B), using an electric scalpel (cutting).

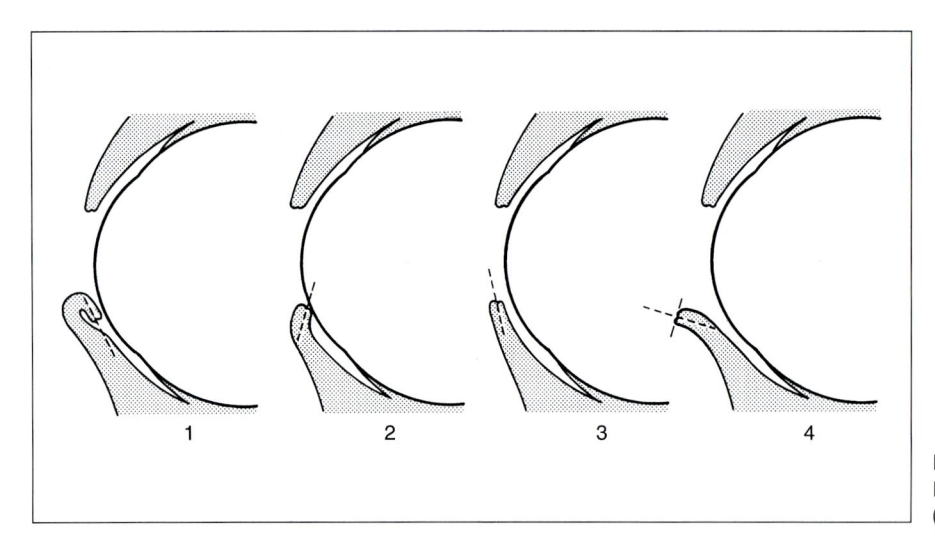

Fig. 7.6:
Positions of the lid margin. Entropion: (1) severe, (2) mild, (3) normal position, (4) ectropion.

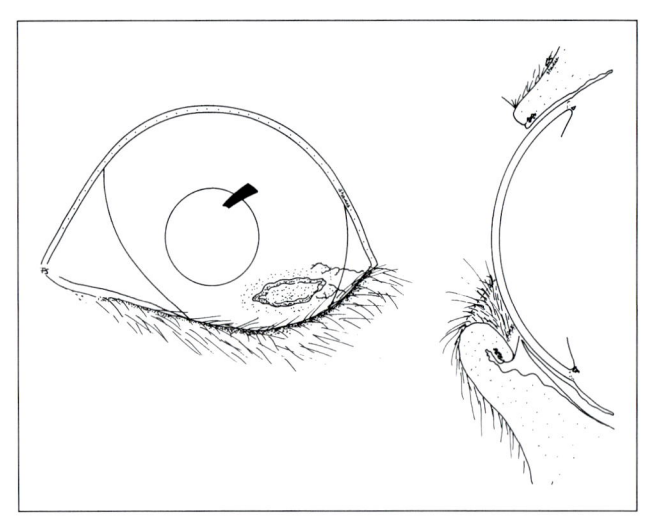

Fig. 7.7:
Entropion, severe and total lower lid margin, with secondary corneal ulceration.

Wound closure is secondary, which may result in irregular scarring. After-treatment consists of topical "initial choice" antibiotic ointment, 4 times daily for 7 days.

Prognosis / prevention: The prognosis is favorable; however, hair follicles may be invisible at the first session or the germinal bud may not be destroyed and the shaft may regrow. Affected animals should not be used for breeding.

7.6   Entropion

Entropion is the inversion of all or parts of the margin of an eyelid (Fig. 7.6, 7.7). The degree of entropion is considered to be mild when the margin is tilted by about 45 degrees, moderate when it is tilted by about 90 degrees, and severe when the margin is turned inwards by about 180 degrees (Plates 7.6–7.9 and 7.10–7.13). Entropion may be medial, angular, or total, and may affect the lower and/or upper lid.

The inverted position of the lid against the cornea results in corneal irritation, extra lacrimation, and blepharospasm. The margin and exterior surface of the eyelid are moist and there may be mucopurulent discharge depending on the severity of the inversion and degree of corneal irritation. Where hairs rub the cornea, corneal defects (Fig. 7.7.; Plate 7.13.) or sequestration is common. Because of the pain there is an enophthalmos, resulting in loss of support of the lid margin and subsequently, an increase of the entropion. This leads to a vicious circle that can only be broken by surgical correction of the entropion. The lesions may heal by granulation tissue or they may deepen until perforation occurs. The final stage is the formation of scar tissue and pigmentation or, sometimes, loss of the eye.

Entropion **79**

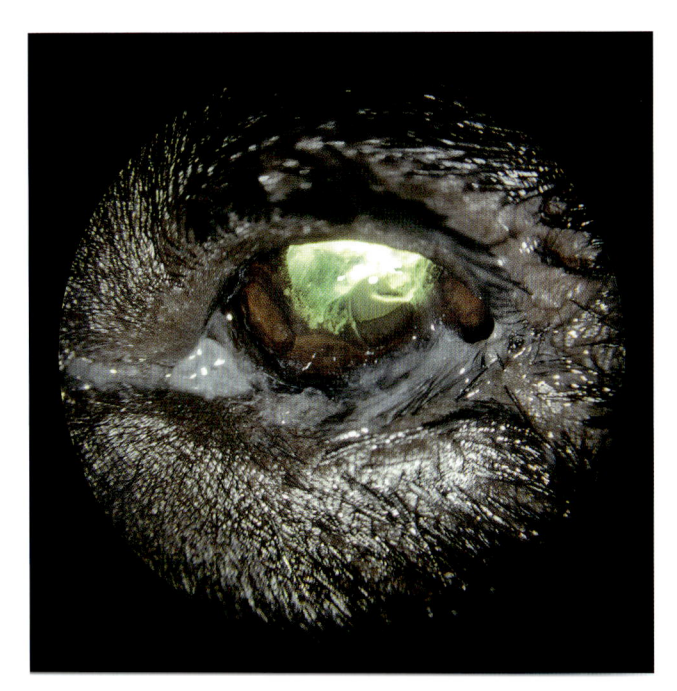

Plate 7.6:
Entropion (total, severe) of the lower lid edge in a Labrador Retriever (OS; see also Plate 7.7).

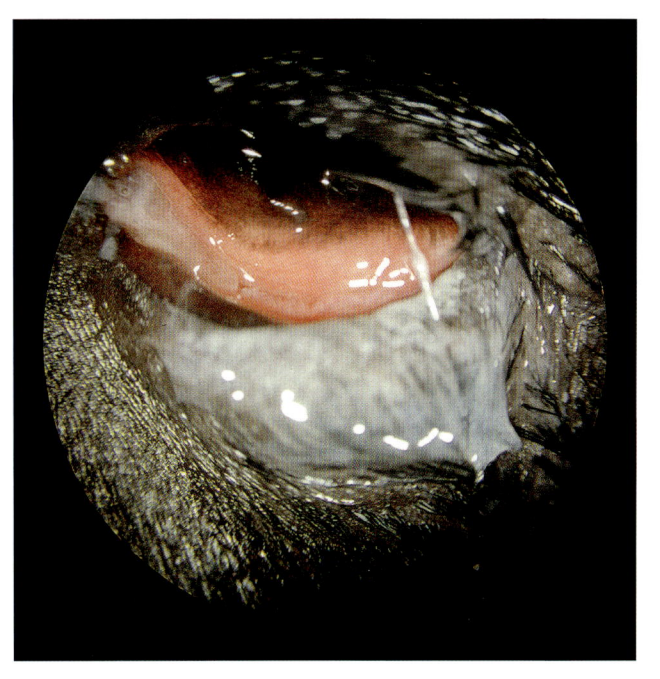

Plate 7.7:
Entropion (total, severe) of the lower lid edge in a Labrador Retriever (OS; same eye as shown in Plate 7.6). The lower lid edge is pulled ventrally. The outside part of the lid, which has been in contact with the tear film/cornea, is wet and depigmented. The outer borderline of mucus is the line where the second incision in the Celsus-Hotz surgical correction procedure with the "blood staining" (Stades) estimation method should be made (see entropion therapy 7.6).

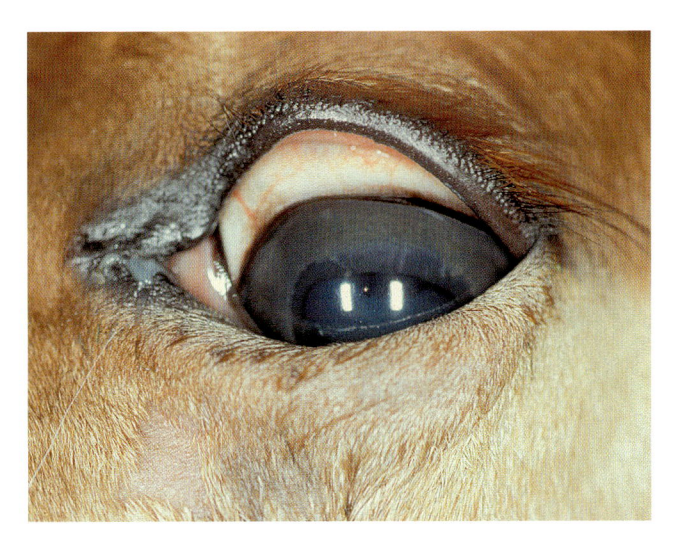

Plate 7.8:
Entropion (total, severe) of the lower lid edge in a foal (OS). Usually manual eversion, several times daily is sufficient for correction, otherwise traction sutures can be used. An "initial choice" antibiotic ointment is used as after-care. Tacking is an alternative.

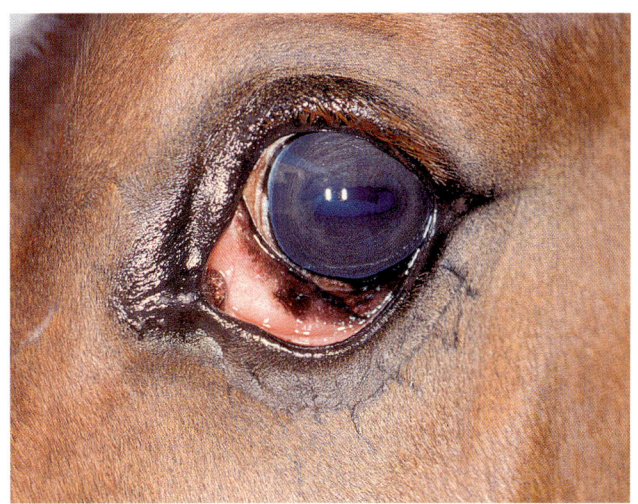

Plate 7.9:
Iatrogenic ectropion of the lower lid in a foal (OS), as the result of an over correction of an entropion. Removal of skin and orbicularis muscle is not indicated in these cases.

Entropion is possibly primarily due to a difference in tension between the orbicularis oculi muscle and the malaris muscle, and it may be influenced by a number of conditions such as conformation of the skull, the orbital anatomy, and the amount and folds of the facial skin around the eyes. Entropion in most cases is due to a hereditary defect and is most likely a polygenic condition.

Severe entropion of the upper lid (usually in combination with trichiasis) occurs in the Bloodhound, Chow Chow, and Shar Pei, while the lower lid is affected in the Chow Chow, Shar Pei, Bouvier, German Pointer, Labrador Retriever, and Rottweiler. Although there is a predisposition in these breeds, this condition can occur in any breed. It is found in the Great Dane and the St. Bernard in combination with an excessively long palpebral fissure. Medial entropion is seen frequently in the English Bulldog, King Charles Spaniel, Pekingese, Pug, Shih Tzu, Toy and Miniature Poodle, and the short-nosed Persian cats (Peke-face).

In some cases, the condition can be secondary (acquired) to severe corneal pain as in primary corneal ulceration. It can also be secondary to a loss of lid support (e.g. in microphthalmos or phthisis of the bulbus).

Symptoms: Signs of entropion include epiphora, moisture on the eyelid margins and eyelids, mucopurulent discharge, blepharospasm, and enophthalmos (Plates 7.6–7.8). There is increased conjunctival vascularity and signs of chronic irritation of the cornea, such as edema, pannus, granulation (Plate 7.13; Fig. 7.7), pigmentation, sequestration in the cat, and ulceration.

Diagnosis: Diagnosis is based on the clinical signs, history, and breed. The patient should be observed without restraint to determine the degree of entropion. After the evaluation has been done at a distance, do not hold the animal too tightly by the nape of the neck during closer examination, as the traction on the skin may evert the entropion. In case of doubt, e.g. when only the outside of the eyelid margin is moist, an entropion test should be performed (Plate 2.8). If the entropion is not blinked off quickly, the existence of at least a habitual entropion must be assumed.

Trichiasis and distichiasis must be considered in the differential diagnosis, but in these conditions the free lid margin can be recognized.

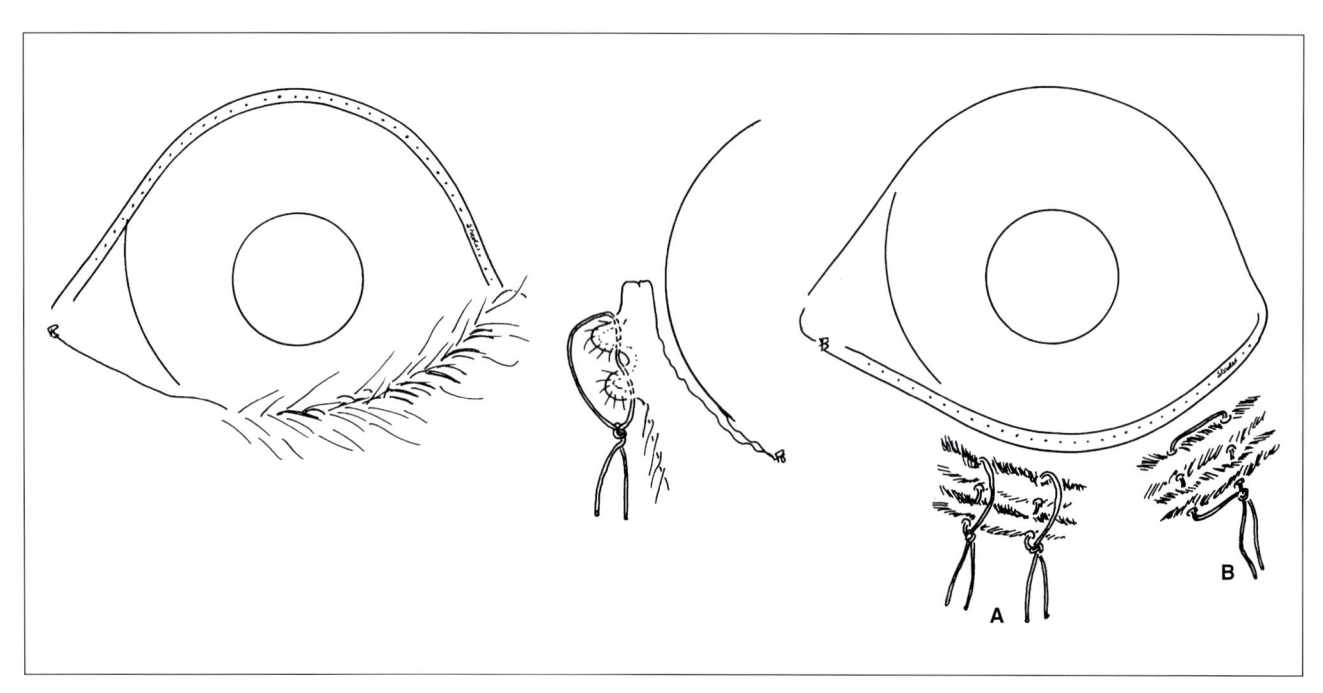

Fig. 7.8:
Surgical correction of severe entropion. Tacking can be performed in puppies. Simple, interrupted suture (A) and U-figure suture (B).

Therapy: In *mild entropion,* the cornea may be protected by a topical lubricant. It is usually best to postpone surgical correction until the head has grown to full size (1–2 years of age). In puppies less than 8–12 weeks old (mainly Shar Peis) with severe entropion, a few sutures ("tacking"; Fig. 7.8; some clinicians use unnecessary irritating staples) can be placed to gather up the skin of the lid and thereby evert the lid, thus preventing corneal lesions.[8] In some cases, the entropion will not require further correction. Tacking causes scar formation, also after removal of the stitches, resulting in correction of the entropion and must thus be considered an operative entropion intervention.

Severe entropion should always be corrected when there are corneal lesions, even in very young animals (within one day). Special care must be taken to avoid overcorrection, particularly in young animals. Before operating, the entropion is evaluated before and after topical anesthesia to determine the extent and degree of entropion. In older lesions, the entropic lid hairs are coated with a mucoid material that appears whitish-tan. This gives the surgeon an indication of the amount of eversion necessary to correct the defect.

Many methods and variations are available for the correction of entropion, mostly based on the Celsus-Hotz procedure (Celsus, 1st century A.D.).[9,10,11,12] There is no "cookbook" method that will fit every patient. Subcutaneous injections using antibiotic emulsions or silicones, or the mechanical crushing of the lid margin using the finger nail all cause an inflammatory reaction resulting in conjunctival swelling, thus correcting the entropion. On technical grounds (unpredictable results, complications), these methods are to be rejected.

Complicated entropion cases, e.g. combinations of upper and lower lid entropion, medial entropion, and combinations with severe corneal lesions (e.g. ulcer, sequestration), should be referred.

Operation: Surgical correction is begun with an incision 2–2.5 mm from and parallel to the margin of the lid (Fig. 7.9), extending at least 1 mm medial and lateral to the entropic part of the lid. If the first incision is too close to the margin, there will not be enough room for suturing, but if it is too far from the margin, the lid will not evert and the result will be difficult to predict (Plates 7.9, 7.10). Overcorrection will cause ectropion, which will itself be difficult to correct (Plates 7.9–7.11). Accordingly, estimating correctly the amount of tissue to be removed is important. The following methods (Fig. 7.10) can be used as an aid:
1. The most entropic part of the skin that lies against the cornea before surgery can be marked. The eyelid is replaced in its entropion position after the first incision has been made. Using forceps, a small amount of blood is applied to mark the margin of the skin of the inverted lid. The second or external, banana-shaped, incision is then made just along the edge of this mark.

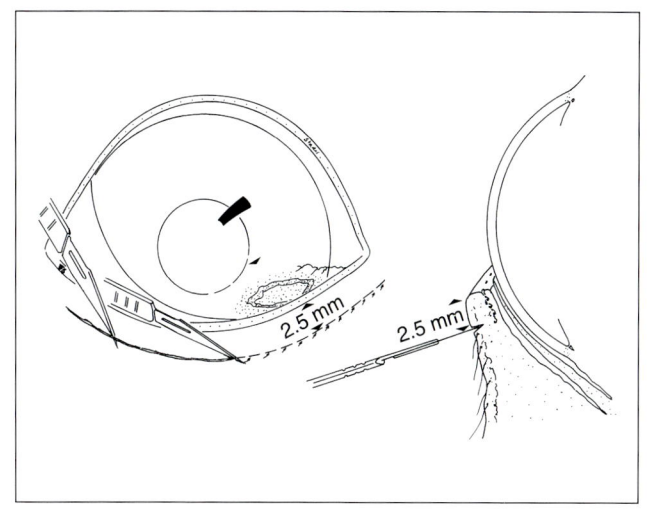

Fig. 7.9:
Entropion correction, Celsus-Hotz procedure. First incision is made perpendicular to the lid skin.

2. The "rule of thumb" technique, which is done by placing digital pressure on the lid skin adjacent to the entropic margin and pulling down until the free lid margin is exposed. The distance the thumb moves to evert the lid is the widest portion of the lid skin excised. The second incision is made in an elliptical fashion joining the two ends of the primary incision.[13]
3. Sufficient skin can be grasped with an Allis forceps until the eyelid returns to its normal position. The resulting fold of skin is removed by cutting with scissors.[14]

The part of the skin around which the incisions have been made is further excised with a scalpel or scissors ("fold" method), including a superficial strip of the orbicularis muscle. The conjunctival sac must not be perforated.

The wound is closed with interrupted sutures of suture material that will effectively reappose the wound edges and should never exceed 5-0 (non-absorbable, e.g. silk, or absorbable [if complications are to be expected during the removal], mono- or polyfilament, fine round-body needle with or without a micropoint). The sutures are placed at intervals of not more than 2 mm (Figs. 7.11, 7.12). A continuous suture is not used because of the risk of rupture of the wound when it is rubbed. The first sutures are placed at the medial and lateral ends and then the rest of the wound is closed by halving. In lateral angle entropion (Fig. 7.11), the first suture is placed at the lateral canthus (Fig. 7.12). Other surgeons use an "arrow pattern", starting in the middle of the wound.[13] Here the first two sutures are placed at an angle of 45 degrees to each other, pointing to the eye. The remaining sutures are placed parallel to each of the first two on the corresponding sides (Fig. 7.10.3 C–D). They should be spaced as described above.

82 Eyelids

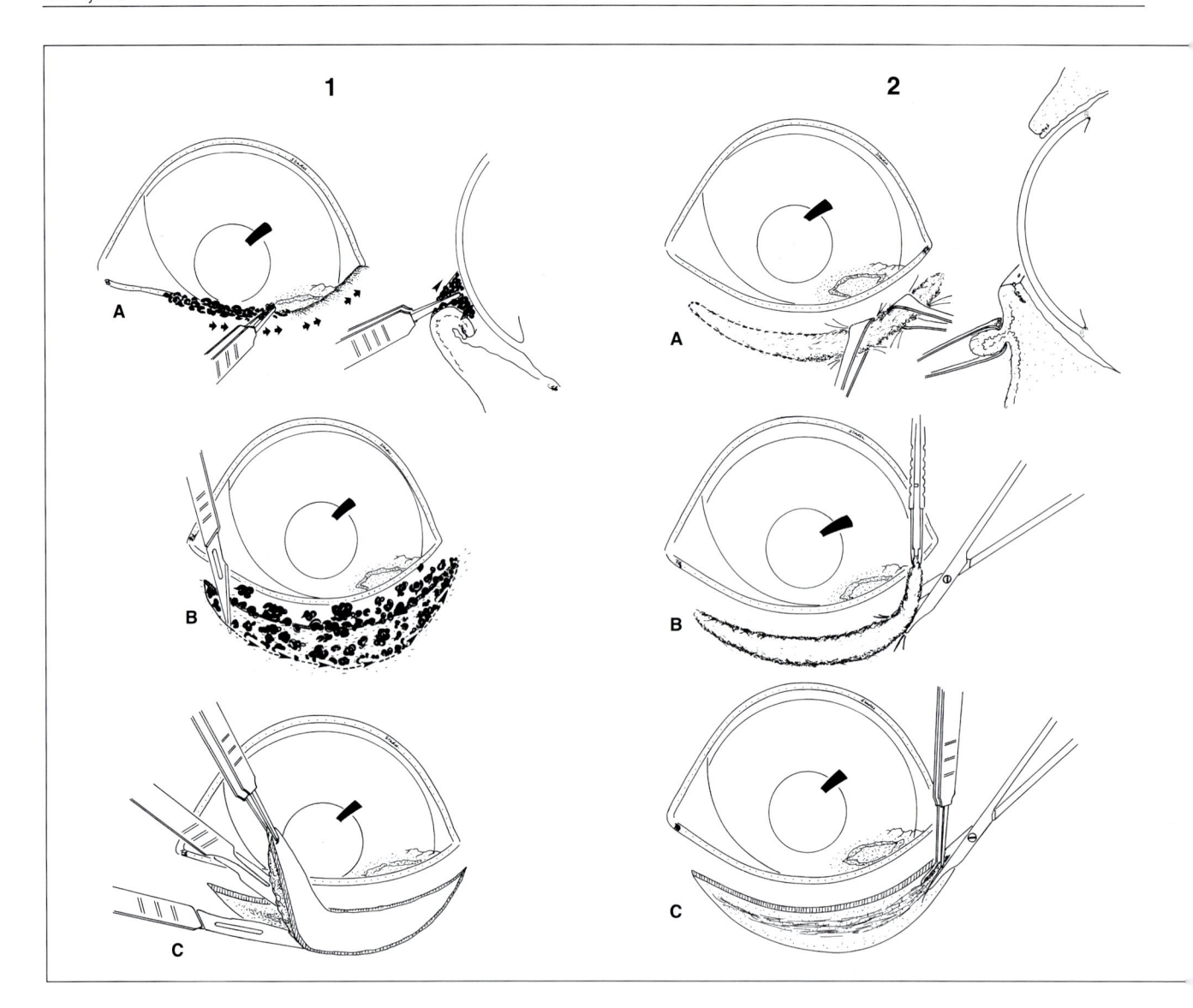

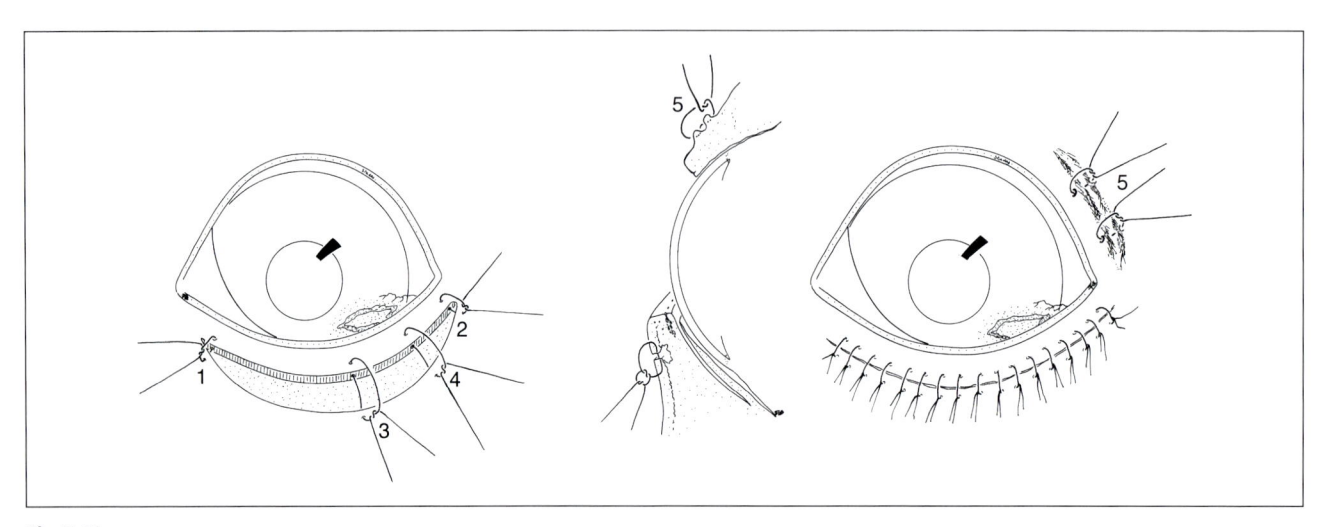

Fig. 7.11:
Suturing sequence in Celsus-Hotz entropion correction (1–4). Further intervals are closed by halving. Tacking stitches (5), preventing possible irritation of upper lid hairs pricking in the postoperatively swollen lower conjunctiva (secondary to entropion correction).

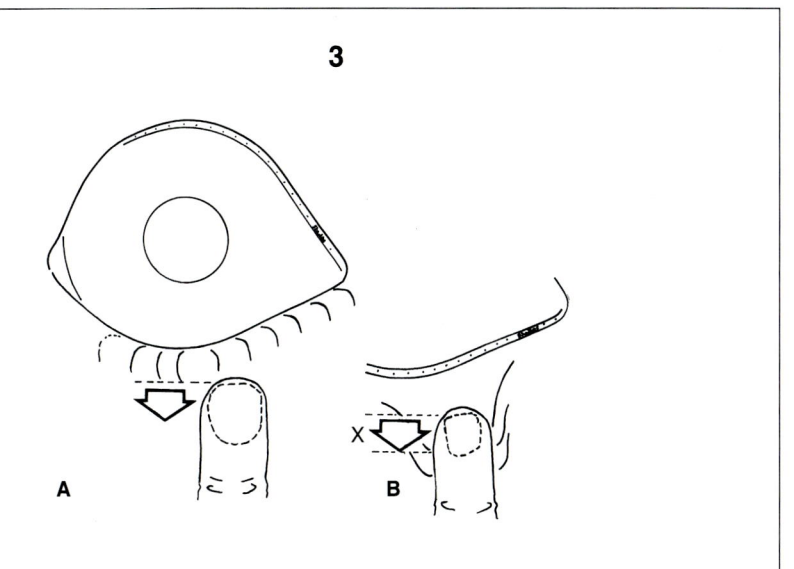

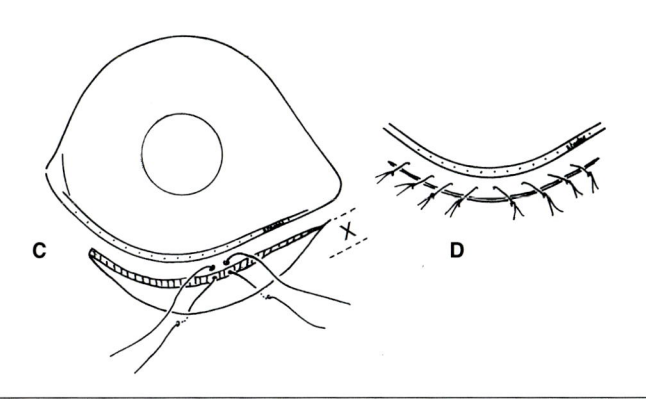

Entropion **83**

Fig. 7.10:
Entropion correction, Celsus-Hotz procedure, estimation methods:
1. (A) "blood staining" (Stades) method; (B) second, external incision; (C) excision of skin plus muscle rim.
2. "folding" method: (A) grasping enough fold to correct the entropion; (B) excision of the fold; (C) excision of the muscle rim.
3. "rule of thumb" (Wyman) method: (A-B) pulling the lid skin down until the lid margin is exposed, then an elliptical part is removed over a distance x; and (C) "arrow pattern" suture method.

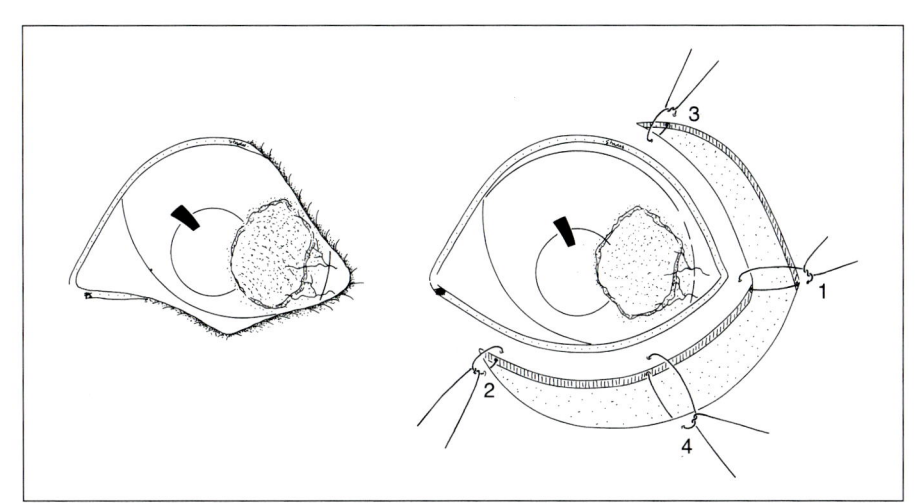

Fig. 7.12:
Surgical correction of lateral angular entropion with a secondary corneal ulcer, and the order of suturing (1–4).

84 Eyelids

Plate 7.10:
Entropion (severe, partial lateral) of the lower lid edge (OD, dog). The scars are due to a non-professional entropion "correction". The incisions were too far away from the lid edges and subsequently the entropion was not corrected. Moreover, excessively thick suture material had been used, resulting in these broad, disfiguring scars.

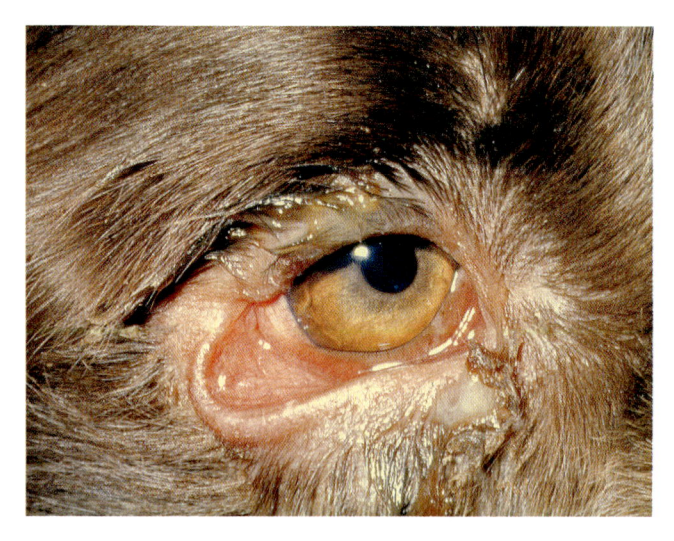

Plate 7.11:
Iatrogenic ectropion due to excessive overcorrection of a severe entropion (OD, dog; see also Plate 7.12). During the correction, strands of scar tissue were found from the scar to the zygomatic arch.

The edges of the wound should be joined together so carefully that no part of an edge remains visible. Some postoperative swelling of the conjunctiva is normal and even desirable because it keeps the eyelid margin off the cornea, which is often still painful, thus allowing the cornea to heal quickly.

In cases of **mild medial entropion** a little more of the skin can be removed to counteract any tendency to develop nasal folds, this without the risk of overcorrection (Fig. 7.13). **Medial canthus entropion** in breeds such as the Pekingese or Shih Tzu should be corrected by medial canthoplasty (Fig. 7.14; see also 7.8.1.2).

After-care consists of applying topical "initial choice" antibiotic ointment (more lubricating), 4 times daily for 14 days. If corneal ulceration is present, 1% atropine is added, 2–4 times daily for 10–14 days. When sutured with great care, a protective collar is generally not necessary. The sutures are removed 10–14 days after surgery. Absorbable materials will not absorb very quickly in the skin, so to prevent itching, they should also be removed.

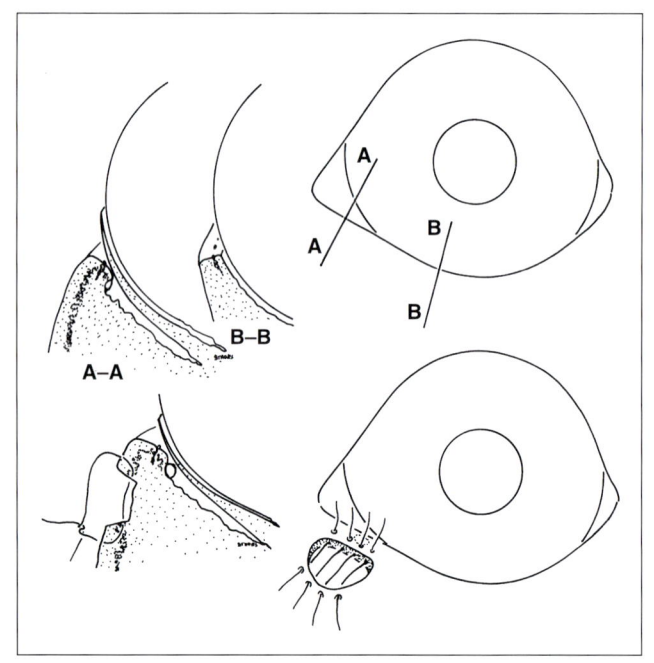

Fig. 7.13:
Surgical correction of a medial lower canthus entropion.

Entropion **85**

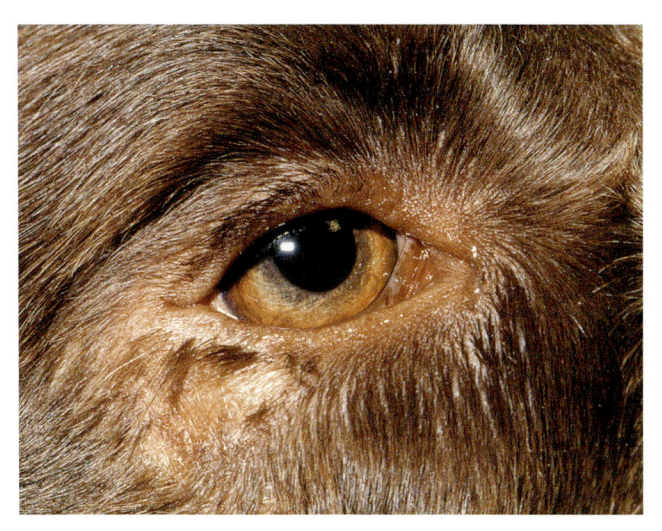

Plate 7.12:
Result of a free transplant blepharoplasty for the correction of iatrogenic ectropion (OD, dog; same eye as shown in Plate 7.11). The banana-shaped transplant, necessary to fill the gap of skin was approximately 25 mm long and 14 mm at its widest point.

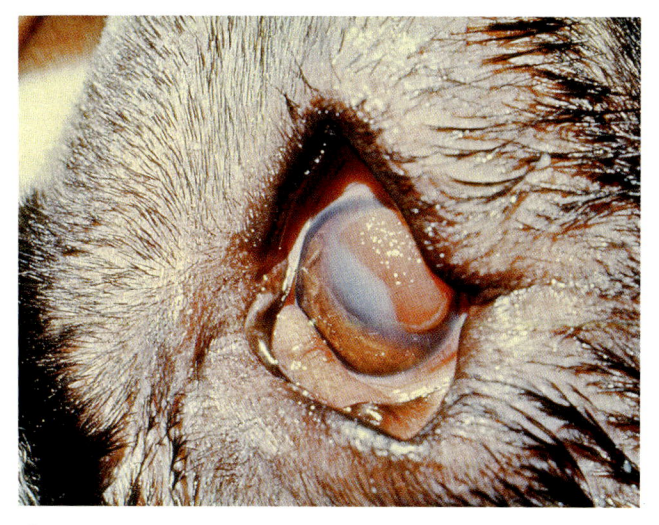

Plate 7.13:
An oversized, diamond-shaped lid fissure, associated with angular entropion and an eversion of the nictitating membrane in a St. Bernhard (OS). Dorsolaterally in the cornea, there is an almost circular, superficial ulcer with undermined edges and granulation from the dorsolateral side.

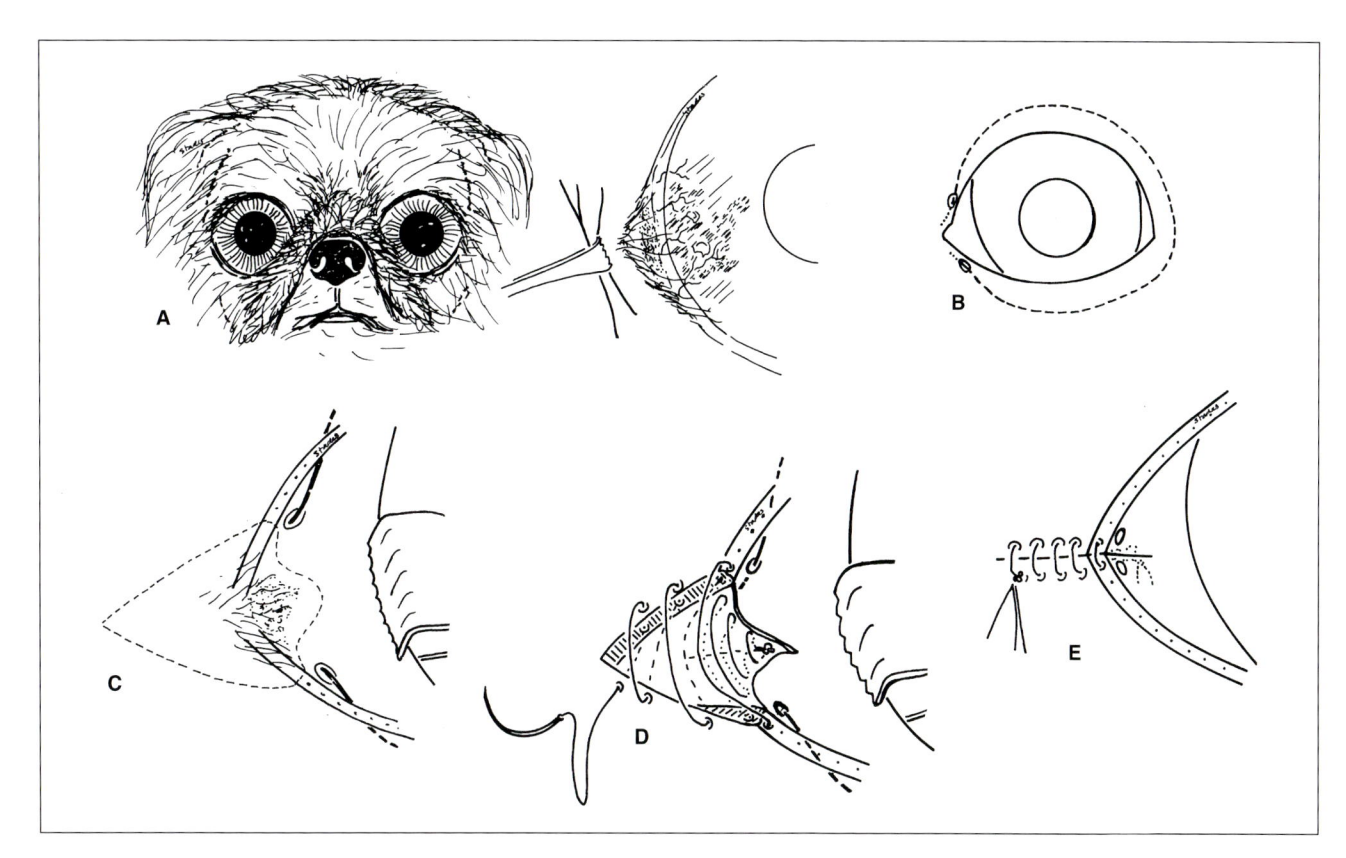

Fig. 7.14:
Surgical correction of a combination of medial entropion, nasal fold trichiasis and oversized lid fissure in brachycephalic animals.

Prognosis / prevention: The prognosis for entropion correction is good when the surgical procedure is performed correctly. In cases of deep corneal damage, corneal scarring is to be expected. Parents and siblings should also be examined. Affected animals should not be used for breeding. Breeding of parents or siblings of affected animals, especially when they are to be mated to animals from an entropion-free line, thus camouflaging the defect, should also be discouraged. Breeding should aim for lids with fissures of normal length. It would be advantageous to have the breed, name, chip or tattoo, and pedigree number of affected animals registered centrally and to persuade owners to report such information to the breed association (see 15).

7.6.1 Entropion in sheep and horses

Congenital, hereditary entropion occurs in sheep and is often seen in significant numbers in lambs within a flock. Entropion in foals is less frequent (Plates 7.8, 7.9) and can also be secondary to dehydration due to serious systemic disease. In mild cases, manual correction, several times a day, and protection of the cornea by a topical lubricant may be sufficient. Traction sutures or tacking (some clinicians use unnecessary irritating staples) can also be performed. Subcutaneous injection of an antibiotic emulsion, silicones or crushing of the lid skin by a finger nail will result in conjunctival swelling, thus correcting the entropion. However, the latter methods are ineffective, unpredictable and ethically undesirable.

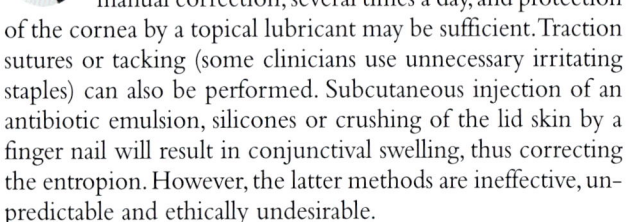

7.7 Ectropion and/or oversized palpebral fissure (macroblepharon) (Ect/OPF)

Ectropion is eversion of the margin of the lower eyelid (Fig. 7.6). It is readily recognized because the orifices of the meibomian glands are visible in the everted margin, the palpebral fissure is often too long, and the lower lid is not adjacent to the globe. In an oversized fissure, the lid margins are distinctly longer (5–15 mm, stretched length over 40 mm) than is necessary to cover the sclera in the opened eye. It is not always easy to differentiate between both entities; for that reason they are discussed below as one abnormality (Plates 7.13, 7.14).

When the lower eyelid is not appropriately apposed to the globe over a distance of 1–10 mm or more, a funnel or sac is formed in the lower eyelid and the lacrimal fluid cannot perform its normal function of cleaning, shielding, and lubricating the globe. The conjunctival sac then becomes chronically inflamed as a result of its permanent exposure to air, dust, bacteria, etc. In more severe cases (e.g. Bloodhound, Clumber Spaniel, Leonberger, St. Bernard, and other breeds), there is often some inversion near both ends when the middle portion of the lid is everted, which will result in a chronic purulent conjunctivitis.

Most forms of Ect/OPF in the dog are congenital and breed-related or hereditary. The genetic transmission is most likely polygenic. Some owners, dog fanciers, and breeders believe Ect/OPF to be normal or even encourage everted lower eyelids (the dog having such a "nice sad and devoted expression"). Some breed standards tolerate or even promote the condition. Breed prescriptions vary from: "not showing much haw" (Sussex Spaniel), "some haw showing but without excess" (Clumber Spaniel); "the haw may sometimes show without excess" (Basset, Artresian Normand); "the lower lid shows a certain looseness" (Grand Bleu de Gascoigne); "red (cryptic description of inflamed conjunctiva) of lower lid appears, though not excessively" (Basset Hound); and in *optima forma* too: "a strongly hanging lower lid, showing the red conjunctiva" (St. Hubertus Hound = Bloodhound), and "a small angular fold on the lower lids with the haws only slightly visible as well as a small fold on the upper lids are permitted" (St. Bernhard). Strangely enough, many kennel clubs do not accept breeding from entropion- or ectropion-affected dogs in their rules.

Ect/OPF is extremely rare in other species. The acquired form is fortunately rare, usually being caused by scar contraction after injuries or being the result of faulty overcorrection of an entropion.

Symptoms: Symptoms of Ect/OPF are a hanging lower lid margin (the openings of the meibomian glands are visible in the free margin), the fissure is often "diamond"- or "pagoda"-shaped (Plates 7.13, 7.14), the conjunctiva is red and swollen, and folded, resulting in increased tear and mucus production and purulent exudate. There is a slight enophthalmos, thus increasing the distance between the lid margin and the globe. When the animal is more active than usual, as at dog shows or on the veterinarian's examination table, and whenever it is held tightly by the nape of the neck, the Ect/OPF may almost "disappear", but there will still be too much sclera visible on the lateral side.

Diseases associated with enophthalmos must be considered in the differential diagnosis (e.g. Horner's syndrome, uveitis).

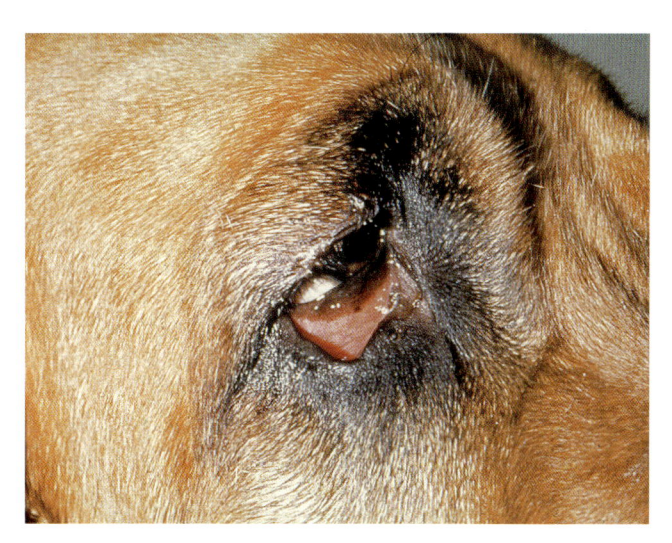

Plate 7.14:
Oversized, diamond-shaped lid fissure with trichiasis/entropion of the lateral upper lid edge in a Bloodhound (OD). The lower lid edge is positioned approximately 15 mm below the bulbus, but is reasonably normal in its upward position. Hence it is not really an ectropion, which would mean a lid edge turned away from the globe.

Therapy: If the defect is slight, no treatment is required apart from irrigating the eyes upon returning from walks and applying a lubricating ophthalmic ointment or solution, particularly in young dogs whose heads have not yet reached adult size. In more severe lesions, corrective measures may be taken. Because these procedures require a high degree of judgment and experience on the part of the surgeon (unwanted scars may be a new "eyesore" to the owner), such patients are usually referred.

7.7.1 Shortening of the lower palpebral conjunctiva

Where there is normal fissure length, a slight correction can be achieved by suturing together (basting) the ventral palpebral conjunctiva with a continuous subconjunctival absorbable suture.

7.7.2 V-Y Method

This method induces scar tissue below the margin of the lower eyelid, which pushes up and supports the lower margin.

These last two methods, however, are only reliable when ectropion is not combined with an overlong palpebral fissure, and so they are only of use in exceptional cases. In most instances, the lower eyelid margin is too long and methods for reducing this, either around the defect in the margin or at the lateral canthus, yield the best results. Other techniques shorten the lower lid at the most ectropic area or in the lateral canthus (simple wedge resection [see 7.7.3] and the method of Kuhnt-Szymanowski, Blaskovic's modification [see 7.7.4]), or the total fissure is shortened.

7.7.3 Simple wedge resection

A full-thickness triangular lower lid section, immediately next to the lateral canthus, is excised. The surgical defect is apposed by one or two layers of sutures. This method is the most simple, but it does not have the benefits of a double-layered staggered wound preventing leakage, and has a greater chance of wound dehiscence and atrophy of the eyelid margin in the long term.

7.7.4 Kuhnt-Szymanowski method, Blaskovic's modification[15]

An incision is made 2–2.5 mm from and parallel to the margin of the lid, similar to the first incision for correcting entropion, starting a few millimeters medial to the worst area of ectropion and ending 5–10 mm lateral to the lateral canthus. From the lateral end of this incision, a 10- to 20-mm incision is made vertically in a ventral direction (Fig. 7.15). The entire flap is loosened by blunt dissection. A wedge-shaped part of the eyelid is excised at the worst area of ectropion, so that the length of the margin is shortened by 5–15 mm. An equally long wedge is removed from the lateral part of the loosened flap. The wound on the eyelid margin is closed very carefully (see 4.5.1). The loosened flap is then sutured after any bleeding has been arrested. This method shortens the eyelid margin to the desired length and draws it upward and laterally.

7.7.5 Kuhnt-Szymanowski method[16]

This basic method for ectropion correction in humans differs from the Blaskovic's modification only in that the incision is not made below the margin of the eyelid but in the margin itself (lid splitting), just in- or outside of the orifices of the meibomian glands. All the meibomian glands are damaged over the operated distance and this technique may easily lead to uncontrolled scarring in the "new" lid margin.

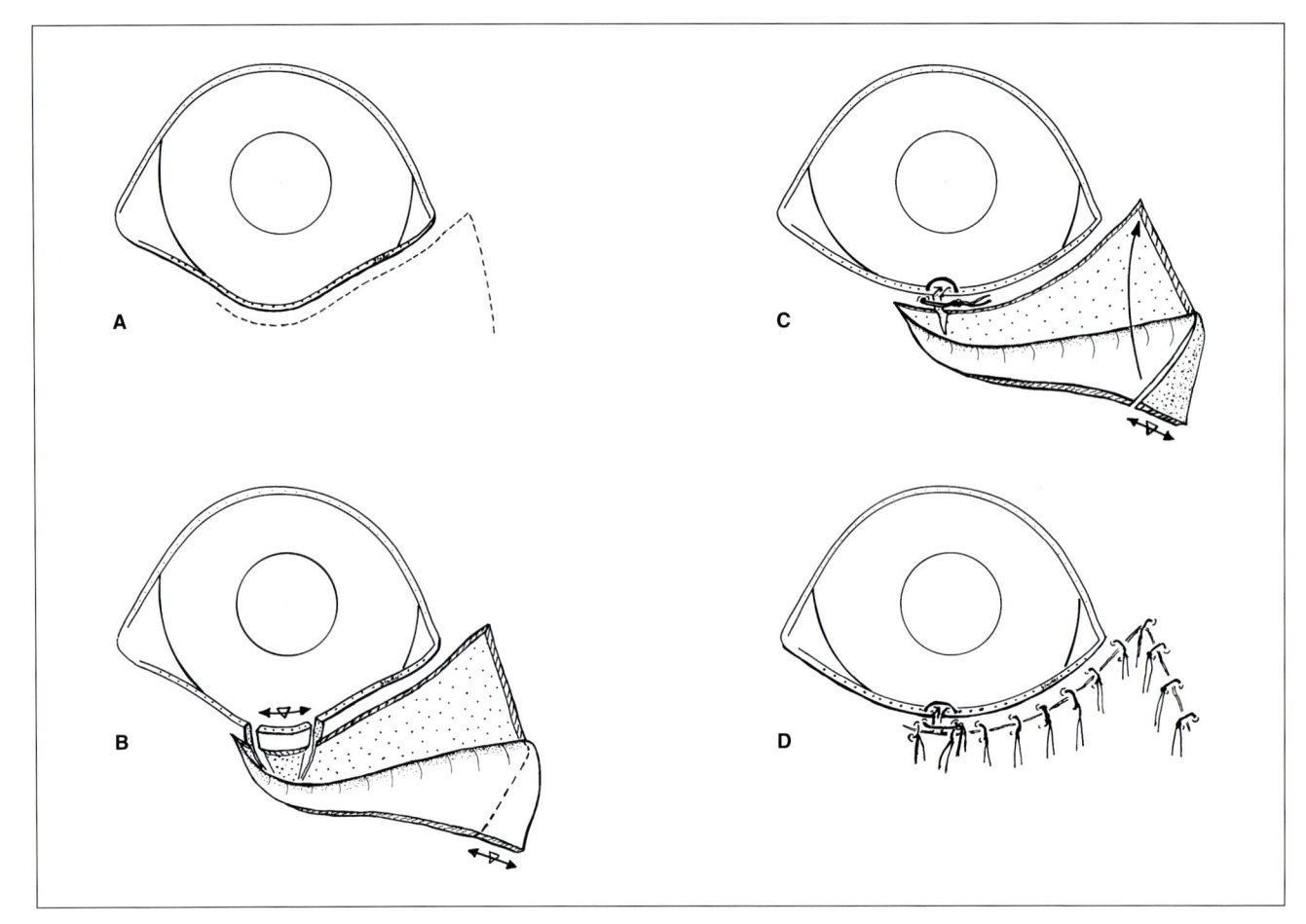

Fig. 7.15:
Surgical correction of an ectropion/macroblepharon (Kuhnt-Szymanowski method, Blaskovic's modification).

7.7.6 Z-plasty/free transplants

These methods are only applied in rare cases to repair iatrogenic ectropion caused by overcorrection of entropion (Plates 7.10–7.12).

7.7.7. Total fissure shortening methods

Many methods are available for shortening the upper and lower lid, and thus the total fissure length. They include, for example, simple lateral tarsorrhaphy, Roberts-Jensen, Fuchs, Wyman-Kaswan, Kuhnt-Szymanowski modification Bedford, Bigelbach, Stades-Diabolo, and Grussendorf (with retraction suture).[17,18,19,20,21] These procedures require a high degree of judgment and experience on the part of the surgeon; such patients are better referred.

After-care consists of applying topical "initial choice" antibiotic ointment (more lubricating), 4 times daily for 14 days. The sutures are removed 10–14 days after surgery. The end result can only be judged after cicatrization, about 6–8 weeks after surgery.

Prognosis/prevention: The prognosis for correction of Ect/OPF, although depending on the cause and the severity of the problem, is good.

Parents and siblings should also be examined and no affected animals should be used for breeding. Breeding should aim for closed lids with fissures of normal length, and also for ears of normal weight and placement, as heavy and low hanging ears will pull the skin forwards and down, causing more Ect/OPF. Breed standards should sustain this and owners should be warned not to "like" these features. It would be advantageous to have the breed, name, tattoo and pedigree number of affected animals registered centrally and to persuade owners to report such information to the breed association (see 15).

7.8 Trichiasis

Trichiasis is the presence of normally located but abnormally directed hairs that irritate the globe and/or conjunctiva. The chronic corneal irritation results in extra lacrimation, blepharospasm, and mucopurulent discharge. Where hairs rub the cornea, corneal defects are common. The lesions are often healed by granulation tissue, but they may also deepen until perforation occurs. The final stage is the formation of scar tissue and pigmentation, or sometimes even the loss of the eye. Trichiasis must usually be corrected surgically. Because the methods available require a high degree of judgment and experience on the part of the surgeon, such patients are usually referred at short notice (in case of corneal defects, within one day).

Trichiasis (Fig. 7.16.) may occur in (1) nasal folds and (2) the upper eyelid, usually dorsolaterally and in combination with entropion in the same area, or (3) in the caruncle or other more rare locations. Aplasia of the lid may also predispose to misdirected hairs irritating the globe (see 7.3). Also, badly healed lid lacerations or blepharoplasties may result in trichiasis. Trichiasis occurs in several dog breeds as a hereditary, most likely polygenic, entity and is a desired characteristic in some breed standards.

7.8.1 Nasal fold trichiasis

Because of breed standards and fashions that disregard the animals' health but are nevertheless supported by breeders, judges, and buyers alike, almost all eyes of prominent-eyed breeds (e.g. Pekingese and Shih Tzu) are chronically irritated and predisposed to luxation. For example, breed standards, which most veterinarians do not agree with, prescribe that the Pekingese should have a short muzzle with a marked stop and heavily wrinkled skin with long and straight hairs, and also that it should have large and protruding eyes. In most patients, nasal fold trichiasis is found in combination with medial entropion, a slightly oversized lid fissure, and lagophthalmos.

The hairs on the nasal fold and of the medial entropion are a source of irritation to the medial quadrant of the cornea (Plate 7.15), resulting in extra lacrimation, slight blepharospasm, edema, vascularization, pigmentation and other corneal defects. The final stage is medial pannus formation with accompanying pigmentation, which may, in the end, cover the entire cornea. Additionally, the prominent eyes and associated lagophthalmos results in drying of the axial cornea and erosion of the epithelium. Ulcers (rounded, crater-like) in these breeds resulting from this insult (without being noticed by the owner) often become lytic and progress to descemetoceles within 24 hours. They may rupture during excitation, which results in pain reactions like whining and moaning, often interpreted by the owner as being traumatic and caused by a cat or dog fight. Traumatic defects, however, are usually scratch-shaped. Finally, the ulcers may end in severe central corneal scarring, often with anterior synechia, or even the loss of the eye.

Therapy: In cases of minor corneal defects, therapy can be started with "initial choice" antibiotic and atropine ointments, 4 times daily. If the defects have healed after 10 days, the cornea may be protected by oil or petrolatum 1–2 times daily, which adheres the hairs together, but this alone seldom resolves the problem (see 7.8.1.2).

7.8.1.1 Removal of nasal folds

Nasal folds can simply be removed. In this operation the fold is lifted, excised with large scissors, and the wound closed with 4-0 to 5-0 absorbable mono- or polyfilament simple interrupted sutures. With some effort, the medial canthal entropion can be corrected in the same procedure. However, this operation does not correct the associated oversize of the lid fissure, which would otherwise prevent lagophthalmia and luxation of the globe.

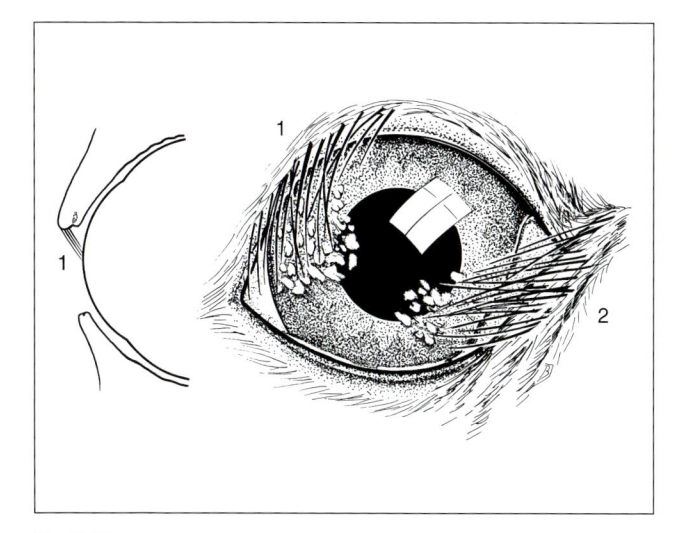

Fig. 7.16:
Trichiasis of the dorsolateral lid edge (1) and nasal fold trichiasis (2).

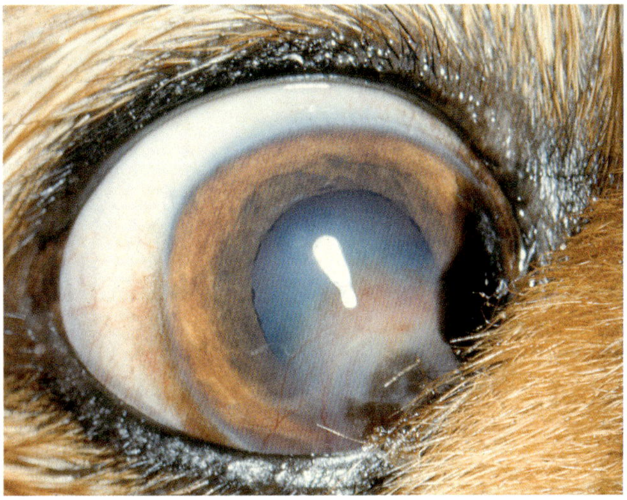

Plate 7.15:
Nasal fold trichiasis and entropion on the medial canthus in a Pekingese (OD). The central, pink granulation suggests chronic irritation by nasal fold hairs. The peripheral pigmentation is due to hairs on the medial canthus itself.

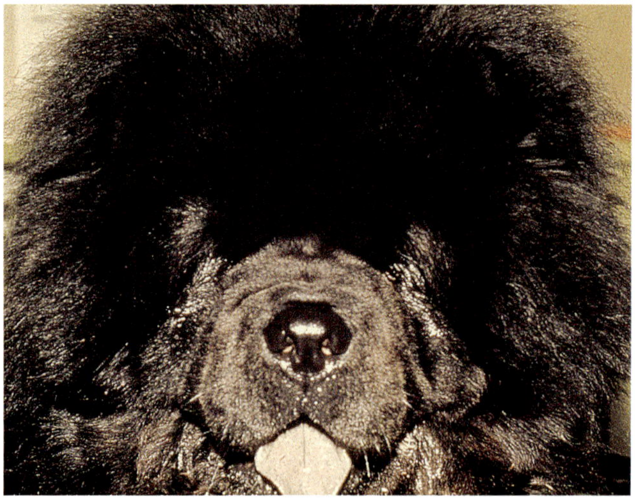

Plate 7.16:
Trichiasis/entropion of the upper lid and entropion of the lower lids in a Chow Chow. Due to the severe blepharospasm, the eyes could not be seen (see also Plate 7.17; by courtesy Drs. G. & F. Kása, Lörrach).

7.8.1.2 Medial canthoplasty

In this operation, the medial canthus skin over about 2 cm, the canthus itself, the first 6–8 mm of the lid edges (without traumatizing the punctae!) and the hairy caruncle in the medial canthal conjunctiva are removed (Fig. 7.14).[22] Care should be taken not to injure the lacrimal puncta and canaliculi. The conjunctiva, the margins of the lid, and the skin are closed with a continuous suture, using 6-0 absorbable material. Postoperative treatment consists of topical "initial choice" antibiotic ointment, 4 times daily for 14 days.

As a result of this operation, the medial canthus is turned outwards, emerges from behind the nasal folds, and is displaced 6–10 mm laterally. Another benefit is the shortening of the palpebral fissure by 6–8 mm, which practically precludes luxation of the globe and diminishes the lagophthalmic complications.

7.8.2 Upper eyelid trichiasis

In this condition, it is the lash-type hairs of the lateral upper eyelid or hairs on the skin folds that irritate the cornea in combination with entropion. These types of hairs droop over the eyes, irritating the conjunctiva and the cornea. Particularly in the Bloodhound, Chow Chow, and Shar Pei (and less severely in the elderly English Cocker Spaniel and Bassets), these hairs may cause very serious lesions of the cornea. In these breeds, the excessive masses of frontal wrinkles press the margin of the upper eyelid inwardly onto the globe (Plates 7.14, 7.16–7.24). In the Bloodhound and English Cocker Spaniel, this is increased by the heavy weight of the dog's ears when the head is turned towards the ground.

The irritation results in extra lacrimation and blepharospasm, which may worsen the situation. The hairs on the upper eyelid are dark and moist with a sticky secretion, and the upper lid margin is slightly entropic. The conjunctiva is red and swollen, and the corneal epithelium is damaged, resulting in ulceration (Plates 7.18, 7.19, 7.22, 7.24), and, in rare cases, also perforation. Finally, the corneal damage often results in scarring and pigmentation.

Therapy: In cases of minor irritation, the cornea may be protected by oil or petrolatum 1–2 times daily, but this alone seldom resolves the problem. A simple entropion correction, as described above, is seldom sufficient. The removal of upper palpebral folds or some of the frontal skin (15–20 cm in Bloodhounds[23] or 6–10 cm in the older English Cocker Spaniel[24]) usually produces only short-term results and does not eliminate the lash-type hairs that cause the irritation. Major

Plate 7.17:
Trichiasis/entropion of the upper lids and entropion of the lower lids in a Chow Chow, after the shaving necessary for a blepharoplasty (method: Kása & Kása). The photograph illustrates the enormous fold formation on the forehead of the modern Chow Chow, which induces trichiasis/entropion of the upper lids (same dog as shown in Plate 7.16; by courtesy Drs. G. & F. Kása, Lörrach).

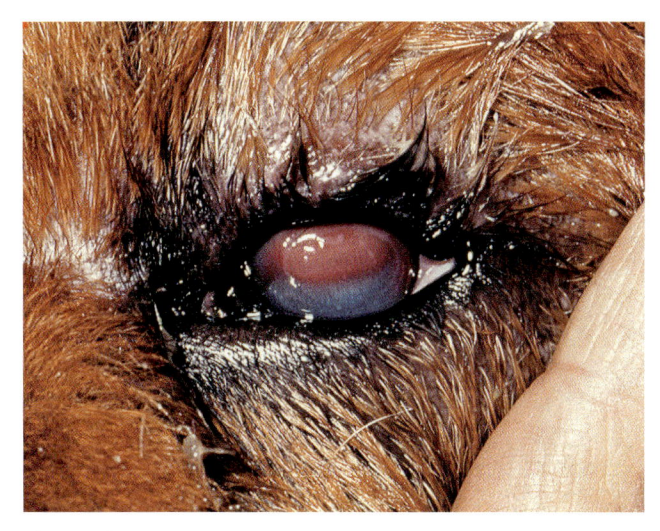

Plate 7.18:
Trichiasis/entropion of the upper eyelid in a Chow Chow with a secondary corneal ulcer (OS). From the 12-o'clock position, the ulcer is filled with granulation and there is an undermined edge.

"facelifts" can be performed in severe cases, as described by Kása and Kása,[25] although the entropion of the upper lid margin itself still has to be corrected. Also a brow-sling, as has been developed by Willis et al.,[26] can be successful, although complications such as recurrences, infections around the implanted sling, and uncontrolled scarring may occur. For these reasons, such methods require the hands of a specialist.

Radical excision of the upper lid skin, including the irritating, eyelash-like hairs, and the forced secondary granulation (Stades' method)[27] can be used in severe cases (Fig. 7.17). The first incision is located 0.5 mm from and parallel to the margin of the eyelid, care being taken not to injure the meibomian glands. A piece of skin up to 25 mm in width is circumcised in the form of a "clown's eyebrow" and removed by blunt dissection (Plates 7.19–7.24). The dorsal edge of the wound is reattached at a distance of 5–6 mm from the margin of the eyelid (absorbable 6-0), at the base of the meibomian glands and edge of the tarsal plate. The open part of the wound is thus forced to heal by secondary granulation (the owner must be warned before surgery). After further scarring, the upper lid is covered by hairless scar tissue, which becomes pigmented after a few months (Plate 7.24). The result of the surgery is that the frontal fold hairs can no longer reach the eye.

Postoperative treatment consists of topical "initial choice" antibiotic ointment, 4 times daily for 14 days.

Prognosis: The prognosis is favorable.

7.8.3 Caruncle trichiasis and trichiasis in other locations

The caruncle normally contains soft hairs, which are directed outwards (Plate 6.1, 6.8). In brachycephalic breeds (Pekingese, Shih Tzu), these hairs may irritate the globe. They may grow very long, up to 10–15 mm. Misdirected hairs irritating the conjunctiva and/or cornea can also be found in other lid skin locations around the eye.

Therapy: The hairs can be epilated first to be sure they are the cause of the irritation. Because the hairs are generally located very near the lid margin, the Celsus-Hotz method will not be effective; instead medial canthoplasty, Stades forced granulation procedure, or electro- or cryodestruction may be indicated. Because of the required experience on the part of the surgeon, such patients are best referred.

Prevention: Affected animals should not be used for breeding. Parents and siblings should also be examined. The desire of breeders and judges, supported by buyers, for very short noses, a marked stop, and heavily wrinkled and abundant facial skin should be discouraged. If the aim for short noses in some Persian cats ("Peke face") is continued, problems as in Pekingese may develop. Breed standards should be corrected. It would be advantageous to have the breed, name, chip or tattoo and pedigree number of affected animals registered centrally, and to persuade owners to report such information to the breed association (see 15).

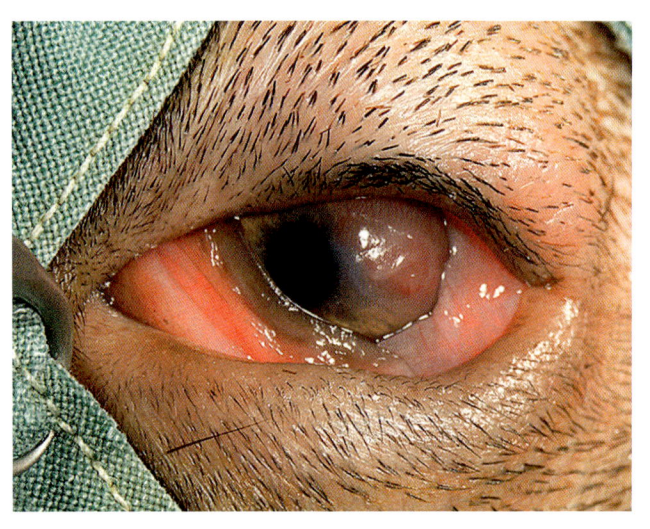

Plate 7.19:
Trichiasis/entropion of the upper lid and entropion of the lower lid in a 1-year-old Shar Pei with a secondary corneal ulcer (OS; same dog as in Plates 7.20–7.22). The ulcer is located dorsally, shows a loose edge and is granulating from the limbus at the 12- to 3-o'clock position.

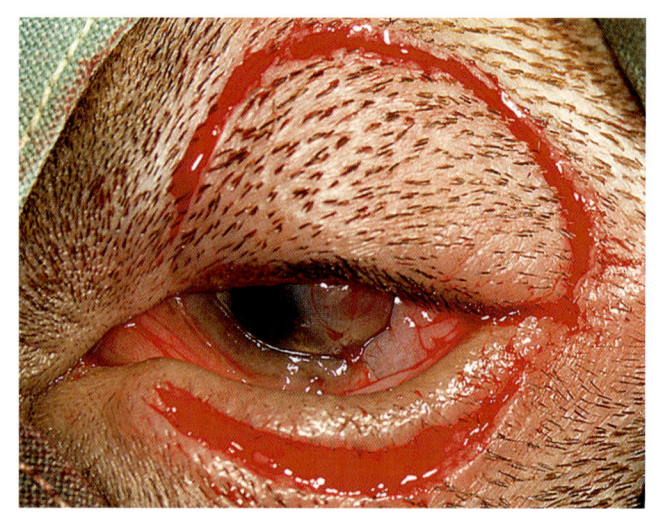

Plate 7.20:
Trichiasis/entropion of the upper lid and entropion of the lower lid in a 1-year-old Shar Pei with a secondary corneal ulcer (OS; same dog as in Plates 7.19 and 7.21, 7.22). In the lower lid, the skin-muscle segment for a Celsus-Hotz entropion correction is removed. The skin incisions for a Stades trichiasis-entropion correction are made in the upper lid.

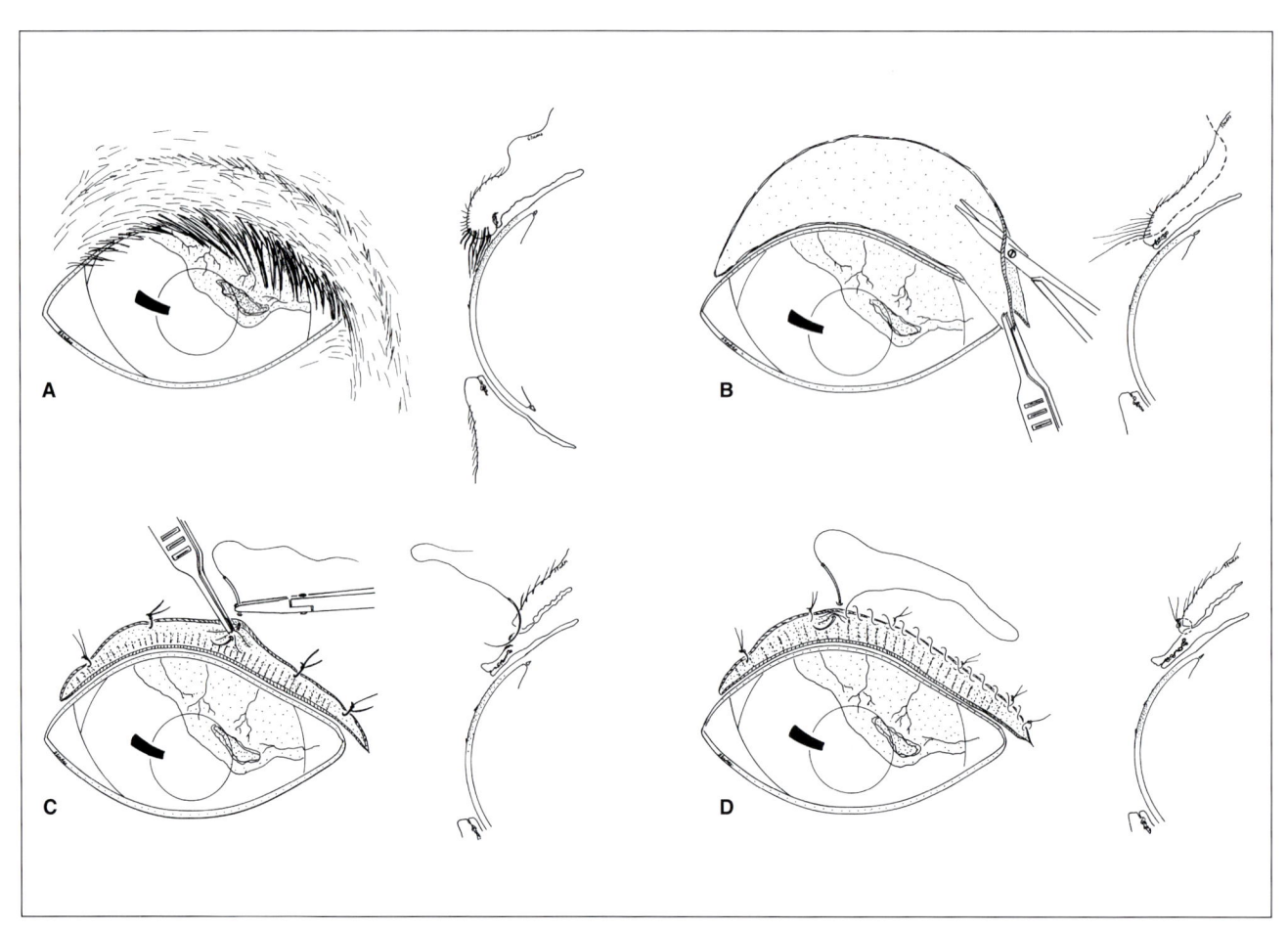

Fig. 7.17:
Trichiasis-entropion of the upper eye lid correction by the forced granulation method (Stades).

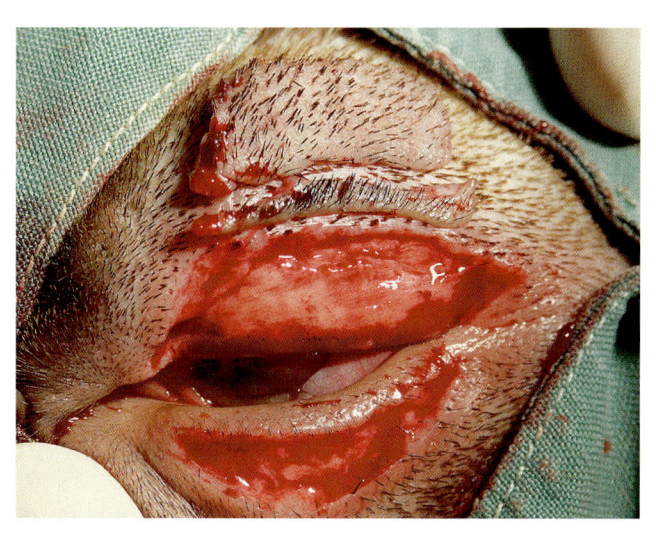

Trichiasis **93**

Plate 7.21:
Trichiasis/entropion of the upper lid and entropion of the lower lid in a 1-year-old Shar Pei with a secondary corneal ulcer (OS; same dog as in Plates 7.19, 7.20 and 7.22). The upper lid skin for the Stades trichiasis-entropion correction has been removed and placed above the wound, in two parts, showing the amount of skin removed.

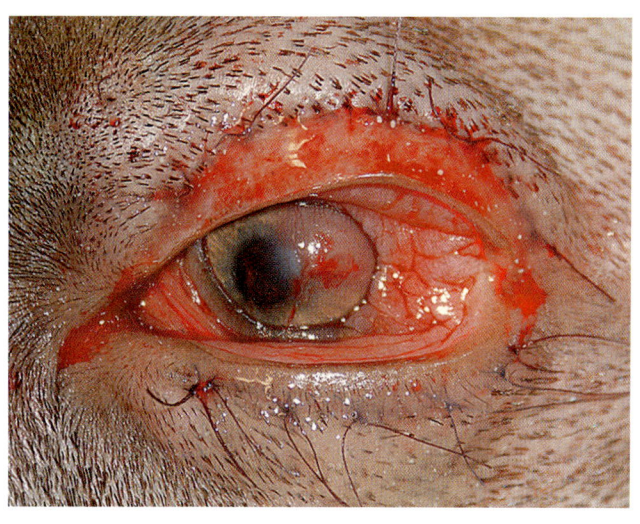

Plate 7.22:
Post-surgical result after a Stades trichiasis/entropion correction of the upper lid and entropion of the lower lid in a 1-year-old Shar Pei with a secondary corneal ulcer (OS; same dog as in Plates 7.19–7.21). The upper lid wound has been left to close by secondary granulation, preventing further hair growth near the lid margin. Both wounds are closed with 5 simple interrupted sutures, covered with a simple continous suture (6-0 absorbable; 4/8 round body needle).

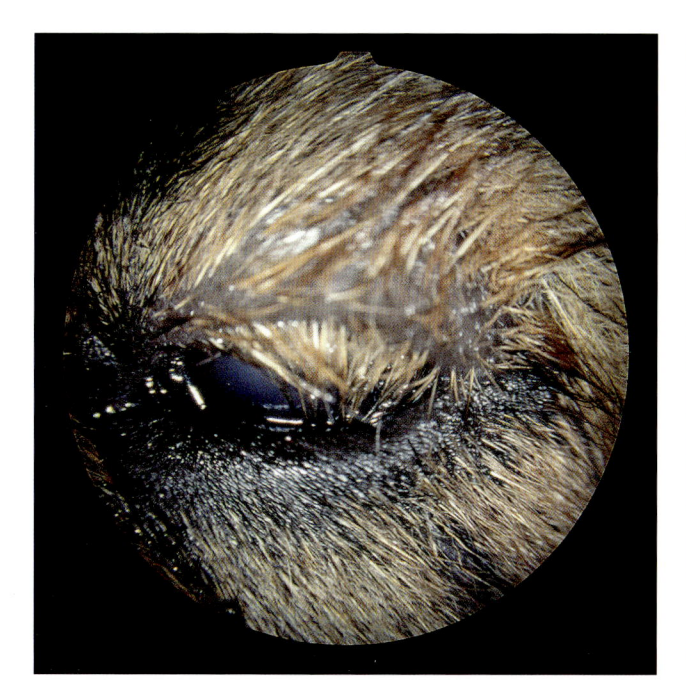

Plate 7.23:
Trichiasis/entropion of the upper eyelid in a Chow Chow of 4 weeks of age (OS). A secondary corneal ulcer is almost covered by the hairs of the upper lid (see also Plate 7.24).

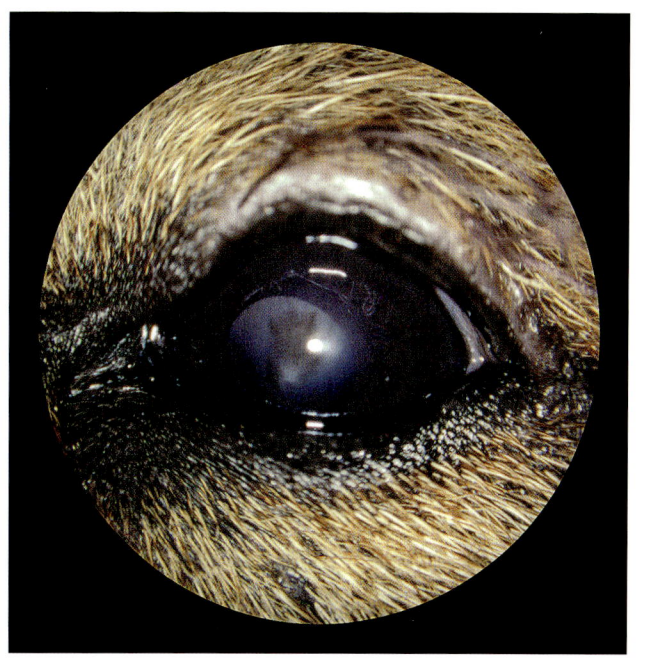

Plate 7.24:
Result of operation 3 weeks after the correction of trichiasis/entropion of the upper eyelid (Stades method) in a 4-week-old Chow Chow (OS; same eye as shown in Plate 7.23).

7.9 Blepharophimosis

Blepharophimosis, or an abnormally small palpebral fissure, usually occurs with entropion of the upper eyelid. It is a rare congenital anomaly in e.g. the Schipperke and Miniature Pinscher. The palpebral fissure appears to be displaced upwards by a few millimeters.

Therapy: Treatment consists of enlarging the palpebral fissure by canthotomy (Fig. 7.18) or, preferably, by lateral canthoplasty (Fig. 7.19). The entropion then relaxes spontaneously. Parents and siblings should also be examined and clients discouraged from breeding from affected animals.

Prevention: Affected animals should not be used for breeding. Parents and siblings should also be examined. It would be advantageous to have the breed, name, chip or tattoo and pedigree number of affected animals registered centrally, and to persuade owners to report such information to the breed association (see 15).

7.10 Oversized/overlong palpebral fissure

(See 7.7, Ectropion and/or oversized palpebral fissure (macroblepharon) (Ect/OPF))

7.11 Injuries

(See 4.5, Penetrating or perforating trauma)

7.12 Ptosis

Ptosis is drooping of the upper eyelid caused by a functional (neural or muscular) disorder of the levator palpebrae (oculomotor nerve) and levator anguli oculi medialis muscles of the upper lid. The causes include Horner's syndrome (see 5.4.2), trauma, paralysis, and other neurologic and hormonal disorders. Treatment must be directed at the primary cause.

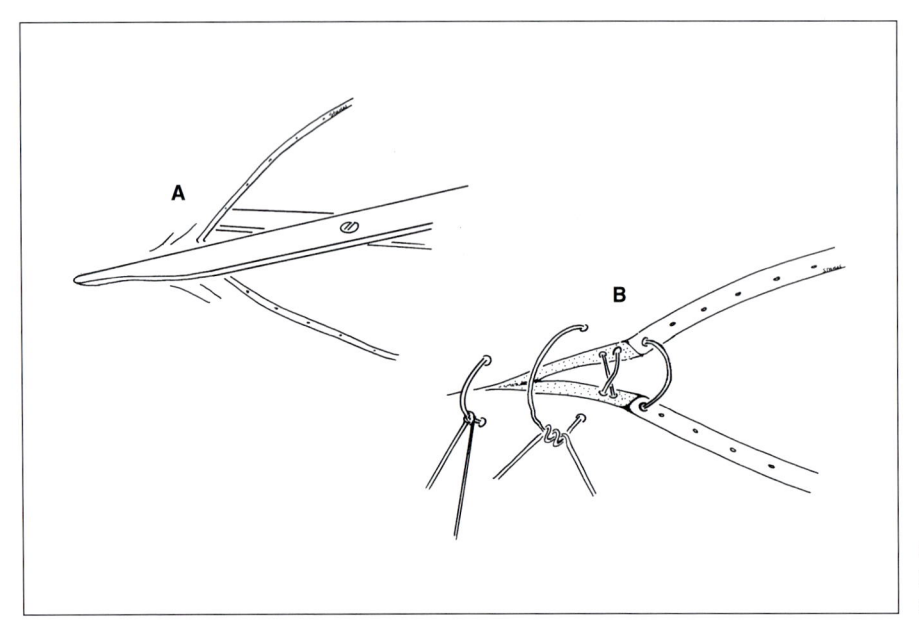

Fig. 7.18:
Lateral canthotomy (A) and a method of suturing (B).

7.13 Lagophthalmos

Lagophthalmos is an inability to close the eyelids. It may be a consequence of disorders of the facial nerve that lead to paralysis of the orbicularis oculi muscle or be congenital in the prominent-eyed breeds (e.g. Pekingese, Persian cat) as previously described. If lagophthalmos persists it predisposes to exposure corneal desiccation, resulting in vascularization, granulation, pigmentation, and in cats, sequestration (see 10.6).

Therapy: Lagophthalmos should be treated medically as a KCS (see 6.2.1) or by temporary tarsorrhaphy (see 4.2) until the cause of the lagophthalmos is found and, if possible, cured. If it is evident that temporary therapy is not sufficient, the lid fissure can be shortened permanently.

7.13.1 Medial canthoplasty

In brachycephalic breeds such as the Pekingese, medial canthoplasty (see 7.8.1.2; Fig. 7.14.) will be helpful. The medial canthus emerges from behind the nasal folds and is displaced laterally, and there will be less corneal irritation caused by the medial canthus entropion and the nasal fold.

In other breeds, the lid fissure should be shortened in the lateral canthus.

7.13.2 Lateral canthoplasty

This is performed by a triangular resection of tissue at the lateral canthus with sliding skin, excising an adequate length of tarsal glands in the lateral upper and lower lid margins, and discarding it. This technique slides conjunctiva in one direction and the lid skin in the opposite direction. This forms a wide scar and prevents postoperative separation. Closure is accomplished by closing the conjunctiva with continuous (8-0 absorbable) sutures, and suturing the lateral canthus wound over it.[28]

These methods require much more experience on the part of the surgeon; therefore it may be best to refer these patients.

7.14 Blepharitis

Blepharitis is an inflammation of the eyelids. When the glands of the margins of the eyelid are also affected, the condition is described as blepharitis adenomatosa, tarsitis, or meibomianitis. Among the causes of blepharitis are direct or indirect hypersensitivity reactions, immune-mediated disease, food allergies, trauma, and infections.

7.14.1 Non-specific blepharitis

Non-specific blepharitis is uncommon in dogs. In most cases, it is a result of demodicosis. In cats, it usually is a result of bacterial infection, secondary to fighting.

In acute cases, pain and swelling (also conjunctival) may develop, sometimes within minutes. The condition may be allergic, e.g. as a result of insect bites or stings, and in exceptional cases as result from topical drugs.

Therapy: Therapy consists of immediate removal of the cause when possible (ticks have to be removed, using specific tick forceps), and the application of wet, cold sponges, antihistamines, and/or corticosteroids.

7.14.2 Chronic blepharitis

In chronic blepharitis, there may be some swelling, loss of hair, exudate, defects, and pustules, with or without pruritus. This type of blepharitis can be difficult to treat. Cytological scraping, biopsy, or sensitivity testing of suspicious areas may be diagnostic.

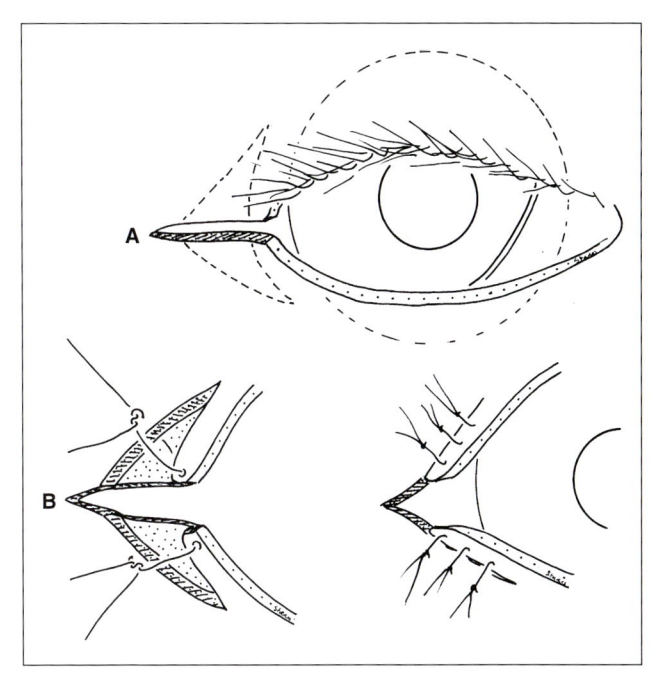

Fig. 7.19:
Blepharophimosis. Canthoplasty for the correction of a too short lid fissure.

Therapy: When the cause is not apparent, a topical "initial choice" antibiotic-corticosteroid combination or broad-spectrum antibiotics given systemically can be administered prior to sensitivity results. Following antibiotic sensitivity testing, an appropriate "specific choice" antibiotic should be administered, together with corticosteroids. Mycotic (e.g. *Microsporon*) and parasitic (*Leishmania, Notoedres, Demodex*) involvement of the lids is usually part of a generalized process and should be treated as such.

7.14.3 Specific blepharitis

7.14.3.1 Chalazion/hordeolum

Chalazion is a localized, sterile inflammation (lipogranuloma) of a meibomian gland or, in rare cases, of a gland of Zeis or Moll (Figs. 7.20, 7.21). Hordeolum (stye) is a localized infection (abscess) in one or more sebaceous glands of the lid margin, frequently due to a staphylococcal infection (Plate 7.25). An external hordeolum is an infection of a gland of Moll or Zeis and an internal hordeolum is an infection of a meibomian gland. In cases of chalazion there is a hard, local, painless swelling, 2–5 mm in diameter, localized just outside the free lid margin. A hordeolum is usually red and painful. After some days, the infection will "point", and may erupt spontaneously. Neoplasms must be considered in the differential diagnosis, but they will often involve the free lid margin as well.

Therapy: Cooperative patients are sedated, others should be given general anesthesia. In cases of chalazion / hordeolum internum, after topical anesthesia, the margin of the eyelid is fixed with a chalazion forceps and the swelling under the conjunctiva is opened parallel to the margin of the lid. The cavity is curetted until it is clean and bleeds a little (Fig. 7.21). In cases of external hordeolum, the abscess should be ripe before opening. This can be speeded by hot compresses, 4–6 times daily, until it "points". The abscess is then incised and drained from the outside. Too early opening or manual expression may spread the infection into the surrounding tissues.

After-care consists of applying a topical "initial choice" antibiotic ointment, 4 times daily for 7–10 days.

7.14.3.2 Blepharitis adenomatosa (meibomianitis)

This condition affects several glands simultaneously. The condition usually occurs in young puppies and may be part of juvenile cellulitis (pyoderma or puppy strangles). It is usually caused by staphylococcal organisms against which the host does not have an adequate immune response.

Therapy: Antibiotics do not penetrate the tarsal glands very well. The margins of the lid should be cleansed regularly with moist swabs and treated with a suitable antibiotic that can also be administered parenterally. Systemic steroids are also needed to facilitate healing. The "specific choice" antibiotic-corticosteroid combination needs to be continued for at least one week after all the signs have abated. The steroids must be discontinued slowly to allow for the animal's endogenous steroids to reach normal levels.

Prognosis: The prognosis is favorable.

7.14.3.3 Juxtapalpebral defects / granulomatous changes

These are slightly thickened, hairless, pinkish, nonpruritic defects, located 5–10 mm from the margin of the lid; they are similar to Collie nose and lick granuloma. They spread very slowly and are probably similar to autoimmune dermatoses such as pemphigus, but usually without defects elsewhere. Sometimes, the cause can be determined by histology or immunofluorescence testing.

Therapy: Affected parts should first be massaged 1–2 times daily with tetracycline-corticosteroid ointment and later with hydrocortisone ointment once every 2–4 days. If not treated, the condition tends to recur. Therapy can be repeated in recurrent cases; in addition, 0.2% cyclosporine can be used.

7.14.3.4 Eosinophilic granuloma

This condition is usually seen as an ulcer, plaque, or linear granuloma of the lips or nose of the cat. In addition, it may manifest itself infrequently in the lids (Plate 8.14) and it can also be seen more commonly in the cornea (see 10.6.1.2). Its etiology is unknown in the majority of cases, though it may be due to infection, atopy and food allergy.

Symptoms: The lesions are well-circumscribed, erythematous, ulcerative, or non-ulcerative plaques that may or may not be pruritic.

Diagnosis: Culturing, cytological scraping or biopsy of suspicious areas, demonstrating eosinophils or, sometimes, mast cells is diagnostic, along with the clinical signs and history.

Therapy: Treat specifically after identifying the cause (see also 10.6.1.2).

Blepharitis **97**

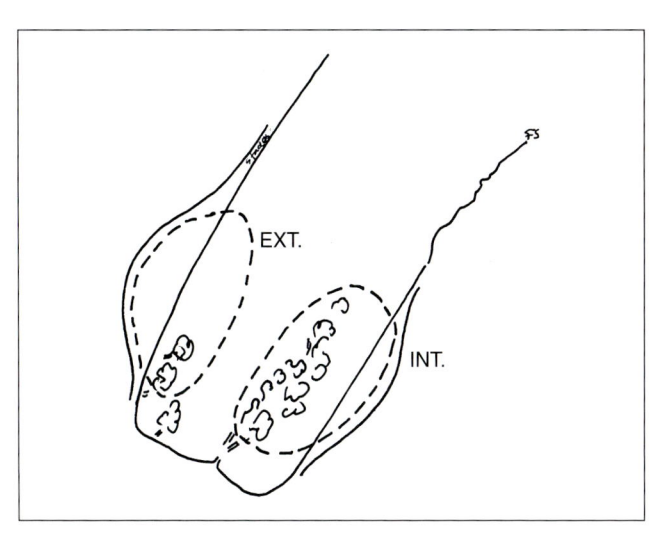

Fig. 7.20:
Chalazion/hordeolum internal/external locations.

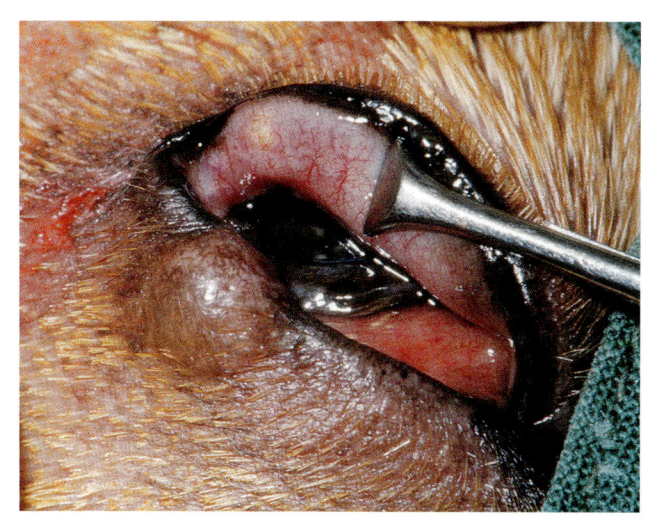

Plate 7.25:
Hordeolum (internal) of some meibomian glands of the upper eyelid, and an external hordeolum in the lower lid (OS, dog).

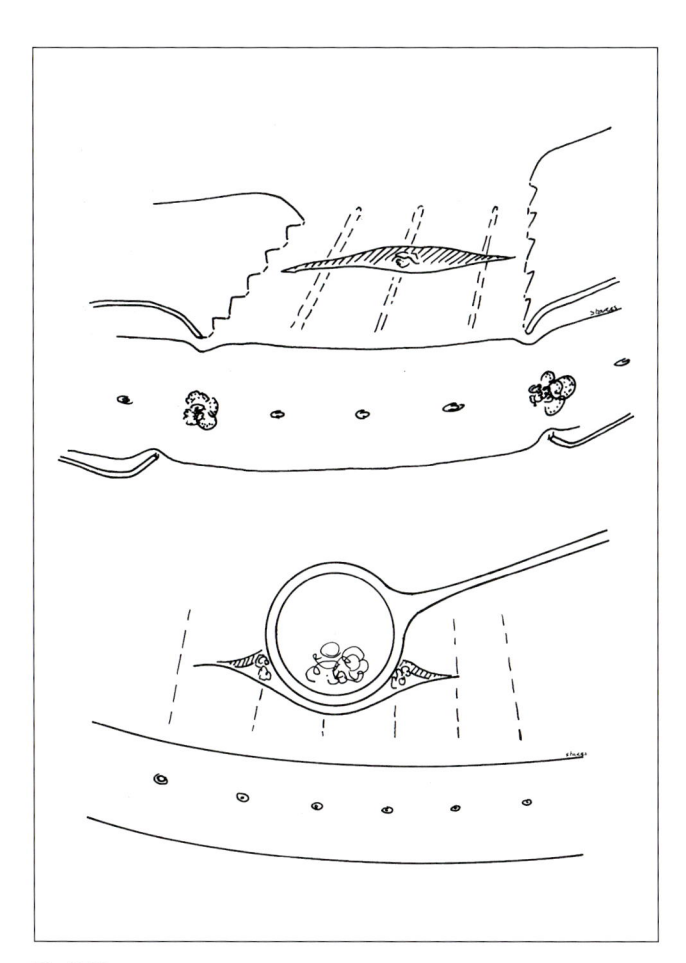

Fig. 7.21:
Curettage of an internal chalazion/hordeolum. Location of the incision in the conjunctiva for opening and curettage.

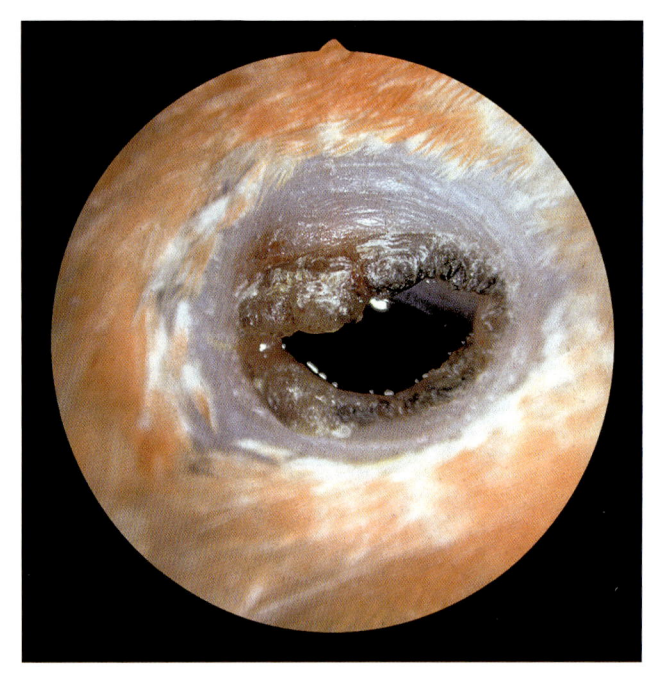

Plate 7.26:
Bird pox on the lid edge of a parakeet (OD).

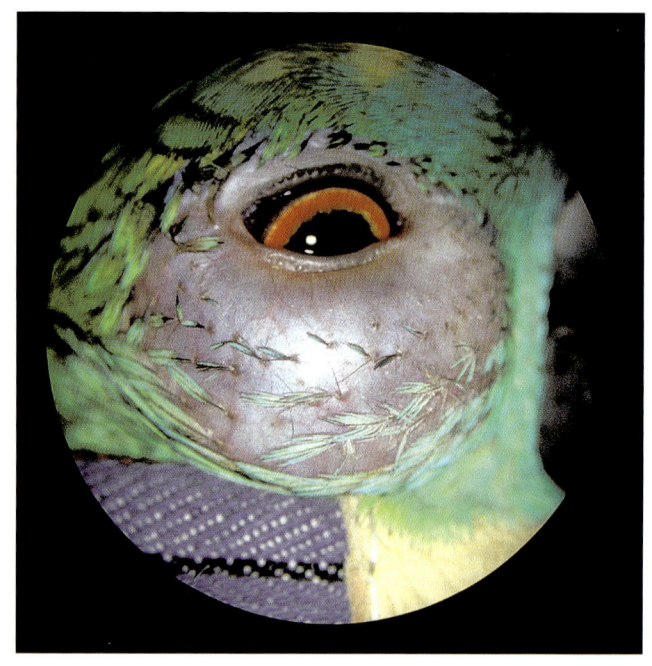

Plate 7.27:
Agapornide showing lower lid swelling due to a lipoma (OD).

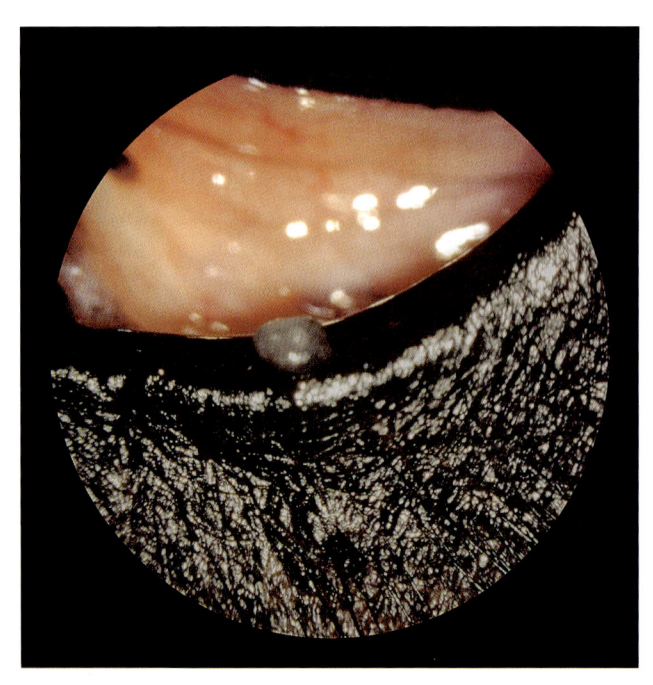

Plate 7.28:
Meibomian gland adenoma (OS, dog). On the free margin of the lid, the top of the tumor coming from the meibomian gland opening is visible (see also Plate 7.29).

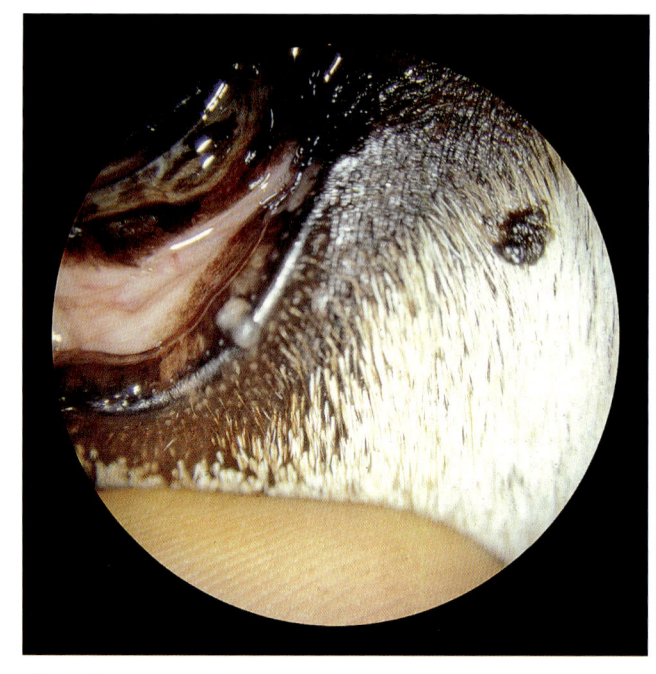

Plate 7.29:
Meibomian gland adenoma of the same type as shown in Plate 7.28, but seen from above (OD, dog). The swelling on the inside of the lid can also now be recognized. On the right is a small papilloma.

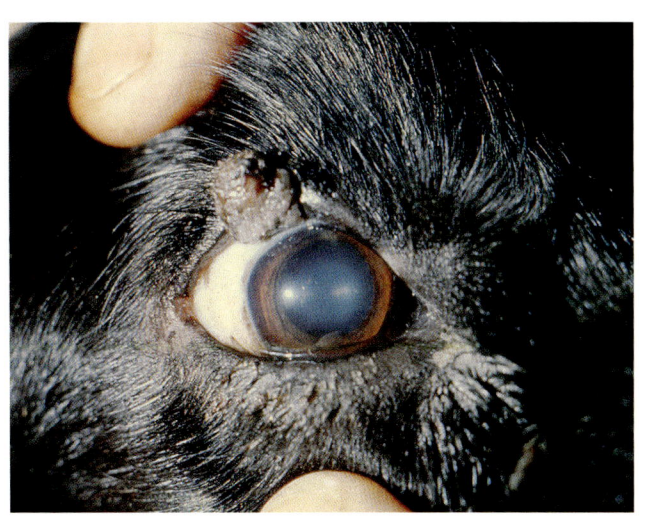

Plate 7.30:
Meibomian gland adenoma on the lid edge (OD, dog). The cauliflower-shaped tumor had a stalk of approximately 2 mm, and had been torn off twice with some bleeding. Because of its location, it irritated the cornea during blinking.

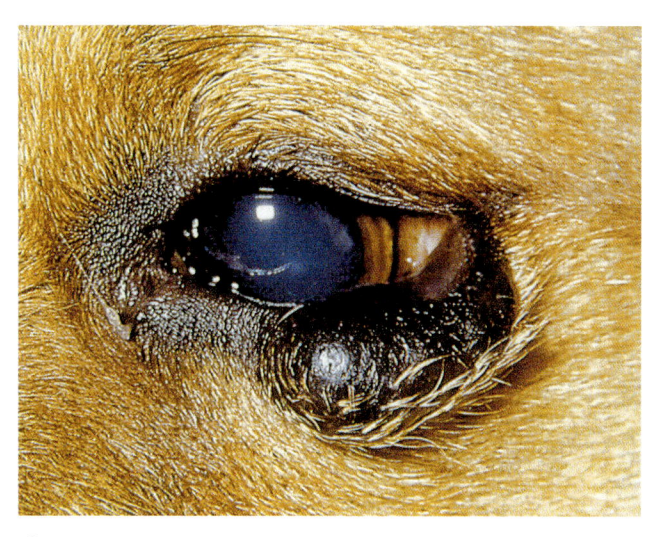

Plate 7.31:
Melanoma of a lower lid edge of a dog (OS). The tumor is relatively broad. In this case, an H-type blepharoplasty could be an appropriate technique to fill the defect after the removal of the neoplasm.

7.14.3.5 Blepharitis in birds

In birds, hyperkeratosis and cauliflower-shaped eruptions can be found on the lid edge, frequently in combination with conjunctival swelling and keratitis. In these cases, vitamin A and pantothenic acid[29] deficiency, ticks, pox, or neoplasms (Plates 7.26, 7.27) must be considered in the differential diagnosis. Bacterial infections have been reported in chickens and turkeys, incriminating *Staphylococcus hyicus*, *Streptococcus* spp., *Escherichia coli* and *Pasteurella multocida*.

Therapy: Vitamin A oil or ointment can be applied topically. In papilloma-like changes, acyclovir, and in pox, 1% mercurochrome solution, can be considered.

7.14.3.6 Blepharitis in horses

Nodular eruptions of the lids and non-healing wounds ventral to the medial canthus or the periocular area characterized by "sulphur granules" especially during the fly season may be caused by *Habronema* spp.[30]

Therapy: Treatment with ivermectin, 0.2 mg/kg and NSAIDs, both administered systemically, as well as topical anti-inflammatory drugs when the conjunctiva is involved, and fly net protection (Plate 3.5) are beneficial (see also 8.11.5).

7.15 Neoplasia of the eyelids

Neoplasms of the eyelids are quite common in dogs, horses, and cattle, but are rare in cats. In dogs, more than 85% are adenomas.[31] Pathologists not experienced in this field can easily misinterpret these as malignant because of the glandular tissue. Small, cauliflower-shaped protrusions on the margin of the eyelid (Plates 7.28–7.30), arising from the meibomian, Zeis or Moll glands (Fig. 7.22), are usually benign adenomas. Papillomas may have a similar appearance, but they tend to hang from the epithelial surface of the outer lid margin. These tumors may irritate the cornea when the eyelid blinks (Plate 7.30); sometimes they may bleed a little when they are rubbed.

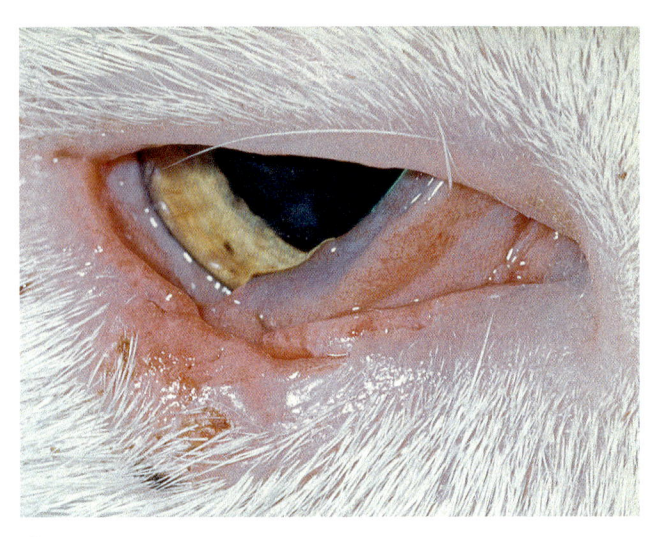

Plate 7.32:
Carcinoma of the lid edge in a (white) cat (OD).

In cats, cattle and horses, neoplasms are usually malignant (squamous cell or basal cell carcinomas and sarcoids; Plates 7.32, 7.33).[32] They are seen more often in white cats (possibly in connection with UV hypersensitivity; Plate 7.32). In cats, eosinophilic granulomas must be considered in the differential diagnosis.

Carcinomas are usually flat, slow-growing, ulcerating defects at or near the margin of the eye lid. They may initially show as a hyperemic area with some dark exudate. They are often accompanied by neoplasms on other parts of the body (e.g. ears, lips). In horses, the ulcerating area will usually slowly progress to a more cauliflower-shaped, granulating deformity.

Diagnosis: Diagnosis is established by means of biopsy or, in the case of small neoplasms, by direct radical excision.

Therapy: Smaller, stalked neoplasia on the margin of the eyelid should never be ligated or pinched out. Under general anesthesia, the lid margin is everted (e.g. with chalazion forceps). In neoplasia involving only one or more glands, radical excision is necessary. If more than approximately 10% of the lid length is involved (normal lid fissure length eye), this is followed by a blepharoplasty (Figs. 7.22–7.26). Cryosurgery is also possible, but may cause long-term depigmentation and leave a lid margin defect. The neoplasia itself should never be squeezed during surgery, as this may cause artifacts for the histopathologist. The neoplasm itself can be stored in 5% formaldehyde, but it is best sent directly for histopathologic evaluation.

The treatment of larger neoplasms or neoplasms with distinct aspects of malignancy, or recurrences consists of a radical removal of the neoplasm. These methods usually require more extensive blepharoplasties, so it may be best to refer these patients. When large or multiple parts of the eyelid margin have to be removed, cryotherapy, laser therapy,[33] or high frequency radiotherapy plus hyperthermia therapy or immunotherapy, e.g. with BCG,[34] can be considered.

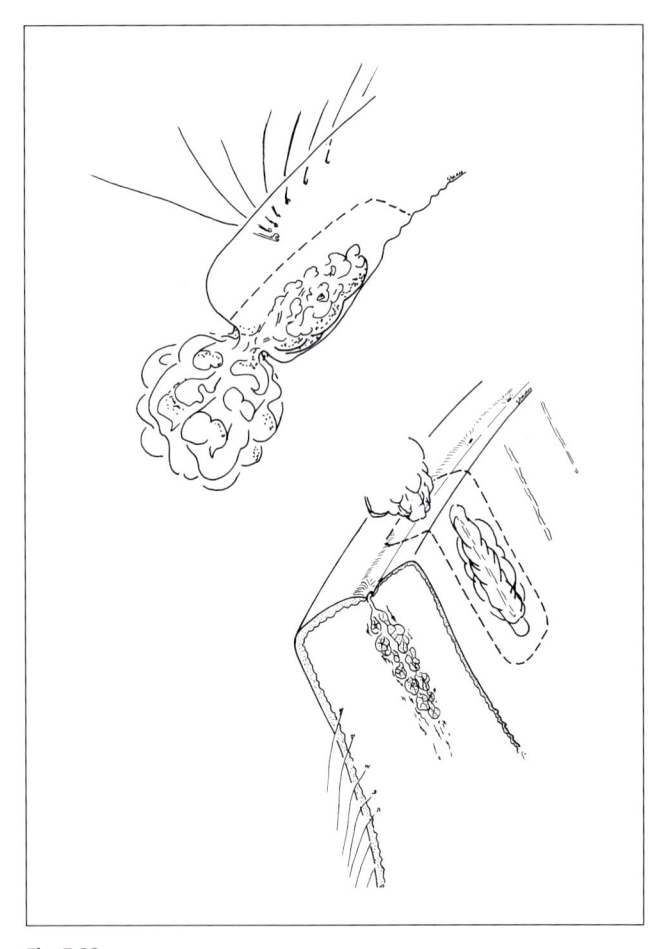

Fig. 7.22:
Location of a meibomian gland adenoma marking the absolute minimal amount of lid margin that has to be circumcised for correction.

Neoplasia of the eyelids **101**

Fig. 7.23:
Triangle (more accurate figure "house"-triangle) blepharoplasty for the correction of small, but relatively deep lid margin defects.

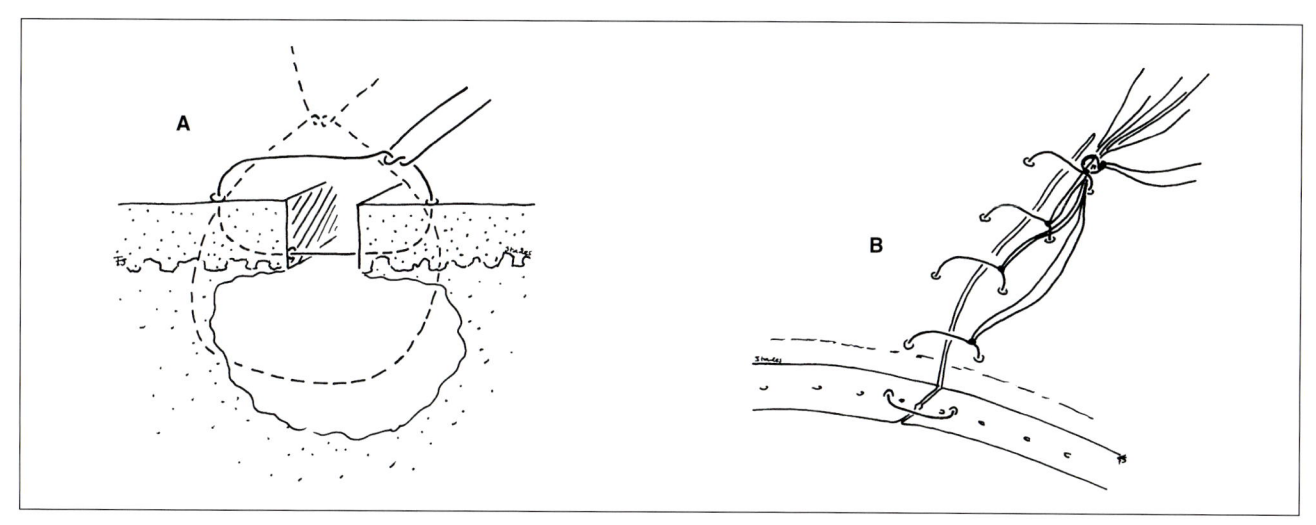

Fig. 7.24:
The wound edges must be closed very precisely (A) and may not be able to move (correct: line; suture too deep: dotted line). The ends of the sutures can be themselves sutured together to prevent irritation of the cornea (B).

102 Eyelids

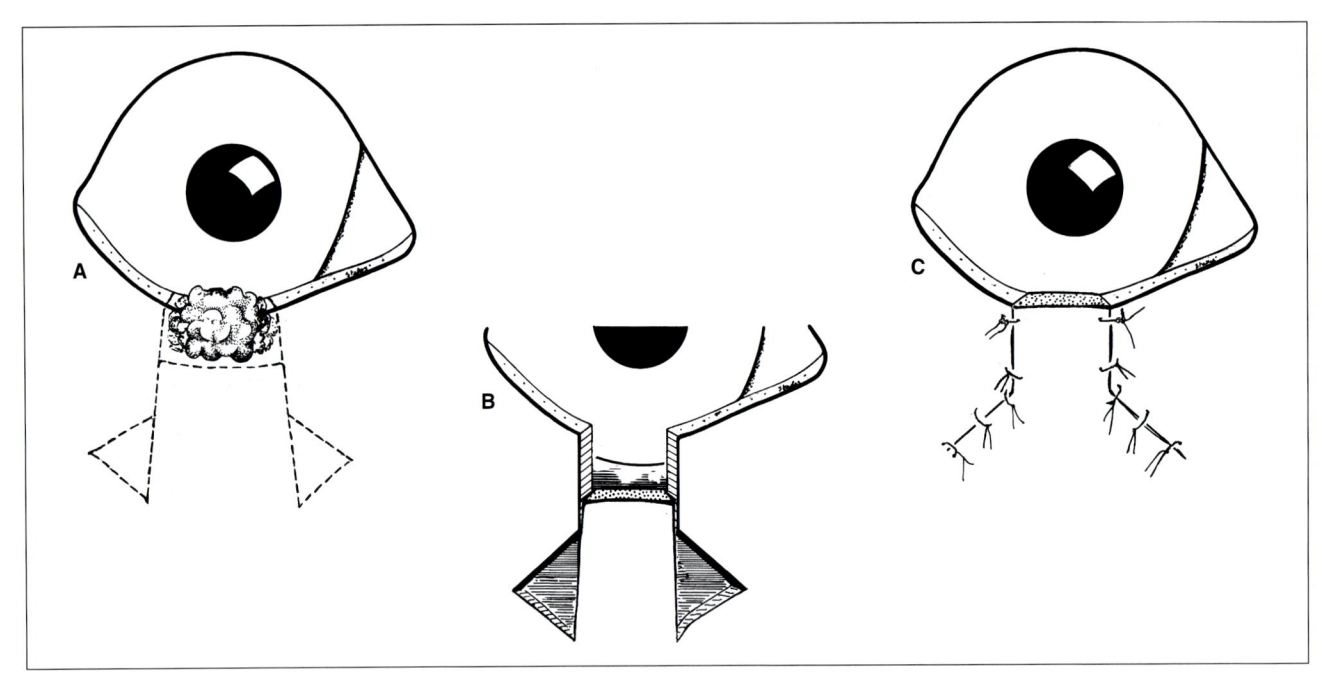

Fig. 7.25:
H-, or sliding graft blepharoplasty for the correction of shallow, relatively broad defects.

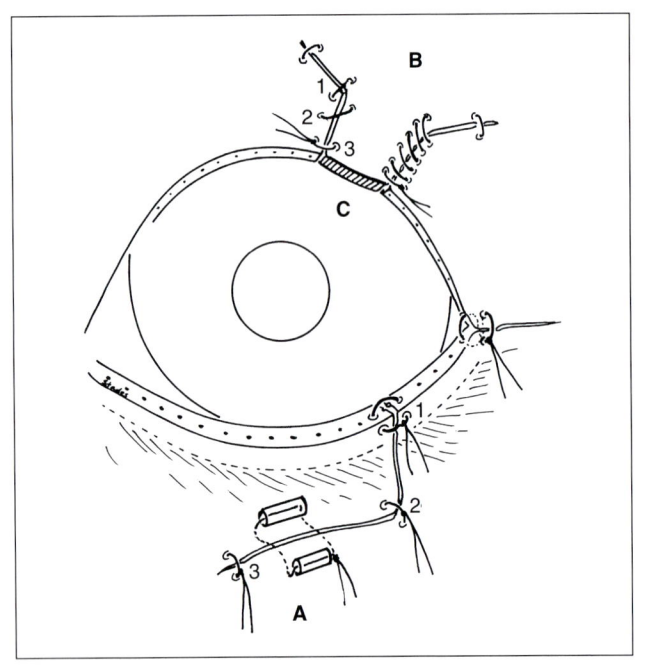

Fig. 7.26:
Lid edge wound apposing methods: (A) relaxation suture; suturing sequence and direction of the sutures (B, 1–3).

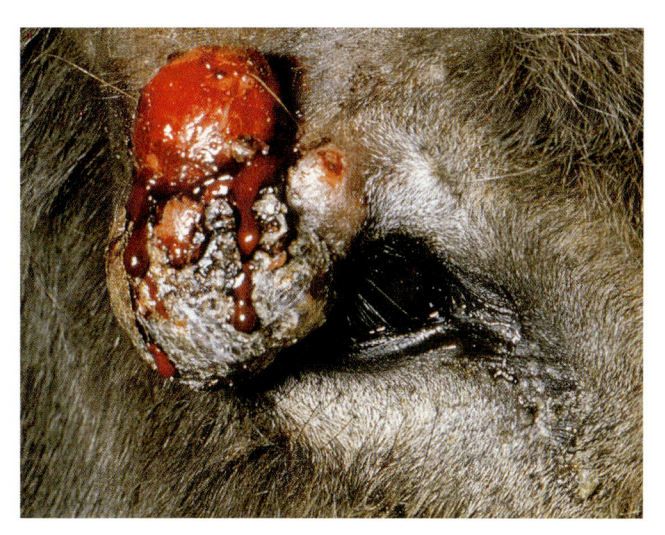

Plate 7.33:
Sarcoid of the upper eyelid of a mule (OD; see also Plate 7.34; by courtesy Dr. W. Klein, Utrecht).

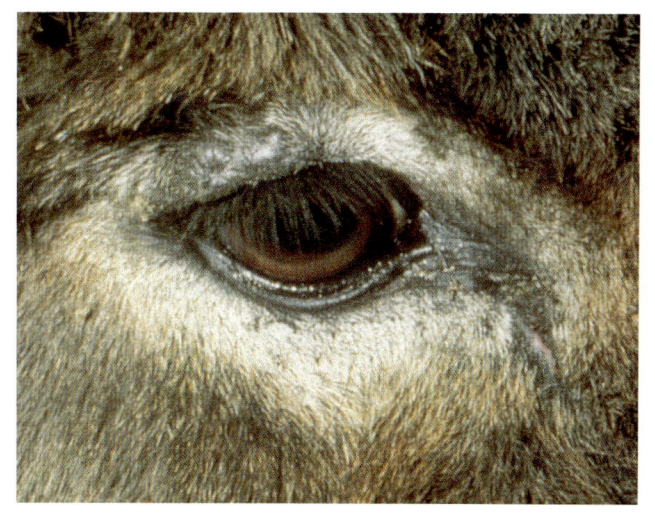

Plate 7.34:
Healed sarcoid of the upper lid of a mule after local injections of 0.25 ml BCG on days 0, 14, 35 and 56 (same eye as shown in Plate 7.33; by courtesy Dr. W. Klein, Utrecht).

7.15.1 Sarcoids in horses

Sarcoids are one of the most common eyelid neoplasms in horses (Plate 7.33). There is growing evidence that the disease is induced by a virus.[35] Clinical characteristics include hyperkeratotic fibropapilloma, fibrosarcoma or fibroblastic fibropapilloma, and mixed forms. The neoplasm can have a "wart-like" aspect, but can also be ulcerative or granulomatous.

Diagnosis: Diagnosis is established on histopathologic evaluation.

Therapy: For radical surgical excision, large areas of tissue have to be removed, and sarcoids do recur frequently. Cryotherapy and immunotherapy with BCG injections (Plates 7.33, 7.34) are currently the most promising treatments.[36]

Literature

1. STADES, F.C., BOEVÉ, M.H. & WOERDT, A. VAN DER.: Palpebral fissure length in the dog and cat. Prog. Vet. & Comp. Ophthalmol. **2**: 155, 1992.

2. ANDERSON, G.B. & WYMAN, M.: Anatomy of the equine eye and orbit: histological structure and blood supply of the eyelids. J. Equine Med. Surg. **3**: 4, 1979.

3. ROBERT, S.R. & BISTNER, S.I.: Surgical correction of eyelid agenesis. Mod. Vet. Pract. **49**: 40, 1968.

4. MILLER, W.W.: Aberrant cilia as an etiology for recurrent corneal ulcers. A case report, Equine Vet. J. **20**: 145, 1988.

5. HALLIWELL, W.: Surgical management of canine distichia. JAVMA **50**: 874, 1967.

6. SCHMIDT, V.: Kryochirurgische Therapie der Distichiasis des Hundes. Mh. Vet. Med., **35**: 711, 1980.

7. WHEELER, C.A. & SEVERIN, G.A.: Cryosurgical epilation for the treatment of distichiasis in the dog and cat. JAAHA **20**: 877, 1984.

8. LENARDUZZI, R.F.: Management of eyelid problems in Chinese Shar Pei puppies. Vet. Small Anim. Clin. **78**: 548, 1983.

9. HOTZ, C.C.: Operation for entropion. Arch. Ophthalmol. **249**: 1879.

10. VEENENDAAL, H.: Eine Modifikation der Entropium-Operation beim Hund. Tijdschr. Diergeneesk. **63**: 299, 1936.

11. WILLIAMS, D.L.: Entropion correction by fornix-based suture placement: use of the Quickert-Rathbun technique in ten dogs. Vet. Ophthalmol. **7**: 343, 2004.

12. VAN DER WOERDT, A.: Adnexal surgery in dogs and cats. Vet. Ophthalmol. **7**: 284, 2004.

13. WYMAN, M. In: Small Animal Surgery, Ed.: Harvey, Newton & Schwartz, Philadelphia, J.B. Lippincott Company, pp 112, 1990.

14. FRÖHNER, E. In: Handbuch der Tierärztlichen Chirurgie und Geburtshilfe, V. Augenheilkunde. Eds.: J. Bayer & E. Fröhner. Wenen, W. Braumüller, 185, 1900.

15. BLASKOVICS, L. & KREIKER, A.: Eingriffe am Auge, 3rd edition. F. Enke Verlag, Stuttgart, p.75, 1959.

16. BLASKOVICS, L. & KREIKER, A.: Eingriffe am Auge, 3rd edition. F. Enke Verlag, Stuttgart, p.71, 1959.

17. JENSEN, H.E.: Canthus closure. Compendium on Continuing Education for the Practicing Veterinarian **10**: 735–741, 1979.

18. KASWAN, R.L., MARTIN, C.L., & DORAN, C.C.: Blepharoplasty techniques for canthus closure. Companion Anim. Prac. **2**: 6, 1988.

19. BEDFORD, P. G. C.: Technique of lateral canthoplasty for the correction of macropalpebral fissure in the dog. J. Sm. Anim. Pract. **39**: 117, 1998.

20. BIGELBACH A.: A combined tarsorrhaphy-canthoplasty technique for the repair of entropion and ectropion. Vet. Comp. Ophthalmol. **6**: 220, 1996.

21. GRUSSENDORF, H.: Outcome of a surgical technique for dogs suffering from macroblepharon, Transactions of the ECVO-ESVO-DOK Meeting Munich. 41, 2004.

22. STADES, F. C. & BOEVÉ, M. H.: Correction for medial canthus entropion in the Pekingese: Transactions of the scientific program of the Int. Soc. Vet. Ophthalmol., New Orleans, USA, 1986.

23. BLOGG, J. R.: Diseases of the eyelids. *In*: The eye in veterinary practice. Ed.: J. R. Blogg, Philadelphia, WB Saunders, 314, 1980.

24. BEDFORD, P. G. C.: Surgical correction of facial droop in the English Cocker Spaniel. J. Small Anim. Pract. **31**: 255, 1990.

25. KÁSA, G. & KÁSA, F.: Exisionsraffung zur Behebung eines Entropiums beim Chow Chow. Tierärztl. Prax. **7**: 341, 1979.

26. WILLIS, M., MARTIN, C., STILES, J. & KIRSCHNER, S.: Brow suspension for treatment of ptosis and entropion in dogs with redundant facial skin folds. JAVMA **214**: 660, 1999.

27. STADES, F. C.: A new method for the surgical correction of upper eyelid trichiasis-entropion: operation method. JAAHA **23**: 603, 1987.

28. WYMAN, M.: Lateral canthoplasty. JAAHA **7**: 196, 1971.

29. KORBEL, R.: Ocular manifestations of systemic diseases in birds and reptiles. ECVO/ESVO, Annual meeting 15–19 June, Oporto, 66, 2005.

30. JOYCE, J. R., HANSELKA, D. W. & BOYD, C. L.: Treatment of habronemiasis of the adnexa of the equine eye. Vet. Med. **67**: 1008, 1972.

31. ROBERTS, S. M., SEVERIN, G. A. & LAVACH, J. D.: Prevalence and treatment of palpebral neoplasms in the dog: 200 cases (197–1983). JAVMA **189**: 1355, 1986.

32. STRAFUSS, A. C.: Squamous cell carcinoma in horses. JAVMA **168**: 61, 1976.

33. JOYCE, J. R.: Cryosurgical treatment of tumors of horses and cattle. JAVMA **168**: 226, 1976.

34. KLEIN, W. R., RUITENBERG, E. J., STEERENBERG, P. A., *et al.*: Immunotherapy by intralesional injection of BCG cell walls or live BCG in bovine ocular squamous cell carcinoma: a preliminary report. J. Nat. Cancer Inst. **69**: 1095, 1982.

35. WATSON, R. E., ENGLAND, J. J. & LARSON, K. A.: Cultural characteristics of a cell line derived from an equine sarcoid. Appl. Microbiol. **24**: 727, 1972.

36. WYMAN, M., RINGS, M. D., TARR, M. J. & ALDEN, C. L.: Immunotherapy in equine sarcoid: a report of two cases. JAVMA **171**: 449, 1977.

8 Conjunctiva and Nictitating Membrane

8.1 Introduction

The space between the eyelid margins and the globe is separated from the ambient environment by a thin, transparent mucosa, the conjunctiva. In the ventral medial canthus, there is a conjunctival fold called the nictitating membrane, third eyelid, or (according to the Nomina anatomica veterinaria) plica semilunaris conjunctivae (Plates 8.1, 8.2, 2.10). The conjunctiva covering the inner surface of the lid and the outside of the nictitating membrane is called the palpebral conjunctiva. The conjunctiva covering the inside of the nictitating membrane is called the bulbar conjunctiva and that covering the sclera is called the bulbar or scleral conjunctiva. The junction of the palpebral and the bulbar conjunctiva is the fornix. The area enclosed by the conjunctiva is called the conjunctival sac. The openings of the primary and accessory lacrimal glands are located in the dorsal lateral fornix, and those of the ventral accessory lacrimal glands, although fewer are present, are located in the ventral fornix. The conjunctiva is firmly attached at the limbus (where it is continuous with the corneal epithelium) and at the mucocutaneous junction, where it covers the meibomian glands and the tarsal plate. The rest is folded and very loosely attached to the subconjunctival tissues. This allows movement of the globe and also enlarges the secretory surface.

The conjunctiva consists of a superficial layer of epithelium and a deeper layer of stroma. The outside stratified epithelium of the conjunctiva (and cornea) is renewed continuously from its basal cell layer. The exfoliated cells gather in the upper and lower fornix within mucus threads. In the medial canthus, the mucus threads join together to form a dry pellet, which is removed when the eyes are rubbed.

The vessels in the stroma are derived from the anterior ciliary and palpebral arteries. These vessels become especially visible when engorged by any conjunctival disturbance. The conjunctiva is rich in lymphatic tissue, which fulfills an important function in the reticuloendothelial system.[1,2]

The superficial epithelial layer contains numerous goblet cells that process the mucus for the mucus layer of the precorneal tear film.[3]

The firmness of the nictitating membrane is derived from a very thin T-shaped cartilage, the base of which is embedded in the superficial gland of the nictitating membrane (an additional deep gland is found in swine, rabbits, and chickens). This gland produces more than 30% of the watery fraction of the tears, and in some species it also secretes some mucus for the precorneal tear film. The outer 2-mm-zone of the palpebral surface of the free margin of the nictitating membrane is usually pigmented. In some white or non-pigmented animals, or those having non-pigmented skin around the eyes, the margins of the nictitating membrane may also be non-pigmented.

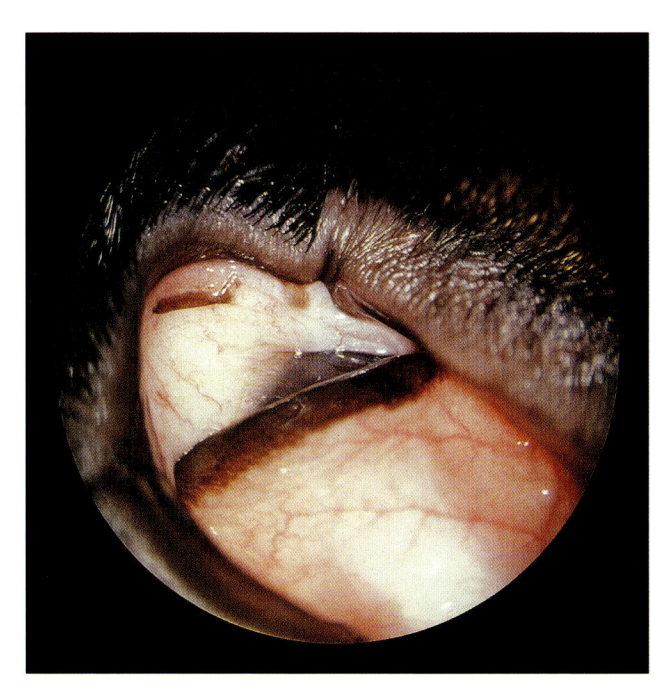

Plate 8.1:
Nictitating membrane, showing the contour of the cartilage in a dog (OD).

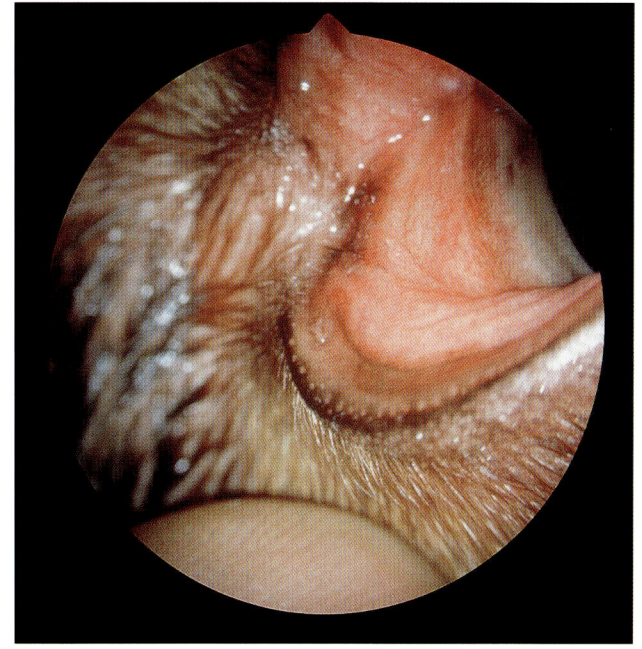

Plate 8.2.
Medial canthus conjunctiva (dog), showing the normal caruncle hair growth.

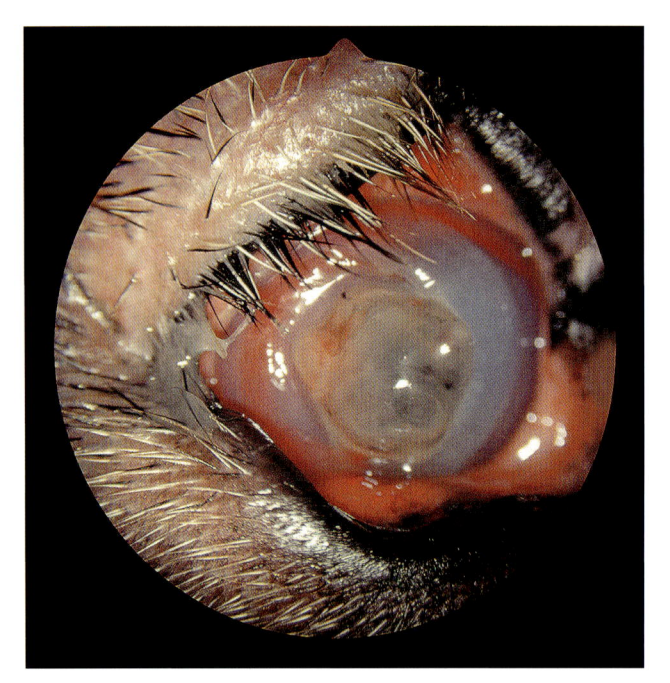

Plate 8.3:
Keratoconjunctivitis sicca with a pre-perforative corneal ulcer (OD, dog) as a result of the total, but contraindicated, removal of a hyperplastic gland of the nictitating membrane.

There are sympathetically-innervated, smooth muscle fibers that actively retract the nictitating membrane in birds. There are only a few such fibers in cats and almost none in dogs, resulting in an almost passive retraction in these species. In birds, the nictitating membrane is almost transparent, originates dorsomedially, and plays a major role in distributing the precorneal tear film and protecting the cornea (Plate 2.10).

Protrusion of the nictitating membrane follows spontaneous or iatrogenic enophthalmos, or may be the result of retrobulbar swelling.

The conjunctiva plays an important role in the production of the tear film, and thus in the direct and indirect protection of the globe. For these reasons, surgical removal of the entire nictitating membrane is only indicated in cases of malignancy of this structure that cannot otherwise be resolved. The removal for other reasons must, therefore, be considered a professional mistake. In addition, the partial removal of an abnormal gland, e.g. because of hyperplasia, should be avoided until all other therapies have failed and the owner has been informed of the consequences. This is mainly because of the risk of inducing secondary entropion or KCS that will require lifelong treatment (Plate 8.3).[4,5]

8.2 Non-pigmented margin of the nictitating membrane

If the free margin of the nictitating membrane is non-pigmented, it may be extremely sensitive to sunlight, resulting in erythema and edema of the margin.

Therapy: If there are only minor symptoms of irritation, treatment consists of topical steroid drops, 1–2 times daily for 2–5 days. In severe cases, black tattooing of the exposed nictitating membrane can be tried or the margin may be shortened by 2–3 mm. The wound is sutured with 8-0 absorbable suture material. The knots are embedded subconjunctivally. Removal of the nictitating membrane for cosmetic effects is not justifiable und must be rejected in favor of the patient's welfare (for the reasons given in the Introduction of this chapter).

8.3 Dermoid

A dermoid or ectopic island of skin located solely in the conjunctiva is rare; usually, the cornea is also involved. For further details, see 10.4.

8.4 Ectopic cilia

Ectopic cilia in the conjunctiva (Fig. 8.1, Plate 8.4) occur singly or in a tuft and grow towards the cornea from a hair follicle below the conjunctiva.[6] In most cases, they are located at the base of the meibomian glands and only rarely are they to be found in the nictitating membrane. As soon as the hair penetrates the conjunctiva, it causes severe irritation of the cornea, soon followed by ulceration. The irritation, which is more severe when the patient blinks, induces epiphora and severe blepharospasm. The abnormality is often associated with distichiasis. It is possible that ectopic cilia, like distichiasis, is a polygenic hereditary anomaly; predisposed breeds are the English Cocker Spaniel, Flat-coated Retriever, Pekingese, and Shih Tzu. This abnormality is found frequently in these predisposed breeds but is quite rare in other dogs, cats, or animals.

Affected animals are usually presented because of a sudden onset of severe blepharospasm; the owner being convinced that trauma was the cause. The hairs are difficult to find, even with x3–5 magnification, especially when they are not pigmented. A circumscribed, pigmented spot about 1 mm in diameter is often the only sign of the existence of an ectopic hair.

Therapy: The hair follicle is either destroyed by electroscalpel or cryotherapy, or is excised under general anesthesia. Magnification of x5–10 is needed. The margin of the lid is fixed by chalazion forceps and the hair follicle is completely destroyed by cutting with the electroscalpel, without penetrating or perforating the skin or is removed by one of the other two methods mentioned. Postoperative treatment consists of topical antibiotic eye ointment or drops, 4 times daily for 7–10 days.

Prognosis / prevention: The prognosis is favorable but the owner must be warned that other hair follicles may have been overlooked or will appear later. Affected animals should be excluded from breeding.

8.5 Protrusion of the nictitating membrane

Protrusion of the nictitating membrane may be caused by many abnormalities. The nictitating membrane will protrude over the globe in cases of
(1) loss of sympathetic innervation (5.4.2, 12.12), as found in Horner's Syndrome or feline dysautonomia;
(2) processes which press the globe into the orbit, such as fractures;
(3) active or passive enophthalmos, as may be caused by pain in the eye, loss of retrobulbar fat, or atrophy of the chewing muscles;
(4) space-occupying processes at the base of the third eyelid; or
(5) swelling or symblepharon of the nictitating membrane itself.

Increased tonus of the muscles, feelings of discomfort, or general illness may, especially in cats, result in a bilateral protrusion of the nictitating membrane. The diagnostic examination should be aimed at differentiating between these causes.

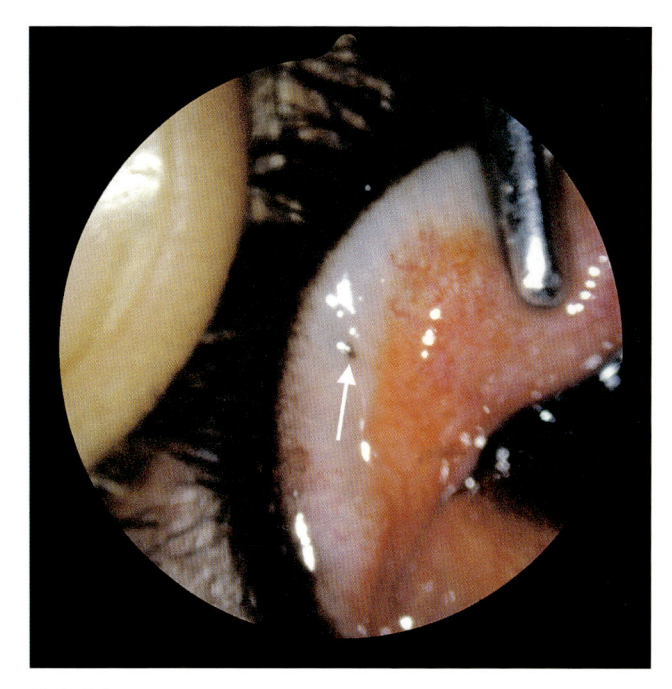

Plate 8.4:
Ectopic cilia (see arrow) in the conjunctiva of the upper lid (OS, dog).

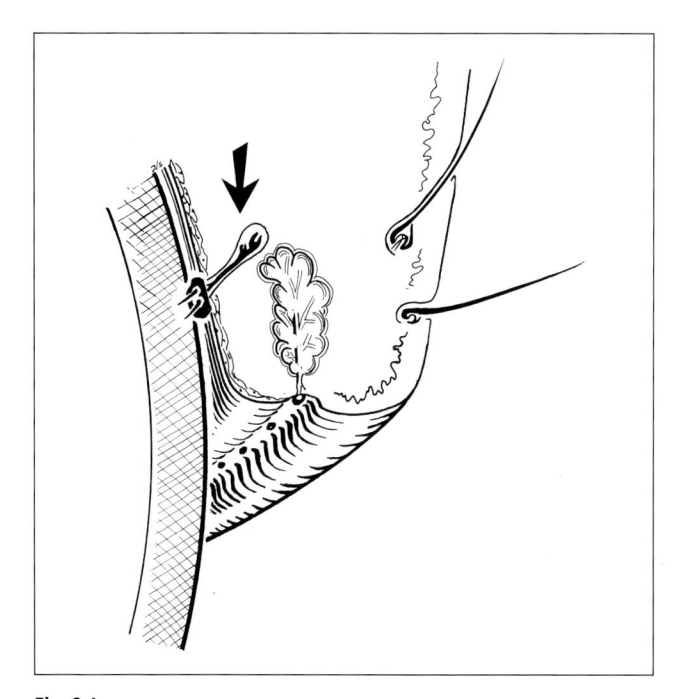

Fig. 8.1:
Ectopic cilia growing through the conjunctiva of the upper lid (arrow).

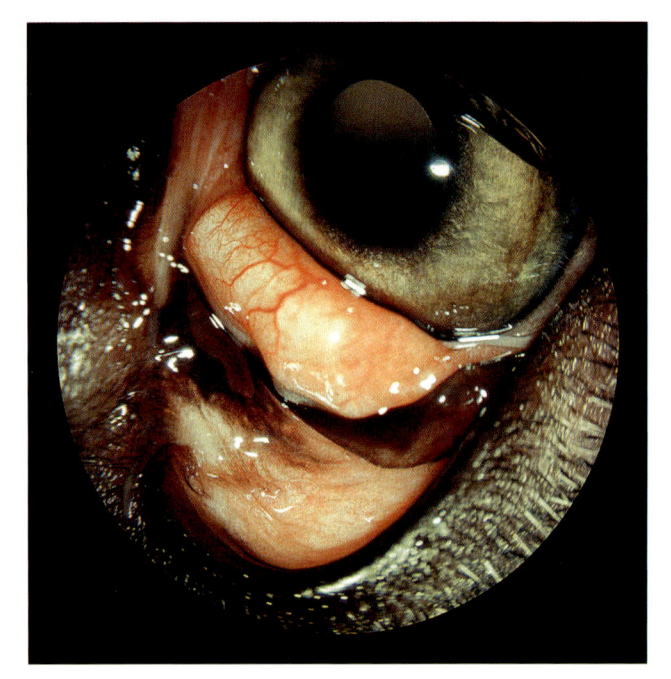

Plate 8.5:
Eversion of the nictitating membrane (OS, dog).

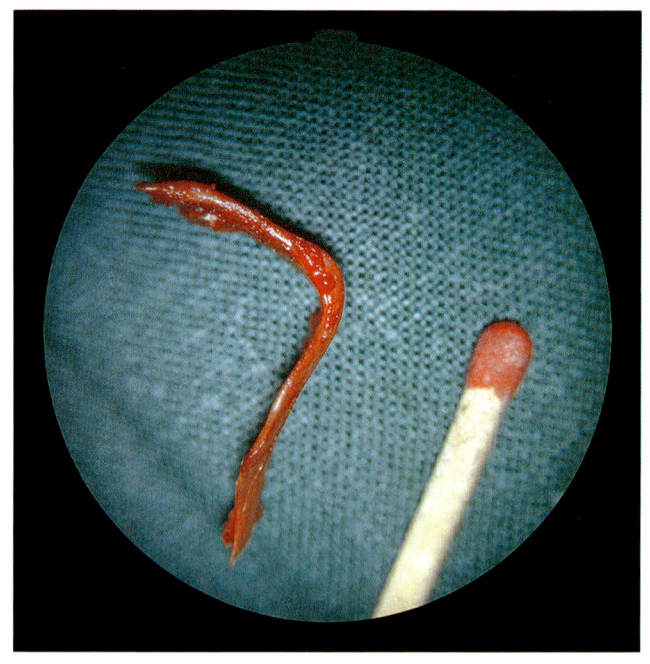

Plate 8.6:
The cartilage removed from an eversion of the nictitating membrane, showing its abnormal curvature.

8.6 Cysts

Cysts of one of the ducts of the nictitans gland, or of other glands elsewhere in the conjunctiva, are rare.[7] They have a glassy blue translucence or are pigmented, vary in size, and occur at the base of the nictitating membrane or elsewhere in the conjunctiva. They may also arise from the lacrimal glands, the zygomatic gland, or ectopic lacrimal tissue. Hyperplasia or neoplasia of the nictitans gland should be considered in the differential diagnosis.

Therapy: Treatment consists of careful, blunt dissection of the mass. The wound can be left open or it may be closed with an absorbable 8-0 continuous buried suture. Postoperative treatment consists of topical "initial choice" antibiotics, used to prevent colonization of bacteria, 4 times daily for 1 week.

8.7 Eversion / inversion of the nictitating membrane

Eversion, or rarely inversion, of the nictitating membrane is caused by a deformed or curled cartilage, usually 2–6 mm from and parallel to the margin of the nictitating membrane (Plates 8.1, 8.5, 8.6). The defect results in eversion or inversion of the distal part of the nictitating membrane. The cause of the deformity may be a difference in the growth rate between the inner and outer surfaces of the cartilage. The deformity usually starts at between 3 and 6 months of age. It is a rare abnormality in the cat. No breed predisposition has been recognized.

The everted part of the nictitating membrane is exposed to wind and dust, which results in erythema and some swelling. The abnormality appears not to cause much discomfort to the animal.

Therapy: Treatment consists of the removal of only the abnormally curved part of the cartilage (Fig. 8.2). Under general anesthesia, the nictitating membrane is retracted laterally over the globe, using a Stades' nictitating membrane forceps or two Allis forceps, exposing the palpebral surface. A small incision is made in the palpebral conjunctiva at the border of the cartilage deformity (on the right side if you are right-handed and on the left side if you are left-handed). The incision should not be made in the ocular conjunctiva, since the resulting scar may irritate the cornea. The curved part of the cartilage is dissected bluntly from the palpebral and ocular conjunctiva using Stevens' scissors. Care must be taken especially to avoid perforating the ocular conjunctiva, which may be weakened by inflammation. When the abnormally curved part of the cartilage has been freed, it is grasped with a Halstead mosquito forceps and cut free with scissors. To prevent sliding of both parts of the cartilage over each other, the two parts can be sutured together using a resorbable, 8-0 continous suture (Fig. 8.2 F). The wound will close by granulation. Postoperative treatment consists of topical "initial choice" antibiotic eye ointment or drops, 4 times daily for 7 days.

Prognosis: The prognosis is favorable.

Eversion/inversion of the nictitating membrane **109**

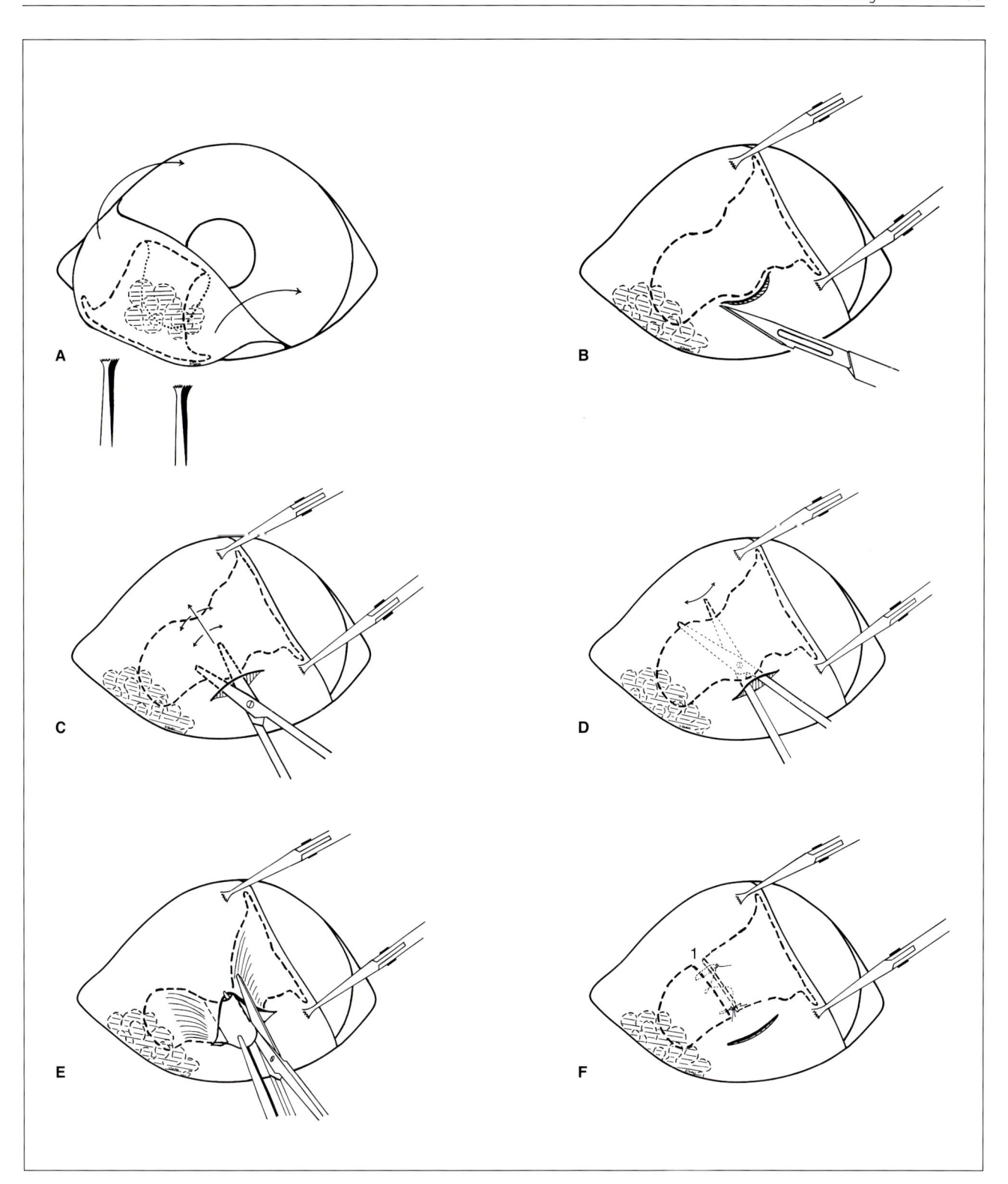

Fig. 8.2:
Surgical correction of an eversion of the nictitating membrane. Only the bent part of the cartilage is freed on both sides bluntly, and dissected. It is preferable to unite both cartilage ends using a resorbable, 8-0 continuous suture (F).

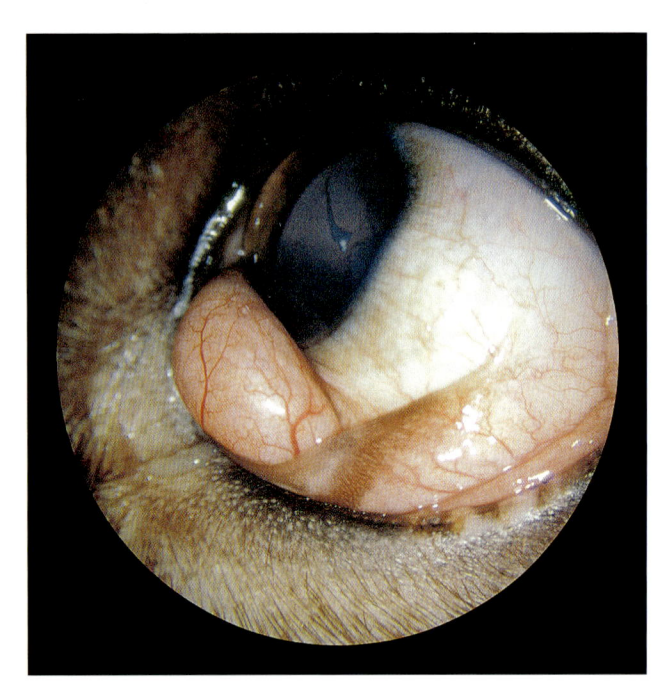

Plate 8.7:
Hyperplastic gland of the nictitating membrane (OS, dog).

8.8 Hyperplasia/hypertrophy of the gland of the nictitating membrane ("cherry eye")

Hypertrophy/hyperplasia of the nictitans gland (Plate 8.7) is thought to result from an inversion of the gland at the base of the cartilage due to a loosening of the attachment of the gland and cartilage to the periorbita, possibly combined with an inversion of the cartilage, although the actual mechanism has not been validated. The gland enlarges and sometimes protrudes from behind the nictitating membrane, but returns to its normal position. When the enlargement is too great, the gland protrudes continuously. The conjunctiva over the protruding gland is exposed to abrasion, dust, and dryness, resulting in inflammatory erythema and swelling. This abnormality is rare in cats, but frequent in dogs 3–6 months of age in breeds which have a distinct stop and abundant loose skin (e.g. American Cocker Spaniel, Cavalier King Charles Spaniel, English Bulldog, Neapolitan Mastiff; though it is also seen in the Shar Pei and Beagle).

The swollen gland protrudes from behind the nictitating membrane. The covering conjunctiva is red and swollen, and there may be some follicular hypertrophy. The results of the STT are either high or normal. There is some mucous discharge. The abnormality is usually unilateral at first, but the other eye is often affected within 1–3 months.

Therapy: Inflammation, with or without infection, is not the primary cause and thus treatment with corticosteroids, with or without antibiotics, is not effective. Also, since it accounts for a significant part of the tear production, neither the gland nor the entire nictitating membrane should be removed. The removal of the entire nictitating membrane because of this indication must be considered a professional mistake.

The purpose of treatment is to relocate the inverted gland in its normal position. Several methods are available (see below), none of which being entirely effective. Some can even introduce a severe risk of perforating the sclera. In all of these methods, the base of the cartilage is anchored to the periosteum of the medial inferior orbital wall; or the gland itself is anchored to the medial canthus on either side of the caruncle; or the gland is repositioned in an orbital pocket and fixed by oversuturing of the conjunctiva; or the base of the nictitating membrane is fixed to the scleral tissues, thus preserving the tear contribution of the gland.

Reposition

Fixation of the base of the cartilage (Fig. 8.3). Under general anesthesia, the nictitating membrane is retracted laterally with Stades' NM forceps. The palpebral conjunctiva at the base of the cartilage is incised. The base of the cartilage is fixed by a suture (20–25 mm, 5/8 curved needle, 4-0 absorbable or non-absorbable) anchored to the periosteum of the rostrolateral orbital wall.[8] The knot can also be placed (sub)cutaneously.

Postoperatively, a topical "initial choice" broad-spectrum ocular antibiotic is applied 4 times daily for 5–7 days. The wound will close spontaneously. The success rate is approximately 60%.

Fixation of the gland in a pocket by oversuturing the conjunctiva (Fig. 8.4). In this method (Morgan et. al.),[9] one incision is made just distal of the gland 5–7 mm from the free margin and another proximal to the gland, which means 6–7 mm towards the base of the third eyelid; both incisions being made parallel to the margin. In the distal wound, a transection of the cartilage is made at the abnormal curvature (modification Boevé). The gland is returned to its normal position in a retrobulbar pocket made from the proximal wound. The two distal and proximal wound edges are sutured together with 5-0 or 6-0 absorbable suture material (round body needle) in a continuous pattern, locking the hyperplastic gland into the pocket. The suture is started from and knotted on the (outer) palpebral surface. To guarantee the escape of the gland secretion, both ends of the wound are left open. The success rate is approximately 90%.[10]

Being less successful and/or more riskful, the other methods mentioned, are not further described.

Extirpation

Partial extirpation of the gland of the nictitating membrane. In cases of recurrence after fixation, the gland may be sacrificed but the owner should be warned in advance of the high risk of KCS. Particularly in patients in which the result of the STT values are low-normal or low, one should be very reluctant to remove the gland, even partially.

Under general anesthesia, the nictitating membrane is everted with Stades' NM forceps. The enlarged portion of the gland is fixed by von Graefe's forceps, slightly lifted, and cut away with scissors. The local arteriole is blocked by bipolar electrocoagulation. The wound will close spontaneously.

Postoperative treatment consists of topical "initial choice" antibiotics, 4 times daily for 7–10 days.

Prognosis: The prognosis is favorable but the risk of secondary KCS, even years later, is still present. It is advisable to repeat the STT in the week after surgery. Additional therapy can then be started immediately if indicated (see 6.2.1).

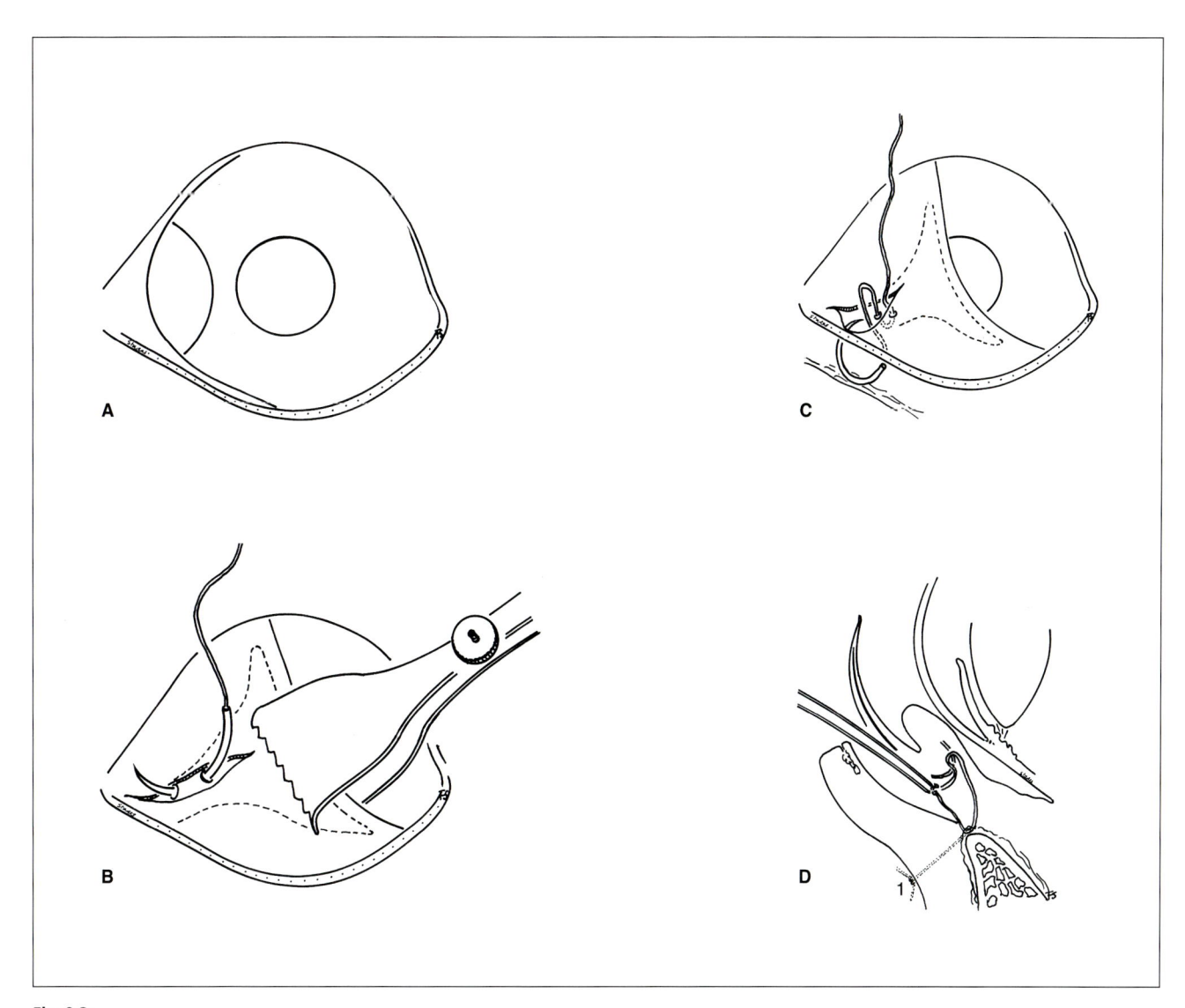

Fig. 8.3:
Surgical correction of a hyperplastic gland of the nictitating membrane by anchoring the base of the cartilage (B) to the periosteum (C) of the orbital wall (after Kaswan & Martin[8]). The knot can also be placed (sub)cutaneously (1).

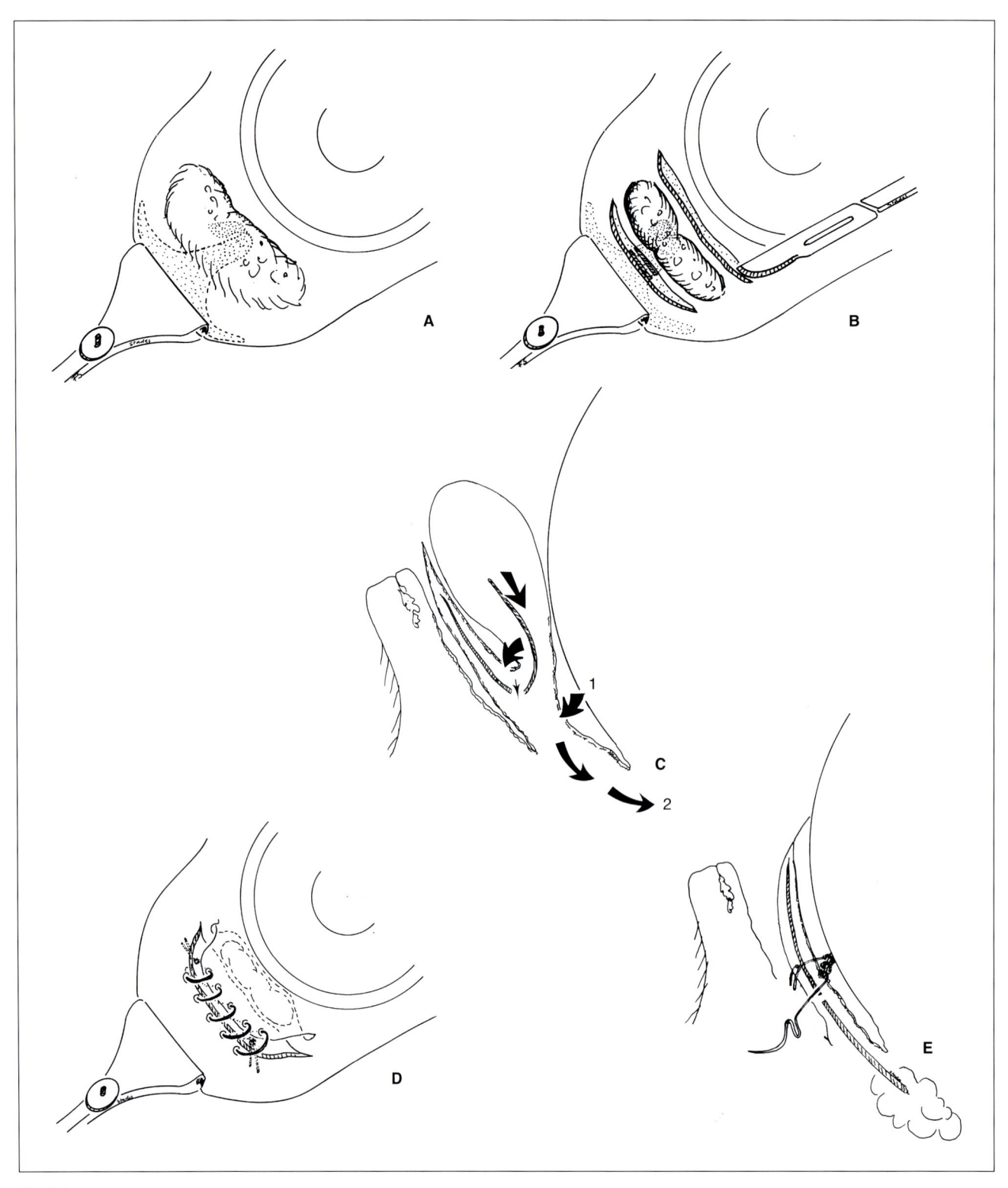

Fig. 8.4:
Surgical correction of a hyperplastic gland of the nictitating membrane by oversuturing the gland with conjunctiva (A–E), after Morgan et al.[9], including cleavage of the cartilage (Boevé modification; B). A retrobulbar pocket is made from the proximal wound by blunt dissection (1–2).

8.9 Subconjunctival hemorrhages

Subconjunctival hemorrhages can develop after leakage (e.g. coagulation disorders) or trauma (see 4) to subconjunctival vessels, resulting in petechiae or larger hemorrhages (suffusions). In cases of coagulation disorders, the examination has to be concentrated on these causes.

8.10 Injuries

(See 4, Ocular Emergencies)

8.11 Conjunctivitis

The conjunctiva and cornea are subjected continuously to noxious environmental agents such as wind, dust and pollen, and infectious agents such as viruses, bacteria, and fungi.[11] For these reasons, the conjunctival sac is usually non-sterile. There are efficient defense systems such as the tear film, the reticuloendothelial system, and the replacement of the conjunctival epithelium. Inflammation of the conjunctiva (conjunctivitis) may have either non-infectious or infectious causes, although often both are involved. Frequently, one factor, such as irritating hairs, dust, or a virus, causes the initial damage, which enables bacteria, fungi, or yeasts to penetrate and colonize the conjunctival sac. A defective defense mechanism may be brought about by a lack of tears, feline autoimmune deficiency syndrome, leukemia/malignant lymphoma, or the long-term use of antibiotics, corticosteroids, or topical anesthetics. Bilateral conjunctivitis is often caused by infections. In cats, the upper respiratory syndrome pathogens are often responsible for conjunctivitis. In dogs, distemper virus can cause bilateral conjunctivitis.

Unilateral conjunctivitis generally has local causes such as foreign bodies, lacerations, or infections, but it may also develop secondary to irritation by hairs, corneal trauma, KCS, dacryocystitis, glaucoma, or uveitis.

Symptoms: Clinical signs of conjunctivitis include:
- **Epiphora,** or overflow of tears, can be caused by irritation of the conjunctiva or cornea. The STT may reach values of over 20–25 mm/min. The lacrimal drainage system is often incapable of draining this overflow and so it will run over the lid margin in the medial canthus, causing a dark brown, wet streak downwards.
- **Serous exudate** may be formed when there is minor irritation of the conjunctiva. This discharge is mixed with the lacrimal fluid, resulting in a higher viscosity of the latter.
- **Mucus discharge** may result from irritation of the mucus cells of the conjunctiva and increased desquamation of epithelial cells. Together, these produce a grayish, glassy, slimy discharge, which generally accumulates in the medial canthus.
- **Purulent discharge** results when leukocytes are mixed in the mucus discharge and the discharge becomes yellow-green. It occurs especially in bacterial and fungal infections. The STT value is high, in contrast to the value found with KCS (Plates 8.8–8.10; see also 8.11.2).
- **Sticky mucus discharge** is produced when leukocytes are mixed in a mucus discharge and there is a lack of the watery fraction of the tear film, which is the case in KCS.
- **Rubor or redness** is caused by hyperemia of the conjunctiva and is a non-specific reaction to conjunctival irritation. There is often an associated conjunctival swelling. Conjunctival hyperemia alone may also be a sign of intraocular disease (i.e. glaucoma or uveitis) or of systemic disease. Redness is usually most distinct in the ventral fornix and can thus escape notice by the owner until the inflammation spreads over the conjunctiva. In rare cases, the reaction is so severe that a vessel ruptures and subconjunctival hemorrhage (suffusion) occurs, although most suffusions are caused by trauma.
- **Tumor or swelling** is usually the result of edema (chemosis), which occurs in almost any type of conjunctivitis. Transudate can easily leave the damaged vessel walls, resulting in a pale, glassy swelling. Because of the very loose attachment of the conjunctiva to the underlying tissues, the swelling may be enormous. In severe chemosis, the conjunctiva may balloon out of the palpebral fissure, completely hiding the globe. In chronic irritation of the conjunctiva, the swelling is more diffuse and contains less fluid resulting in a more solid swelling and folding, especially of the ventral conjunctiva. In rare cases, localized swellings or papules of fibrovascular tissue develop. These are pink-red, firm, and up to a few millimeters in diameter.
- **Follicle** formation (Plate 8.11) is a reaction to chronic inflammation of the conjunctiva; for example, due to viral (e.g. upper respiratory infection in cats) or bacterial infections. They are pale, glassy vesicles, 0.5–2 mm in diameter, with a red base. Each is located at the end of a capillary and encloses a concentration of lymphocytes. Severe inflammation causes more follicles to develop and their bases are redder, resulting in a red field with yellow-pink eruptions (see 8.11.3).
- **Red-pink, papillary/nodular/granulomatous infiltrates** with a smooth, glassy surface may be granulation tissue (e.g. eosinophilic granuloma in cats, leishmania granuloma in dogs (Plate 12.9), or thelaziasis and habronemiasis in horses) or be caused by autoimmune processes (see 8.11.5 and 8.12).
- **Blue-red, bilateral, focal infiltrates** (Plate 8.12) spreading over the (UV-)light-exposed outer surface of the nictitating membrane suggest plasmacellular conjunctivitis (see 8.11.4).

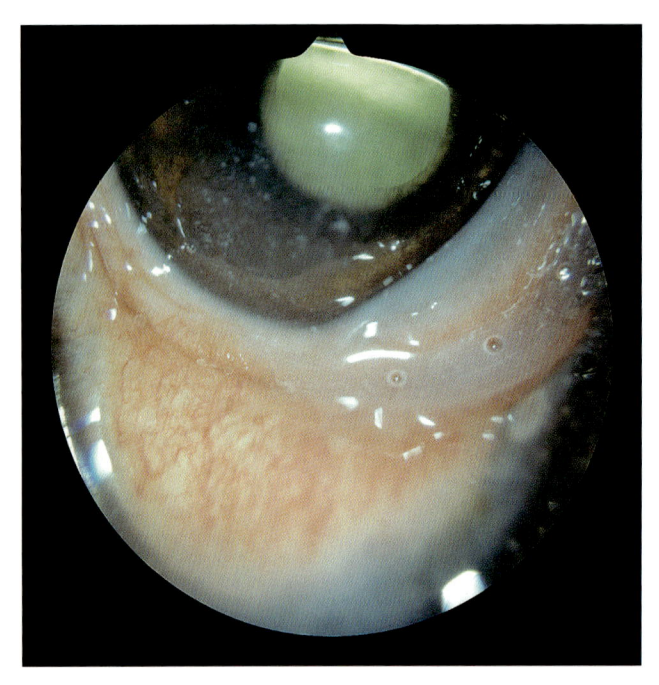

Plate 8.8:
Acute purulent conjunctivitis (OD, dog). There is an overproduction of tears containing little flecks of pus (see also Plate 8.10).

8.11.1 Catarrhal (or serous) conjunctivitis

In catarrhal conjunctivitis, serous exudate is mixed with the tear film. The film's viscosity increases and lacrimal drainage decreases, resulting in epiphora and tear stripe formation below the medial canthus. The serous reaction may be caused by wind, dust, ammoniac from dirty cage bottoms or allergens. Other causes are acute infections such as upper respiratory disease or infectious rhinitis in cats caused by FHV-1, *Mycoplasma* spp., and *Chlamydia* spp.[12,13,14] The serous reaction is followed by the production of more mucus and more desquamated epithelial cells.

Catarrhal conjunctivitis is characterized by epiphora, redness, slight swelling, and mucus discharge. In the acute phase, epiphora is especially prominent, while in the chronic phase (after 1–2 weeks), redness, swelling, and discomfort increases.

Conjunctivitis usually causes more itching than pain. The predominance of pain is a sign of corneal involvement. The pruritus may result in rubbing and a minor blepharospasm. Often, some follicular activity will follow, increasing when the conjunctivitis persists. Epithelial defects in the conjunctiva and cornea, which may occur in upper respiratory disease in cats, have much more serious consequences for the eye. When two opposite layers are affected, the surfaces may adhere and grow together (symblepharon). This process is often found in the lacrimal canaliculi, between the palpebral conjunctiva of the nictitating membrane and the lids, and between the palpebral conjunctiva and the cornea (see 8.14.1).

- **Membranes** may occur after very severe processes in which there is rejection of larger areas of epithelium. If these are removed, the underlying tissues bleed easily.
- **Pseudo-membranes** develop following formation of crusts consisting of exudate and detritus.
- **Symblepharon** is an adhesion of conjunctival surfaces or of conjunctiva to the cornea and may develop after epithelial defects caused by infections, such as upper respiratory disease in cats (Plate 8.15; see 8.14.1).

Based on the most distinct signs, the following types of conjunctivitis can be distinguished:

8.11.2 Purulent conjunctivitis

In purulent conjunctivitis, inflammatory cells are mixed with the serous exudate and the tear film (Plates 8.8–8.10). This results in an increased amount of tear fluid with aggregates of pus that accumulate in the medial canthus. As the process continues, more epithelial cells and mucus are produced, resulting in larger, yellow-green accumulations of pus.

In the rabbit, the pus in general will be white and have a caseous consistency. Production of purulent material is usually more prominent in bacterial and fungal infections. Purulent conjunctivitis often follows catarrhal conjunctivitis caused by mechanical or infectious agents.

Diagnosis: Diagnosis of catarrhal or purulent conjunctivitis can be made on the basis of the following criteria:
1. History (e.g. distemper / upper respiratory disease).
2. Examination of the eyes, including the STT, sensitivity testing, conjunctival smear or scraping, and rose bengal staining.

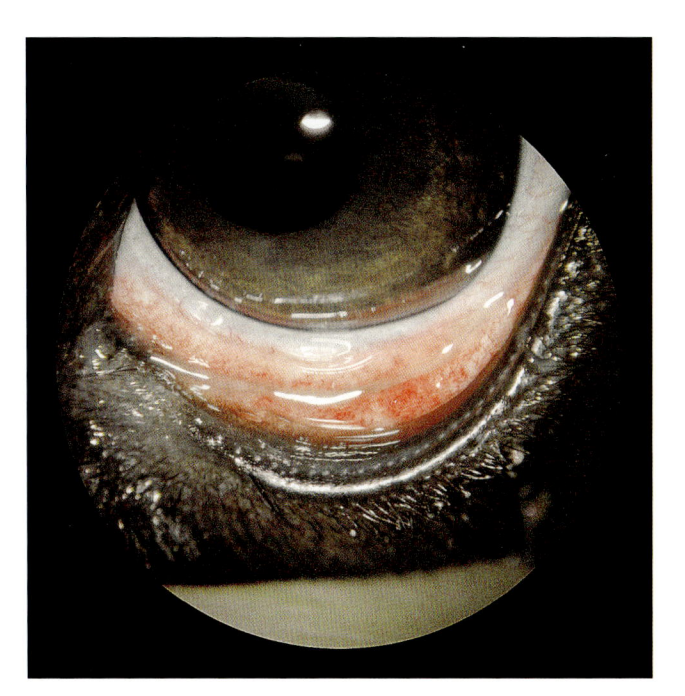

Plate 8.9:
Acute mucopurulent conjunctivitis (the lower eyelid is slightly ectropionized; OS, dog). Abundant tears, rubor and swelling of the conjunctiva are distinct. Mucopurulent material *appears* not to be present (see also Plate 8.10).

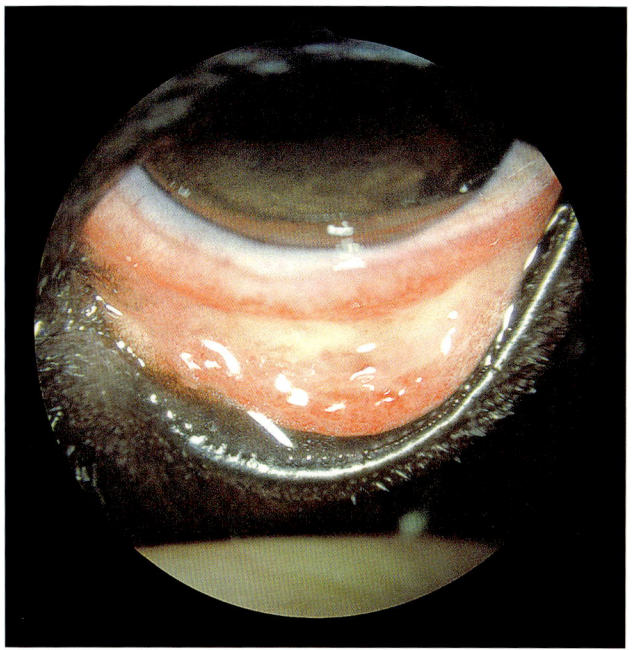

Plate 8.10:
Acute mucopurulent conjunctivitis (OS, dog; same eye as shown in Plate 8.9; the lower lid is more ectropionized now). The signs of inflammation are distinct. It is clear now that there is a large lump of exudate in the ventral conjunctival sac. Before any drugs are instilled, this has to be removed by the use of acetylcysteine and/or an eyewash, otherwise the drug will not fully reach the conjunctiva.

3. General physical examination for signs of infectious diseases, such as upper respiratory disease in cats or distemper in dogs and the ferret, and pasteurellosis or myxomatosis in rabbits.
   Unfortunately, confirming a viral etiology is time-consuming and costly. Distemper inclusion bodies or *Chlamydophilia felis* organisms may be found in a Giemsa-stained smear during the first month of infection.
4. Exclusion of other eye diseases causing secondary conjunctivitis, such as dacryocystitis, KCS, glaucoma, or uveitis.

Therapy: The therapy in acute catarrhal conjunctivitis consists of removal of the mucous discharge by irrigation, 1–4 times daily. The conjunctiva usually begins to regenerate in a matter of days. If there is no spontaneous improvement, "initial choice" ocular antibiotic drops or ointment can be applied 4 times daily for 5–7 days in dogs. In cats, oxytetracycline or chlortetracycline ointment are the "specific choice" antibiotics to be used.

In acute purulent conjunctivitis, the therapy consists of dissolution of the purulent exudate by acetylcysteine, followed by irrigation, at least 4 times daily. "Initial choice" ocular antibiotics may be applied 4–6 times daily for 7–10 days.

In acute conjunctivitis due to upper respiratory disease in cats, or pasteurellosis in rabbits, topical therapy consists of acetylcysteine (diminishing the risk for symblepharon), irrigation, oxytetracycline or chlortetracycline, 4–6 times daily for 10–14 days, and doxycycline orally.

In chronic conjunctivitis, the clinical examination should be repeated and initial treatment intensified. Irrigation with 0.1% $ZnSO_4$ and a vasoconstrictor/antihistamine may be indicated. The choice of antibiotic is made on the basis of an antibiogram. In infections caused by a fungus or yeast, treatment for 4–6 weeks with an antimycotic drug (see 3.2.5.2) is indicated.

8.11.3 Follicular conjunctivitis

Lymphoid follicles may develop as a reaction to primary infections (e.g. feline upper respiratory disease), chronic irritation (dust), or hypersensitivity (pollen). They are 0.5–3 mm in diameter, pale, glassy, and red at the base. Almost every follicle has its own capillary. Follicles are most frequently located on the ocular conjunctiva of the nictitating membrane, between the outer margin of the nictitating membrane and the gland.

> The area adjacent to the edge of the cartilage is most often affected in folliculitis in cats.

The presence of a few small follicles, especially in young animals, is normal. More follicles are often seen as a consequence of an earlier episode of irritation (pollen, viral infection). If many follicles develop, they may become a confluent field on the ocular conjunctiva of the nictitating membrane as well as throughout the rest of the conjunctiva.

Clinical signs may vary from none to minor enophthalmos, blepharospasm, mucus discharge, some redness and swelling of the conjunctiva, and the presence of follicles (Plate 8.11.).

Therapy: If there are no signs of infection or other obvious causes, treatment consists of topical ocular steroid drops, 4 times daily for 2–3 weeks. If the result is unsatisfactory or there is recurrence after 3–4 weeks, surgical intervention may be indicated.

Operation: In young animals, surgery should be postponed until 1–1½ years of age. Under general anesthesia, every follicle is cauterized separately by electrocoagulation. Coagulation near the cornea and the lid edges should be done with great care, since the current may arc to the tear film. The Stades' NM forceps facilitates surgery by providing good exposure. If the follicles are located in only one field on the ocular conjunctiva of the nictitating membrane, curettage may be a satisfactory alternative, but recurrences are more frequent with this method. Etching methods, e.g. using $CuSO_4$, are less selective and have an unacceptable risk, since remnants of the etching material may damage the cornea. Postoperatively, topical "initial choice" antibiotic-corticosteroid eye drops or ointment are applied 4 times daily for 7–10 days.

8.11.4 Plasmacellular conjunctivitis

This specific form of conjunctivitis is characterized by nests of plasma cells in the palpebral conjunctiva of the nictitating membrane. It is mainly found in the German Shepherd Dog and the offspring of crossings with this breed. It is rare in cats. It is immune-mediated and is associated with chronic superficial keratitis or pannus in the German Shepherd Dog (10.6.1.1). It may be similar to the proliferative keratoconjunctivitis syndrome in Collies, for both disorders are activated by UV light.

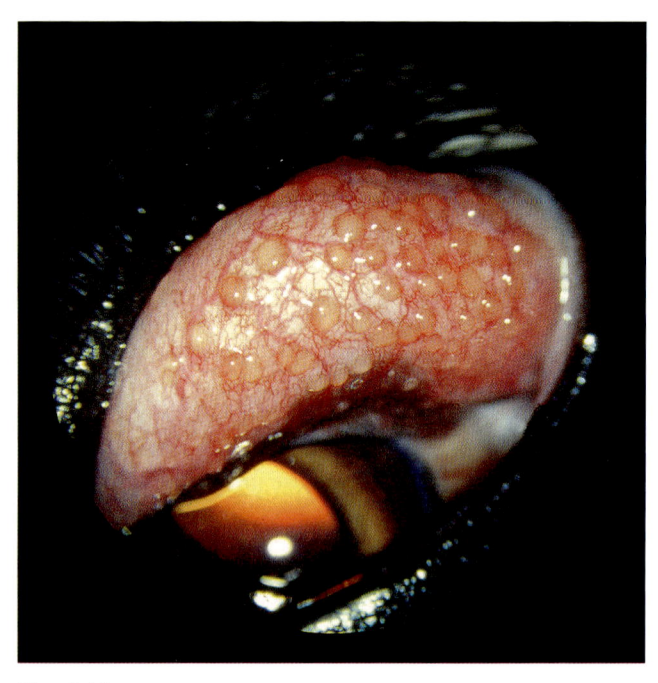

Plate 8.11:
Severe follicular conjunctivitis in the upper lid conjunctiva (OS, dog).

Symptoms: There are chronic, blue-red, painless focal swellings in the conjunctiva of the outside margin of the nictitating membrane (Plate 8.12). There may be some protrusion of the nictitating membrane and mucous discharge. The process spreads slowly to all areas of the conjunctiva. Cytological scraping or biopsy of the suspicious area is usually diagnostic.

Therapy: Treatment consists of the lifelong administration of topical corticosteroids. Initially, one drop of topical ocular steroid solution is administered 4–6 times daily and ocular steroid ointment is applied at night. The administration of topical steroid is decreased to twice daily and then to alternate days. On days of abundant or intense sunlight, especially when the animal is near water or snow, or at a high altitude, the treatment should be increased at once. If there is significant deterioration, injections of a depot-corticosteroid solution can be administered subconjunctivally. If there is continuing deterioration, treatment with cyclosporine (0.2%) is a possible alternative. Also, the local application of 500 rads of β-radiation can be tried or 3–5 mm of the margin of the nictitating membrane can be excised. The wound is sutured with 8-0 absorbable suture material. Knots should be embedded subconjunctivally or completely avoided if possible, thus preventing corneal irritation.

Also the use of sunglasses will be helpful (see 10.6.1.1)

Conjunctivitis **117**

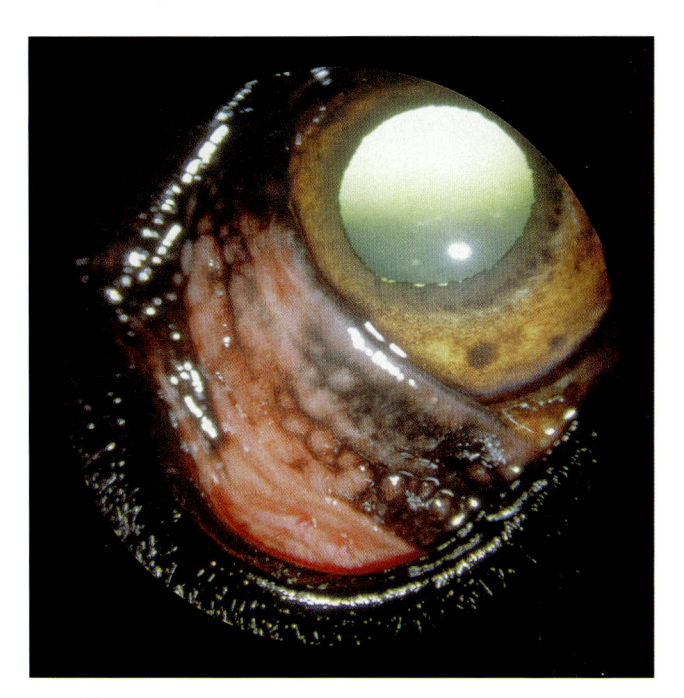

Plate 8.12:
Plasmacellular conjunctivitis (OS, dog).

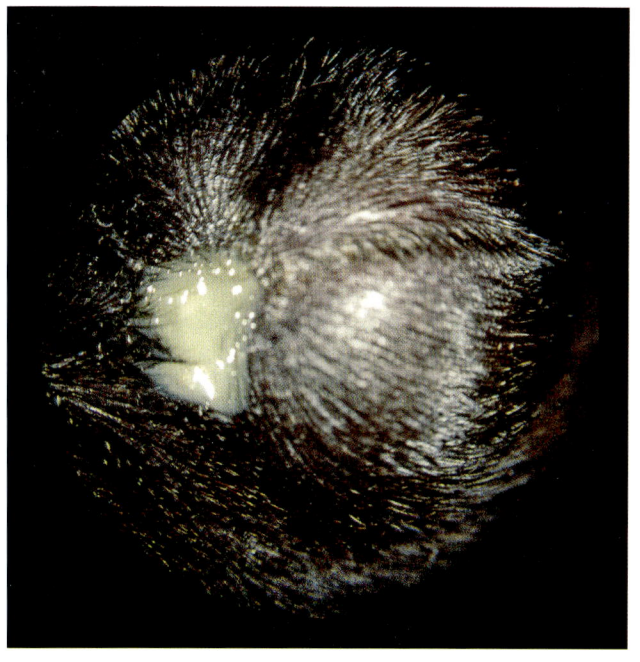

Plate 8.13:
Conjunctivitis neonatorum in a 3-day-old Great Dane (OS). Some pus has escaped through a minimal opening in the lid fissure.

Prognosis: The prognosis is favorable if treatment is continued lifelong.

8.11.5 Papillary / nodular / granulomatous conjunctivitis

These forms of chronic conjunctivitis are mainly characterized by fibrovascular, inflammatory infiltrates in the conjunctiva, resulting from chronic irritation caused, for example, by *Leishmania* spp. in dogs and *Thelazia* spp., *Habronema* spp., or *Onchocerca* spp. in horses (mainly in the USA).[15]

Symptoms: The granulomatous lesions can be massive, red, glassy, pink, nodular, etc. The nodules themselves may be a new source of irritation, thus causing a chronic mucopurulent conjunctivitis. They can be found scattered over the conjunctiva or they can be concentrated near the limbus, the lid margins, or the tear ducts.

Sometimes, adult parasites (*Thelazia*) can be seen moving under the conjunctiva or found in the fluid from nasolacrimal irrigation. Caseous, necrotic nodules (*Habronema*) or depigmented areas near the limbus (*Onchocerca*) can be recognized. Often, the diagnosis is only confirmed by biopsy and histology.

Therapy: If the cause can be diagnosed, the disorder can be treated in an appropriate way. *Thelazia* larvae can be killed by parenteral levamisole (5 mg/kg) or topical ecothiophate iodine[15], 1% levamisole, fenbendazole, or ivermectin.[16] The conjunctival sac is thoroughly irrigated and the adult parasites (*Habronema*) may be picked out with forceps. Re-infestation can be prevented by adequate antiparasitic control of the larvae and flies. Chronic granulomatous conjunctivitis can be treated with topical "initial choice" antibiotic-corticosteroid eye ointment, 4 times daily.

8.11.6 Conjunctivitis neonatorum

This type of "conjunctivitis" is caused in general by a bacterial infection (especially *Staphylococcus* spp.) in the conjunctival sac (Plate 8.13) occurring just after birth. The infection is most probably acquired intrauterine. The still closed lids bulge and the overfilled conjunctival sac fluctuates. If there is some opening of the palpebral fissure, purulent exudate will escape. If the condition persists, there will be severe and permanent damage to the cornea.

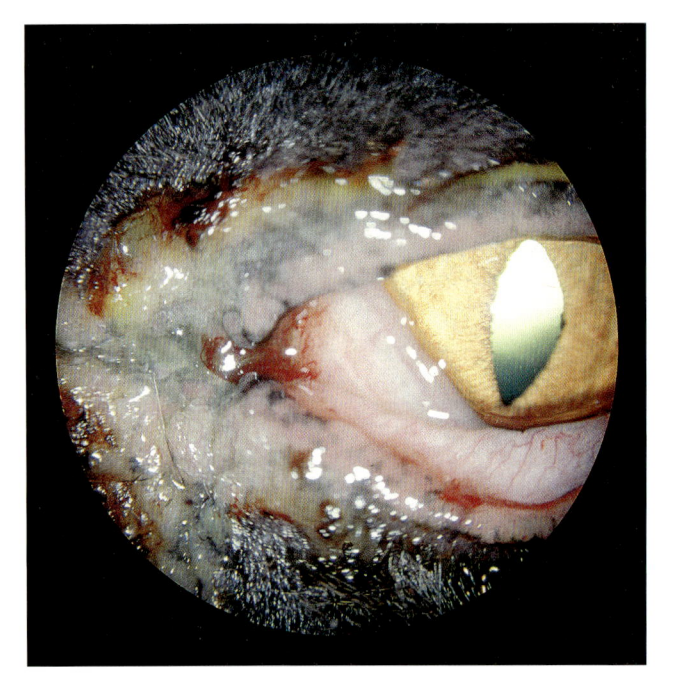

Plate 8.14:
Eosinophilic granuloma of the medial lid margin and conjunctiva in a cat (OS).

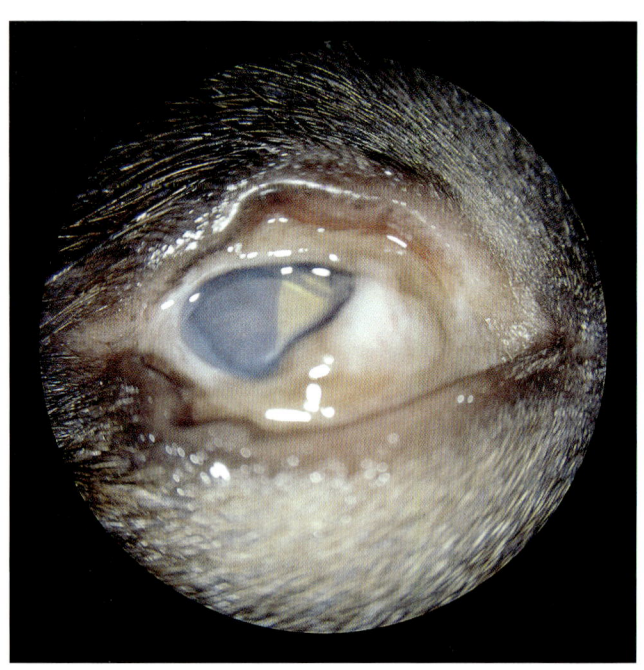

Plate 8.15:
Symblepharon as a scar, after upper respiratory disease in a Siamese cat (OD).

Therapy: Therapy consists of an immediate opening of the palpebral fissure. The rim is opened by massage or bluntly with a Mosquito-Halstead clamp. In this way, the fissure is "zipped" open and the exudate can escape. The subsequent treatment consists of acetylcysteine 10%, irrigation and "initial choice" ocular antibiotics, 4–6 times daily for 7–10 days.

Prognosis: The prognosis is favorable if treatment is instituted promptly.

8.11.7 Infectious bovine / ovine keratoconjunctivitis (pinkeye)

This is the main eye disease found in herds of cattle and flocks of sheep. The infection in cattle is caused mainly by *Moraxella bovis* and in sheep and goats by *Mycoplasma* spp., but Chlamydia (*Chlamydophilia*), other bacteria (e.g. *Pasteurella* spp.) and viruses also contribute to the disease. The infection is spread through the herd or flock by contact, but flies are also an important vector.[17,18] There is an acute, mucopurulent keratoconjunctivitis, bladder-like corneal ulceration, edema, and corneal vascularization.

Therapy: There will be a rapid resolution of the problem if the condition is recognized early, affected animals isolated immediately (in a stall, with fly control), and treatment instituted promptly. If treatment is delayed, deep corneal ulcers can develop, sometimes resulting in anterior uveitis, corneal perforation, and loss of the eye. Sometimes, it is impossible to isolate the affected animals or to treat them at frequent intervals. In such cases, additional subconjunctival "specific choice" antibiotics and/or systemic long-acting oxytetracyclines (20 mg/kg, I.M., repeated after 72 hours) can be beneficial and will result in fewer carriers. In sheep and goats, some immunity will develop.[19]

8.12 Eosinophilic granuloma

This condition in cats, which occurs most often on the lip and cornea, may, in rare cases, also affect the conjunctiva. Chronic, slowly spreading, red, painless, focal swellings develop in the conjunctiva or even on the lid margins (Plate 8.14; see 10.6.1.2).[20]

8.13 Allergic conjunctivitis

Allergic conjunctivitis is occasionally seen in dogs with atopic dermatitis after contact with, or absorption of allergens. Allergic/atopic-based conjunctivitis is generally bilateral. This conjunctivitis is the result of a T-cell-mediated and an IgE-associated inflammation. Pruritus and other clinical manifestations are caused mainly by histamine and leukotriene release. Causative allergens may be the pollens of grasses, weeds and trees, or less likely house dust mites, food components, or spider and insect bites, etc. The conjunctivae are bilaterally swollen, more or less red, and itchy.

Allergic conjunctivitis as the result of drugs is usually associated with an irritant reaction (rapid response) or a delayed-type hypersensitivity. Examples are benzalconium chloride, cyclopentolate, neomycin, and pilocarpine. As stated before, the bites or stings of spiders or insects may also cause this type of conjunctivitis, although the actual area of the sting or bite can rarely be identified. In such cases, the chemosis will usually be more acute, often bilateral, and quite intense.

Therapy: Therapy consists of stopping the contact to the presumed allergen if recognized, and topical corticosteroid ointments or drops, 3–4 times daily for 1 week. Additional intravenous or intramuscular corticosteroids may be necessary in acute, severe cases. Cyclosporine A treatment may be an option in case of a persistent allergic response.

8.14 Conjunctival adhesions

8.14.1 Symblepharon

Symblepharon is an adhesion between parts of the conjunctiva or between the conjunctiva and the cornea. It is especially found in young cats as a complication of upper respiratory disease. The primary viral/mycoplasmal/chlamydial infection and the secondary bacterial infection destroy the superficial layers of the epithelium. In conjunction with the mucus discharge, this results in the conjunctival layers adhering to each other and subsequently growing together. In particular, there are frequently adhesions between the walls of the lacrimal canaliculi and/or the palpebral conjunctiva of the nictitating membrane and the rest of the conjunctiva (Plate 8.15). Symblepharon is usually unilateral.

Symptoms: Signs of symblepharon are epiphora, tear stripe formation, permanent protrusion of the nictitating membrane, and blepharospasm (Plate 8.15). The adhesions are found during examination with von Graefe's forceps. If the cornea is involved, there may be membranes of scar tissue spreading over and loosely attached to the cornea.

Therapy: Treatment consists of loosening the adhesions. This should only be performed after the underlying infectious disease has run its course. The adhesions to the cornea may be loosened (Fig. 8.5). The flap of tissue should not be cut away but sutured back in the direction of the fornix, thus preventing the possibility of recurrence due to adhesions of two adjacent surfaces without covering epithelium. Larger defects should be covered by conjunctivoplasty. Complete adhesion of the palpebral surface of the nictitating membrane will often recur after loosening. In these cases, the margin of the nictitating membrane may be trimmed away over several millimeters. Adhesions of lacrimal canaliculi are difficult to open and readily recur.

Further treatment consists of topical corticosteroids (be aware of the risk of reactivating the infection) and a "specific choice" antibiotic (e.g. oxytetracycline) at least 4 times daily, combined with doxycycline orally at a dose of 2 mg/kg/day for 7–10 days. Installation of a large contact lens will facilitate re-growth of the epithelium and thus prevent recurrence of the adhesions.

Prevention/prognosis: The prognosis is not very favorable as recurrence is possible. Adhesions may be prevented if, during the acute phase of upper respiratory disease in cats, the adhesive mucus discharge is removed very thoroughly by topical acetylcysteine and irrigation.

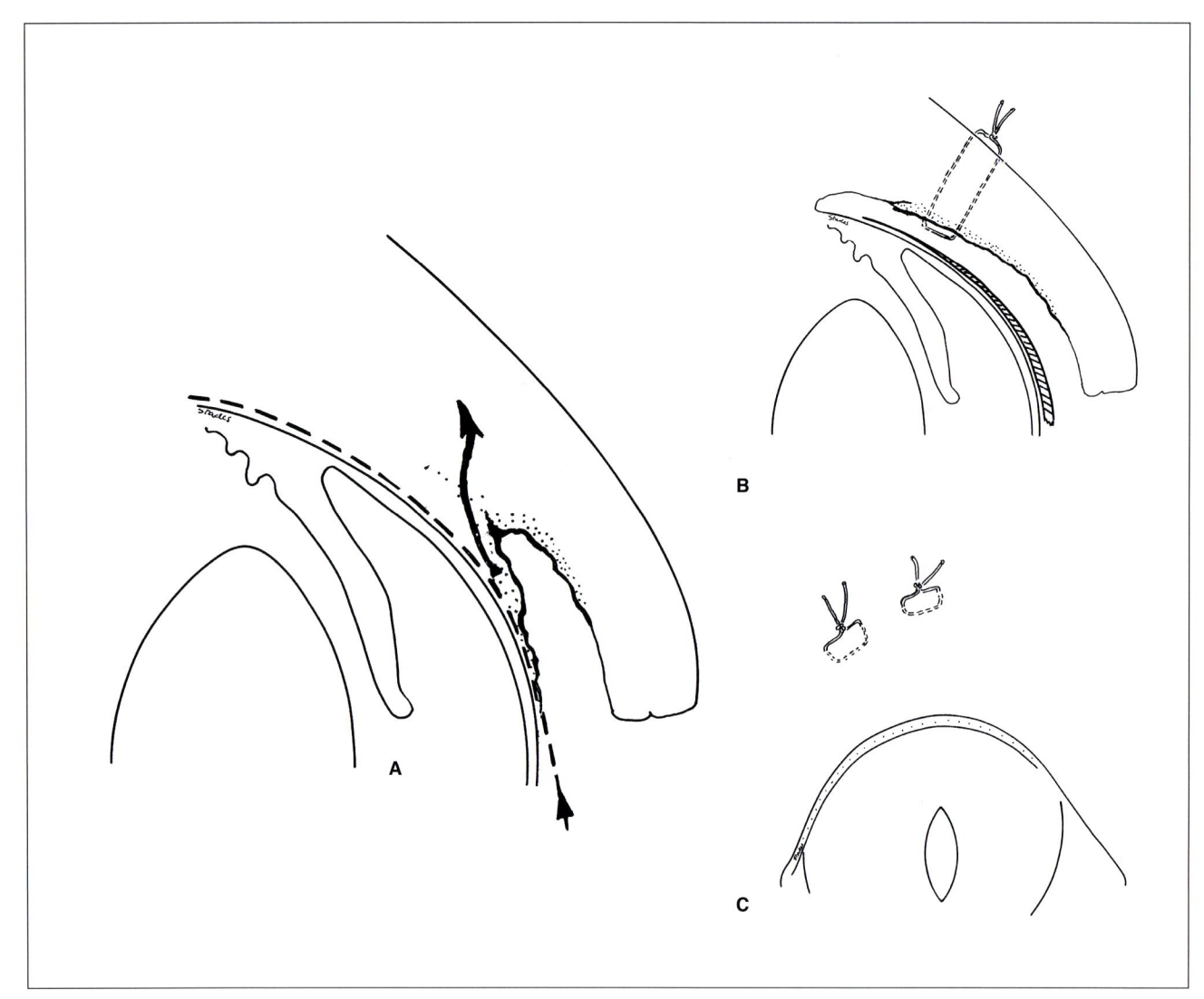

Fig. 8.5:
Surgical correction of a symblepharon (A). The conjunctiva-like corneal overgrowth is bluntly dissected (B) and re-attached in the fornix with 2–3 sutures (C).

8.14.2 Conjunctival stricture in the rabbit (Plate 8.16)

In the miniature rabbit, the bulbar conjunctiva can retract circularly over the corneal surface until only a pupil-like opening of a few millimeters in diameter remains centrally, showing an edematous cornea. Total overgrowth is also possible. The etiology is unknown.

Therapy: The overgrown conjunctiva can be split medially and laterally, and the doubled conjunctival layers can be relocated to the upper and lower "fornix" and fixed to the outside skin (U-sutures, resorbable, 6-0) (Fig. 8.6, Plate 8.17).

Conjunctival adhesions **121**

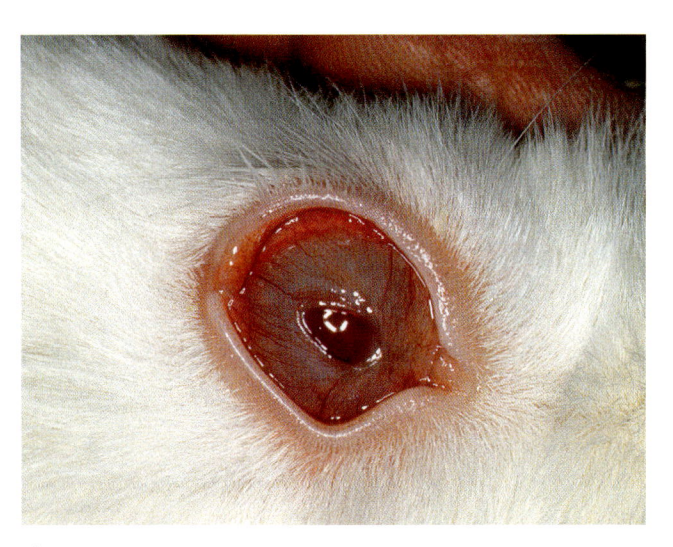

Plate 8.16:
Circular contraction of conjunctiva over the cornea in a miniature rabbit (OD; see Plate 8.17).

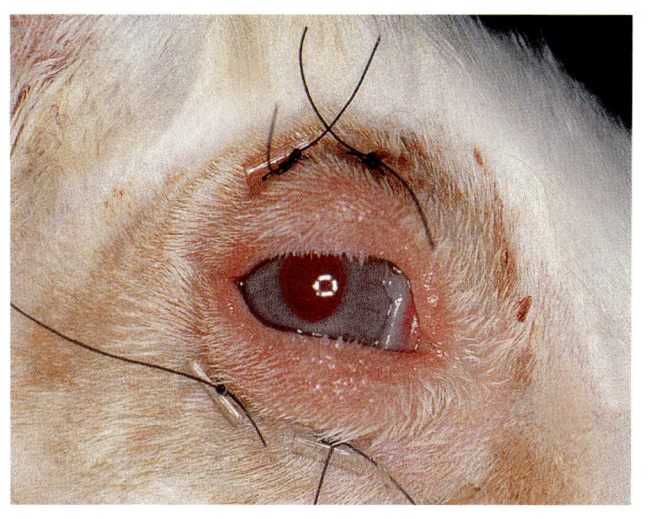

Plate 8.17:
Circular contraction of conjunctiva over the cornea in a miniature rabbit, after surgical correction (OD; same rabbit as in Plate 8.16). The overhanging conjunctival stricture is split medially and laterally (see Fig. 8.6). The upper and lower doubled conjunctival layers are relocated to the upper and lower "fornix" and fixed to the outside skin.

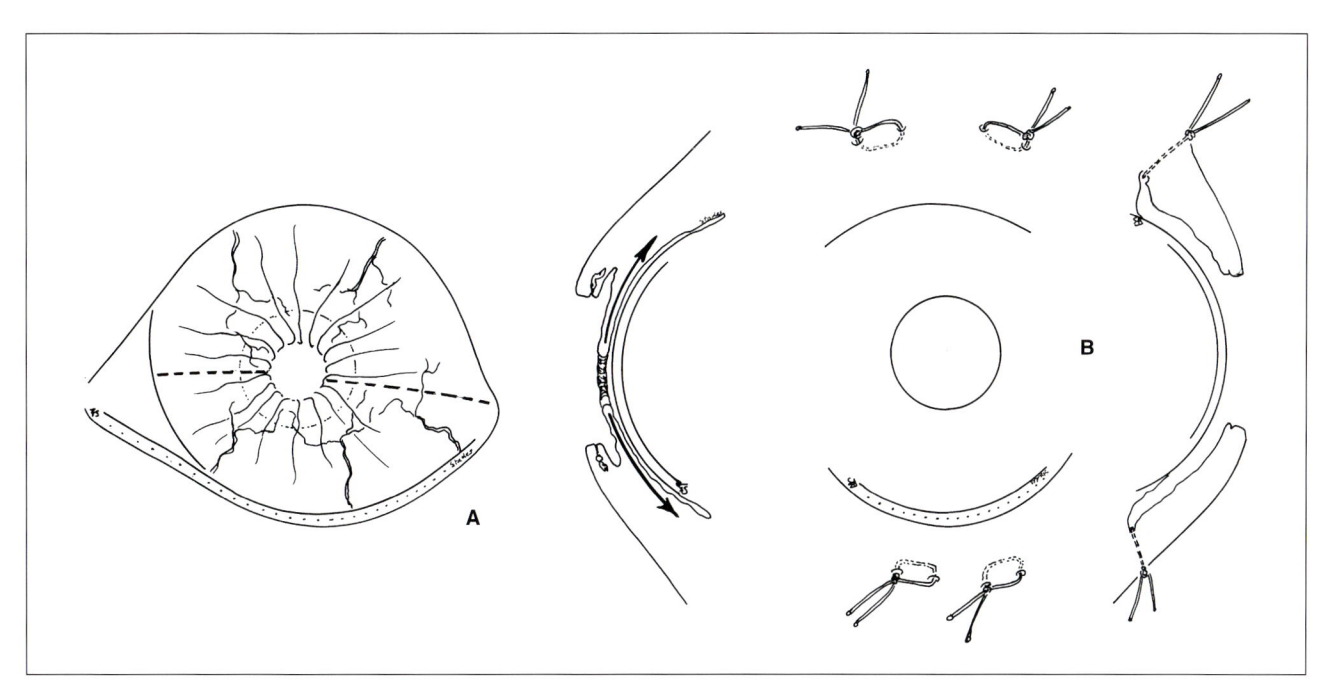

Fig. 8.6:
Conjunctival stricture in a miniature rabbit. The overhanging conjunctival stricture is split medially and laterally (A). The doubled conjunctival layers are relocated to the upper and lower "fornix" (B) and fixed to the outside skin.

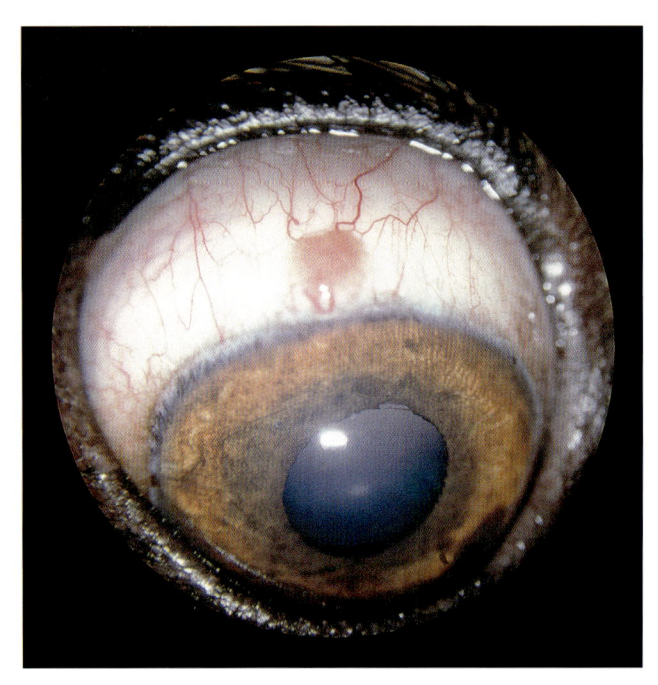

Plate 8.18:
Papilloma, resembling a mini jellyfish, originating from the scleral conjunctiva in a dog (OD).

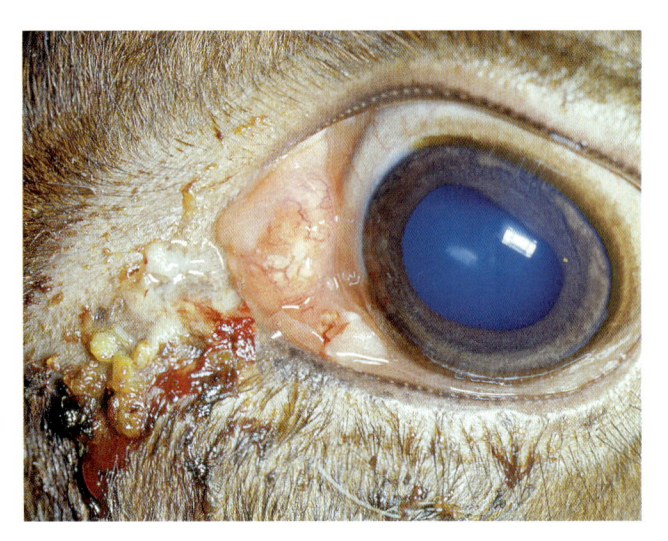

Plate 8.19:
Squamous cell carcinoma originating from the nictitating membrane in a cow (OS). (By courtesy Dr. W. Klein, Utrecht.)

8.15 Neoplasia of the conjunctiva

Neoplasms of the conjunctiva are rare.[21] Papillomas often take the form of pinkish-red, cauliflower-shaped nodules, about 5 mm in diameter, which appear almost to drift on the surface of the conjunctiva (Plate 8.18). The treatment consists of surgical removal of the neoplasm together with the conjunctiva at its base.

Malignant neoplasms often cause more diffuse swelling, especially at the base of the nictitating membrane and are frequently accompanied by exophthalmos. The most frequent neoplasms are squamous cell carcinomas (Plate 8.19), but lymphosarcoma, mastocytoma, and other neoplasms also occur. Bilateral involvement is most likely to be due to lymphosarcoma.

Unexplained pigmented or non-pigmented swellings should be examined microscopically by means of fine needle aspiration biopsy, or by surgical biopsy, or excision. They may also be further localized by MRI or CT scanning.

Therapy: Radical excision should be performed if feasible, but an attempt must be made to spare as much as possible of the nictitating membrane and the rest of the conjunctiva. Malignant neoplasms deep to the base of the nictitating membrane usually have to be removed by orbitotomy or, in the most extensive cases, by exenteration of the orbit. Such patients should be referred to a specialist. If a major loss of tissues is to be expected, cryotherapy[22] and/or hyperthermotherapy[23] or combinations of both can be considered.

Immunotherapy using an injection of BCG locally appears to be the most promising therapy in (conjunctival) carcinomas in cattle.[24]

Literature

1. BANIS, J.: Microflora of normal and diseased conjunctiva in horses and dogs. Acta Vet. Belgrade, **9**: 97, 1959.

2. SAMUELSON, D.A., ANDRESEN, T.L. & GWIN, R.M.: Conjunctival fungal flora in horses, cattle, dogs, and cats. JAVMA **184**: 1240, 1984.

3. MOORE, C.P. et al: Density and distribution of canine conjunctival goblet cells. Invest. Ophthalmol. Vis. Sci, **28**: 1925, 1987.

4. PEIFFER, R.L. & HARLING, D.E.: Third eyelid. In: Textbook of small animal surgery. Ed.: D.H. Slatter, Philadelphia, Lea & Febiger, 1501, 1985.

5. DUGAN, S.J., SEVERIN, G.A., HUNGERFORD, L.L., WHITELEY, H.E. & ROBERTS, S.M.: Clinical and histologic evaluation of the prolapsed third eyelid gland in dogs. JAVMA **201**: 1861, 1992.

6. HELPER, L. & MAGRANE, W.G.: Ectopic cilia of the canine eyelid. J. Small Anim. Pract. **11**: 185, 1970.

7. LATIMER, C.A. & SZYMANSKI, C.: Membrana nictitans gland cyst in a dog. JAVMA **183**: 1003, 1983.

8. KASWAN, R.L. & MARTIN, C.L.: Surgical correction of third eyelid prolapse in dogs. JAVMA **186**: 83, 1985.

9. MORGAN, R., DUDDY, J. & MCCLURG, K.: Prolapse of the gland of the third eyelid in dogs: a retrospective study of 89 cases (1980–1990). JAAHA **29**: 56, 1993.

10. HUVER, I.M.G. et al.: Comparison of four techniques used in the surgical approach of protrusion of the gland of the nictitating membrane in dogs, Proceedings FECAVA-Voorjaarsdagen, Amsterdam, p.305, 2005.

11. URBAN, M. et al.: Conjunctival flora of clinically normal dogs. JAVMA **161**: 201, 1972.

12. CAMPBELL, L.H., FOX, J.G. & SNYDER, S.B.: Ocular bacteria and mycoplasma of the clincally normal cat. Feline Pract. **3**: 10, 1973.

13. CRANDELL, R.A. et al.: Experimental feline viral rhinotracheitis. JAAHA **138**: 191, 1961.

14. STUDDERT, M.J., STUDDERT, V.P. & WIRTH, H.J.: Isolation of *Chlamydia psittaci* from cats with conjunctivitis. Aust. Vet. J. **57**: 515, 1981.

15. LAVACH, J.D.: Large animal ophthalmology. St. Louis, C.V. Mosby, pp 252, 1990.

16. RIIS, R.C.: Equine ophthalmology. In: Veterinary ophthalmology, Ed.: K.N. Gelatt. Philadelphia, Lea & Febiger, 569, 1981.

17. PUGH, G.W., HUGHES, D.E. & PACKER, R.A.: Bovine infectious keratoconjunctivitis: interactions of *Morexella bovis* and infectious bovine rhinotracheitis virus. Am. J. Vet. Res. **31**: 653, 1970.

18. BARILE, M.F., GUIDICE, R.A.D. & TULLEY, J.G.: Isolation and characterization of *Mycoplasma conjunctivae* from sheep and goats with keratoconjunctivitis. Infect. Immun. **5**: 70, 1972.

19. SMITH, J.A. & GEORGE, L.W.: Treatment of acute ocular *Moraxella bovis* infections in calves with a parenterally administered long-acting oxytetracycline formulation. Am. J. Vet. Res. **46**: 804, 1985.

20. PENTLARGE, V.W.: Eosinophilic conjunctivitis in five cats. Trans. Nineteenth Ann. Sci. Prog. Am. Coll. Vet. Ophthalmol, 107, 1988.

21. WILCOCK, B. & PEIFFER, R.: Adenocarcinoma of the gland of the third eyelid in seven dogs. JAVMA **193**: 1549, 1988.

22. JOYCE, J.R.: Cryosurgical treatment of tumors of horses and catte. JAVMA **168**: 226, 1976.

23. GRIER, R.L., BREWER, W.G., PAUL, S.R. & THEILEN, G.H.: Treatment of bovine and equine ocular squamous cell carcinoma by radiofrequency hyperthermia. JAVMA **177**: 55, 1980.

24. KLEIN, W.R., RUITENBERG, E.J., STEERENBERG, P.A. et al.: Immunotherapy by intralesional injection of BCG cell walls or live BCG in bovine ocular squamous cell carcinoma: a preliminary report. J. Nat. Cancer Inst. **69**: 1095, 1982.

9 Globe

9.1 Introduction

The eyes in predatory species such as dogs and cats are frontally located and the axes of their eyes lie almost parallel. This position affords a wide field of binocular vision, which is important for catching prey. In prey species such as horses, cattle, and rabbits, the eyes are usually placed more laterally, providing constant surveillance of the surroundings, including the rear, leaving only a very small blind area.

The globe is fairly spherical, with the exception of the cornea, which has a smaller curvature. The diameter in Beagle fetuses and puppies increases from roughly 3 mm in day 37 post coitus fetuses to respectively 5 mm (D 44), 9 mm (D51), 10 mm (partum), 12 mm (week 1), 13 mm (week 3), 15 mm (week 5), up to 18 mm in puppies of 7 weeks of age.[1] The diameter of the globe in the adult is about 20–25 mm in dogs and cats, 50–54 mm (laterolateral) to 45–50 mm (anteriorposterior) in horses, 36–40 mm in cattle, 27–30 mm in sheep, and 25–26 mm in swine. With the eye in place, the only reliable way of measuring the diameter of the globe is by the use of either ultrasonography, MRI or CT scanning. By measuring the mediolateral diameter of the limbus with calipers, an impression of the diameter of the total globe can be obtained. This diameter is about 17 mm in the dog (dorsoventral [dv]: 16), 18 mm in cats (dv: 17), 33 mm in horses (dv: 26), 30 mm in cattle (dv: 23), 22 mm in sheep (dv: 16), and 17 mm in swine (dv: 15).[2]

The diameter of the globe is relatively large in birds. The diameter of the avian cornea varies enormously and is large, e.g. in night birds, compared with the scleral part of the globe. To obtain an impression of the diameter of the relatively large globe in birds, the examiner must realize that the scleral part of the two globes is separated only by a very thin bony septum; the globes almost touch each other in the medium plane, and fill a major part of the volume of the skull.

The globe is comprised of three tunicae. The protective and form-determining outer fibrous tunica consists of the cornea and sclera. In birds, the form of the globe is largely maintained by a scleral bony ring and bone plates. The middle, vascular tunica is formed by the uvea, which provides nutrients to the various structures in the eye and removes their waste products. The inner, nervous tunica is formed by the retina. About three-quarters of the globe's structure is maintained by the production and removal rate of the aqueous humor.

The globe is held in place and moved by the retractor bulbi muscles and the four straight and two oblique eye muscles. The dorsal, medial, and ventral rectus muscles and the ventral oblique muscle are innervated by the oculomotor nerve (CN III). The dorsal oblique muscle is innervated by the trochlear nerve (CN IV). The abducens nerve (CN VI) innervates the retractor and the lateral straight muscle. Loss of sympathetic activity results in enophthalmos and protrusion of the nictitating membrane (see 5.4.2).

The axons of the retinal ganglion cells form the retinal nerve fibers, which join to make the papilla or optic disc, and pass from there together as the optic nerve (CN II) to the brain. Fifty to seventy percent of the nerve fibers cross in the optic chiasm to the contralateral side of the brain, except in Siamese cats in which nearly all of the fibers may cross over.

During clinical examination of the globe as a whole, attention should be given to its position in the orbit and its position during movements of the head and of the eye itself, and to the size and tension of the globe.

9.2 Exophthalmos, enophthalmos

These positional changes are caused by abnormalities of the tissues around the globe or neurologic conditions elsewhere, i.e. Horner's syndrome (see 5).

9.3 Pseudo-exophthalmos / pseudo-enophthalmos

The globe can appear to be displaced rostrally because of enlargement due to glaucoma or an intraocular neoplasm, or because of abnormalities such as episcleritis or a color difference between the eyes due to corneal cloudiness or cataract. Similarly, the appearance of enophthalmos can be due to an undersized eye (see 9.7, 9.8; Plates 9.4, 13.6), a difference in color, or a lid opening that is too short (see 7.9).

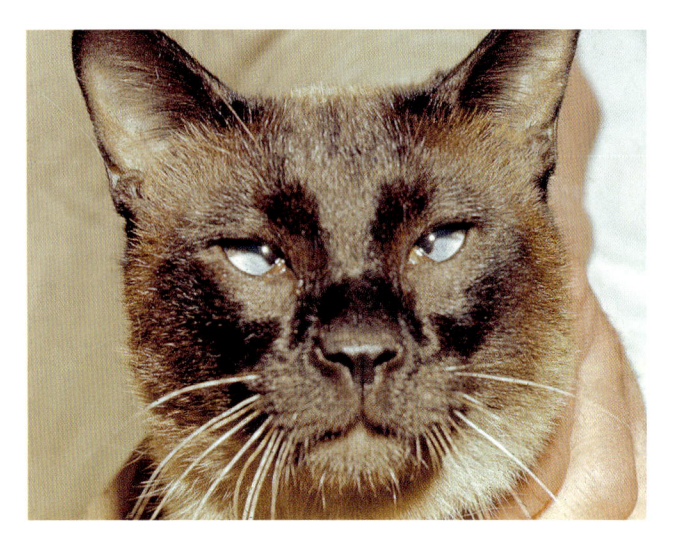

Plate 9.1:
Strabismus (convergent) in a Siamese cat.

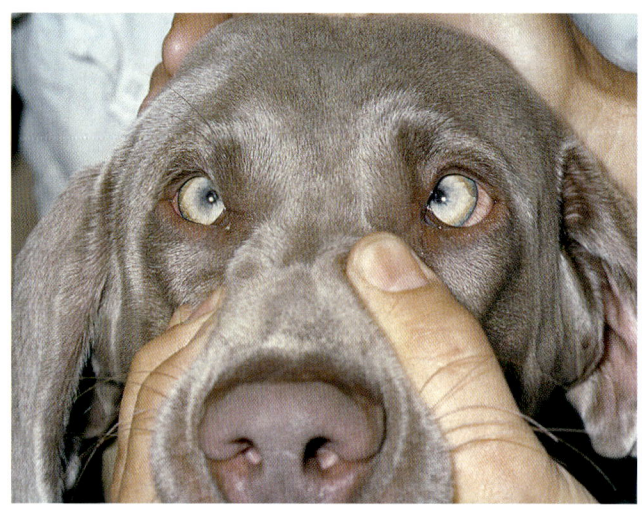

Plate 9.2:
Acquired strabismus convergens in a Weimaraner dog due to inflammatory scarring of the extraocular muscles.

9.4 Setting sun phenomenon

The globes can be abnormally placed in the orbits as a result of abnormal development of the skull due to hydrocephalus. Because of this, the pupils seem to disappear behind the lower eyelids.

9.5 Strabismus

The term strabismus is understood to include every abnormal placement of the visual axes. The abnormality can be due to the inability to function as a result of opacities in the eye (usually congenital), or it can be due to displacement of the eye muscles on the globe or disturbed muscle function (Plate 9.1), muscle trauma (secondary to luxation of the globe), or muscle degeneration. In the latter form, the globes can follow each other at a fixed angle of squinting in all directions (concomitant strabismus), or the angle can vary (paralytic) depending on the direction in which the eyes are looking.

Convergent or divergent strabismus in animals is rare. In dogs, strabismus may be due to atrophic degeneration of the straight eye muscles (Plate 9.2). Only in Siamese cats does concomitant strabismus with convergent axes (esotropia) occur with some frequency (Plate 9.1). It can be associated with a fluttering nystagmus. This convergent strabismus is an inherited disorder, probably recessive, which is often encountered in the Siamese and very rarely in other cats. It is associated with an abnormal crossover pattern in the nerve pathways in the Siamese. Cats with this abnormality show no obvious visual problems (e.g. in catching birds or mice), but it must be assumed that their stereoscopic vision is distorted.

Surgical replacement, shortening, or cutting of the abnormal eye muscle(s) in the Siamese is contraindicated, but in other animals it can be beneficial, although recurrence is certainly possible.[3]

Divergent strabismus secondary to luxation of the globe is usually due to a partial or total rupturing of the medial straight muscle from the globe. If some muscle fibers are still in contact with the globe, there may be spontaneous restoration of the normal position after a period of 6–8 weeks. If all the fibers have been torn, the muscle will retract deep into the orbit and lose all contact with the globe, which will result in a permanent divergent strabismus (see 4.2). This situation is frequently found in Pekingese after luxation of the globe.

9.6 Nystagmus

Nystagmus is involuntary, rhythmic movements of the eye. The movements can be pendular, jerky, rotary, or fluttering. The jerky movements are usually due to a vestibular disturbance in which the slow component is the corrective movement. Because the fast movement is recognized more easily, it is used to name the nystagmus. Fluttering or flickering movements are sometimes seen in Siamese cats with strabismus. If the cat fixes its sight on an object, the nystagmus disappears. This form of nystagmus does not appear to cause problems in affected cats.

Pendular, jerky, or rotary nystagmus can sometimes be seen as a secondary sign in severe congenital eye disorders in which the patient is blind and has, therefore, not learned to fix the eyes. In such cases, the prognosis depends on the severity of the other congenital abnormalities present.

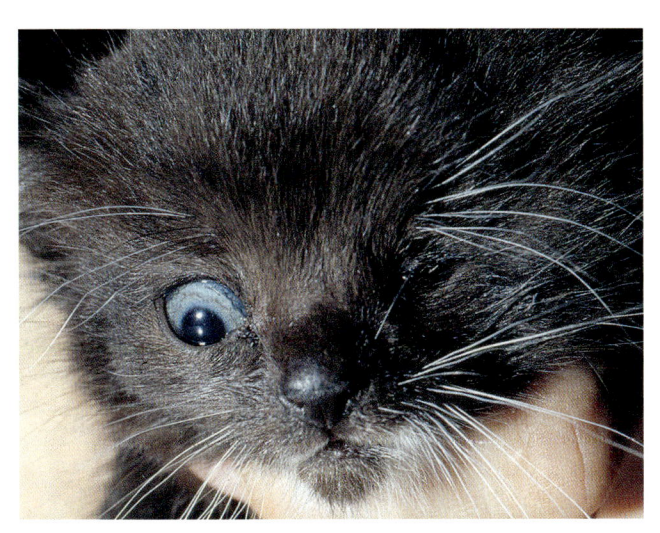

Plate 9.3:
Anophthalmia in a 3-week-old kitten.

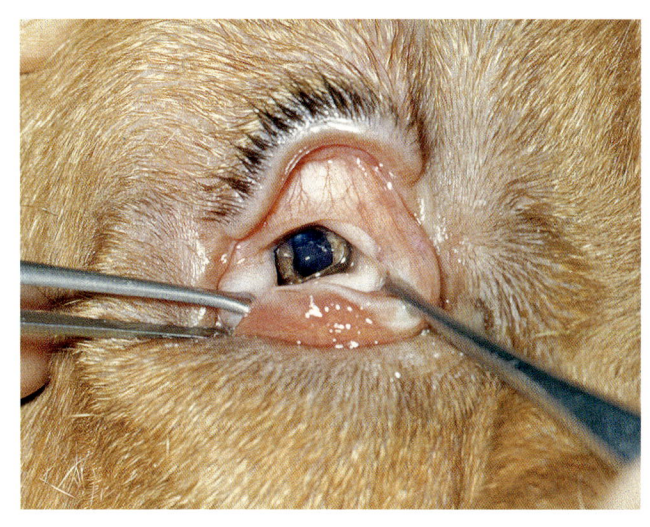

Plate 9.4:
Microphthalmos in a 6-month-old Bloodhound (OD). The diameter of the entire bulbus was only 11 mm.

A rare form of nystagmus is found in photoreceptor dysplasia in the Abyssinian cat (see 14.9).

An acquired nystagmus often originates from the organs of balance or is the result of trauma.

9.7 Anophthalmia, cyclopia, microphthalmia

The congenital absence of one eye (anophthalmia; Plate 9.3), a single centrally-located eye (cyclopia), or a congenitally small eye (microphthalmia; Plate 9.4) can be the result of a chance congenital accident, e.g. a prenatal infection.[4] Usually, however, these abnormalities are the result of a (presumably recessive) hereditary defect.[5] They often occur in combination with other developmental disorders such as palpebral aplasia, iris coloboma, persistent pupillary membrane, persistent hyperplastic tunica vasculosa lentis, cataract, and retinal dysplasia.[6] Recently a marker for microphthalmia has been found in Texelaar sheep.*

Diagnosis: The diagnosis of unilateral microphthalmia is usually not difficult, but when there is doubt, the corneal diameters (mediolateral limbus) can be measured and compared. When bilateral microphthalmia is suspected, the corneal diameters must be compared with those of the animal's littermates. At 7 weeks of age, the corneal diameter is about 7–10 mm in both the dog and cat. If the diagnosis is uncertain, the measurement should be repeated when the head is well-developed and the diameter of the cornea can be compared with the normal diameter of an adult animal of the same breed. In cases of confirmed or suspected microphthalmia, a complete examination of the eye should be carried out because of the probability of other developmental disorders. The littermates and parents should also be examined.

Therapy: There is no effective treatment for any of these disorders. If the eyelids lose their support from the globe and secondary entropion develops, it must be corrected surgically. If the lids and globe cause continuing irritation to the animal, enucleation is indicated (see 5.6).

Prognosis / prevention: The prognosis must be based on the other abnormalities that are present. Eyes with pronounced microphthalmia sometimes appear to have normal visual ability. Close relatives should be examined for the anomaly. Affected animals and their close relatives should not be used for breeding.

9.8 Phthisis bulbi

Phthisis bulbi refers to a shrunken, blind globe as the result of severe damage to the ciliary body, usually caused by post-traumatic or primary uveitis. The aqueous humor production is inadequate and the normal tension of the eye cannot be maintained. If inadequate pressure (usually <10 mm Hg) persists for months, the eye gradually becomes smaller.

Therapy and prognosis: Treatment is the same as for microphthalmia. If the lids and globe cause continuing irritation to the animal, enucleation is indicated (see 5.6).

---
* Marker test for microphthalmia in Texelaar scheep. Ovita® Limited, Dunedin, New Zealand.

9.9 Macrophthalmia

Macrophthalmos is a congenitally large eye, usually as a result of a chance congenital error, and is very rare.

If young birds are held in continuous light or dark, the globe may enlarge.

Therapy: There is no effective treatment for this disorder. If the globe is non-functional and a discomfort to the patient, enucleation will be beneficial.

9.10 Buphthalmos / hydrophthalmia

Buphthalmos (Gr: ox eye; every enlarged globe) or hydrophthalmos (Gr: water; enlarged by water) is an enlarged globe as the result of a continuous (one week, but usually weeks), elevated intraocular pressure (IOP). Enlargement of the globe, in exceptional cases, can also occur as the result of an intraocular neoplasm that fills the eye. Glaucoma can be primary or it can be the result of processes that close off the drainage angle, such as lens luxation, uveitis, or intraocular neoplasms (see relevant sections).

Symptoms: The globe is enlarged. If there is uncertainty, the globe should be compared to the other eye or ultrasonography should be performed. In general, the cornea will be stretched and show edema. If the IOP continues for a longer period of time, tearing of the Descemet's membrane and endothelium will develop. Water enters through these defects to the stroma, resulting in irregular lines of edema. When the IOP declines to normal, the endothelial cells will repair the defect. Sharp white lines (like cracks in ice) remain and are known as striae of Haab (Plate 11.7).

Neoplasia may be recognized in the anterior chamber or deeper in the eye. Ultrasonography, CT or MRI are important diagnostic instruments.

Diagnosis: Diagnosis is based on clinical signs, ultrasonography, CT and MRI.

Therapy: If the eye is non-functional and the globe is a discomfort to the patient (less active patient), enucleation will be very beneficial, even if bilateral enucleation is necessary (see 5.6). An alternative is the use of an intrascleral prosthesis, which has a better cosmetic effect but is not in the interest of the animal and is a risk for the patient that is ethically not outweighed by the cosmetic appeal to the owner (see also 5.7).

9.11 Endophthalmitis, panophthalmitis

Endophthalmitis is an inflammation of all the tissues lying within the globe, while panophthalmitis is an inflammation of all the tissues of the globe, usually resulting from trauma or an infection (see 12.10).

Literature

1. BOROFFKA, S.A.E.B.: Ultrasonographic evaluation of pre- and postnatal development of the eyes in beagles. Vet. Radiol. & Ultrasound **46**: 22, 2005.

2. BAYER, J.: Augenheilkunde, Braumüller, Wien, 1914.

3. GELATT, K.N. & MCCLURE, J.R.: Congenital strabismus and its correction in two Appaloosa horses. J. Equine Med. Surg. **3**: 240, 1979.

4. GELATT, K.N., PEIFFER, R.L. & WILLIAM, L.W.: Anophthalmia / Microphthalmia. In: Spontaneous Animal Models of Human Disease. Vol. 1. Eds.: E.J. Andrews, B.C. Ward & N.H. Altmann, New York, Academic Press, 145, 1979.

5. GELATT, K.N., POWELL, N.G. & HUSTON, K.: Inheritance of microphthalmia with coloboma in the Australian Shepherd dog. Am. J. Vet. Res. **42**: 1686, 1981.

6. PEIFFER, R.L. & FISCHER, C.A.: Microphthalmia, retinal dysplasia and anterior segment dysgenesis in a litter of Dobermann Pinchers. JAVMA **183**: 875, 1983.

10 Cornea and Sclera

10.1 Introduction

The cornea covered with the tear film forms a window through which light enters the globe. The cornea is about 0.6–0.8 mm thick and consists of 4 layers (Fig. 10.1).[1] The epithelium which forms the outer layers is 7–12 cells thick in the center and slightly thinner at the periphery where it merges with the conjunctival epithelium. Its basal cell layer consists of continuously dividing cuboidal epithelial cells. As the cells mature and progress to the surface (about 7 days), they become progressively flatter.[2] The outermost cells of the epithelium are large, flat, polygonal cells with microvilli. The mucus layer of the tear film is firmly attached to these cells. Vitamins A and C are important for the intercellular cement.[3] The basal cell layer is separated from the stroma by a thin basement membrane that is attached to the basal cell layer by hemidesmosomes.

The stroma constitutes about 90% of the thickness of the cornea. It consists of bundles of collagen fibers, fibroblasts, and cement substance. The fibers lie precisely parallel within the bundles, while the bundles themselves crisscross each other. Posterior to the stroma lies the elastic membrane of Descemet (posterior limiting membrane). The inner side of the cornea is covered by a single layer of cells which, because of its endothelial properties, is called the corneal endothelium.

The cornea is provided with a network of nerves (nonmyelinated, sensory branches from the long ciliary nerve, which is a branch of the ophthalmic division of the trigeminal nerve) that pass into the stroma from the sclera. Small branches, having neither a myelin sheath nor Schwann cells, penetrate between the epithelial cells.

The shape of the limbus in most animals is circular to horizontally oval as observed in ungulates. In horses, the perilimbal cornea frequently appears white; some authors attribute this to the pectinate ligament/trabecular system not being totally covered by the sclera. The opaque sclera (tunica fibrosa), which is white except for a slight pigmentation in the limbal area, forms the rest of the outer tunica of the eye. The sclera is thickest (1.5 mm) in the area of the venous plexus, 3–10 mm behind the limbus, and is thinnest (0.2 mm) at the equator, becoming thicker again as it approaches the exit of the optic nerve.

In order to function as a window and as part of a strongly refractive medium, the cornea must be transparent. It is clear because of the regularity of the collagen fibrils of the stroma at about 81% hydration, and its avascularity. A stable hydration of the cornea is maintained mainly by a pumping mechanism in the endothelium. The cornea is still relatively "dehydrated"; when the endothelium is damaged the cornea takes up a great amount of water, which increases its thickness 3–4 times. When there is epithelial damage, the thickness may double and the edema is restricted to that area. The uptake of water also distorts the regularity of the fibrils, resulting in a cloudy cornea. Some parts take up more water than others, resulting in irregular cloudiness and a somewhat undulating surface. Because of the avascularity of the cornea, the delivery of nutrients and removal of wastes take place at the limbus and via the tear film and aqueous fluid.

Corneal reactions, reaction patterns, and symptoms

10.1.1 Symptoms of corneal disease
(Plates 10.1–10.34)

Pain and photophobia: Pain can be caused by stimulation (mechanical or light or other radiation) of nerve endings, which are mainly located in the superficial layers of the cornea. Consequently, pain is generally greater with superficial than with deep disease processes affecting the cornea. Stimulation of the cornea is often increased by the blinking mechanism of the lids when there are defects in the surface. Irritation of the nerve endings can also result in reflex hyperemia, transudation from the iris, and a very painful spasm of the ciliary muscle.

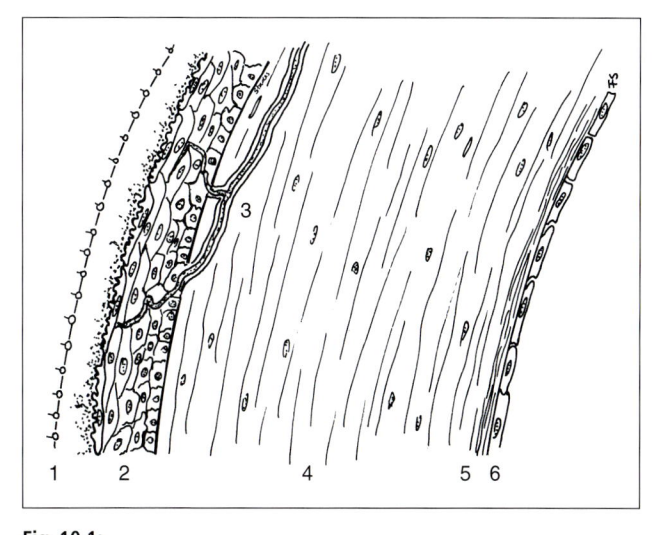

Fig. 10.1:
Section of the tear film (1) and cornea, (2) epithelium, (3) nerve, (4) stroma, (5) Descemet's membrane, (6) endothelium.

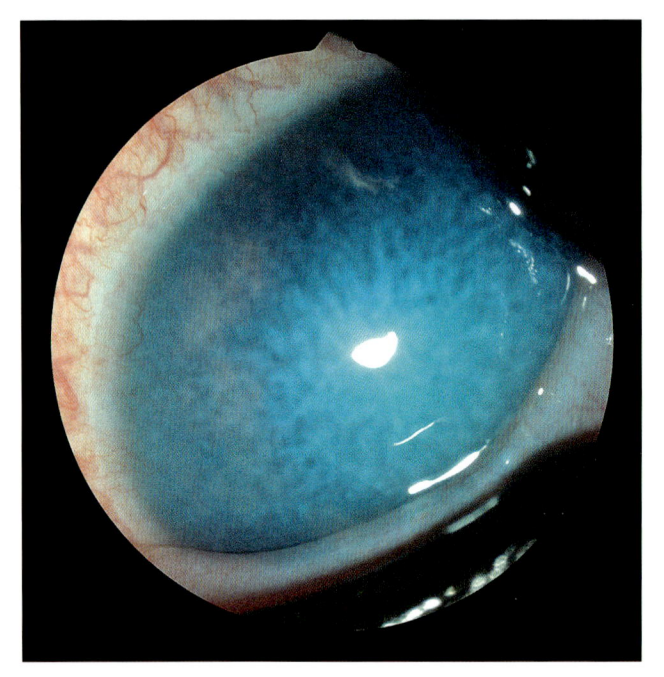

Plate 10.1:
Corneal edema (OD, dog). Diffuse, blue-white, in an island pattern, due to disruption of the geometric structure and the irregular leakage of water into the cornea.

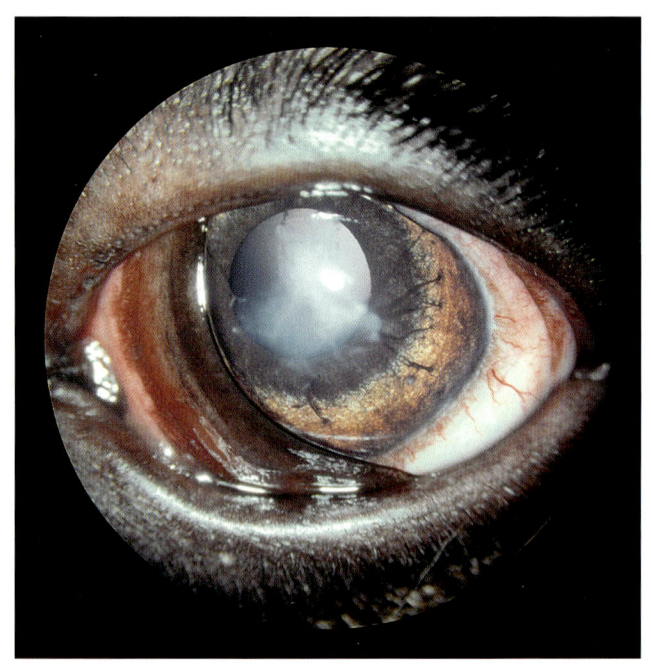

Plate 10.2:
Dense white scar due to a persistent pupillary membrane (OS, dog). The strands are attached to the corneal endothelium, causing an area of dense white tissue that has the appearance of the animal's own sclera.

- ■ **Excessive lacrimation:** The production of tears is reflectorily stimulated by irritation of the cornea.
- ■ **Blue-white opacities:**
  - **Bluish-white, irregular, variably opaque "island pattern":** characteristic for edema. In dysfunction of or damage to either the epithelium or the endothelium, the cornea takes up water and becomes edematous (Plate 10.1). Edema leads to an irregular thickening of the cornea, and as a result the reflected image on the cornea (e.g. of the window or examination lamp) is slightly deformed, although the contour on the overlying tear film remains sharp.
  - **Irregular bluish-white lines (like cracks in ice;** Plate 11.7): characteristic for tearing of the Descemet's membrane (Striae of Haab). During enlargement of the globe (buphthalmos), the Descemet's membrane can be torn and the underlying endothelium damaged. Water enters through the defect, resulting in lines of edema. After normalization of the IOP, the endothelial cells expand and repair the defect. The elasticity of Descemet's membrane results in "recoil" and in the scars, which are referred to as "striae".
  - **White-blue band-like streaks** in the cornea in horses: possibly because of a thinning of the Descemet's membrane of unknown cause.[4]
  - **Dense white or opaque** like fibrous tissue and therefore closely resembling the structure of the sclera (Plate 10.2): characteristic of scar formation. After a deep defect is filled by granulation tissue, a scar is formed (cicatrization).
  - **Glittering white, crystal-like or angel's hair-like structures:** characteristic for precipitates (Plates 10.26–10.31) of cholesterol, calcium, proteins, or polysaccharides in the superficial or deeper layers of the cornea (see 10.7).

- **Corneal defects staining with fluorescein:** edema develops at the periphery of superficial defects. The defect will be stained by fluorescein which can penetrate into and between the damaged epithelial and stromal cells (Plates 10.9–10.11). Descemet's membrane is a lipid-rich (hydrophobic) structure which will not stain with fluorescein. The neurologic effects of corneal damage include reflex hyperemia and transudation from the iris, and a spasm of the ciliary muscles.
  - **Irregular rounded to oval fluorescein staining, frayed epithelial defects** with undermined edges: characteristic for ulcers (Plate 10.9, 10.10). This is a more specific defect involving loss of substance of the cornea. There are often frayed, irregular edges that are undermined.
- **Yellow-green discoloration:** inflammatory cell infiltration of the stroma may color the cornea yellowish to green, especially in horses. If the area is also swollen, there may be bacterial proteolytic enzymes active, resulting in melting of the stroma (see 10.6.3.2).
- **Grayish-white dots:** characteristic for an exudate of fibrin and leucocyte aggregations clotted against the endothelium (keratitic precipitates) (see 12.10; Plate 12.5).
- **Grayish-white, granular cloudiness** only visible with a slit-lamp microscope at higher magnifications: typical for infiltrates of leukocytes penetrating the cornea.
- **Vascularization:** superficial or deep vessels can grow into the cornea (about 1 mm/day maximum). Superficial vessels are usually more undulating and branched, and are joined to the conjunctival vascular system. Deep vessels are straighter and at the limbus, they disappear under the sclera in the direction of the uvea (Plates 10.3, 10.8, 11.5).
- **Pannus:** This is cellular and fibrovascular subepithelial tissue that infiltrates the cornea from the limbus, while the surface remains intact (see also 10.6.1, 10.6.2; Plates 10.5, 10.6).
- **Granulation:** This term is used to describe newly formed (usually fluorescein-negative) fibrovascular tissue that is pinkish-red and slightly vesicular (Plate 10.3). It is formed to fill deeper defects but also superficial defects under the influence of chronic stimulation, such as entropion or infection.
- **Pigmentation:** Some superficial pigmentation can develop during chronic irritation or after repair of defects by granulation or scar formation. This pigment migrates along the course of vascular ingrowth and arises from the melanocytes at the limbus.

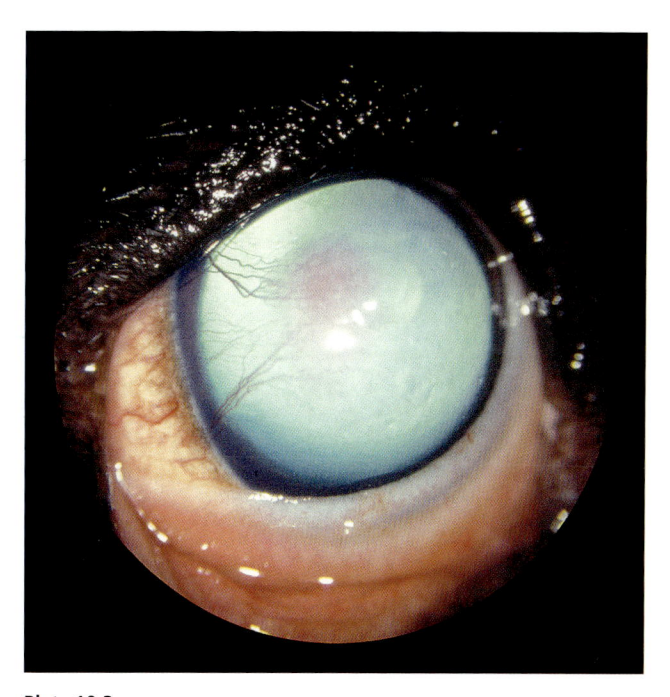

Plate 10.3:
Vessel ingrowth (superficial) ending in granulation, as a result of reparation of a corneal defect (OD, dog).

- **Black-brown, smooth, shiny, circumscript "plaque":** In cats, superficial parts of the cornea can become sequestered (see 10.6.4; Plates 10.22–10.24). Also, foreign bodies (dark plant material, especially bud leaves) may look similar (see 4.5.3).
- **Keratoconus:** Thinning and weakening of the central part of the cornea can result in it becoming conical. The cornea can also become conical if local dense edema develops.
- **Corneal irritation reactions:** In general, if irritated chronically, the cornea will react with edema, vascularisation, and pigmentation (low in cat), as well as epithelial keratinization, resulting in a "skin-like" appearance. In acute and more severe irritation, the cornea lacks the time to adapt, resulting in loss of tissue, such as ulceration.

10.1.2 Localization and causes of corneal abnormalities

The localization of a corneal abnormality (Fig. 10.2) often gives an indication of where to look for a cause, as follows:
- **Peripheral-medial** can indicate such causes as medial entropion, nasal fold trichiasis, abnormalities of the nictitating membrane, or a foreign body behind the nictitating membrane.
- **Peripheral-dorsolateral:** can indicate such causes as palpebral aplasia, distichiasis, ectopic cilia, or ptosis / trichiasis / entropion of the upper eyelid.
- **Peripheral-ventrolateral** can indicate such causes as abnormalities of the lateral canthus, entropion, distichiasis, or a foreign body in the conjunctival sac.
- **Central** can indicate such causes as a foreign body, burns, or drying due to paralysis of the eyelids or KCS.
- **Involvement of the entire cornea** can indicate such causes as burns, infections, KCS, or processes in the cornea such as deposition of cholesterol, or processes in the eyeball such as glaucoma and iritis.

10.1.3 Corneal regeneration

- **Superficial defects:** In very superficial defects of the cornea, such as a scratch by a grain of sand, there is excessive tear production, slight edema, and pain. The superficial epithelial cells become flattened and slide and migrate over the defect. After 8–10 hours the defect is covered. It can then no longer be demonstrated by fluorescein staining and infectious agents can no longer penetrate easily. The pain and edema also disappear. Within a few days, the epithelium returns to its original thickness by the outwards progression of epithelial cells produced by the basal cell layer. Within a week, the cornea is completely healed, without any scar formation.
- **Moderately deep defects:** In moderately deep defects, to about 1/3 of the thickness of the cornea (Fig. 10.3), the signs are somewhat more severe but the healing process is essentially the same as that for very superficial defects. The defect in the basal cell layer is, however, filled by mitotic reproduction of the epithelial basal cells from the edges of the defect. The cornea becomes fully transparent again but a scar remains visible microscopically as a very shallow dip of irregularly positioned basal cells.
- **Deep defects:** In deeper defects, edema is especially prominent. Within a few hours, the defect is covered with a gray layer of leucocytes mainly from the perilimbal vascular arcade and delivered via the tear film. The epithelial cells of the wound edges attempt to cover the defect, resulting in rounding off of the edges. The epithelialization alone is, however, insufficient to fill the deep defect. Superficial vessels grow out to the defect from the closest part of the limbus. Thus the defect becomes filled from the bottom up, with pinkish-red, vesicular, fibroangioblastic tissue (Plate 10.3). After the cicatrization phase, a white scar remains.
- **Descemetocele / Descemetal hernia:** In defects extending to Descemet's membrane, the bottom of the defect will not be edematous and will not stain with fluorescein (Plates 10.12, 10.14). Thus, an edematous area in the cornea with a clear center indicates that only Descemet's membrane and the endothelium of the cornea protect against perforation. If the membrane becomes thinner or the pressure in the eye increases, the membrane bulges out to form a hernia (descemetocele) which makes the crater look less deep. Very slight trauma, even manual measurement of the pressure in the eye, will then be enough to cause perforation.
- **Perforation:** If the cornea is perforated, the aqueous humor escapes through the opening. It coagulates within a short time and thus closes the opening. If the defect is larger, a piece of the iris usually lodges in the opening and closes it (staphyloma; Plates 4.19, 10.15). The piece of iris becomes covered with exudate and later with epithelium. Fibroangioblastic tissue forms directly via the vessels of the iris and eventually also from vessels growing in from the limbus, and this closes the perforation. The end result is a corneal scar that is adherent to the iris (anterior synechia, adherent leukoma).

The regeneration of the cornea only proceeds optimally if nutritionally complete food is provided. Among other factors, vitamins A and C play important roles in the growth of keratocytes.

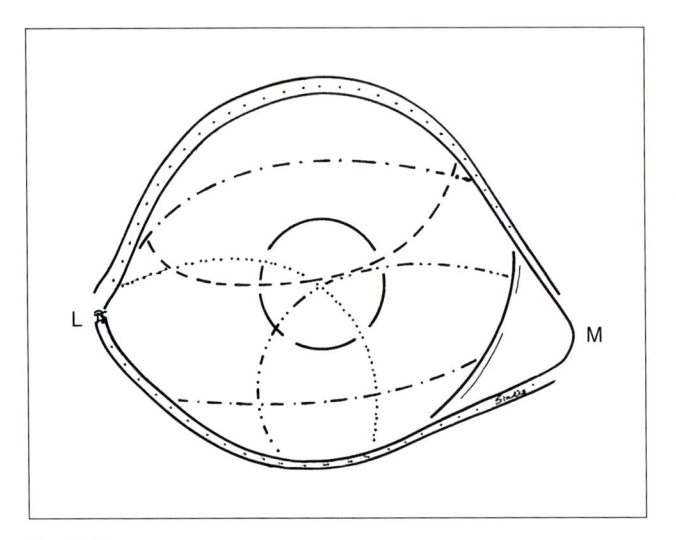

Fig. 10.2:
Locations of corneal entities often betray the cause or the location of the abnormality. Medioventral area (– ·· line, e.g. irritation due to med. entropion/nasal fold); central area (between both – – lines, e.g. sicca syndrome); peripheral-dorsolateral (dorsal of – – line, e.g. trichiasis upper lid ulcer); peripheral (· ·· line, e.g., lower lid entropion).

10.1.4 Retardation of healing

Morphologic changes in the basal lamina and especially a lower number of hemidesmosome anchorages are possibly responsible for indolent corneal ulceration in the dog (see 10.6.3).

Caution: Regeneration is retarded by mechanical irritants such as hairs, follicles, scars, exudates, dust, sand, microorganisms, lytic enzymes, materials with a non-physiologic pH or osmotic tensions, and some medications and diagnostic agents. Certain antibiotics, such as ciprofloxacin, cause a distinct retardation of corneal epithelial growth in vitro, while polymyxin, neomycin und gentamycin induce a moderate retardation, and chloramphenicol a mild one.[5] In particular, the use of corticosteroids and local anesthetics must be considered with great care, for both cause a definite retardation of epithelialization. Corticosteroids also have a retarding effect on vascularization, the transport of inflammatory cells, fibroblastic activity, and the mechanisms of resistance against infections in general. In addition, they cause a reduction in the firmness of the healed tissue. Corticosteroids also increase the activity of the collagenases released by damage to keratocytes, such as occurs in ulcers; therefore, corticosteroids should be used only if these retarding effects are particularly desired, the side effects are weighed against the advantages, and the side effects prevented if possible.

Local anesthetics not only retard epithelialization but also reduce the lid closure reflex and can cause a very painful hypersensitivity (dolorific or painful neuritis); therefore, they should be used only for diagnostic purposes.

10.2 Microcornea

Microcornea, which is a cornea of too small a diameter, occurs almost exclusively in microphthalmia (see 9.7).

10.3 Persistent pupillary membrane (PPM)

If remnants of the embryonal pupillary or epipupillary membrane adhere to the endothelium of the cornea and are not absorbed, they will lead to scars on the inner side of the cornea (Plates 4.18, 10.2, 12.1, 12.2). This material is usually dense and white, comparable to scleral tissue or boiled egg-white. There may also be threads of tissue between the scar and the iris (1–2 mm outside the edge of the pupil). During changes in the size of the pupil, these can cause traction on the endothelium. The traction and scar influence the normal functioning of the endothelium, resulting in local edema of the overlying cornea. Often, patients with these problems are presented because of corneal cloudiness, which the history suggests has been caused by trauma during the period before weaning. Tissue threads, often still visible from the periphery and seen to extend to the surface of the iris (to the collarette), are indicative of PPM. In the differential diagnosis, PPM can occasionally be confused with an acquired anterior synechia after a local penetrating trauma. In contrast, inflammatory strands usually arise from the pupillary margin, and in the cornea the overlying corneal layers show scar tissue (see 12.2).

10.4 Dermoid

A dermoid is an ectopic piece of skin on the cornea or conjunctiva, sometimes extending to the eyelids (see 7.4). In the Wire-haired Dachshund this defect is possibly inherited recessively. In other breeds of dogs and in cats, it is not yet certain whether there are hereditary factors involved.

Dermoids are usually located at the limbus (Plate 10.4), partly on the cornea and partly on the conjunctiva, and in rare cases they can extend into the skin of the eyelid. The hairs are almost always pointed towards the center of the cornea. The more they grow, the more they irritate the cornea. This results in a zone of edema progressing towards the center, followed by

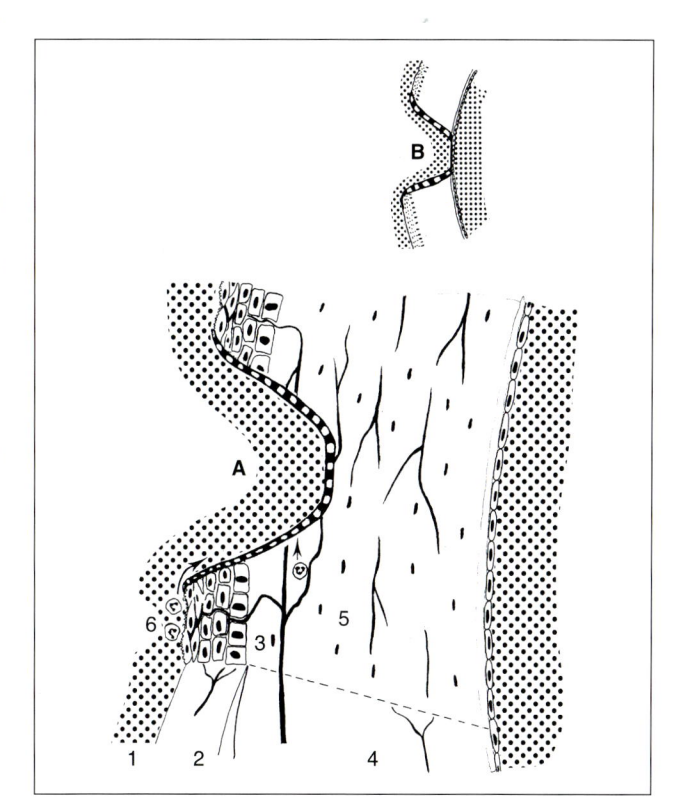

Fig. 10.3:
Section of a corneal defect deeper than approximately 1/3 of the thickness of the cornea (A) and a defect up to the Descemet's membrane (B), which itself does not stain with fluorescein. (1) Tear film, (2) scleral conjunctiva, (3) epithelium, (4) sclera, (5) stroma, (6) leucocytes. ⊙ leucocytes ▬ fluorescein

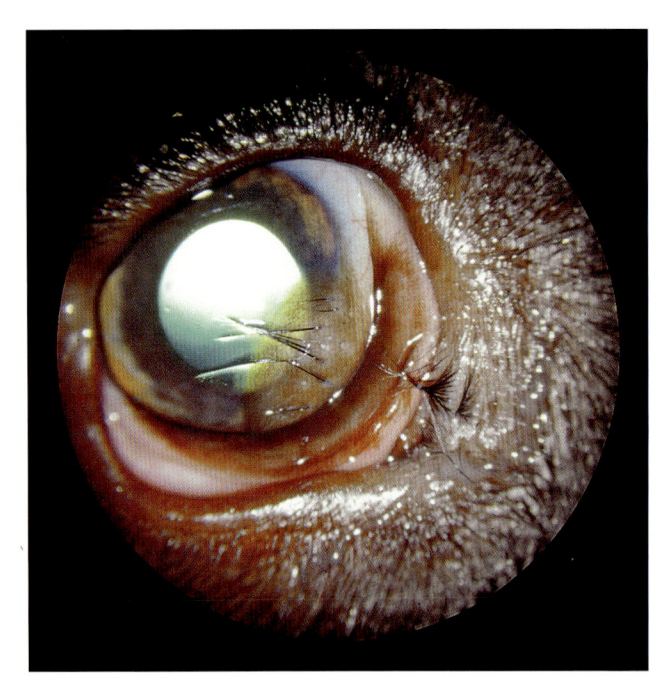

Plate 10.4:
Dermoid at the limbus in a puppy (OD, dog). Irritating hairs have caused an area of corneal pigmentation and edema.

pigmentation of the cornea. There is also epiphora, slight blepharospasm, and slight conjunctival hyperemia.

Therapy: Treatment consists of a very precise keratectomy with a rounded diamond scalpel, beginning at the center and removing the dermoid and the most superficial layers of epithelium (superficial keratectomy). Magnification of x5–10 is necessary to be certain that no hair follicles remain and that the cornea is not incised too deeply. The appropriate anesthesia must be used, i.e. inhalation anesthesia in combination with a muscle relaxant (e.g. (cis)atracurium or norcuronium) to prevent rotation and enophthalmos, but this also necessitates artificial respiration (see 3.3.1).

The operation should preferably not be performed before the 12th week of life (better liver function, thus less anesthesia risk). If the veterinarian lacks the necessary facilities or experience in these very young animals, the patient should be referred. Before surgery, the cornea is protected by a neutral oil or ointment, such as one containing vitamin A.

Treatment following surgery consists of prophylactic "initial choice" antibiotic ointment, 4 times daily. Corticosteroids may be added later to suppress excessive granulation during healing.

Prognosis / prevention: The prognosis is good. The parents and littermates should be examined. Affected animals and, ideally, members of the immediate family should be excluded from breeding (see 15).

10.5 Trauma

(See 4, Ocular Emergencies)

10.6 Keratitis

The outer cornea and conjunctiva are continuously exposed not only to noxious materials such as wind, dust, and microorganisms, but also to other sources of irritation such as hairs of the animal itself (e.g. trichiasis, entropion, distichiasis), especially in dogs. This type of problem often provides the port of entry for other factors (e.g. bacteria or fungi) to colonize and cause disease. Iatrogenic problems can also develop as a result of surgical trauma or the use or misuse of medication.

Keratitis can arise not only from primary corneal or corneal-conjunctival problems, but is often secondary to such causes as irritation by hairs, a foreign body, insufficient tear production, glaucoma, or iritis.

Note: It is of great importance to differentiate the many forms of "keratitis", because the management of the disease demands identification of the underlying cause(s); alas, the etiology can not always be clarified.

In a number of patients, there is no indication of the cause of secondary keratitis, and in addition it is also not possible to be always definite about the local cause of a keratitis. One can then only determine whether the process is superficial keratitis or deep (interstitial / profunda) keratitis, and whether the keratitis is associated with a more or less definite increase in tissue (granulation, pannus) or with loss of tissue (ulceration); the fluorescein staining test is most helpful in this determination. On the basis of such immediately apparent characteristics, the following clinically relevant forms of keratitis can be differentiated:

10.6.1 Superficial keratitis (without ulceration)

Superficial keratitis is characterized by edema, superficial ingrowth of vessels, granulation, scar formation, and finally pigmentation. Many microorganisms (viruses, bacteria, fungi, yeasts, mycoplasmas) can cause such a form of keratitis. The

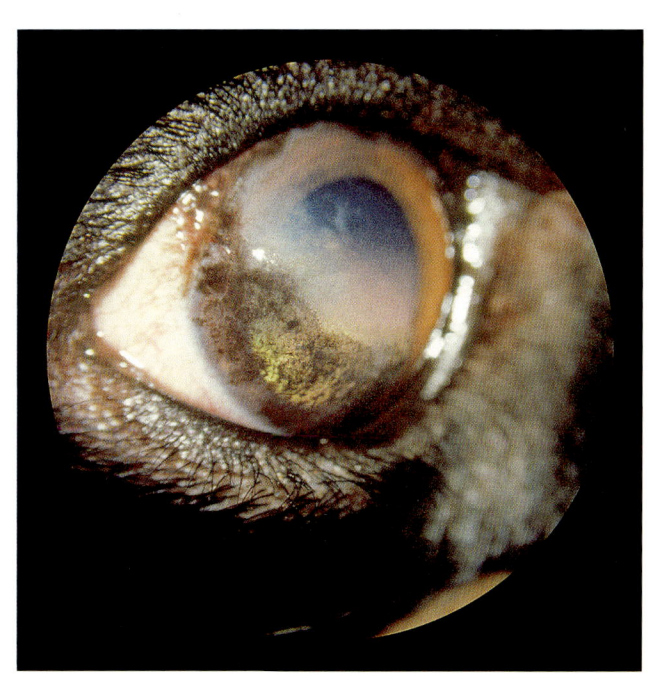

Plate 10.5:
Pannus at the limbus of the right eye of a German Shepherd. Vessel ingrowth and edema, followed by pigmentation, are more prominent in this active case.

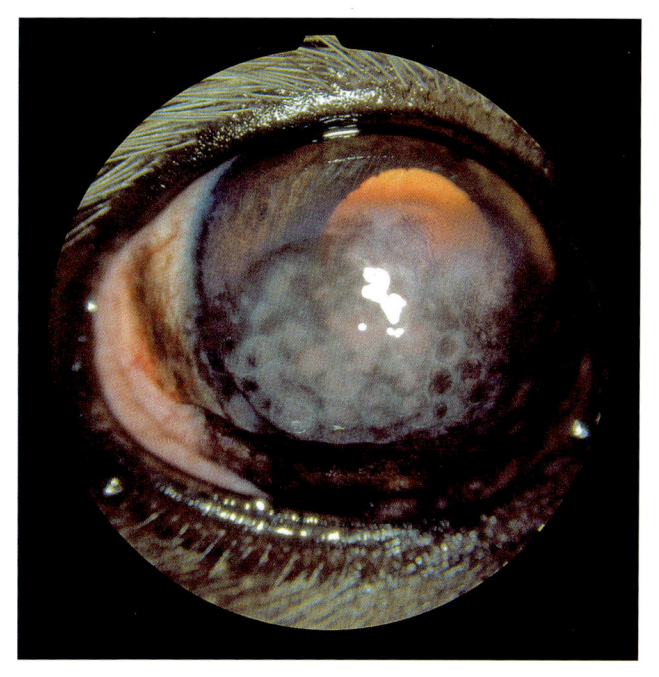

Plate 10.6:
Pannus at the limbus of the right eye of a German Shepherd. In this case, the edema, granulation and pigmentation are more prominent.

most important causes in cats are the etiologic agents of the "upper respiratory disease complex". Autoimmune-related causes are also possible. In some cases there is mainly granulation, with remarkable numbers of plasma cells (see 10.6.1.1) or with many eosinophils (see 10.6.1.2). Superficial keratitis is often seen in dogs and cats and can occur unilaterally or bilaterally.

> Keratitis is often associated with handling or caging, lid margin abnormalities, trauma or foreign bodies in birds.

Diagnosis: The diagnosis is made primarily on the basis of the history and by exclusion. An attempt at a more specific diagnosis can be made by means of microbiologic or histologic examination.

Therapy: Treatment is symptomatic and consists of an "initial choice" antibiotic ointment 4–6 times daily and a corticosteroid ointment 2–4 times daily (provided that the cornea is fluorescein negative) for about 10 days. The corticosteroid therapy can then be decreased gradually. There should be a definite improvement within 2–4 days after the start of treatment. If there is no improvement, the examination should be repeated and extended, or the patient should be referred.

Prognosis: The prognosis is guarded. It is often possible to do no more than arrest the process, particularly if the abnormalities have developed during or just following an upper respiratory tract infection and are associated with symblepharon formation (see 8.14.1).

10.6.1.1 Chronic superficial keratitis (Überreiter)/ pannus/keratitis pannosa/photoallergic keratitis/vascular and pigmentary keratitis/ German Shepherd dog keratitis[6]

This is a chronic, superficial, proliferative immune-mediated keratitis that is activated by UV light.[7] The bilateral abnormalities almost always start on the lateral side, where the cornea is most exposed to light, and if there is no treatment, the proliferation covers both corneas usually within a year. The abnormality occurs mainly in the German Shepherd dog and the offspring of crossings with this breed, the Belgium Shepherd dog, and in a less severe form in the Long-haired Dachshund. There is almost certainly a hereditary predisposition. Very infrequently, a similar picture is seen in other breeds (Cairn Terrier; Groenendaler; Collies, associated with Collie nose syndrome).

Symptoms: (Plates 10.5, 10.6). Initially, there is a slight superficial corneal opacity along the ventrolateral limbus of both eyes, with slight conjunctival vascular injection and pigmentation. The abnormality can be combined with plasmacellular conjunctivitis (see 8.11.4). The disease is not associated with signs of pain or ocular discharge and fluorescein staining is negative. Superficial corneal vascular injection develops, followed by granulation and pigmentation. If the pannus proceeds very aggressively (excessive exposure to sun in the summer, on water, in snow, or in the mountains), granulation is more severe and pigmentation is less apparent. In the area of granulation, there are bluish-purple foci with many plasma cells. The pannus spreads slowly towards the center of the eye and finally (after 1–2 years) over the entire cornea.

Diagnosis: Diagnosis is made on the basis of the clinical picture. The plasma cells and lymphocytes can be demonstrated by cytologic examination of corneal scrapings.

Therapy: Treatment is based on continual suppression of the inflammatory process. Initially, dexamethasone eye drops are administered 6 times daily and prednisolone ointment at bedtime. Once the cornea is fairly clear, the dose can be reduced to 1 drop 3 times daily, eventually only on alternate days. Cyclosporin 0.2% can also be used.[8] On sunny days or when the dog is on water or in snow, the owner should increase the number of administrations per day. The treatment must be continued life-long. If treatment is stopped, the process will soon recur with greater severity and there will often be a poorer response to therapy. If the dog is presented with severely affected corneas, supportive treatment with subconjunctival administration of a corticosteroid depot preparation should be considered. The time that the dog spends in high-UV (snow, water reflection) environments should be reduced. On sunny days, affected dogs are better kept inside. Avalanche rescue dogs with this disorder are sometimes fitted with highly protective sunglasses. Nowadays, special dog-fitting sunglasses (Cabriobrille® or www.doggles.com) and also dark contact lenses are available. In addition, Vitamin A eye gel/ointments are supposed to give UV-protection. When the abnormalities are very severe, referral for β-irradiation (strontium-90) is possible. Some ophthalmologists advocate the use of superficial keratectomy. This can, however, only be performed once or twice because of the marked thinning of the cornea that results.

Prevention: Affected animals should be eliminated from breeding. When German Shepherd dogs are presented for annual vaccinations, it is advisable to check the lateral limbus area for signs of this disorder.

10.6.1.2 Eosinophilic keratitis

This is a superficial keratitis in the cat in which granulation over the cornea is prominent.[9] The etiology is not known but this disorder may be part of the eosinophilic granuloma complex. It occurs fairly infrequently and can be unilateral or bilateral. A zone of opacity followed by pink granulation tissue invades the superficial layer of the cornea, usually from the lateral side (Plates 10.7, 10.8). Sometimes, the granulation is covered locally by white-yellow necrotic plaques (staining fluorescein positive).

Diagnosis: Diagnosis is made on the basis of the finding of large numbers of eosinophils and mast cells among other inflammatory cells on cytologic or histologic examination, and seldom by the presence of increased circulating eosinophils.

Therapy: Therapy consists of dexamethasone drops (0.1%), 3–6 times daily until the signs disappear, after which maintenance administration to effect is adequate. Treatment with β-irradiation (about 500 rads) or cyclosporin (0.2–2%) is also possible. In addition, megestrol acetate can be used (0.5 mg/kg daily for 3 days, decreasing to the lowest effective frequency), but the progestin and glucocorticoid side effects could lead to more problems than do locally administered corticosteroids.

Prognosis: The prognosis is favorable, even if recurrences have to be repeatedly suppressed.

10.6.2 Deep or interstitial keratitis or keratitis profunda (without defects)

A deep keratitis is characterized by a rapidly progressive dense opacity, superficial and deep ingrowth of vessels, and scar formation.[10] The disorder seldom occurs as a separate entity.

Therapy: If a primary cause cannot be discovered, treatment as for superficial keratitis can be started, but it would be preferable to repeat the diagnostic examinations or to refer the patient for a more definitive diagnosis.

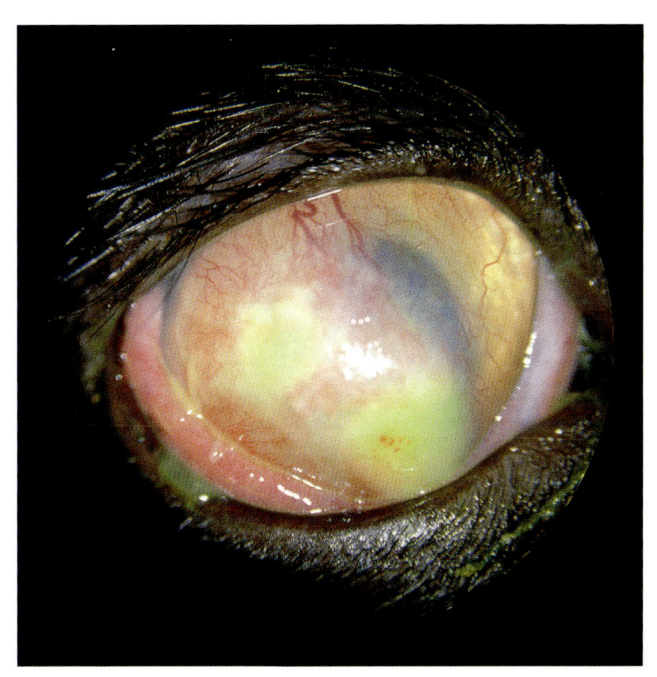

Plate 10.7:
Eosinophilic granuloma in a 5-year-old cat (OS; see also Plate 10.8). Two areas within the granulation are stained with fluorescein. This could lead to the false conclusion that it is a corneal defect.

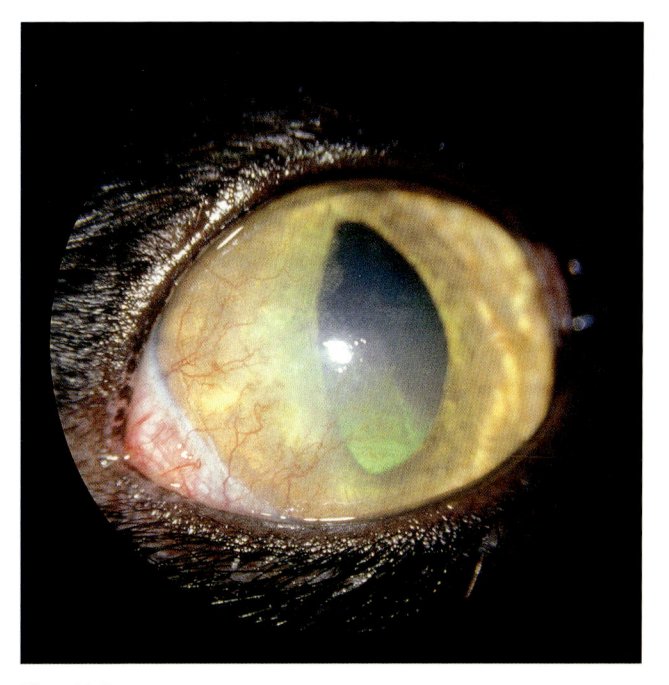

Plate 10.8:
Eosinophilic granuloma in a 5-year-old cat (same eye as in Plate 10.7) after 14 days of treatment with topical dexamethasone 0.1%, 4 times daily.

10.6.3 Ulcerative keratitis

Ulcerative keratitis, or a corneal ulcer, is characterized by superficial or deep erosive processes in the cornea with disruption or loss of tissue (Plates 10.9–10.15).

Clinical differentiation between (1) uncomplicated, circumscript ulcerations, with local, superficial edema and minimal secondary iritis; and (2) deep, complicated ulcers with melting, necrotic, colored edges; generalized, deep edema; and distinct iritis, with or without hypopyon (Plate 10.13) is of great importance.

> Keratitis is often due to handling or caging, lid margin abnormalities, trauma or foreign bodies in birds.

10.6.3.1 Superficial ulcers
Superficial ulcers can have causes such as:
- **mechanical irritation:** own hairs, entropion, distichiasis, ectopic cilia, palpebral aplasia, foreign bodies, trauma.
- **infections:** especially viral, such as the upper respiratory disease complex, and in companion animals and the horse: rare fungi[11]
- **drying out** of the cornea (KCS: large-eyed and short-nosed cats and dogs; atropine treatment and [ketamine] anesthesia).

In ulcers due to the above three causes, the corneal epithelium is damaged and/or infiltrated, and a superficial, fluorescein-positive defect develops. The edges of the defect consist of reasonably healthy tissue and there is a healthy support system. In such processes; the tendency for spontaneous healing is usually high (see 10.1.3). It is usually only necessary to remove the source of irritation and prevent serious secondary infection. Further primary causes should be prevented or treated, and the ciliary spasm suppressed.
- **"degenerative" processes:** such as a degenerative reduced attachment between the basal cells and the basal membrane (rodent ulcer or Boxer ulcer in the Boxer or indolent ulcer in older dogs), or the sequestration tendency in cats (see 10.6.4).[12] Other possible factors in the development of ulcers include reduction in resistance by malignant lymphoma or feline "AIDS", or the suppression of resistance by corticosteroids or local anesthetics. In such processes, the tendency towards healing is much lower, and in order to activate healing the loose or sequestered parts should be removed.

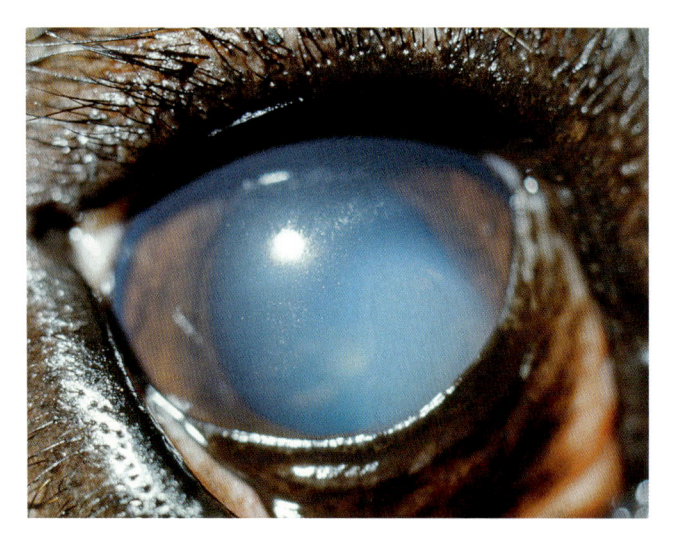

Plate 10.9:
Indolent, superficial corneal ulcer in a Boxer, with an approximately 2-mm undermined edge (OD; see also Plate 10.10).

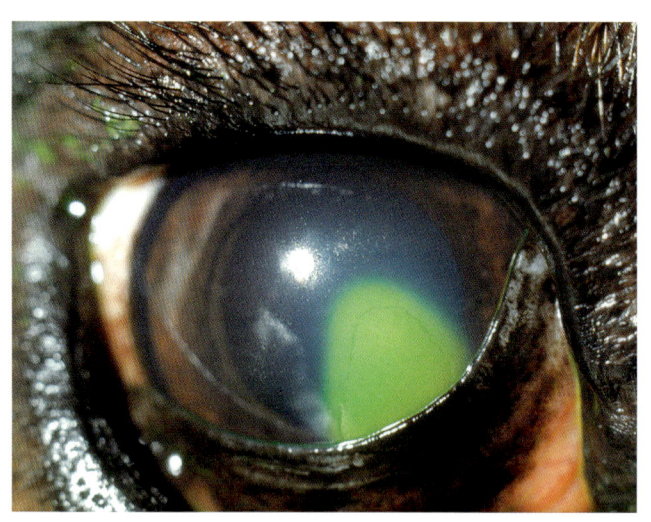

Plate 10.10:
Indolent, superficial corneal ulcer in a Boxer, with an approximately 2-mm undermined edge, now stained by fluorescein (same eye as shown in Plate 10.9). Compare the form of an ulcer to the form of a traumatic defect as shown in Plate 10.11.

Symptoms: (Plates 10.9, 10.10). The signs are blepharospasm, increased tear production (except in KCS), more or less clear mucus discharge, conjunctival hyperemia, and corneal edema. The irregularly circumscribed corneal defect is undermined at the edges, is fluorescein positive, and has no ingrowth of vessels. If the defects are multiple punctae or are dendritic, they are probably a specific form of corneal ulcer, namely keratitis punctata (see 10.6.5). There can be signs of anterior uveitis present at the same time, such as miosis and photophobia.

These superficial ulcers are usually quite indolent. Spontaneous healing mainly occurs only after vessel ingrowth via fibroangioblastic tissue, and this often requires weeks to take place. Secondary infections with protease-producing bacteria can occur and sometimes lead to very aggressive, deep ulcers (see 10.6.3.2).

The differential diagnosis should include corneal defects caused by trauma (often in the form of a scratch [Plate 10.11] or a right angle) or early deep ulcers with soft "melting" edges.

Therapy: The goal of treatment is to eliminate the initial cause, and to potentiate and stimulate spontaneous corneal regeneration, prevent infections, and suppress the ciliary spasm. Since epithelialization is retarded by corticosteroids, and very strongly so by local anesthetics, their use in both superficial and deep ulcers is contraindicated, even though the process appears to be "so nicely calmed down" or the pain (initially) "so nicely killed".

Medical therapy

Therapy is started by eliminating all mechanical factors causing corneal irritation, such as foreign bodies, ectopic cilia, entropion, trichiasis, distichiasis, etc. This is followed by "initial choice" antibiotic ointment 4–6 times daily, vitamin A oil 4 times daily, and 1% atropine (if signs of anterior uveitis are manifest) 2–4 times daily (preferably as an ointment as in liquid form it has shorter contact with the cornea and increases salivation, especially in the cat).

If the ulcer has loose edges, their spontaneous disappearance will be very slow. When there is an obvious indolent ulcer, the edges should be removed and the ulcer activated. If the veterinarian lacks the facilities or experience, the patient should be referred for surgical therapy.

Surgical therapy

Removal of the loose edges and epithelium: The eye is anesthetized locally and animals that are difficult to handle are sedated or anesthetized. After staining the ulcer with fluorescein, the loose portions of the edges and the loose epithelium are curetted away with a curette or a special corneal rust-ring remover (Fig. 10.4 A). Also, a sterile dry cotton applicator can be used to remove the redundant border by rolling the cotton applicator to "lift" the epithelium. The removal is done firmly but gently until the epithelium resists removal. *Caution:* overzealous pressure can also remove too much of the epithelium from a normal cornea, which is not necessary.

Activation: Activation is possible using curettage or phenol, but also direct grid or stab keratotomy or lamellar keratectomy can be performed. These last three methods are disadvantageous in inexperienced hands and in uncooperative patients, due to the risk of deep insults to the cornea or even perforation.

Caution: Activation of the cornea is to be performed only in superficial ulcerations and chronic epithelial erosions. It should never be performed in severely infected, lytic, deeper ulcers. In these cases, a dramatic deterioration of the process is to be expected.

- **Curettage activation**: (Fig. 10.4 A). The ulcer and its edges are curetted firmly, working from the periphery to the center, breaking the basal layer.
- **Phenol activation:** (Fig. 10.4 B). The ulcer, including the edge, is etched by the use of a small cotton swab dipped in a saturated solution of phenol or iodine tincture. Directly after etching, the eye is thoroughly washed with 0.9% NaCl and the medical treatment described above is started.
- **Grid / stab keratotomy activation:** Grid keratotomy (Fig. 10.4 C) is performed with a 0.45-mm cannula attached to a small syringe or held in a Mosquito artery clamp (or by using a diamond knife with depth control) by drawing the needle over the surface of the defect (or stabbing), extending at least one millimeter into the normal epithelium and going all the way across the defect to a similar position on the opposite side. This procedure is continued at one millimeter intervals across the entire lesion and then a second group of similar cuts are made at 90 degrees to the original "scratches". These should remain superficial and just barely visible. Caution: this procedure may induce sequestration in the cat.
- **Keratectomy activation:** The whole ulcer is removed by superficial lamellar keratectomy (using an operation microscope).

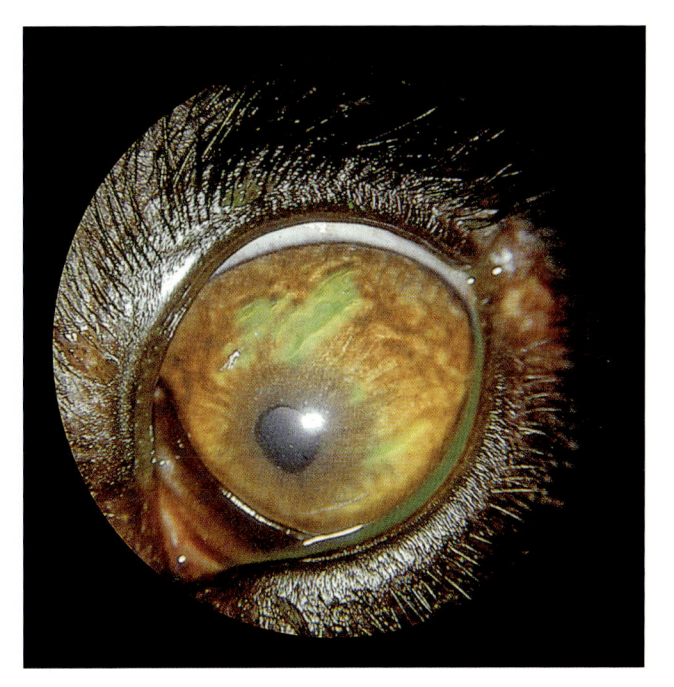

Plate 10.11:
Corneal defect due to scratch trauma (OS, dog). Compare this with the roundness of an ulcer as shown in Plates 10.9 and 10.10.

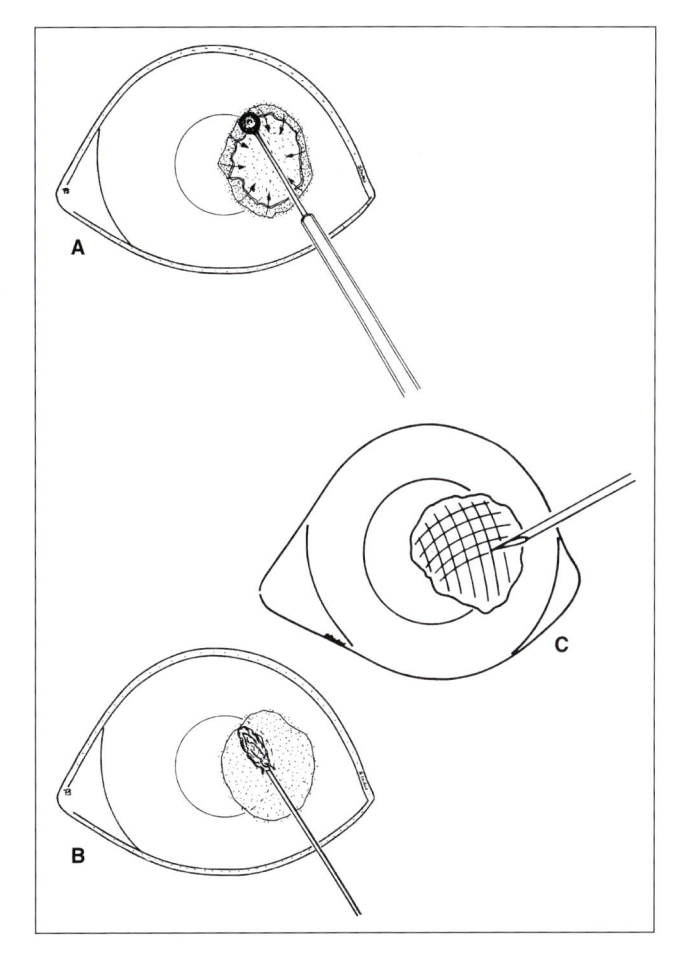

Fig. 10.4:
Curettage (A) and phenol activation (B) or grid-keratotomy activation (C) of an indolent corneal ulcer.

After-care: Medical treatment should be continued for at least 1–3 weeks. At the follow-up examination after about 10 days, fluorescein staining is used to determine whether superficial epithelialization has occurred. There should at least at this time be vessel growth into the cornea in the direction of the ulcer. If the effect is not adequate, the curettage and activation are repeated. When total mydriasis has been induced, the atropine can be stopped. If there is no fluorescein staining, the antibiotic can also be stopped. The vitamin A lubricant is continued for at least 2 weeks longer.

The owner should be instructed to bring the dog promptly for re-examination if the center of the ulcer becomes cloudy or, even worse, clear, or if there is more pain or a definite production of pus (see 10.6.3.2). Clearing from the periphery is a sign of healing. The administration of corticosteroids to suppress scar tissue formation is contraindicated because of the risk of retarding epithelialization and as the tendency to form scars in superficial defects is very small.

If an ulcer shows no sign of healing in spite of repeated removal of loose epithelium and activation, the nictitating membrane can be sutured over the defect, or contact lenses or other conjunctival or corneal covering techniques, or superficial lamellar keratectomy can be used (see 10.6.3.5).

Prognosis / prevention: Uncomplicated defects or ulcers will heal within 8–10 days, after the initial cause is eliminated. Prognosis for indolent ulcers is generally favorable, although complete healing may take 4–6 weeks. The owner should be informed that recurrence can occur in the affected eye or in the opposite eye, since it has been demonstrated that there is a defect in the basement membrane of these animals. After healing, the corneas of both eyes (Boxer, Persian cat) can be protected permanently with neutral, oil-based eye drops, such as vitamin A, administered once daily.

10.6.3.2 Deep ulcers

Deep ulcers are usually the result of a secondary bacterial infection in a defect that is already present (see above), usually in combination with reduced resistance. Bacterial proteases, produced by bacteria such as *Pseudomonas* spp. and hemolytic *Streptococcus* spp., as well as endogenous collagenases, can very rapidly soften and liquefy the stromal proteins. In the Pekingese, nasal fold irritation and lagophthalmos are very often the primary cause. In all short-nosed animals, microtrauma to the less protected exophthalmic eyeballs can also be an important initiating factor. These more complicated ulcers can very rapidly become deeper and wider (Plates 10.12–10.15). The edge of the ulcer softens and swells considerably and acquires a syrupy, yellow-green appearance. Other signs of inflammation, such as blepharospasm, photophobia, episcleral and conjunctival redness and swelling, pain, the production of purulent exudates, and signs of anterior uveitis (hypopyon), increase in severity. Without very rapid intervention, such aggressive ulcers can progress within one or more days to perforation, panophthalmitis, and often to loss of the eye.

Therapy: Treatment for superficial ulcers should be started and the patient referred immediately for further examination and treatment. This will consist of collection of material for culture and antibiotic sensitivity testing, and then treatment 6–8 times daily with acetylcysteine, careful irrigation, and administration of "specific choice" antibiotics, such as neomycin/polymyxin and/or gentamycin (or one following sensitivity testing) and atropine (if signs of anterior uveitis are manifest; better to use drops and 6–8 times daily). A protective collar is often used to prevent injurious contact with the eye. The ulcer will subsequently be covered by means of one of the oversuturing methods (see 10.6.3.5). If the therapy is effective, the severity of the clinical signs decreases rapidly. The edge of the ulcer becomes rounded and less swollen, and fluorescein staining remains positive only in the depth of the ulcer. If vessels reach the ulcer, fibroangioblastic repair, granulation, and finally scar formation will follow.

Because corticosteroids or topical anesthetics retard epithelialization, these drugs are especially contraindicated in deep ulcers (although the cornea initially appears more comfortable).

Prognosis: At the moment of onset of the process, the prognosis is guarded.

10.6.3.3 Hernia of Descemet's membrane (descemetocele)

If the corneal epithelium and stroma are destroyed due to trauma or enzymatic collagen dissolution, the transparent Descemet's membrane is exposed (Plate 10.15) and, depending on the size of the defect, it bulges out. The dark iris is often quite clearly visible under the transparent hernia. A descemetocele often is the result of initial (micro)trauma and secondary bacterial infection or keratomalacia, with the development of a subsequent rapidly deepening corneal ulcer, usually due to melting of the stroma. It is a rare occurrence; however, it is more frequent in brachycephalic breeds such as the Pekingese, Pug, and French Bulldog. The risk of perforation is great.

Therapy: Treatment consists of the same medications as for a deep ulcer, but in combination with oversuturing of the open conjunctiva as a conjunctival pedicle flap or strip, or with the circular bulbar conjunctiva oversuturing procedure, or with a free transplant of conjunctiva or cornea (see 10.6.3.5; Plates 10.16–10.21). The use of the nictitating membrane in these cases is generally insufficient. The method chosen depends on the instruments available, the experience of the surgeon, and the extent of softening of the edge of the defect.

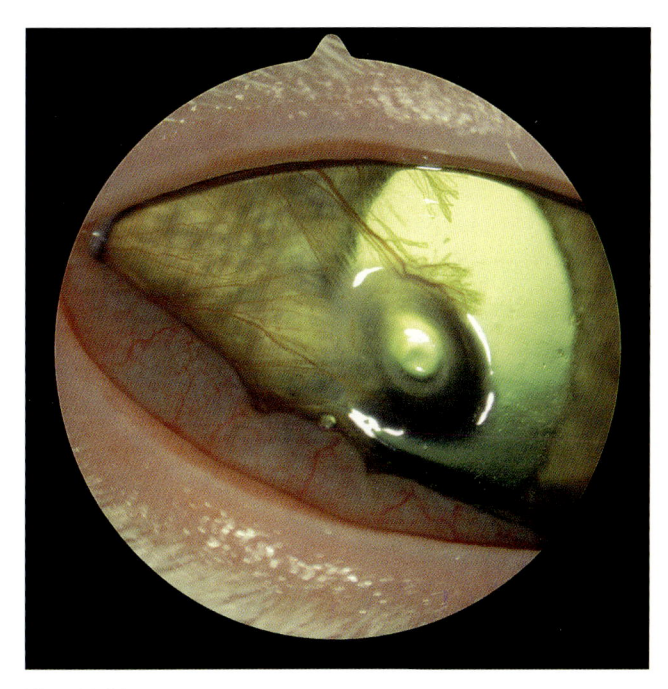

Plate 10.12:
Deep, lytic corneal ulcer in a cat (OD). The ring and edge of the deep crater are edematous, but the center is clear. This is pathognomonic for a defect reaching Descemet's membrane.

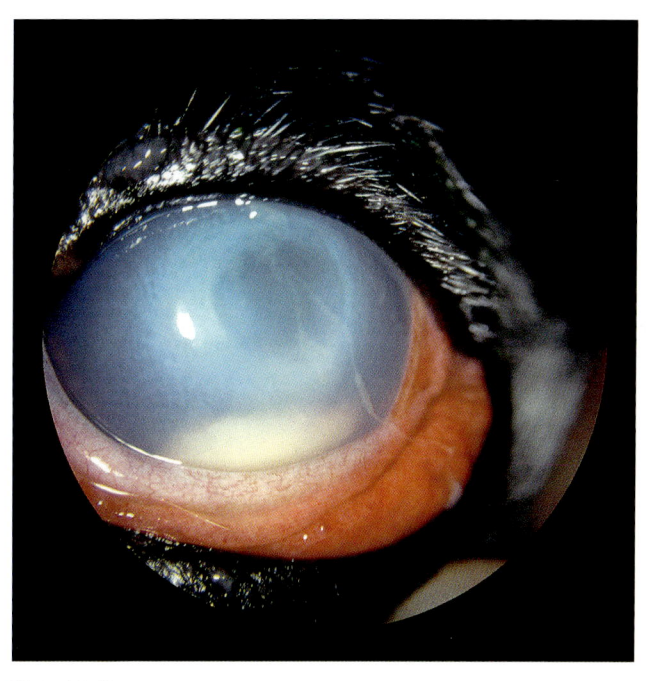

Plate 10.13:
Deep corneal ulcer, with melting edges due to proteolytic enzymes, and a hypopyon (OS, dog).

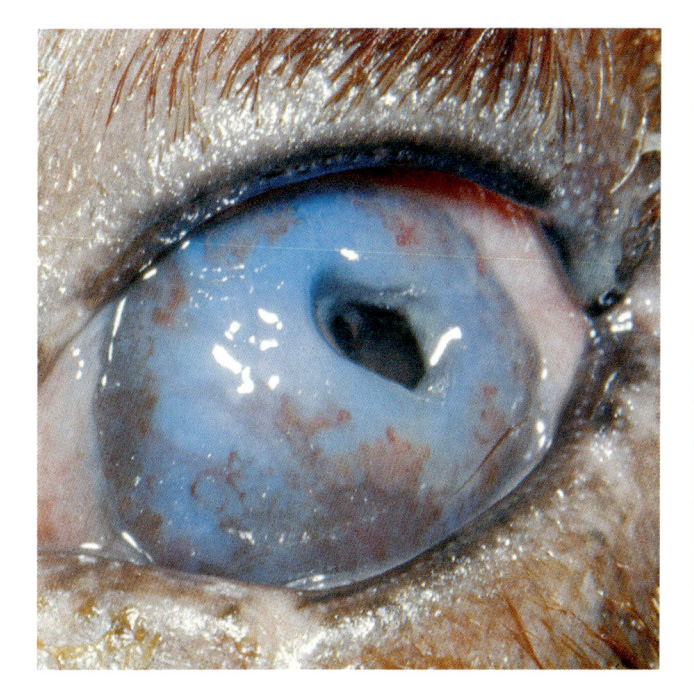

Plate 10.14:
Severe corneal edema and vessel ingrowth into a crater reaching the Descemet's membrane, which itself is not edematous otherwise it would be stained by fluorescein.

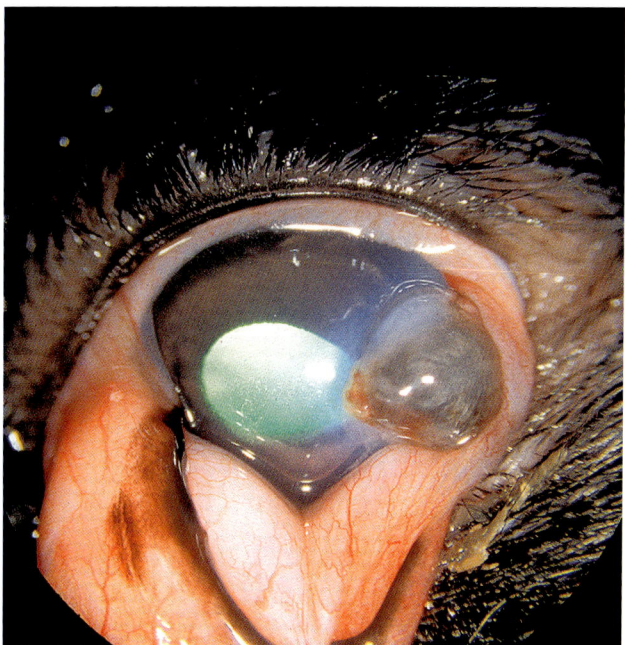

Plate 10.15:
Staphyloma after rupture of a deep lytic corneal ulcer. Because a piece of the iris is caught in the defect, the pupil has the shape of a pear (OS, dog).

10.6.3.4 Corneal perforation (staphyloma)

Corneal perforations are usually the result of stab or slicing wounds and, infrequently, the result of a perforated melting corneal ulcer. When the defect is small, some aqueous escapes, coagulates, and closes the perforation. When the defect is larger, the iris prolapses and appears as a black bladder-shaped bulge (Fig. 10.5, Plate 4.19, 10.15). In scleral staphylomas the defect is filled directly by uveal tissue. If the pain in this stage is severe, it causes blepharospasm. After a few hours, the staphyloma is covered by blood clots and exudate.

Therapy: Patients with corneal perforation should as a general rule be referred directly. The immediate treatment that can be given consists of administration of neomycin-polymyxin and atropine eye drops (not ointments) and putting a protective collar on the animal. If the perforation has been caused by trauma, it must usually be sutured (see 4). A perforation resulting from an ulcer cannot usually be closed satisfactorily by suturing because its diameter is too large and the edges are of poor quality. In this case, preference must be given to removal of the herniated part of the iris by electrocautery and closure of the defect with a conjunctival flap or a transplant.

10.6.3.5 Nictitating membrane, conjunctival, and corneal oversuturing techniques

After luxation of the globe, after a traumatic corneal defect, or in the case of a poorly healing corneal ulcer, the eye can be "bandaged" by using the nictitating membrane, which covers the defect with intact conjunctiva. The defect can also be provided with blood vessels by means of oversuturing of freed conjunctiva, in which case the subconjunctival side of the conjunctiva comes to lie against the defect and is intended to grow together with it. A defect can also be treated by a lamellar (partial thickness) keratoplasty or by filling it with a free conjunctival or corneal transplant or an ocular adhesive. The latter methods in particular require x5–10 magnification, special instruments, and considerable surgical skill. The oversuturing techniques are carried out under general anesthesia.

The nictitating membrane in birds is unsuitable for oversuturing. Here, a temporary tarsorrhaphy is more effective.

Nictitating membrane oversuturing methods or flaps
- **Attachment to the upper eyelid** (Fig. 10.6)
  The nictitating membrane is sutured over the eyeball with two mattress sutures anchored to the upper eyelid and to the cartilage of the nictitating membrane, but without perforating its ocular conjunctiva. This method is simple and effective though it allows movement of the eyeball under the conjunctival membrane.

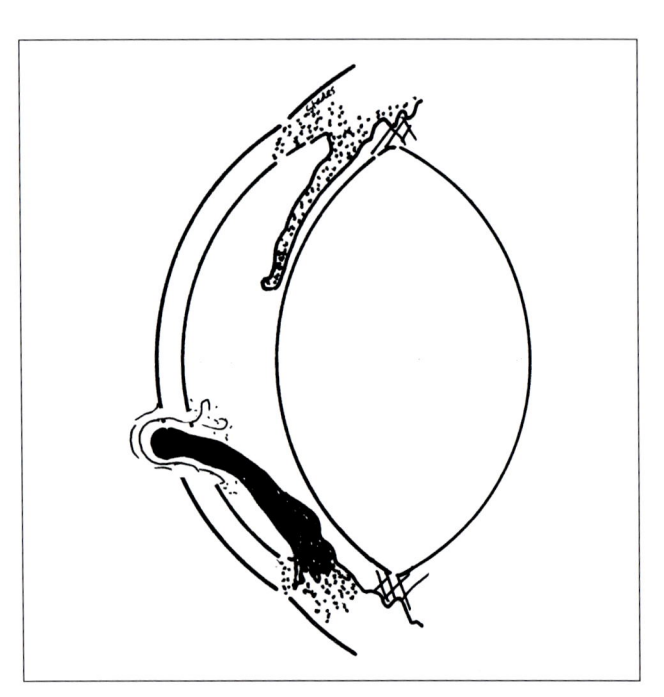

Fig. 10.5:
Staphyloma. A piece of the iris bulges through the defect.

The suture material is 4-0 or 5-0 polyfilament nylon with a 4/8 circle, 20–30 mm long, round, micropoint needle. The first suture is placed slightly medial to the middle of the upper eyelid. The second is placed about 10 mm closer to the lateral canthus. The upper lid is held with surgical forceps. One end of the forceps is, therefore, in the conjunctival sac and the other on the skin of the lid, 10–15 mm from the edge of the lid. The needle is inserted at the tip of the forceps through the eyelid into the fornix. The edge of the nictitating membrane is held with a Graefe's forceps at a point where the central part of the cartilage ends. The needle is passed through from the palpebral side at a point 2–3 mm from the edge of the nictitating membrane, just inside the edge of the cartilage. It penetrates the conjunctiva and is passed below the cartilage but does not perforate the ocular conjunctiva. It is passed along the ocular surface of the cartilage for 3–5 mm, parallel to the edge, and is returned through the cartilage and conjunctiva to the palpebral side. The needle is then returned via the fornix through the upper eyelid to the lid skin. The ends of the suture are brought through a small button or a piece of thin tubing, to prevent the suture from cutting through the skin. Both mattress sutures are placed before either is tightened and tied. The second suture is placed in the same manner, a few millimeters closer to the lateral canthus. No folds should be allowed to form as the nictitating membrane is drawn over the eye, therefore careful attention must be given to the placement of the sutures and the distance between them. Before the sutures are tightened, liberal amounts of chloramphenicol, or those antibiotics initially used for treatment of the ulcer, and 1% atropine eye ointment are deposited under the nictitating membrane.

Postoperative treatment consists of once daily application of the same ointments in the lateral canthus. If the sutures are well anchored in the cartilage, they can remain in place for 10–14 days. They are removed under local anesthesia.

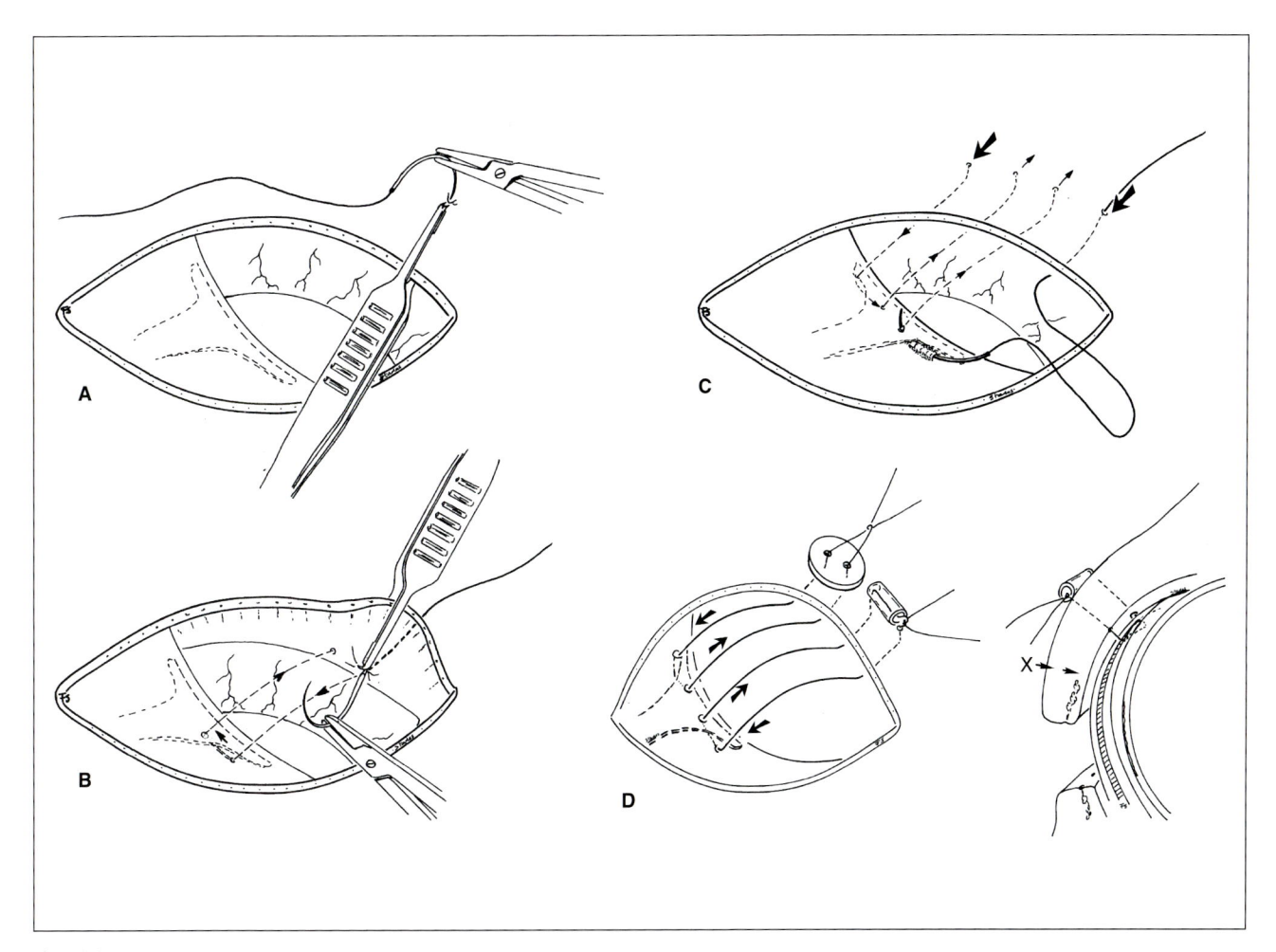

Fig. 10.6:
Nictitating membrane to the upper lid flap covering method. X = suturing too near the lid margin.

After-care: See under the appropriate indication for oversuturing of the nictitating membrane (corneal ulcer, luxation of the globe, etc.).

- **Attachment to the dorsolateral conjunctiva**
(Fig. 10.7)
The edge of the nictitating membrane is fixed to the dorsolateral bulbar conjunctiva using two or three mattress sutures. This method is, therefore, not suitable for preventing a recurrence of globe luxation. Suturing is done with 5-0 or 6-0 monofilament or polyfilament material with a 15- to 20-mm, 4/8 circle, round needle. Two mattress sutures, about 5 mm wide, are placed through the nictitating membrane, about 2 mm from the margin. The suture is continued in the matching segment on a line 2–3 mm from the limbus of the dorsolateral conjunctiva, and inserted through the nictitating membrane again. Each suture can be tied immediately. Before the last suture is tied, broad-spectrum antibiotic and atropine ointments are deposited under the nictitating membrane.

Conjunctival tissue oversuturing methods
(Figs. 10.8, 10.9; Plates 10.16–10.21)
In these techniques, part of the bulbar conjunctiva is freed or a free transplant of conjunctiva is prepared and sutured over the corneal defect.[13]

The remaining conjunctival defect is sutured in horses, if possible, to prevent retrobulbar fat prolapse.[14]

It is intended that the open subconjunctival tissue will grow together with the surface of the defect and thereby seal it.

After-care: consists of an antibiotic (preferably after culture and sensitivity testing) and 1% atropine (ointment or drops, 4–6 times daily). After the defect has firmly healed, the surrounding conjunctiva is cut free. It usually retracts and attaches itself again along the limbus. The portion which has adhered to the cornea is transformed into a scar, but after a few months this will have often become remarkably small and transparent.

- **Conjunctival pedicle flap oversuturing**
(Fig. 10.9 AB)
In this method, the conjunctiva is cut free along the limbus over a distance of 10–15 mm. The bulbar conjunctiva is freed in such a way that the flap can be laid over the defect without tension. Only the conjunctiva should be freed and not the underlying Tenon's capsule. This means that the tips of the scissors must remain visible through the conjunctiva. The free edge of the conjunctival flap is sutured to the healthy edge of the defect with simple interrupted sutures about 1 mm apart, using 8-0 or 9-0 monofilament nylon with a 6–8 mm spatulate needle.
- **Conjunctival strip oversuturing** (Fig. 10.9 CD; Plate 10.21) In this method, the conjunctiva is freed along the limbus from 12 to 6 o'clock on the same side of the cornea as the defect. A second incision is made in the conjunctiva parallel to the first over an arc of about 150 degrees. The width of the resulting conjunctival strip should be 5 mm wider than the corneal defect. After the conjunctiva has been freed, the result is a vertical strip that is only attached at the top and bottom. The free edges of the strip are sutured to the medial and lateral edges of the defect (suture material of 8-0 or 9-0, as in the previous method).

The remaining conjunctival wound edge may be attached at the limbus with a continuous suture, especially in horse (risk for retrobulbar fat prolapse). Alternatively, it is possible to loosen the strip over a smaller circle (e.g. 100 degrees) and to cut the strip loose at one end, thus creating a pedicle less broad based than in the previous technique (Plates 10.19, 10.20).

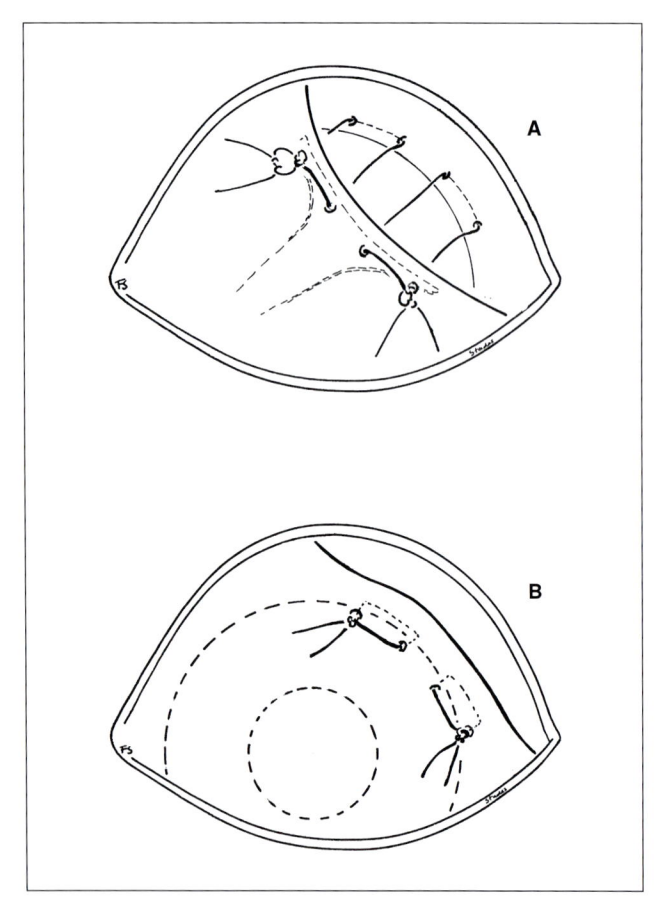

Fig. 10.7:
Nictitating membrane to the dorsolateral conjunctiva covering method.

Keratitis **145**

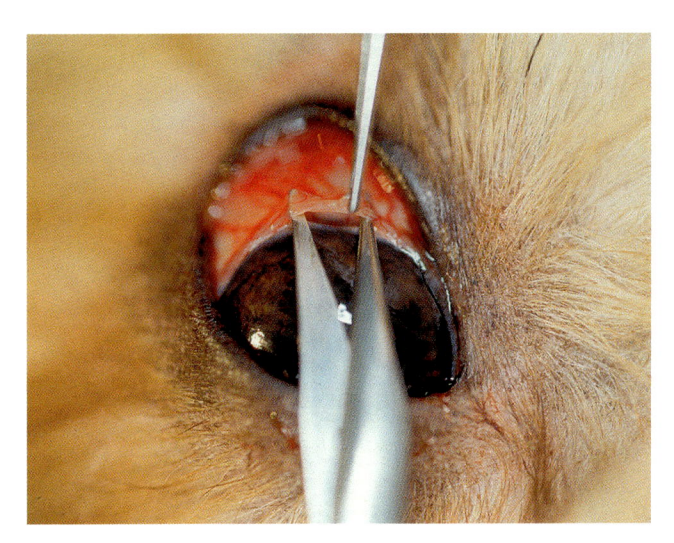

Plate 10.16:
Start of blunt dissection of the conjunctiva at the limbus for the covering of a large, deep corneal ulcer.

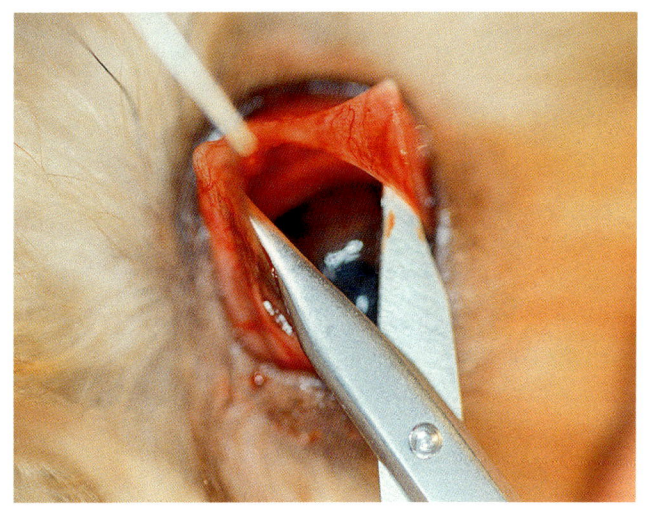

Plate 10.17:
Further blunt dissection of conjunctiva at the limbus for the covering of a large, deep corneal ulcer.

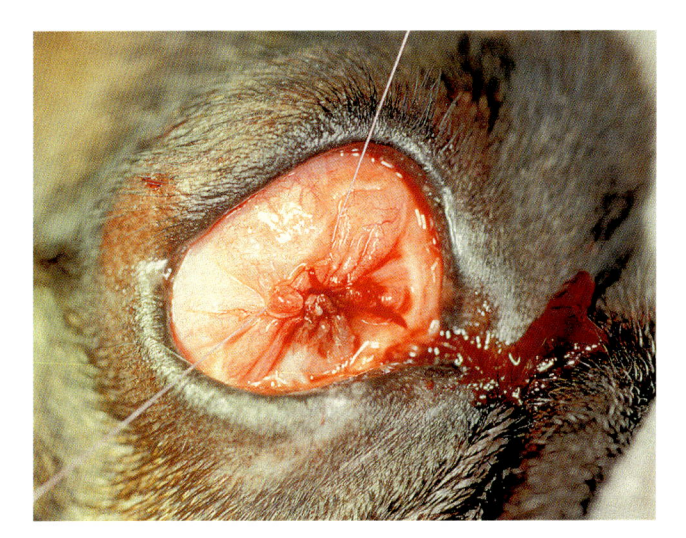

Plate 10.18:
Total circular covering with scleral conjunctiva of a large, deep corneal ulcer closed with a sack suture.

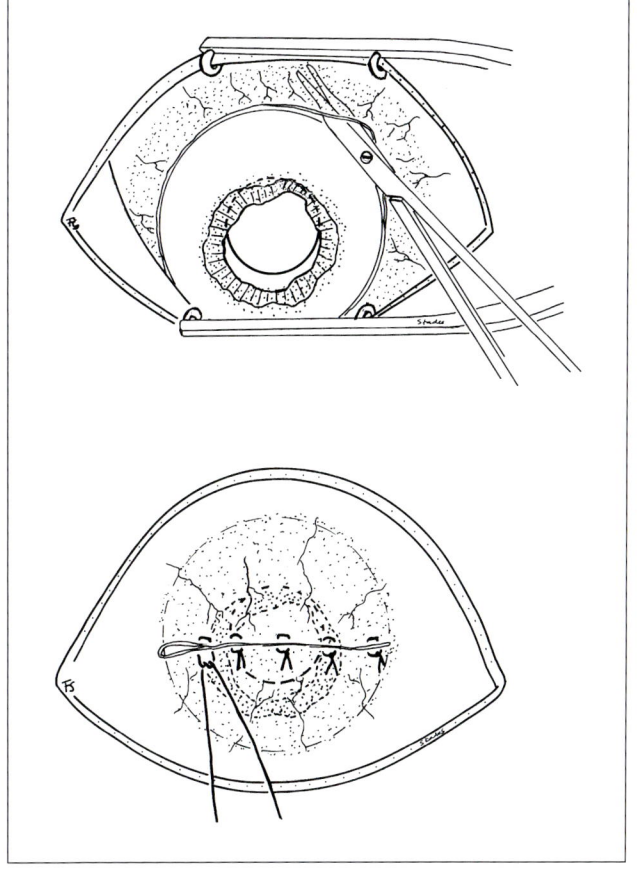

Fig. 10.8:
Conjunctival total circular oversuturing method for the covering of a deep corneal defect or ulcer.

10

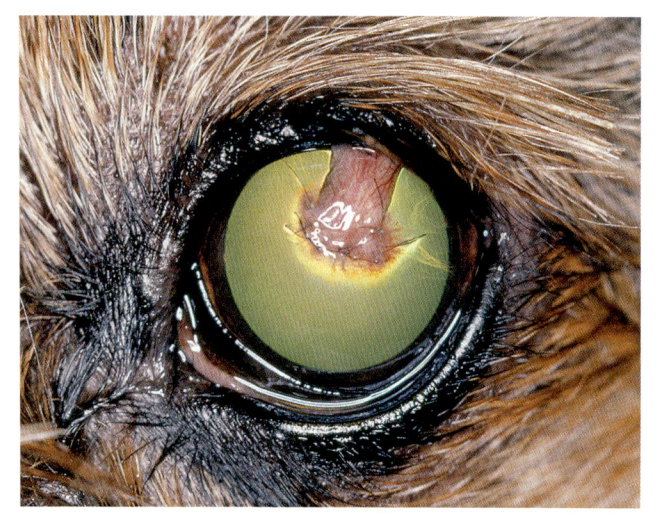

Plate 10.19:
Pedicle graft for the covering of a deep, small corneal ulcer (OS, dog; nylon 9-0 sutures; pupil in mydriasis because of the use of atropine; see also Plate 10.20).

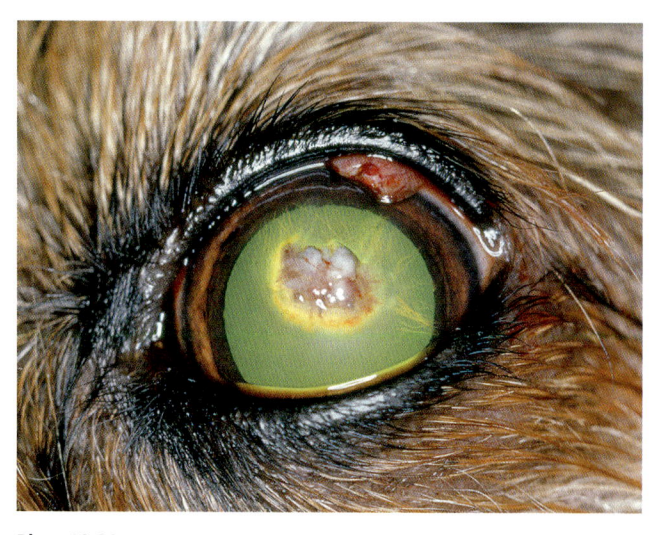

Plate 10.20:
Rest granulation after dissection on both sides of the pedicle graft, which was used to cover a deep corneal ulcer (same eye as in Plate 10.19).

- **Bulbar conjunctiva oversuturing**
  (Fig. 10.8; Plates 10.16–10.18)
  The conjunctiva is cut all along the limbus for 360 degrees and freed from the Tenon's capsule. The conjunctiva at 12 o'clock and 6 o'clock is brought together and attached with a flat mattress suture (5-0 or 6-0 silk or nylon, round body needle) or one circular suture. The remainder of the conjunctiva is joined with a few mattress sutures so that a mediolateral seam results. This method is simpler than the first two and can cover large defects, but is less specific and more traumatic.

- **Conjunctival free autotransplant**
  A piece of conjunctiva, a little larger than the corneal defect, is freed and excised, e.g. from the outside of the nictitating membrane. This conjunctival transplant is attached with simple interrupted sutures (9-0 nylon) to cover or fill the defect. This method is more likely to be successful if the ulcer is already distinctly vascularized.

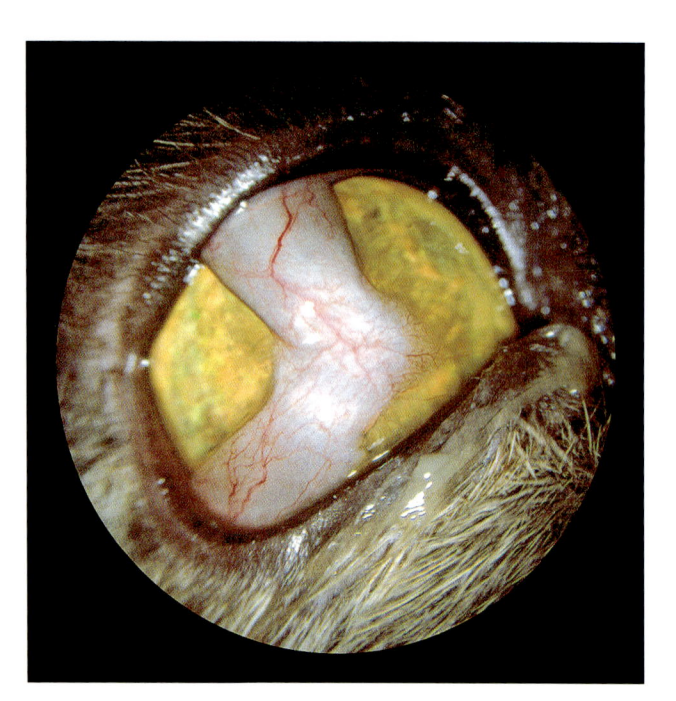

Plate 10.21:
Conjunctival strip grown together with, and thus covering, a deep corneal ulcer (OD, Persian cat, 6 weeks after surgery).

Corneal oversuturing methods[15]

- **Lamellar corneal graft oversuturing**
  In this technique, a lamellar strip (slightly divergent) of the animal's cornea and sclera, including the covering conjunctiva, is freed, pulled over the defect, and sutured (9-0 or 10-0 monofilament nylon) to the defect.
- **Corneal free transplant**
  A lamellar or full penetrating part of a donor cornea can be used to cover or close the defect. The donor cornea is sutured (9-0 or 10-0 monofilament nylon) in a continuous pattern.

Covering with tissue glue

Small corneal defects, ulcers or recurrent erosions can be covered using cyanoacrylate tissue glue (e.g. Histoacryl®, Braun). The ulcer bed must be dried thoroughly, and a minimum amount of glue is applied as a fine layer (edges may be most irritating, anesthesia required). The glue has an antibacterial effect and stops the destruction of stromal collagen. After re-epithelization, 2–4 weeks later, the glue layer will be rejected.[16]

10.6.4 Corneal sequestration / cornea nigrum / corneal necrosis / corneal mummification[17]

These terms refer to a glistening, black-brown pigmented area or plaque of amorphous, necrotic material in the superficial layers of the cornea of cats. Whether this lesion should be considered one of the degenerative diseases of the cornea is not certain. In cats, chronic irritation caused by hairs (e.g. in palpebral aplasia, entropion, distichiasis, or trichiasis) or irritation resulting from the deficient tear film in KCS, or infection with feline herpes virus (FVH-1), often leads to sequestration. There are also cases in which no direct irritating factors can be found. These chiefly involve cats with exophthalmia, such as the short-nosed Persian, which is predisposed to this condition. It is probable that infrequent lid closure, the prominent eye and hereditary factors, resulting in a too rapid a breaking up of the center of the tear film play a role in this disease.

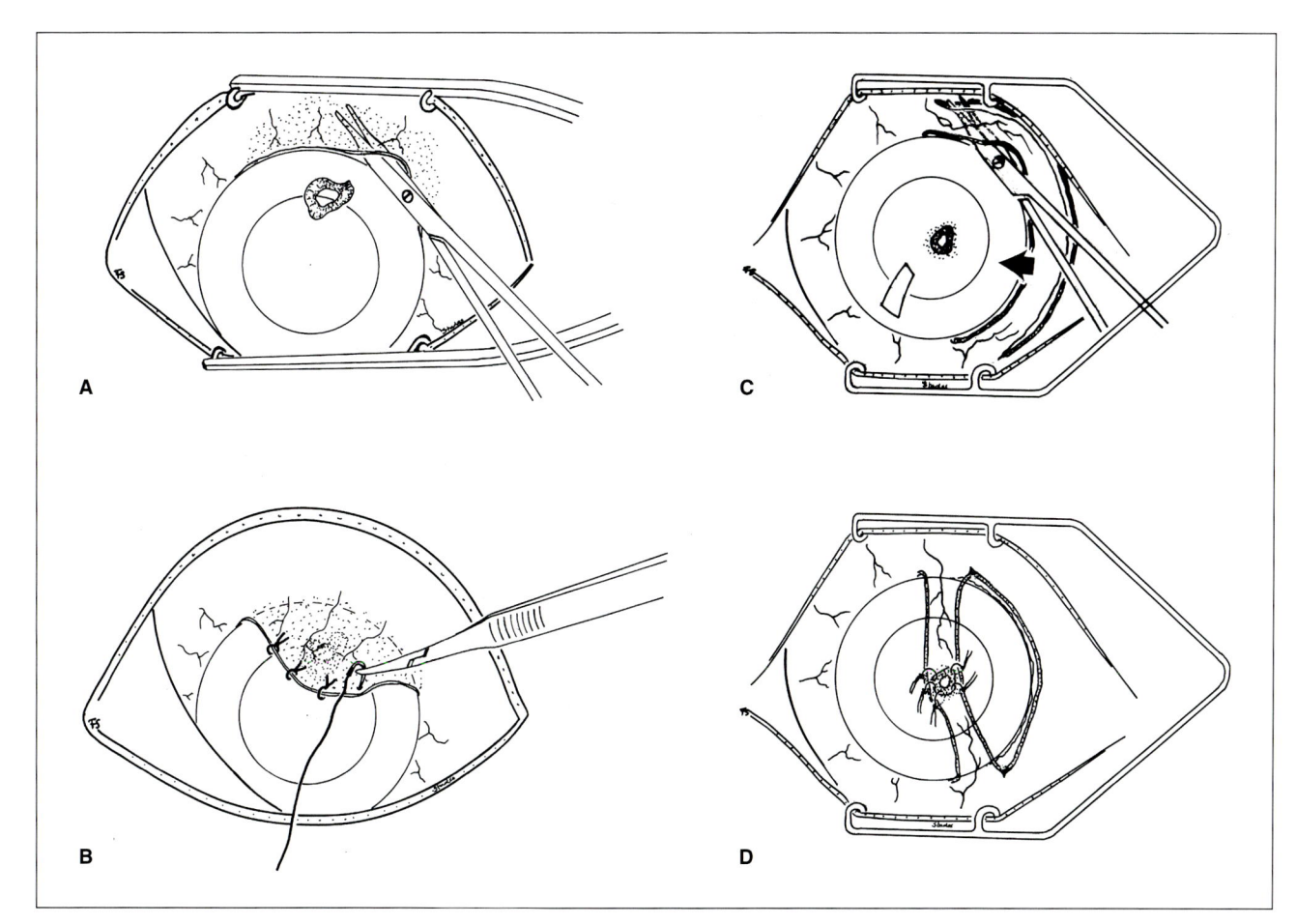

Fig. 10.9:
Conjunctival (A–B) flap, and (A, C–D) strip oversuturing methods for the covering of deep corneal defects or ulcers.

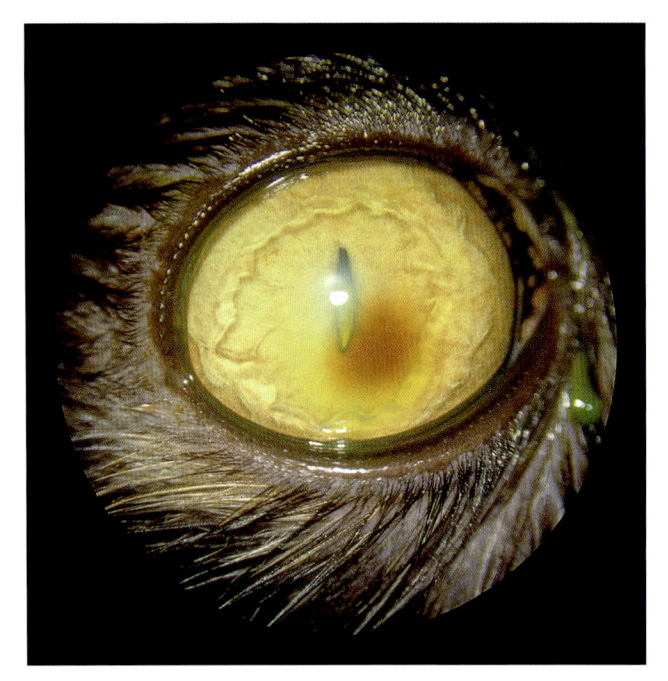

Plate 10.22:
Corneal sequester in a cat, start of pigmentation (OD).

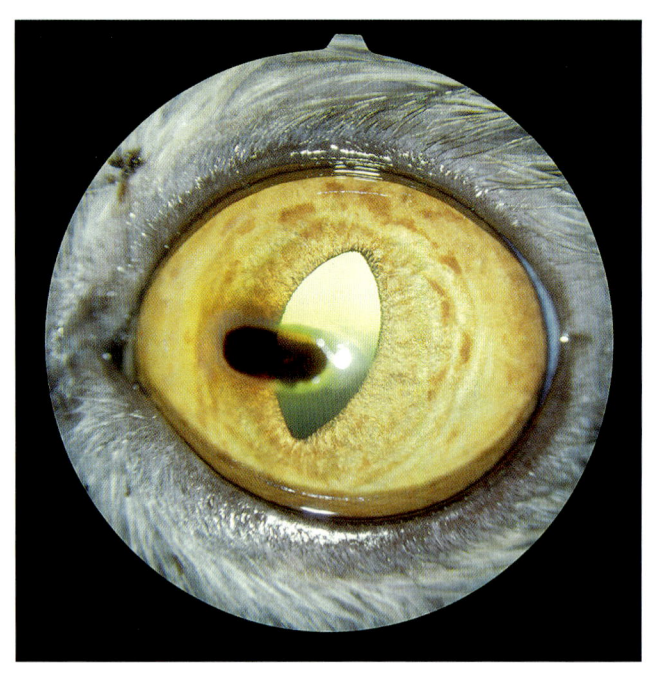

Plate 10.23:
Corneal sequester in a cat without any vessel activity.

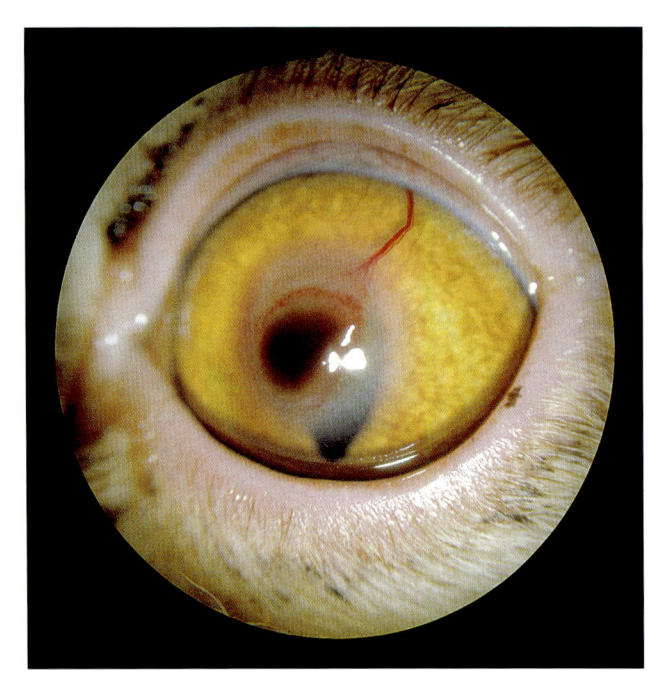

Plate 10.24:
Corneal sequester in a cat. The sequestrum has been undergrown by a vascular bed (OS).

Symptoms: The abnormality usually begins with diffuse pigmentation in the central epithelium of the cornea. Gradually, a thick, glistening, black plaque is formed in the center of the corneal surface (Plates 2.7, 10.22–10.24). This plaque consists of amorphous material which has yet to be identified. Whether it arrives via the cornea or the tear film alone is also not clear. Over the course of weeks more reaction develops in the form of opacification and necrosis of the underlying and surrounding corneal epithelium and stroma. The pain reaction in cats is usually not very severe but there is overproduction of tears and protrusion of the nictitating membrane. Superficial ingrowth of vessels develops slowly. Over the course of many months to a year, most sequestrums are extruded very gradually by means of granulation under the plaque. The sequestration process may also go deeper until perforation occurs, indicating the need for early surgical intervention. A corneal scar usually remains.

Diagnosis: The superficial, more or less central, black plaque is so characteristic that it can hardly be confused with other abnormalities. Foreign bodies, such as leaves from plant heads, that can be found adhered to the cornea of dogs, are extremely rare in cats and can be removed directly by irrigating and removing them with forceps (compare: Plates 4.13 and 10.23).

The sequestrum does not stain with fluorescein (although it does with rose bengal), but the necrotic ring around the plaque may be lightly stained.

Therapy: Treatment is with an "initial choice" antibiotic-Vitamin A ointment. Because spontaneous extrusion of the sequestrum requires a very long time, the authors prefer referral for lamellar keratectomy (some clinicians wait for spontaneous healing).

A keratectomy is carried out under both general and local anesthesia, the latter reducing the depth of the former. It is necessary to use at least x5–10 magnification, a capsule forceps, and a special round-tip diamond knife. A more complete set of instruments should be readily available for complications such as perforation. The incision is directed under the sequestrum from the healthy corneal tissue just outside it. The plaque is then loosened from the underlying stroma using spatula dissection.

After removal of the sequestrum, the wound edges are checked to ensure that they lie in vital cornea and that they slope gradually. If the pigmentation extends almost to Descemet's membrane, it is better not to remove the deepest part of the sequestrum, because of the risk of perforation. This pigment will either be removed spontaneously or will be raised to the surface by granulation and can then be removed in a subsequent operation. Full thickness sequestrums do occur, but are rare. In such cases, the defect has to be filled by conjunctiva or donor cornea.

The postoperative treatment is as described above. If there is evidence of anterior uveitis, the addition of 1% atropine ointment (no drops for cats) 2–4 times daily is indicated. The filling of the defect usually requires 1–4 weeks. Eventual scar formation is mainly dependent on the depth of the previous sequestration. The lesion recurs occasionally, more often in Persian cats, and must then be treated in the same way.

Prevention: To help prevent recurrence it is advisable to continue protecting the cornea with vitamin A oil, 1–2 times daily. In addition, efforts should be made to stop the breeding of cats with such "lovely great" eyes, and buyers must be convinced as well.

10.6.5 Keratitis punctata

This has a specific appearance, characterized by multiple, dendritic fluorescein-positive corneal defects (Plate 10.25). The defects slowly become deeper but are usually filled in again after 1–2 months, with or without vessel ingrowth towards the defect. The defect usually recurs a few months after recovery.

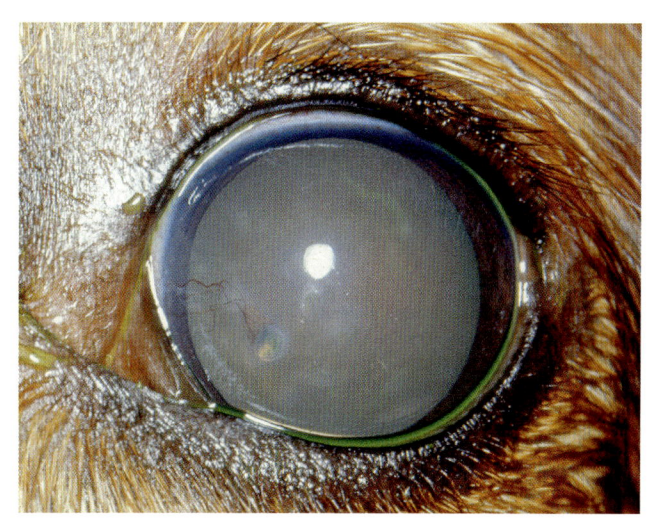

Plate 10.25:
Punctate keratitis in a Long-haired Dachshund (OS). The punctate- and dendritic-shaped defects are stained with fluorescein.

The abnormality is mainly found in the Long-haired Dachshund. It may be due to a herpes virus infection in the dog, but the virus has never been demonstrated. However, the lesions resemble very closely those of herpes virus infection of the cornea in humans. Also, such an illness has been described in horses, caused by equine herpes virus 2 and 5.

Symptoms: There are multiple, small, punctate or dendritic, fluorescein-positive, superficial or deeper defects in the cornea. During the first few days, the dog is usually somewhat listless, with a slight blepharospasm of the affected eye and a slight discharge. In the recovery phase, there is usually superficial vessel ingrowth towards the defects and the depth of the defects decreases.

Diagnosis: Diagnosis is made on the basis of the clinical picture. In the differential diagnosis, all forms of ulcers should be considered. In the Long-haired Dachshund, the main differential diagnoses are KCS and keratitis pannosa.

Therapy: In the early stages, when small punctate fluorescein-staining spots are present, treatment consisting of topical corticosteroids or cyclosporin A ointment may be prescribed.[8]

Prognosis: The prognosis is favorable. Recurrence can be expected, but if the owner immediately resumes treatment at the first signs of recurrence, there is usually recovery again within a week.

10.6.6. Keratitis herpetica

Viral keratitis is frequent in the cat and horse. In the cat, it is mainly caused by feline herpes virus I (FVH-1), calici virus, and chlamydia (Chlamydophilia felis). In the horse, two types of equine herpes viruses (EHV-2 und EHV-5) have been recognized.

Symptoms: Ocular FHV-1 infection is very variable in the cat (see also 8.11). In the kitten, the signs of upper respiratory disease, associated with agressive, necrotizing keratoconjunctivitis prevail. In the end phase, there may often be unilateral adhesions between the layers in the tear ducts, resulting in obstruction: between parts of the conjunctiva including the nictitating membrane, and between the conjunctiva and cornea (symblepharon; Plate 8.15; see 8.14.1).[18]

In the adult cat, a FVH-1 infection manifests as a chronic, frequently recurrent keratoconjunctivitis. The infection is characterized by linear branching, so called dendritic lesions in the superficial corneal layers, as seen in human herpes virus infections. Especially in the brachycephalic cats, a third type of herpes keratitis may manifest as superficial erosions, with subsequent sequestration (see 10.6.4)

Diagnose: Diagnosis is made on the basis of the clinical picture. Further proof is possible using PCR; however, the diagnosis is often difficult due to the carrier status and ubiquitous nature of this herpes virus. The demonstration of intranuclear inclusion bodies by cytologic examination of corneal scrapings is often negative.

Therapy: In the kitten, therapy is started against the secondary bacterial invasion using topical acetylcysteine (diminishing the risk for symblepharon), irrigation, oxytetracycline or chlortetracycline 4–6 times daily for 10–14 days, and doxycycline orally (see also 8.11.2).

Adult cats are treated with virustatic agents: trifluorothymidine (TFT), minimum 4 times daily.[19] Also famcyclovir 30 mg 2 times daily, orally and lysine supplementation could be helpful in chronic cases.[20,21] Moreover, interferon is considered clinically useful.

Corticosteroids should not be used in the case of an affirmative Herpes PCR because of a possible viral relapse and ulceration. A high number of infected cats will become carriers and may spread the virus.[22]

Prophylactic vaccination is possibly helpful, though quarantine of new cats for several weeks, optimal hygiene, good ventilation, segregation and removal of cats with signs of upper respiratory disease from the colony are very important.

Prognosis: Prognosis in proven cases is guarded. Chronic or recurrent keratoconjunctivitis is likely.

10.6.7 Infectious bovine / ovine keratoconjunctivitis

This is the most important eye disease in herds of ruminants. In cattle, the infection is mainly caused by *Moraxella bovis*, and in sheep and goats by *Mycoplasma* spp. However, Chlamydia (*Chlamydophilia*), bacteria (e.g. *Pasteurella* spp.) and viruses are also possible factors. A mucopurulent conjunctivitis develops with "bladder"-like areas in the cornea and uveitis. These areas deepen and may lead to perforation and loss of the eye. The ulcers can become vascularized and granulation tissue develops, giving the name "pink-eye" (for therapy, see 8.11.7).

10.6.8 Corneal cysts[23]

This is thickening of the cornea due to a vesicle, usually a few millimeters thick and filled with a yellowish fluid. The cyst is the result of secretory epithelium within the corneal stroma.

Diagnosis: Diagnosis is made on the basis of the clinical picture, which can be confused with that of local granulation, abscesses, or a neoplasm.

Therapy: Treatment consists of the surgical removal of the thickening and eventual curettage of the cyst wall. The removal requires x5–10 magnification, special instruments, and sufficient experience; for which reasons the patient should usually be referred.

10.6.9. Corneal abscess[24]

Corneal abscesses in companion animals are rare, but more frequent in the horse. They appear as painful infiltrations of inflammatory cells in the corneal stroma, without encapsulation. They cause considerable inflammatory reactions. They can result from stab wounds, infected (incompletely removed) suture material, implanting microorganisms into the corneal stroma, and are rapidly closed by re-epithelization.

Diagnosis: Diagnosis is made on the basis of the clinical picture, which can be confused with that of local granulation, cysts, or neoplasms. It can be confirmed by cytology, culturing and antibiogram.

Therapy: After lamellar keratectomy and curettage, topical "initial choice" antibiotics and atropine ointment are administered. Deep abscesses may be covered using a conjunctival flap.

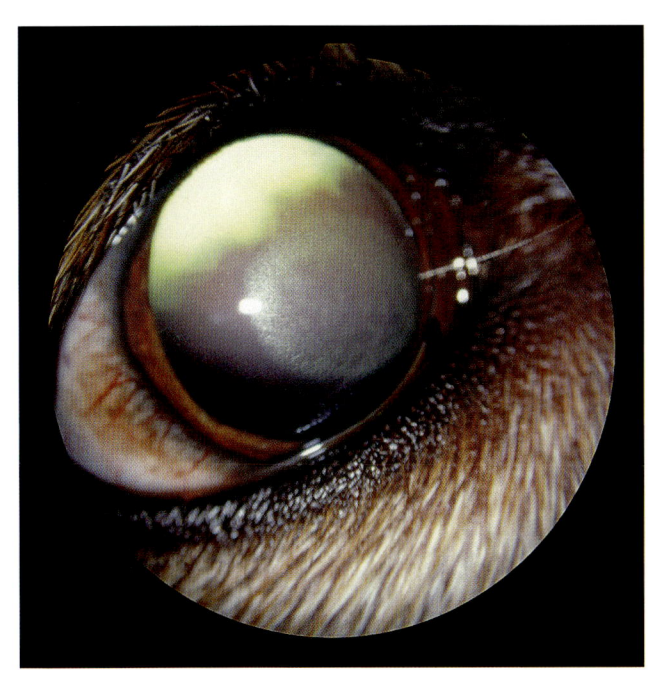

Plate 10.26:
Epithelial/stromal corneal lipidosis in a Labrador Retriever (OD). The crystals of cholesterol with the appearance of sugar or glass fiber crystals are located superficially in the cornea.

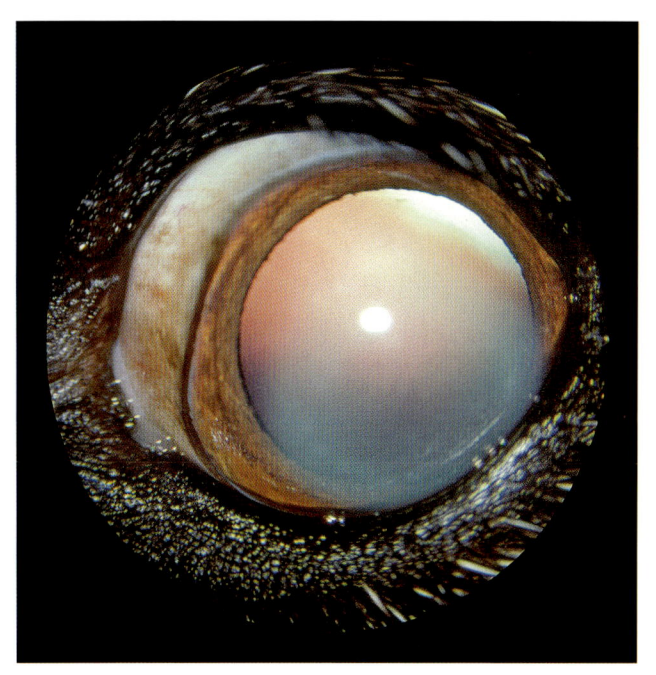

Plate 10.27:
Hereditary epithelial/stromal corneal dystrophy in a Siberian Husky (OD).

10.7 Dystrophic/degenerative deposits in the cornea

Dystrophic or degenerative deposits in the cornea can be separated into the bilateral, familial, and/or hereditary forms, which are usually called the real dystrophies, and local degenerative deposits, e.g. corneal lipidosis, and deposits which can occur secondary to other local or systemic disorders.[25] The borderline between these forms is sometimes difficult to define exactly.

10.7.1 Corneal dystrophies

These are familial or hereditary, bilateral degenerative metabolic disturbances. They occur mostly in the central parts (greatest distance from the limbal blood vessels) of the cornea, where they accumulate as crystalline deposits of cholesterol or other lipids. At least two forms can be distinguished according to their depth of localization in the cornea: epithelial/stromal and endothelial. Possibly the indolent ulcer of the Boxer (see 10.6.3.1) and corneal sequestrum of the cat (see 10.6.4) may belong to this group; they have been discussed previously under corneal ulcer (see 10.6.3).

10.7.1.1 Epithelial/stromal dystrophy

In these disorders the deposits are located centrally in the superficial layers of the cornea. The process usually begins at 1–2 years of age and enlarges slowly to a more or less glistening area with a diameter of 5–7 mm, in the center of the cornea (Plate 10.26). This dystrophy occurs as a hereditary disorder in the Siberian Husky, Samoyed and Beagle (Plate 10.27),[26] and is familial in such breeds as the Collie, Afghan, and Cavalier King Charles Spaniel.

In the rabbit, hereditary dystrophies and also high cholesterol diets may cause lipid deposits in the cornea.

Diagnosis: Diagnosis is made on the basis of the fluorescein-negative, centrally-located, hazy area in the cornea, consisting of crystalline structures. When examined with a loupe, they resemble sugar crystals or glass fibers.

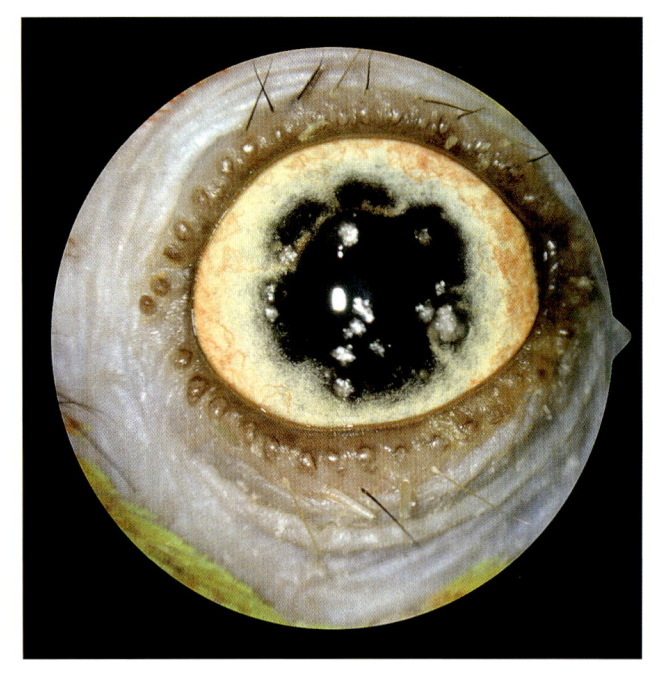

Plate 10.28:
Epithelial/stromal corneal lipidosis in a parakeet (OD). The cholesterol crystals with the appearance of sugar crystals are found *in/on* the corneal surface. They could be removed by curette, as loose grains.

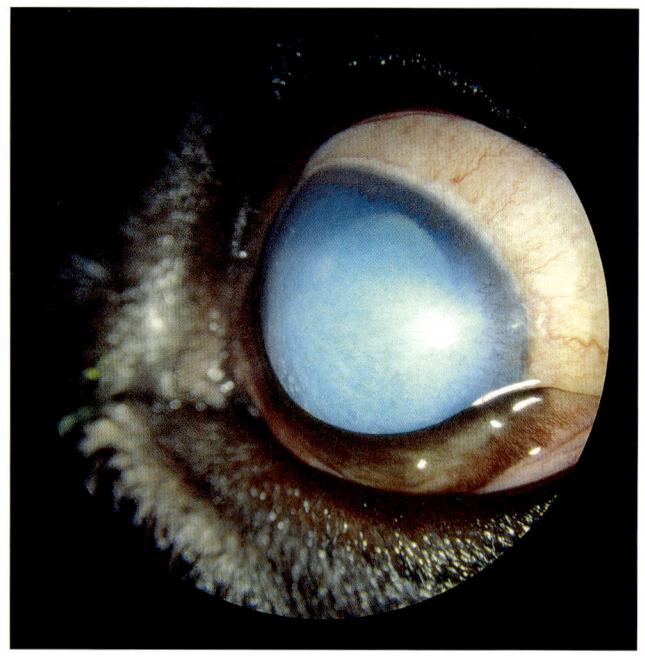

Plate 10.29:
Senile endothelial corneal degeneration in an 11-year-old Boston Terrier (OS).

In birds (Plate 10.28), these structures may possibly be induced by vitamin A deficiency. The deposits may appear like sugar crystals, irregularly spread in the corneal surface.

There are no other abnormalities such as pain or exudate or signs of inflammation. The serum lipid levels are almost never abnormal.

Therapy: Treatment consists of reducing the level of saturated fats in the diet. This sometimes halts the process or even reverses it (mainly in the non-hereditary forms). In more severe cases, referral for keratectomy or, in exceptional cases, for corneal transplantation, is possible, but there is a high probability of new and more severe recurrence.

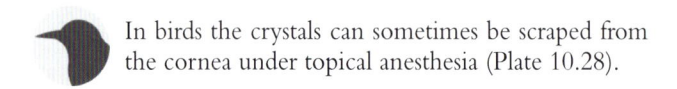

In birds the crystals can sometimes be scraped from the cornea under topical anesthesia (Plate 10.28).

Severe visual disturbance rarely occurs. It is wise to exclude hereditarily affected animals from breeding.

10.7.1.2 Endothelial dystrophy or senile endothelial degeneration[27]

In this disorder, the dystrophic-degenerative processes occur near the endothelium. Dysfunction of the endothelium allows aqueous to escape into the cornea and deep, dense, usually central, corneal edema develops (Plate 10.29). This occurs with an intact corneal surface. Sometimes, however, there is also a certain degree of loosening of the layers above the endothelium, via which bullae (bullous keratopathy) or ulcers can form. The abnormality is mainly seen in older dogs of brachycephalic breed, such as the Boxer, Boston Terrier, and Chihuahua. Because of the central location of the lesion, blindness generally develops after a few months.

Diagnosis: Diagnosis is made on the basis of the characteristic bilateral, central corneal edema. On examination with the slit-lamp biomicroscope, very fine crystals can sometimes be recognized just above the endothelium.

Therapy: An attempt can be made to reduce the edema by means of a hypertonic eye ointment (such as 3–5% NaCl). Corticosteroids often bring initial improvement, but they increase the risk of ulceration. If an ulcer develops, it is treated as an indolent, superficial ulcer (see 10.6.3). In the case of a painful bullous keratopathy, coagulation of the superficial stromal layers by thermokeratoplasty may reduce

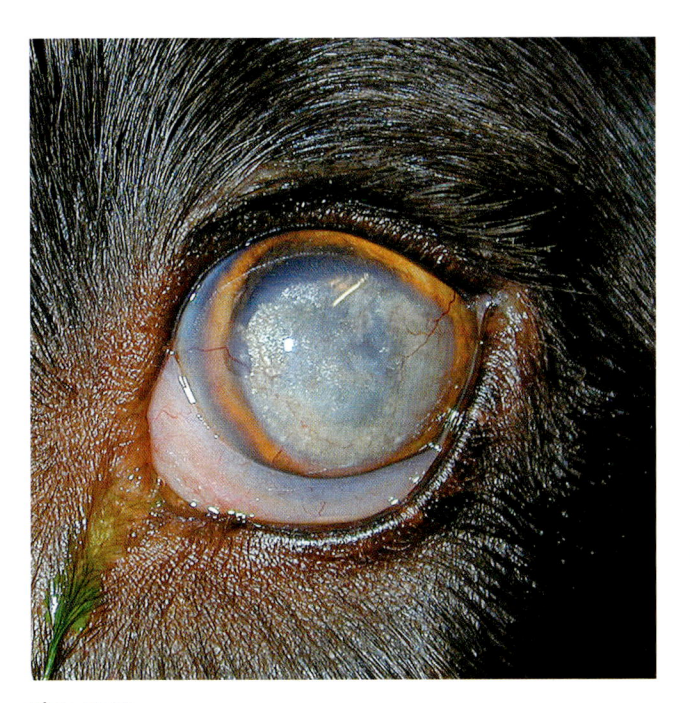

Plate 10.30:
Idiopathic, local crystal deposits in the cornea of a dog.

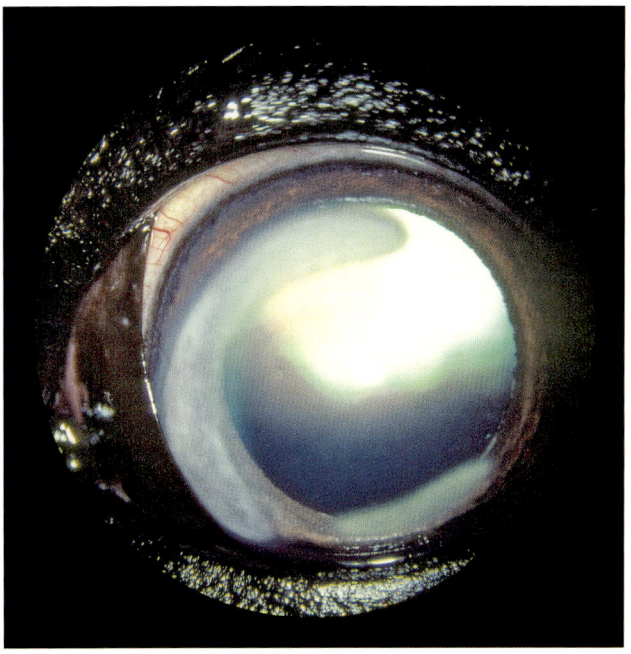

Plate 10.31:
Deposits in the cornea as an arcus lipoides in a dog, typical for hypothyroidism.

the edema.[28] Penetrating corneal transplants have also been advocated.

Prognosis: The prognosis for regaining sight is usually poor.

10.7.2 Local degenerative crystal deposits

Local crystalline deposits can have an idiopathic cause and have a clinical appearance similar to the familial or hereditary dystrophies (e.g. corneal lipidosis). Other causes to be considered include inflammatory processes, ulcers, etc., as a result of which there is a disturbance in the normal corneal metabolism at the edge of the process, resulting in the deposition of lipids or calcium salts, for example, forming a local, glistening area of crystals in the cornea (Plate 10.30) Treatment is directed at the primary process. Deposits, when present, are not usually resorbed.

10.7.3 Deposits resulting from systemic diseases[29]

Crystals can deposit in the cornea as a result of hyperlipidemia, hypercholesterolemia, or hypercalcemia. An arcus lipoides can develop as a result of hypothyroidism (Plate 10.31). This is a more or less circular deposit of crystals in the cornea as a 1- to 3-mm wide band, 1–2 mm from the limbus.

10.7.4 Corneal edema in the Manx cat

A nowadays rare, specific vesicular corneal edema has been described in the Manx cat, caused by changes in the stromal collagen and Descemet's membrane. It begins at about 6 months of age with a bilateral central superficial edema. The edema slowly becomes denser and has a vesicular appearance. The vesicles can occasionally lead to formation of superficial erosions.[30] The cause of the abnormality is not yet certain. Treatment as for superficial corneal ulcers, can be considered.

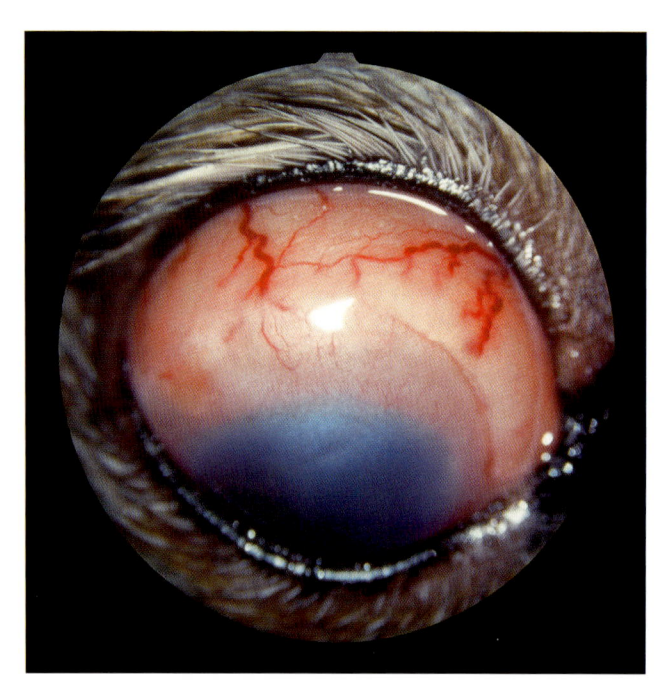

Plate 10.32:
Episcleritis (diffuse type). The pinky red tissue has partly overgrown the sclera and cornea (OD, dog).

10.7.5 Mucopolysaccharidosis[31]

In cats, this rare metabolic disturbance has been found to be associated with diffuse corneal cloudiness, flattening of the head, dwarfism, and possibly retinal atrophy. The abnormalities appear to be due to congenital enzyme deficiencies. A positive toluidine blue test in the urine is indicative of such a disorder. The diagnosis can only be confirmed by means of extensive investigations of the possibly affected enzymes. There is no known therapy.

10.7.6. GM1 and GM2 gangliosidosis[32]

In gangliosidosis, complex lipids accumulate, for example, in the brain. A congenital disturbance in the metabolism of these substances has been described in kittens with progressive corneal cloudiness. The associated rapidly-developing tremors, followed by ataxia, are much more significant than the ocular lesions and often lead to euthanasia.

10.8 (Epi)scleritis

(Epi)scleritis is a benign, sterile, proliferative inflammation that causes one or more nodular, or more diffuse, swellings in the episcleral tissue.[33] (Epi)scleritis occurs particularly in middle-aged or older dogs.

Symptoms: One or more pink, nodular or diffusely circular, smooth, painless swellings occur on or adjacent to the limbus (Plate 10.32). In general, the conjunctiva can easily be moved over the swelling. There is usually some corneal opacity along the limbus adjacent to this process, sometimes followed by a glistening white band of superficial corneal lipidosis.

Diagnosis: Diagnosis is made on the basis of the clinical picture, supported if necessary by histologic examination of an excised nodule or a biopsy.

Differential diagnosis: If there is a diffuse extension of the inflammation around the eye, the entire globe is enlarged, while the "scleral" globe is not increased in size. As a result, such an eye can very strongly resemble buphthalmos, especially if the corneal opacity also increases. The nodular swellings can also lead to misdiagnosis. When there is doubt, or when consideration is being given to enucleation of the eye or even euthanasia, histologic examination (by an ophthalmic pathologist) should be performed.

Therapy: Treatment consists of injecting 1–3 deposits (0.2–0.4 ml) of a corticosteroid depot preparation around the lesion. Further lifelong treatment consists of dexamethasone eye drops 3–6 times daily (provided that fluorescein staining is negative and the eye is held open). When there is inadequate improvement, treatment with cyclosporin 0.2–2%, azathioprine, or beta irradiation and local surgical removal is possible, for which the patient is usually referred. However, topical treatment cannot be stopped.

Prognosis: The prognosis is favorable, although the lesion will only be suppressed and not healed. Recurrences have to be suppressed by repeated deposits of corticosteroids (every 3–6 months).

10.9 Neoplasms

Primary or secondary neoplasms arising from the cornea and/or sclera occur sporadically. They should not be confused with benign processes such as (epi)scleritis or eosinophilic keratitis. If any process in this area does not appear to correspond with the disorders described above, neoplasia should be considered. Abnormalities that are associated with irregular, strongly pigmented or pinkish-white, firm or lardaceous tissue proliferation are particularly suspect. In dogs, limbal melanomas (Plate 10.33) are found infrequently, and they are usually relatively benign.[34]

In horses and cattle, carcinomas may also spread to the cornea and sclera (Plate 10.34). Careful slit-lamp microscopic examination and biopsy are then necessary.

Therapy: Treatment depends on the type of neoplasm and its location, and can vary from a superficial excision (keratectomy) to perforating keratoplasty,[35] enucleation of the globe, or exenteration of the orbit, for which the patient can be referred. Limbal melanomas can be successfully removed by keratectomy, eventually combined with cryotherapy, or by perforating keratoplasties.[34]

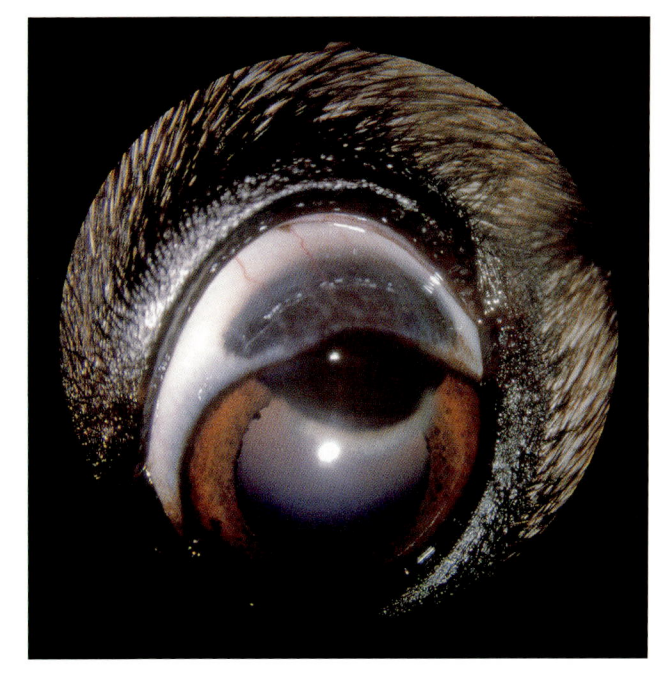

Plate 10.33:
Limbus melanoma in the cornea-sclera of a dog (OD).

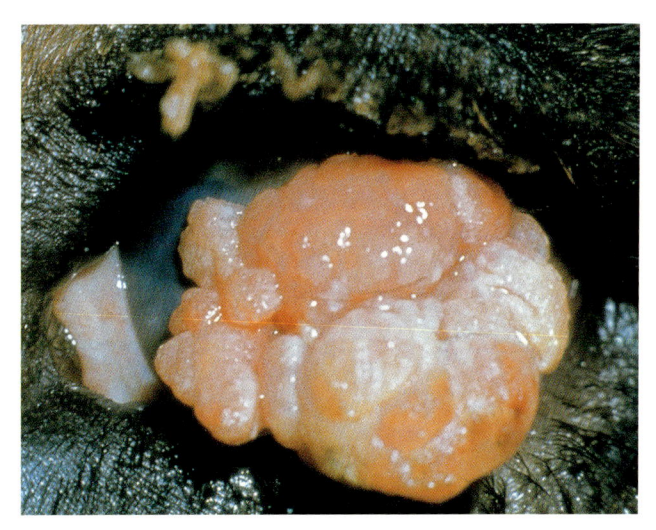

Plate 10.34:
Squamous cell carcinoma in a cow (OS). (By courtesy of Dr. W. Klein, Utrecht.)

Literature

1. GILGER, B.C., WHITLEY, R.D., MCLAUGHLIN, S. A. *et al.*: Canine corneal thickness measured by ultrasonic pachymetry. Am J. Vet. Res. **52**: 1570, 1991.

2. HOFFMANN, F. & SCHWEICHEL, J.U.: The microvilli structure of the corneal epithelium of the rabbit in relation to cell function: A transmission and scanning electron microscopic study. Ophthalmic Res. **4**: 175, 1972/1973.

3. RASK, L., GEIJER, C., BILL, A. & PETERSON, P.A.: Vitamin A supply of the cornea. Exp. Eye Res. **31**: 201, 1980.

4. WALDE, I.: Bandopacties. Equine Vet. J. Suppl. **2**: 32, 1983.

5. HENDRIX, D.V.H., WARD, D.A. & BARNHILL, M.A.: The effects of antibiotics on canine corneal epithelial wound closure in tissue culture. Trans. Am. Coll. Vet. Ophthalmol, Santa Fe, New Mexico, USA, p. 99, 1997.

6. ÜBERREITER, O.: Eine besondere Keratitisform (Keratitis superficialis chronica) beim Hund. Wien. Tierärztl. Monatschr. **48**: 65, 1961.

7. SLATTER, D.H., LAVACH, J.D., SEVERIN, G.A. & YOUNG, S.: Überreiter's syndrome (chronic superficial keratitis) in dogs in Rocky Mountain area. J. Small Anim. Pract. **18**: 757, 1977.

8. BOLLIGER, J.O.: Die lokale Applikation von 1%igen Cyclosporin Augentropfen bei der Keratokonjunktivitis sicca, der Keratitis superficialis chronica und der Keratitis punctata. Veterinär-Chirurgische Klinik. Diss. Zürich, Universität Zürich, 1997

9. PAULSEN, M.E. *et al.*: Feline Eosinophilic keratitis: A review of 15 clinical cases. JAAHA **23**: 63, 1987.

10. CARMICHAEL, L.E., MEDIC, B.L.S., BISTNER, S.I. & AGUIRRE, G.D.: Viral antibody complexes in canine adenovirus type 1 (CAV-1) ocular lesions: leukocyte chemotaxis and enzyme release. Cornell Vet. **65**: 331, 1975.

11. WYMAN, M. *et al.*: Experimental *Pseudomonas aeruginosa* ulcerative keratitis model in the dog. Am. J. Vet. Res. **44**: 1135, 1983.

12. GELATT, K.N. & SAMUELSON, D.A.: Recurrent corneal erosions and epithelial dystrophy in the boxer dog. JAAHA **18**: 453, 1982.

13. PEIFFER, R.L., GELATT, K.N. & GWIN, R.M.: Tarsoconjunctival pedicle grafts for deep corneal ulceration in the dog and cat. JAAHA **13**: 387, 1977.

14. GELATT, K.N.: Herniation of orbital fat in a colt. Vet. Med. **65**: 146, 1970.

15. LAVIGNETTE, A.M.: Lamellar keratoplasty in the dog. Sm. Anim. Clin. **2**: 183, 1962.

16. BROMBERG, N.M.: Cyanoacrylate tissue adhesive for treatment of refractory corneal ulceration. Vet. Ophthalmol. **5**(1): 55–60, 2002.

17. VERWER, M.A.J.: Partial mummification of the cornea in cats. The corneal sequestrum. Oric. Am. Anim. Hosp. Assoc: 112, 1965.

18. SPIESS, B.: Symblepharon, Pseudopterygium und partielles Ankyloblepharon als Folgen feliner Herpes-Keratokonjunktivitis. Kleintierpraxis **30**: 149–154, 1985.

19. STILES, J.: Treatment of cats with ocular disease attributable to Herpes virus infection – 17 Cases (1983–1993). JAVMA **207**(5): 599–603, 1995.

20. MAGGS, D.J., NASISSE, M.P. *et al.*: Efficacy of oral supplementation with L-lysine in cats latently infected with feline herpesvirus. Am. J. Vet. Res. **64**(1): 37–42, 2003.

21. NASISSE, M.: Manifestations, diagnosis, and treatment of ocular Herpes virus infection in cats. Comp. Cont. Educ. **4**(12): 962–968, 1982.

22. NASISSE, M.P.: Feline herpesvirus ocular disease. Vet. Clin. North Am. Small Anim. Pract. **20**(3): 667–80, 1990.

23. KOCH, S.A., LANGLOSS, J.M. & SCHMIDT, G.M.: Corneal epithelial inclusion cysts in four dogs. JAAHA **164**: 1190, 1974.

24. WHITLEY, R.D. & GILGER, B.C.: Diseases of the canine cornea and sclera. *In*: Veterinary Ophthalmology. Ed.: K. Gelatt. Philadelphia, Lippincott Williams & Wilkins, 1999.

25. CRISPIN, S.M. & BARNETT, K.C.: Dystrophy, degeneration and infiltration of the canine cornea. J. Small Anim. Pract. **24**: 63, 1983.

26. WARING, G.O., MACMILLAN, A. & REVELES, P.: Inheritance of crystalline corneal dystrophy in Siberian Huskies. JAAHA **22**: 655, 1986.

27. GWIN, R.M., POLACK, F.M., WARREN, J.K., SAMUELSON, D.A. & GELATT, K.N.: Primary canine corneal endothelial cell dystrophy: specular microscopic evaluation, diagnosis and therapy. JAAHA **18**: 471, 1982.

28. GELATT, K.N., & GELATT, J.P.: Small Animal Ophthalmic Surgery. Boston, Butterworth & Heinemann, 2001.

29. CRISPIN, S.M. & BARNETT, K.C.: Arcus lipoides corneae secondary to hypothyroidism in the Alsatian. J. Small Anim. Pract. **19**: 127, 1978.

30. BISTNER, S.I., AGUIRRE, G.D. & SHIVELY, J.N.: Hereditary corneal dystrophy in the Manx cat: A preliminary report. Invest. Ophthalmol. Vis. Sci. **15**: 15, 1976.

31. JEZYK, P.F. *et al.*: Mucopolysaccharidosis in a cat with arylsulfatase B deficiency: A model of Maroteaux-Lamy syndrome. Science. **198**: 834, 1977.

32. CORK, L.C., MUNELL, J.R. & LORENZ, M.D.: The pathology of feline GM2 gangliosidosis. Am J. Pathol. **90**: 723, 1978.

33. BELLHORN, R.W. & HENKIND, P.: Ocular nodular fasciitis in a dog. JAVMA **150**: 212, 1967.

34. STADES, F.C., BOEVÉ, M.H., LINDE-SIPMAN, J.S. VAN DE & EN SANDT, R.R.O.M. VAN DE: MEM-Dextran stored homologous grafts for the repair of corneal-scleral defects after the removal of limbal melanomas in four dogs. Trans. Am. Coll. Vet. Ophthalmol./Int. Soc. Vet. Ophthalmol. Scottsdale, Arizona, USA, **24**. 24, 1993.

35. MARTIN, C.L.: Canine epibulbar melanomas and their management. JAAHA **17**: 18–90, 1981.

11 Intraocular Pressure and Glaucoma

11.1 Introduction

The aqueous humor (humor aqueous) plays an essential role in the delivery of nutrients and the removal of metabolites from the cornea, uvea, lens, and possibly also the anterior vitreous and fundus. It also maintains the pressure necessary for the conformation of the eye and for refraction. In birds, the globe achieves its extra sturdiness by the existence of a bony ring and/or bony plates in the sclera. Aqueous differs from plasma in its very low protein and lipid concentrations[1] and its other constituents, all of which confirm the fact that it is secreted by active as well as passive mechanisms. As passive secretion will not produce aqueous against a gradient pressure, it is the active portion of the production of aqueous that is mainly responsible for the turgidity of the globe in health and the elevated pressure in glaucoma. Most of the aqueous is produced actively and continuously by the epithelium of the ciliary processes (Fig. 11.1). This active secretion is based on complex enzymatic processes in which the enzyme carbonic anhydrase (among others) plays an essential role. Passive transport is by ultrafiltration, diffusion, and dialysis of plasma. The aqueous production in cats is most likely similar to that in rabbits (3–4 ml per minute) and slightly less in the dog.[2,3,4,5] In inflammatory disease, the blood-aqueous barrier is broken down; this means that the tight junctions between the nonpigmented and the pigmented epithelium (which comprise the secretory organ) are compromised. There is also a dilatation of the episcleral vessels, with a secondary drop in episcleral venous pressure. These together result in a decreased intraocular pressure (IOP) or hypotony. In contrast, when there is obstruction to flow and the active secretory process is functional, there is a marked increase in IOP (glaucoma). The important facts are that aqueous production is dynamic and aqueous humor is in a state of constant turnover.

Once it is produced by the epithelium of the ciliary processes, the aqueous passes into the posterior chamber and through the pupil into the anterior chamber to the peripheral junction of the cornea and iris (irido-corneal angle). This area, via which the aqueous is removed from the globe and returned to the general circulation, is referred to as the drainage

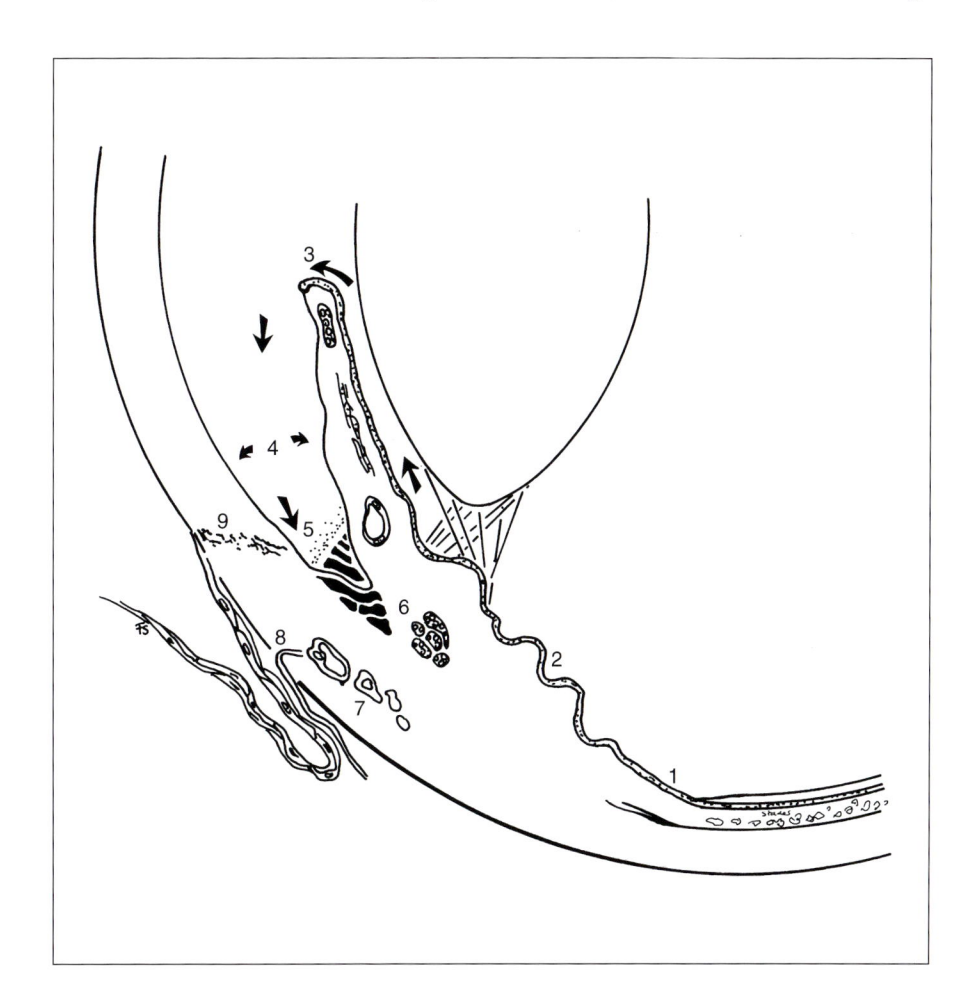

Fig. 11.1:
Aqueous production.
(1) Pigment epithelium,
(2) ciliary body,
(3) pupil,
(4) iridocorneal angle,
(5) pectinate ligament,
(6) drainage angle/ciliary cleft,
(7) scleral venous plexus,
(8) conjunctival vessel anastomosis,
(9) limbus.

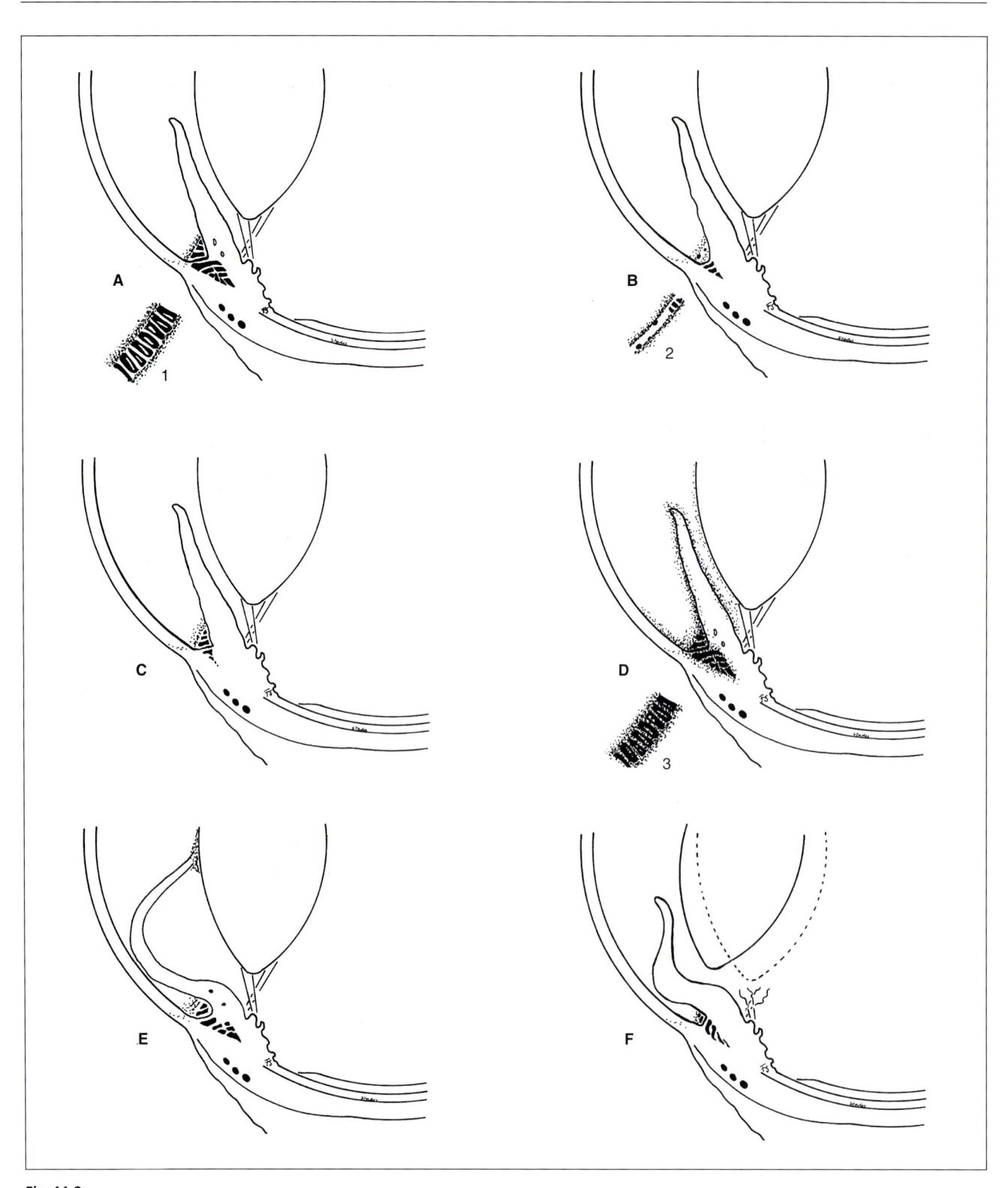

Fig. 11.2:
Anterior chamber irido-corneal angle sections (A–F), gonioscopic view on the pectinate ligament (1–3), and the drainage angle/ciliary cleft in the different forms of glaucoma. A. Normal pectinate ligament (1); B. pectinate ligament abnormality, goniodysplasia or dysgenesis; occlusion [2]); C. narrow/closed drainage angle; D. exudate blockage of the irido-corneal angle/pectinate ligament (3); E. Posterior synechia resulting in an iris bombé and a less open iridocorneal angle; F. narrow/closed irido-corneal angle due to e.g., luxation of the lens.

angle. The drainage angle starts with the pectinate ligament.[6,7] This structure originates from the periphery of the iris base and inserts into the inner peripheral surface of the cornea. It consists of numerous fibers, which are usually the same color as the iris and are larger and more numerous in dogs than in cats. The pectinate ligament occurs in large domestic animals as well. The pectinate ligament and its individual fibers can be examined using a special contact lens (gonioscopy). Immediately behind these ligaments lies the finely pored trabecular meshwork. This provides the resistance to aqueous outflow which maintains the globe turgid in contrast to the surrounding tissue pressure. The trabecular meshwork is composed of the extension and insertions of the accommodation muscles. This arrangement is similar in all mammals but with minor variations, e.g. the canal of Schlemm is present in primates and absent in domestic animals. The aqueous is removed from the globe via the drainage angle, partly to the scleral venous plexus (main part) by a process based on pinocytosis, and partly by leakage through the interstitial spaces of the ciliary cleft to the veins of the uvea, sclera, and scleral conjunctiva.

The IOP ("tension" would be more correct because it measures the combination of the IOP and the rigidity of the cornea) varies between 10–20 mmHg in dogs, cats, and horses. One has to realize that in excited animals IOP may spontaneously rise by 10–20 mmHg.

Elevated pressure can in principle arise because of an elevated production of aqueous (which has not yet been found in animals) and/or obstruction to its removal (Fig. 11.2).

11.2 Glaucoma (Plate 11.1)

Glaucoma can be defined as a pathological process of varying etiology, characterized by decreased retinal ganglion cell sensitivity and function, and by ganglion cell death, optic nerve axonal loss, and optic nerve head cup enlargement, incremental reduction in the visual field, blindness, and in animal is associated with an increase in IOP.[8,9] In the pathogenesis of glaucoma, glutamate (neurotransmitter) may play a role as it is toxic for the ganglion cells.[10]

Glaucoma is not curable but can be better controlled if diagnosed early in the course of the disease. An IOP of between 20–30 mmHg are considered to be moderately elevated, whereas IOP elevations in individual animals of over 20–30 mmHg should result in "prophylactic" therapy. Irreparable damage occurs in the eye if the pressure is elevated above 40 mmHg for as little as 48 hours. The eye will accommodate if the pressures are elevated above 20 mmHg but less than 40 mmHg over a prolonged period of time, but even in these instances, irreversible damage does occur, but not as drastic. With this information, it becomes evident that early recognition of the condition is needed, thus producing better results in prolonging vision without the development of pain that accompanies overt glaucoma.

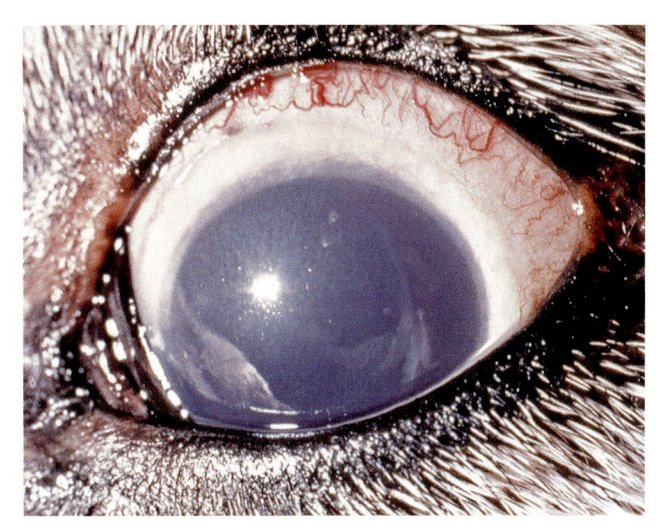

Plate 11.1:
Acute, primary glaucoma. The bulbar conjunctival vessels are congested, there is diffuse corneal blueing (edema), and the mydriatic pupil is non-reactive (OS, Siberian Husky; the iris is white).

Elevated IOP is only the result of obstruction to aqueous flow and not the actual disease, which must be classified further with regard to its cause. Much glaucoma research has been done in animals and humans, and many classification schemes have been suggested without any real information regarding the mechanism. Regardless of the classification, one of the most important criteria for successful management of this enigmatic manifestation is early recognition. This is true in humans as well as in animals, and is, alas, much more difficult to accomplish in animals than humans.

Glaucoma can be classified as follows (see also Fig. 11.2):
- Etiologically as primary, secondary, or absolute.
- According to the condition of the irido-corneal angle, i.e. open, narrow, or closed irido-corneal angle glaucoma.
- According to the condition of the drainage angle, i.e., open or primary morphologically abnormal.
- According to the length of time it has taken to develop, i.e., acute or chronic glaucoma.

11.2.1 Etiology

11.2.1.1 Primary glaucoma
Primary glaucoma is defined as a glaucoma not accompanied or preceded by another detectable eye disease.

Primary glaucoma occurs regularly in dogs and is rare in cats.[11] Frequently, dogs are presented with acute congestive episodes of primary glaucoma because the owner is not aware of the incipient changes that have occurred previously. Such cases are very refractive to effective medical therapy and this is why early recognition is so important in the management of this disease.

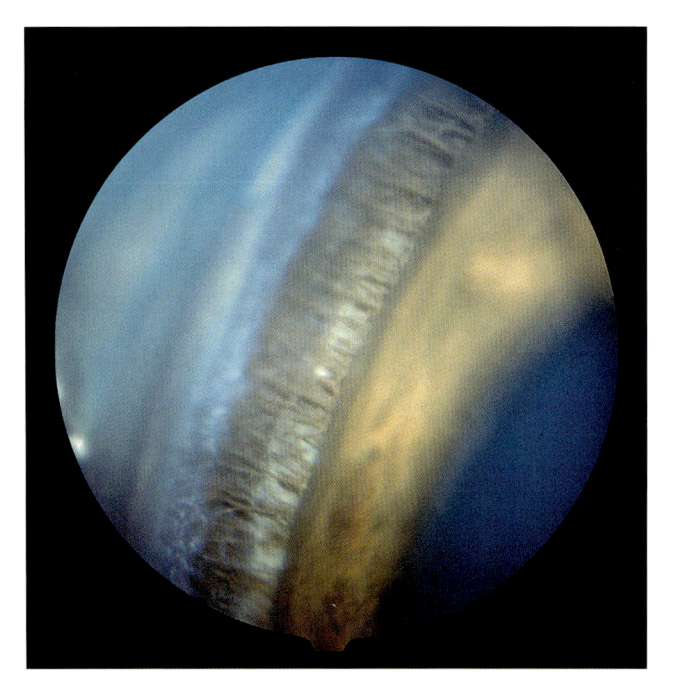

Plate 11.2:
Gonioscopic view of a normally developed pectinate ligament (2×).

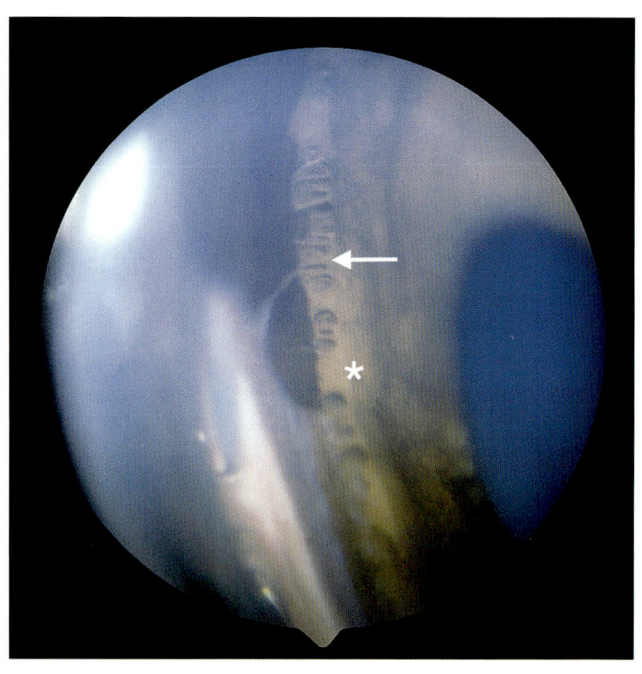

Plate 11.3:
Gonioscopic view of moderate pectinate ligament abnormality in a Flat-coated Retriever. The fibers are broad (fibrae latae, arrow) and there are plate-like deformities (laminae, asterix)

11.2.1.2 Secondary glaucoma
The secondary forms can occur as a result of abnormalities connected with the lens (lens luxation, secondary to uveitis as a result of the release of lens' proteins, postoperatively after lens extraction), the uvea (trauma, uveitis, i.e., resulting in angle-spanning fibrovascular membrane formation, and neoplasia), or the use of medication such as atropine or as corticosteroids in humans.

11.2.1.3 Absolute glaucoma
In a fairly large proportion of cases, the changes due to glaucoma are already so severe (buphthalmos, cupping of the optic disc, retinal degeneration, ingrowth of vessels, scars in the cornea, and blindness) that it is no longer possible to determine whether the glaucoma is primary or secondary. Such cases are described as absolute glaucoma.

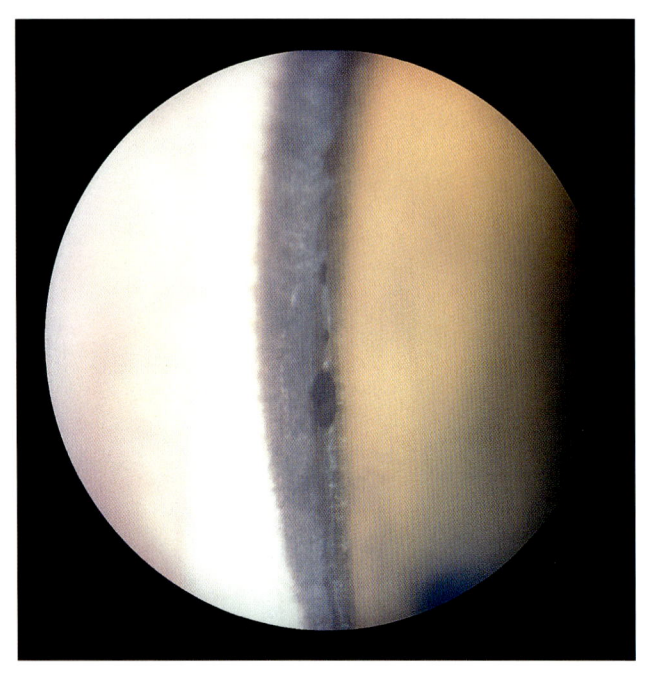

Plate 11.4:
Gonioscopic view of severe pectinate ligament abnormality. The ligament is totally closed, except for some very small flow holes in a Bouvier des Flandres with acute primary glaucoma of the other eye.

11.2.2 Irido-corneal angle abnormalities

11.2.2.1 Open irido-corneal angle glaucoma
This form of glaucoma occurs without demonstrable changes in the width of the irido-corneal angle. The depth of the anterior chamber is also normal. This is true "primary" glaucoma. Little is known of the etiopathogenesis of this condition; however, it is assumed that the cause is in the trabecular meshwork, the collecting tubules, or in the intrascleral plexus. Unfortunately, in the literature the terms narrowed, closed, or open angle, chamber angle, or drainage angle are used interchangeably.

11.2.2.2 Narrowed or closed irido-corneal angle glaucoma
In this form of glaucoma, the base of the iris is displaced in the direction of the cornea. The anterior chamber is shallow. In severe cases, the lens-iris diaphragm is displaced anteriorly to completely obliterate the anterior chamber and thus completely close the angle. The passage to the trabecular meshwork is then compromised and the IOP rises. This is another reason for obtaining as much information as possible, or referring the patient if doubt exists regarding the nature of the angle. The narrowing or closure can occur as a result of swelling of the base of the iris (e.g. neoplasia) or because the iris is pressed forward by the lens (lens luxation), by vitreous (lens luxation in which the vitreous bulges anteriorly or after intracapsular lens extraction), or by aqueous (in iris bombé). Almost without exception, these are secondary forms of glaucoma.

11.2.3 Conditions of the drainage angle

11.2.3.1 Open pectinate ligament glaucoma
This term is used for glaucoma in which gonioscopic examination reveals no abnormality in the pectinate ligament. In general, it also implies that the irido-corneal angle is not abnormally narrow and that there are no symptoms indicative of a secondary glaucoma.

Open pectinate ligament glaucoma appears to be the most frequent form of primary glaucoma in cats and is found in the Persian, Siamese, and European Shorthaired cat.

11.2.3.2 Primary morphologically abnormal pectinate ligament
In this form of glaucoma, gonioscopic examination of the pectinate ligament reveals inadequate and/or very small drainage openings, or is almost totally closed (Plates 11.2–11.4).

Three predominant types of involvement of the pectinate ligament can be distinguished:
1. the normal part of the pectinate ligament fiber is too short (fibrae latae); the abnormal parts are broad;
2. plates or sheets (laminae) of continuous tissue (i.e. without flow holes), with very short remaining fibers;
3. totally closed (occlusion) pectinate ligament, with small flow holes, and a narrowed irido-corneal angle and/or shallower anterior chamber.

The abnormality is caused by a developmental proliferation of tissues of the pectinate ligament (starting as a dysplasia or dysgenesis), which increases with ageing. It leads to inadequate and/or very small drainage openings to parts of the ligament in which there are no openings at all. In such eyes, the drainage often appears to remain undisturbed for a long time. However, in a small percentage of cases the drainage becomes obstructed and there is an acute increase in IOP. Additional conditions such as inflammatory swelling, compression, and/or plugging can cause blockage of the remaining drainage pores.

According to some authors, goniodysplastic glaucoma should be referred to as congenital glaucoma. It has been documented that the pectinate ligament abnormality occurs at birth but glaucoma is rarely manifested early in the animal's life. There are other primary defects that are congenital and the term can be applied to those defects, e.g. aniridia with drainage angle deformity, as an additional descriptive word.

Pectinate ligament abnormality, (dysplasia or dysgenesis) is known to be hereditary in the American Cocker Spaniel, the Bassets (English and French), the Bouvier des Flanders, Flat-coated Retriever, Great Dane, Samoyed, and in the English Cocker Spaniel and the Welsh Springer Spaniel in Great Britain.[12,13,14,15,16,17]

11.2.4 Length of time of development and progression of glaucoma

11.2.4.1 Acute glaucoma
In this disorder, there is a sudden (within hours) and sometimes episodic increase in IOP. The symptoms of glaucoma, such as pain, diffuse corneal blueing, mydriasis, and loss of vision, are prominent. If treatment is not started promptly, the retina and optic nerve may be damaged, leading to irreparable blindness within 2–7 days. Continued elevation of the IOP results in stretching of the fibrous tunic, thus causing buphthalmos. Acute primary glaucoma occurs primarily in breeds of dogs with pectinate ligament abnormality.

11.2.4.2 Chronic glaucoma (Plates 11.5, 11.6)

In this disorder there is a chronic, sometimes episodic, mild increase in IOP (30–40 mmHg). The first symptoms are scarcely noticed by the owner. The increase in IOP is often very difficult for the veterinary practitioner to diagnose because he / she lacks the index of suspicion for the disease (i.e. there are no direct/specific signs of this problem).

11.2.4.3 Hydrophthalmia or buphthalmos
(Plates 11.7, 11.8)

Because the normal globe of animals is elastic (especially in the adolescent), it can be stretched by increased IOP and thus become enlarged. This is termed hydrophthalmos (enlarged by water) or buphthalmos (Gr.; bous: ox; enlarged in general). During this process there can be tearing of the Descemet's membrane, via which water leaks into the corneal stroma. This results in curvilinear streaks in the cornea due to the elastic recoil that accompanies the tearing (Plate 11.7). The resulting stripes (striae) resemble cracks in ice. They remain visible as scar striae, even after the IOP has been normalized.

As a result of enlargement of the globe, the suspensory ligaments of the lens can break and thus a secondary luxation of the lens can occur (Plates 11.7, 11.8). If a patient is presented with a buphthalmic eye, including lens luxation, it is often no longer possible to determine whether there has been a primary or secondary glaucoma.

Another aspect of the occurrence of hydrophthalmos (buphthalmos) is that it indicates that the retina and the optic nerve fibers must have already been exposed to an increased pressure for a long time. The increased IOP causes direct damage (pressure damage to the nerve fibers) and / or indirect damage (pressure ischemia of the microcirculation of the optic disc) to the retina, optic nerve, and nerve fibers at the level of the optic disc. A definite buphthalmos thus implies that the nerve fibers are irreversibly damaged, the functional connection with the brain is interrupted, and the eye is therefore blind and will remain blind. One exception is that if the pressure rise has been subclinical over a long period of time, the eye can stretch and the retina and optic nerve accommodate, and the patient may still be able to see. Vision is compromised because of the associated increase in axial length of the eye and the displacement of the lens. Acute manifestation of buphthalmos is definitely blinding.

11.3 Clinical aspects of glaucoma

In practice, it is of great importance to identify subtle elevations of IOP prior to the first "signs" of glaucoma. These signs are more easily recognized in the usually acutely developing primary glaucoma in dogs. In the more chronically developing forms (especially in cats), recognition is much more difficult.

Note: If a patient is suspected of glaucoma but no reasonably reliable method of measuring the IOP is available, then it is emphatically recommended that the patient is referred promptly for tonometry and further ophthalmic evaluation in order to confirm the diagnosis.

Further examination will reveal whether there are indications of other eye abnormalities and hence, whether the glaucoma is secondary. Treatment should be started immediately.

11.3.1 Acute glaucoma

In the primary forms, acute cases are usually caused by pectinate ligament abnormalities in predisposed dog breeds. The drainage is blocked suddenly, with the result that aqueous cannot escape. For example, about 10–20% of the Bouviers in the total population in the Netherlands probably have severe pectinate ligament abnormalities. Yet, roughly estimated, probably only 0.2% of these dogs develop actual glaucoma.[18] It is likely that these cases are mainly related to an inflammatory reaction, thus causing the definitive blocking. Because of the acutely developing and usually obvious increase in IOP (40–120 mmHg), the signs (such as corneal edema and episcleral vascular injection) are usually quite noticeable but not very specific. The eye is painful and causes headache, so the animal is usually listless. The optic disc and the area around it come under great pressure, which results in ischemia and / or inflammation with an acute and usually complete loss of vision. If intervention is not immediate, vision will be irreversibly lost within 2–7 days.

History: The patient is often presented with a very acute, diffuse, dense, bluish-white edema of the entire cornea (Plates 10.1, 11.1) and listlessness. The owner usually believes, and suggests, that is has been caused by trauma. The animal has reduced appetite, is less active ("sleeps all day"), and may also object to being patted on the head. This aversion is caused by patient discomfort from the acute rise in IOP and anxiety that the diseased eye will be touched. In humans, acute congestive glaucoma is accompanied by severe continuous pain. The episcleral vascular injection is usually not noticed by the owner.

Symptoms: Acute glaucoma is seldom presented initially as a bilateral disease but it is possible. The IOP is usually high and is thus, even without a tonometer, reasonably easy to determine by bilateral, digital tonometry going from the normal to the abnormal globe. Because the bulbar conjunctival vessels are distended, they give the appearance of a marked **hyperemia** (Plate 11.1) of these vessels. Especially at the beginning of the elevated IOP, the diffuse redness and swelling typical of conjunctivitis or uveitis are missing in glaucoma. There is **diffuse corneal bluing**. This is due to derangement of the collagen fibers and edema. The collagen fibers of the normal cor-

Clinical aspects of glaucoma **163**

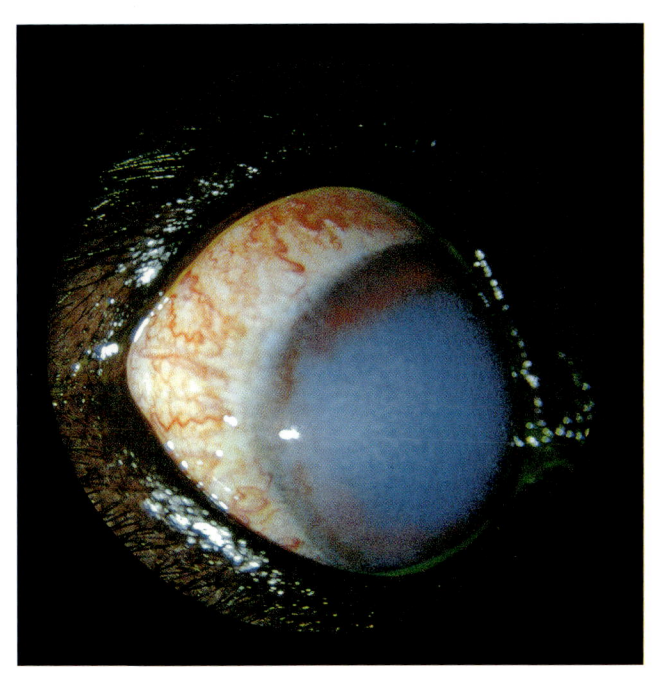

Plate 11.5:
Chronic primary glaucoma (dog). The bulbar conjunctiva shows severe hyperemia, there is circular superficial vessel ingrowth in the cornea, and a dense, diffuse corneal edema. The pupil cannot be judged.

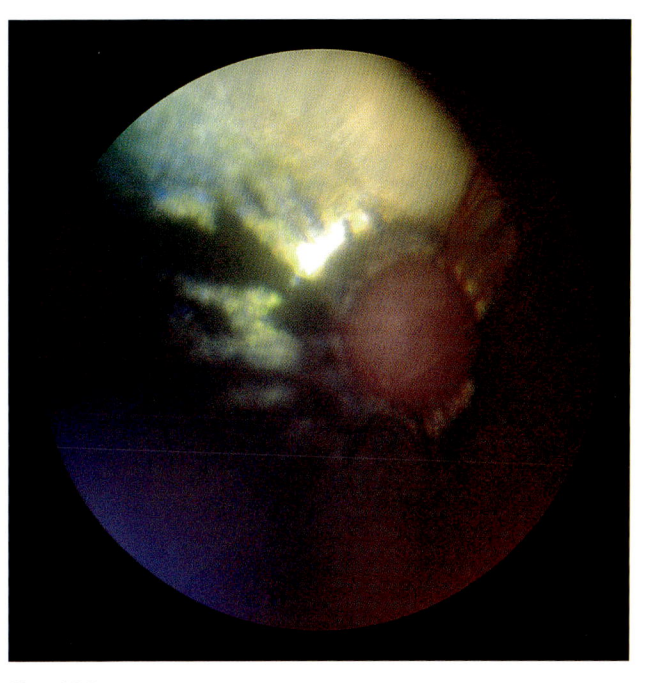

Plate 11.6:
Chronic primary glaucoma (OD, dog). The fundus shows hyperreflection, hyperpigmentation, retinal vessel atrophy, and a dark, atrophic excavated optic disc as a result of some weeks of increased IOP.

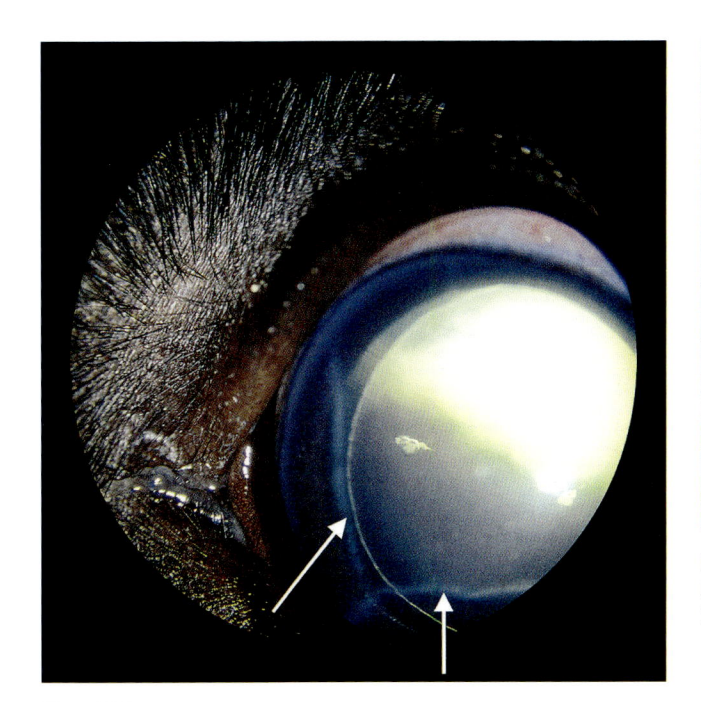

Plate 11.7:
Descemet's tears (striae of Haab, see arrows) after a long period of high IOP (OS, dog). There is also a secondary lens luxation.

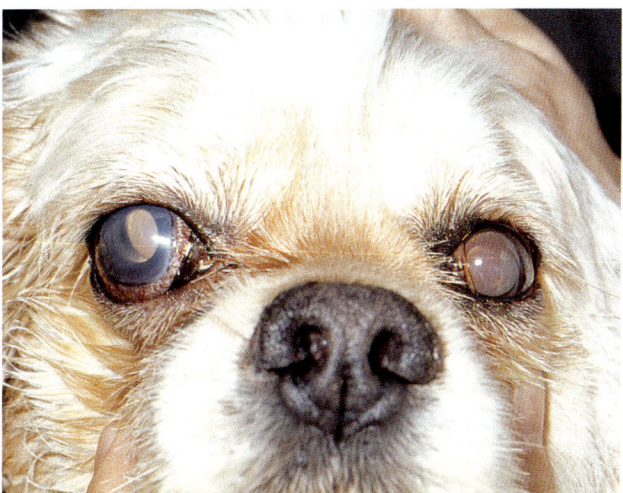

Plate 11.8:
Buphthalmos (OD) as a result of chronic primary glaucoma in an American Cocker Spaniel. There is also is a secondary lens luxation.

neal stroma are arranged in a very geometric form and the normal cornea contains a stable, relatively high percentage of water (75–80%), resulting in corneal clarity. When the geometric structure is disrupted by stretching etc., the refraction is altered and clarity is compromised. One can simulate this phenomenon by applying external pressure to the normal eye. The endothelial cells are primarily responsible for corneal deturgescence, and as long as they are functional, edema is less prominent. However, during glaucoma water is pressed and leaks into the cornea, resulting in an increase in corneal thickness up to 30–50%. The corneal changes can be misinterpreted as a primary "keratitis". The anterior chamber is usually normal with respect to contents and depth. The pupil is unresponsive to light and there is **mydriasis** (8–12 mm). On monocular, direct ophthalmoscopy, excavation of the papilla is scarcely recognizable. The retinal vessels may be a little thinner and the edge around the papilla and the papilla itself may be a little darker than normal.

If glaucoma persists, the changes in the cornea become more severe. The tension and infiltration result in vascularization, and with continuous exposure the cornea may become eroded resulting in granulation tissue proliferation. Mydriasis may only be demonstrable by the use of retrograde illumination. The globe enlarges (hydrophthalmos / buphthalmos) and pseudo-exophthalmos occurs with a greater chance that the eye will be injured. The stretching of the globe continues to cause pain, a fact that must be appreciated by the veterinarian, even though the patient accommodates to this pain with time. This is very obvious to the owner and the veterinarian when the eye is removed, since the dog becomes much more active and appears to be "happier" without the pain. Eventually, if left untreated the ciliary body ceases to function due to degeneration of the epithelium and the pressure gradually decreases. The globe still remains enlarged for a long time but the edema, vascular injection, and pain decrease. Because of pressure atrophy, the retina can no longer absorb light and thus it becomes hyperreflective, starting around the optic disc in a flame-like pattern (Plate 11.6). The excavated optic disc and a ring around it are usually darkly pigmented and the eye is completely blind.

The differential diagnosis must include all the causes of conjunctival vascular injection and/or corneal edema, as well as causes of exophthalmos. The most important disorders to be considered are conjunctivitis, primary forms of keratitis, and anterior uveitis. In conjunctivitis and keratitis, the anterior uvea may not be affected and there is a lively pupillary reaction. When there is secondary anterior uveitis associated with keratitis, all the signs of uveitis may be present including exudate in the anterior chamber and an abnormal iris, and, in contrast to glaucoma, miosis and a lowered or normal IOP are to be expected. Secondary glaucoma can occur after healing due to the sequelae of an inflammatory insult, i.e. posterior synechia or compromised angle. Exophthalmos is generally caused by a retrobulbar mass, which does not increase the IOP but rather the retrobulbar pressure.

Buphthalmos can also occur as a result of a massive intraocular neoplasm.

11.3.2 Chronic glaucoma

Glaucoma in cats is rare and almost always chronic. If acute glaucoma in dogs becomes chronic, the chronic signs will become more prominent. However, primary chronic glaucoma in dogs occurs in Siberian Huskies and only sporadically in other breeds.

A chronically recurring increase in IOP, usually mild in the beginning, results in few noticeable signs. The size of the globe increases very gradually and, because of the great elasticity of Descemet's membrane, there may be very little tearing. Excavation of the papilla and atrophy of the surrounding retina develop gradually and thus there is a gradual but irreversible loss of vision.

History: There are few noticeable symptoms in the beginning. Patients are often presented because of anisocoria (inequality in the size of the pupils) or because of a minor, diffuse corneal edema and slight injection of the episcleral vessels.

Symptoms: Chronic glaucoma seldom occurs bilaterally. The IOP usually increases moderately and may remain between 30 and 40 mmHg, and is thus very difficult to determine without a tonometer. There is hyperemia because the conjunctival vessels drain the additional aqueous fluid (Plate 11.5). At least at the beginning, there is an absence of the redness and swelling of the conjunctiva that are typical of conjunctivitis or uveitis. Signs of pain are not very noticeable. There is a diffuse subtle corneal "haziness" and there can be ingrowth of vessels into the cornea from all around the limbus, giving a ring-like appearance. In exceptional cases, there are tears in Descemet's membrane or keratoconus formation. These corneal changes can be erroneously interpreted as "keratitis". Ophthalmoscopy reveals the retinal vessels to be slightly thinner than normal and the edge of the papilla and the papilla itself is slightly darker.

Eventually, there is often a ring of irregular, increased reflection (retinal atrophy) around the papilla in radial retinal infarctions (appearing somewhat like flames around the optic disc). The size of the globe and thus the diameter of the cornea gradually increase, resulting in buphthalmos (Plates 11.7, 11.8).

As in acute glaucoma, the differential diagnosis must include all causes of conjunctival vascular injection and/or corneal edema, as well as the causes of exophthalmos.

11.3.3 Therapeutic possibilities in glaucoma

The purpose of glaucoma therapy must be to keep the IOP below 20 mmHg as even pressures between 25 and 30 mmHg will result in a slow loss of ganglion cells. If medical treatment is insufficient, the patient has to be referred for surgical treatment possibilities.

The initial therapy for acute and chronic glaucoma is the same. Chronic glaucoma generally responds better to treatment, so the doses and concentrations can be reduced more quickly to maintenance levels and surgical therapy is less frequently indicated.

Medical treatment

Medical treatment is most effective when the diagnosis of increased IOP can be made before the advent of clinical signs. This requires early recognition and education of the owner by the veterinarian is the key to successful management. Glaucoma is still incurable; it can only be controlled so that it must be monitored constantly in order for the treatment to be effective. Animals, regardless of the species, presented with advanced signs of glaucoma rarely respond effectively to medical therapy and are therefore candidates for those procedures which ameliorate pain rather than restore or maintain vision.

The basic principals of glaucoma therapy include:
1. Reduction of aqueous production.
2. Improvement of outflow.
3. Reduction of intraocular volume.

1. Reduction of aqueous production. Drugs which result in decreased aqueous production include both topical and systemic carbonic anhydrase inhibitors (CAI), e.g. dorzolamide, brinzolamide, dichlorphenamide, methazolamide, and acetazolamide; and beta-adrenergic blockers, e.g., timolol, detaxolol, and others.

All CAIs decrease aqueous production and it has been reported that they can reduce active secretion by as much as 20–30%, which is clearly potentially helpful.[19] The agents that have proved most effective and are better tolerated are topical 2% dorzolamide and 2% brinzolamide (no effect in cats), 2–3 times daily. Systemic CAIs are adjunctive to topical drugs and are instituted when topical drugs can no longer manage the IOP and should not be used independently. Systemic CAIs are dichlorphenamide, methazolamide and acetazolamide.

The initial dose for dichlorphenamide is 2–2.5 mg/kg, 4 times daily for 5–10 days and thereafter 1.25 mg/kg, 3–4 times daily. Methazolamide is the CAI available in the USA and is administered at 4–6 mg/kg, 2–3 times per day. The frequency is determined by the response to therapy. Although dichlorphenamide is usually well tolerated, if it is to be used for extended periods, there should be periodic measurement of plasma Na and K levels and correction (e.g. KCl) as required. Alternative drugs (e.g., acetazolamide) more frequently cause vomiting and diarrhea as side effects. An advantage of acetazolamide is that it can also be administered intravenously in the acute stage, which may result in a rapid reduction in IOP. The combination of local and parenteral CAIs appears not to result in additional effects.

Note: It is worth noting that diuretics such as furosemide (Lasix®, Dimazon®) or aminophylline do not lower IOP at all.

The beta-adrenergic blocking agents are most effective in control of occult (potential) glaucoma and can be used successfully in delaying the advent of overt glaucoma. These are employed most effectively in the normotensive eye in animals of breeds predisposed to glaucoma. It is imperative that when presented with a patient that has overt glaucoma in one eye and is apparently normal in the opposite eye, both eyes are treated. However, it is not necessary to use the more potent and reactive drugs, therefore beta-blockers can be helpful. Timolol and other beta-adrenergic blocking agents such as levobunolol, optipropanol, metipranolol, and betaxolol, etc. can be used. They all seem to work similar to timolol.[20] The beta-blockers available at present only decrease IOP by about 5%, therefore their use in overt glaucoma is questionable. Stronger concentrations of 4–6% are more effective, but are not yet commercially available.

2. Improvement of outflow. Drugs which mimic the effect of acetylcholine on parasympathomimetic postganglionic nerve endings within the eye improve the outflow. These agents are either direct-acting (cholinergic agents; e.g. pilocarpine and carbachol), or indirect-acting (anti-acetylcholine-esterase agents; e.g. ecothiophate iodide, physostigmine, demecarium, and isoflurophate). In addition, sympathomimetic drugs also facilitate outflow. These drugs include epinephrine and the prodrug, dipivefrin.

Very strong miosis can be induced with ecothiophate iodide. Because of its side effects, mainly caused by resorption via the nasopharynx, and the very high costs for very specific drugs such as this for small groups of patients (minor species), ecothiophate iodide is not available at the moment. Possibly a gel will be available in the near future.

Pilocarpine is available in concentrations from 1–10%; however, concentrations above 4% have no additional benefit and cause more adverse reactions. Concentrations of 2% are most effective and best tolerated after a period of accommodation. It is imperative that the clinician explains the reactions produced by these agents and the importance of continuing medication in this disease. For example, 2% pilocarpine in a normal eye will produce initially lesions that simulate Horner's syndrome. Clients may believe their pet is in pain and discontinue the medication. Similar signs can be manifested by any of the drugs that mimic acetylcholine. The chosen drug should be administered 3–4 times a day and IOP re-evaluated and the frequency of application being modified as the condition changes. The objective is to use the least frequent and the lowest concentration that effectively controls the IOP.

The new prostanoids such as 50 µg/ml latanoprost, bimatoprost (not in cats) and travoprost, have shown to be effective, when applied once daily in the human eye. These agents improve the posterior uveal outflow. They have been demonstrated as being effective in the dog (questionable in cat) and can be administered 1–2 times daily. They do produce a highly miotic pupil and should be used with extreme caution in anterior uveal inflammation when present with glaucoma.

Epinephrine, or the prodrug dipivefrin, can be used as an adjunct to the anti-acetylcholine agents in patients with refractive glaucoma. There are medications available that combine pilocarpine and epinephrine for the convenience of the client.

Note: Atropine, in general, is contraindicated in glaucoma. In normotensive horse eyes atropine does not influence the IOP. It may even lower the IOP in glaucomatous horse eyes by improving the uveo-scleral outflow. However, it should only be used when strictly monitored.

3. Reduction of intraocular volume. Hyperosmotic agents, e.g. glycerin, mannitol, and urea, reduce the intraocular volume. Recently, in the USA, a new agent (isosorbide) has been marketed. All these agents decrease IOP by creating an osmotic gradient in which the blood is hypertonic to the intraocular fluid, particularly of the vitreous, causing this fluid to move out of the eye into the bloodstream. They are used to reduce IOP safely and rapidly in emergency conditions, and are not advocated for continual maintenance. Glycerin can be given orally, although it often predisposes to gastric irritation and emesis. It is given at 0.2–0.3 ml/kg orally, 4–6 times daily, followed by withholding of water for one hour, for 1–2 weeks. The purpose of the glycerin should be explained to the owner, who may otherwise think that it is intended as a laxative and may fail to administer it.

To produce an immediate decrease in IOP, mannitol can be used (an alternative is acetazolamide, I.V.). It reduces the tension more rapidly than glycerin and there are also fewer side effects. It is administered strictly intravenously, by slow injection at a dose of 1–5 ml/kg/24 hours of a 20% concentration. These drugs produce a rebound reaction which can result in greater than pretreatment IOP if adequate ancillary therapy is not undertaken. The anterior chamber is widened after effective administration of hyperosmotic agents. The lens-iris diaphragm moves posteriorly resulting in increased depth and widening of the irido-corneal angle. This allows for a more effective control of outflow and provides an opportunity to re-establish homeostasis in the aqueous dynamics.

The owner must be warned in advance that all the medications used to counteract glaucoma can have side effects of anorexia, vomiting, and diarrhea.

The veterinary practitioner who does not have access to use of a reliable tonometer is advised to refer the patient immediately or by the following days for tonometry, gonioscopy, and further treatment. The initial therapy should be started immediately.

If the pressure becomes stabilized at a normal level after 1–2 weeks, a maintenance dose must then be determined that is well tolerated by the patient and which the owner will find easy to continue. However, it must be emphasized to the own-

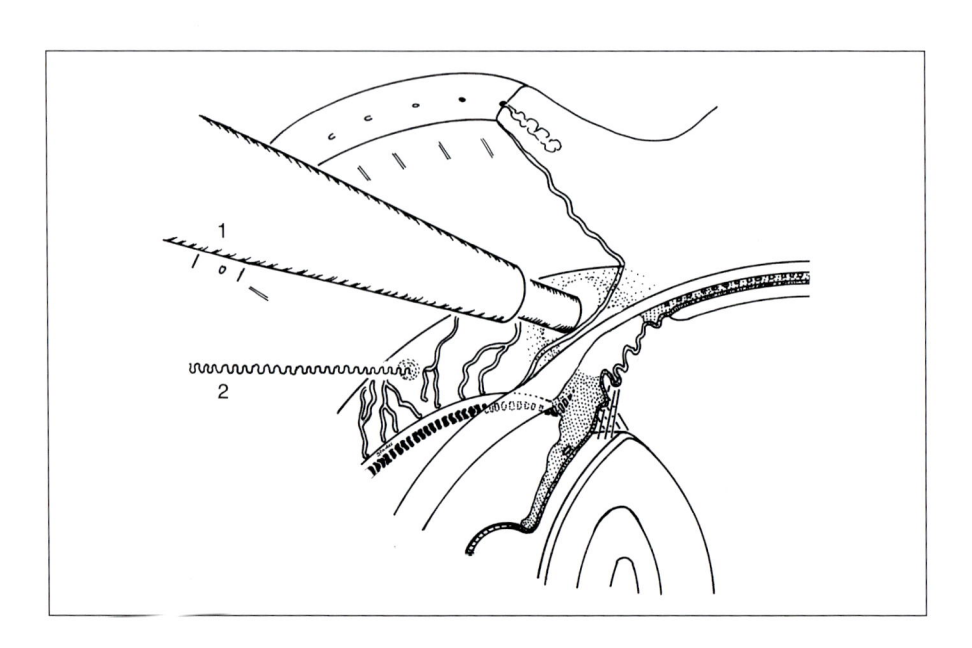

Fig. 11.3:
Cyclodestruction: by (1) cryo or (2) laser. The ciliary epithelium is locally destroyed via the scleral conjunctiva, causing a permanent decrease in aqueous production.

er that there can be new episodes of glaucoma, which must be immediately controlled by returning to high doses of the medications.

If chronic glaucoma is recognized early, and the anterior chamber angle and pectinate ligament are open, the pressure can often be kept under control with timolol alone (0.5%, 1–2 times daily).

Surgical treatment

If glaucoma cannot be controlled satisfactorily by medical treatment, the patient is usually referred for surgical treatment. Unfortunately, none of the various surgical methods have proved to be optimal.

1. Cyclodestruction. Although it is no panacea, this is one of the best methods of controlling glaucoma in an eye that is sighted and poorly controlled by medical therapy. If pressures continue at the 30 mmHg level while the animal is on maximum medical therapy, then surgical intervention is a rational option. The object in this procedure is the controlled destruction of the epithelium of the ciliary processes causing a permanent decrease in aqueous production, and an opening of a part of the drainage angle. This is a non-invasive procedure performed transclerally either with a freezing probe[21,22] or contact laser photocoagulation (Fig. 11.3).[23] An Olympic ring configuration is performed starting approximately 1.5 mm from the limbus in the inferotemporal region (which will prevent damage to the retina), or 3–6 locations about 5 mm posterior to the limbus are frozen (2 min/location). Laser treatment is done in a similar fashion with 20–40 points. However, the cost of the necessary instrumentation is prohibitive and not economically feasible at this time. These procedures are less effective in the acute phase of glaucoma.

2. Drainage with the aid of an implant. In this procedure, very thin silicone tubing with approximately a 0.7-mm outer and 0.3-mm inner diameter (Plate 11.9), or a device provided with a valve (Molteno, Joseph), is placed at a right angle or parallel to the limbus, from the subconjunctival space to the anterior chamber angle. The implant drains the aqueous fluid to the subconjunctival / retrobulbar space, where it is absorbed by the (conjunctival) vessels. This method can also be performed in combination with cyclodestruction. Unfortunately, the tubing sometimes becomes blocked or there is inadequate absorption of aqueous fluid in the subconjunctival space, resulting in recurrence of the glaucoma. The cost of the valve devices and the frequency of failure make the procedure questionable at this time.

3. Fistula methods. Examples of these are trepanation-iridectomy and iridencleisis, or variations of these. In trepanation-iridectomy, the conjunctiva is loosened and lifted. Then an opening of 2-mm diameter is trephined through the sclera into the anterior chamber. Following this, an opening is made in the base of the iris so that the aqueous can drain from the posterior chamber. It can reach the space under the conjunc-

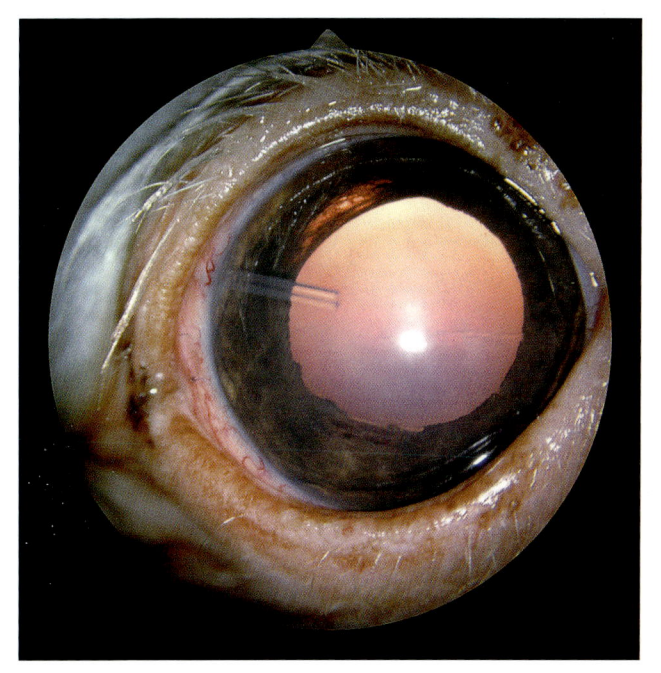

Plate 11.9:
Possible surgical therapy in acute primary glaucoma, using an implant (at the 10-o'clock position; silicone tubing 0.3 mm internal and 0.7 mm external diameter). The tube (or valve) can be placed at a right angle to the limbus, through the subconjunctival space to the anterior chamber angle. The implant drains the aqueous fluid to, for example, the retrobulbar space. There is some iris atrophy.

tiva via the opening in the sclera. In iridencleisis, the iris at the edge of the pupil is pulled through a similar opening and attached to the sclera so that the fistula remains patent. Initially, the fistulas function, but in animals they usually close within weeks.

Prognosis: The residual vision can usually be evaluated 1–2 weeks after restoration of normal IOP. The good eye can be shielded to evaluate the vision of the treated eye. In spite of therapy, the prognosis concerning vision over the long term must be reserved. In more than 50% of patients the affected eye becomes blind, despite all therapeutic efforts. In such cases, enucleation of the globe is beneficial to the patient. Even permanently blind patients, in which an uncontrollable bilateral glaucoma makes bilateral enucleation necessary, manage quite well, and they are then *without* pain.

Prevention: When primary glaucoma occurs in one eye it is advisable to perform gonioscopic examination of the other eye. The owner should check the eyes daily, or at least whenever there is the slightest indication of a problem. This involves measuring the pressure by palpation and stimulating miosis with a strong light. In addition, the eye that is not (yet) affected can be treated prophylactically as discussed previously. Affected animals should not be used for breeding. If the number of animals available for breeding allows it, parents or siblings of affected animals should also be excluded from breeding, because of their higher risk of being carriers.

Distinguishing the predominant type and the degree of involvement of the pectinate ligament gonioscopically gives the owner and/or the breed club/society the opportunity to select animals with less chance of developing glaucoma.[24]

11.4 Secondary glaucoma

In secondary glaucoma, the increase in IOP is the result of another disorder of the eye. The abnormality is usually one that affects the drainage of aqueous and involves the pupil or the drainage angle. The symptoms of secondary glaucoma are in principle the same as those of primary glaucoma, with the understanding that there are also changes involving parts of the eye not involved in the regulation of IOP.

11.4.1 Secondary glaucoma associated with the lens or vitreous

11.4.1.1 Dislocation of the lens
If a large number of zonular fibers are broken, the vitreous can escape and the posterior chamber of the eye and/or the drainage angle can become blocked (Fig. 13.11). If the lens luxates into the anterior chamber, the lens and/or the vitreous that is dragged with it can block the drainage of aqueous fluid via the drainage angle. If the lens is luxated posteriorly, the vitreous that is thereby displaced anteriorly can hinder the flow of aqueous through the pupil. In dogs, secondary glaucoma due to lens luxation usually occurs very soon after the luxation.

Secondary glaucoma occurs less often in cats. Cats may have a luxated lens moving freely, even anteriorly, for a considerable period of time without developing glaucoma, yet lens luxation is still the most frequent cause of glaucoma in this species.

Therapy: A posteriorly luxated lens can be trapped behind the pupil by means of a miotic drug such as latanoprost (50 μg/ml, once daily, in the evening) until the eye is operated. In the case of an anteriorly luxated lens, only CAIs are administered. This is often a good method (for example, in animals in poor condition) of temporarily preventing or delaying the development of glaucoma in the short term. However, secondary glaucoma develops in almost all cases, even in cats. Since the onset of glaucoma cannot be predicted, it is preferable to perform an intracapsular lens extraction before it occurs, if the condition of the patient allows it (see 13.4).

11.4.1.2 Lens proteins
If lens proteins escape, via changes in permeability (lens resorption) or defects in the capsule (trauma, extracapsular lens extraction), they can give rise to anterior uveitis and affect the drainage of aqueous, resulting in glaucoma (see 11.4.2). However, lens resorption and lens trauma seldom occur.

11.4.1.3 Cataract
In exceptional cases, the development of a cataract is associated with such a marked swelling of the lens that this leads to secondary glaucoma via narrowing of the irido-corneal angle.

11.4.2 Secondary glaucoma associated with uveal changes

11.4.2.1 Uveitis
Inflammation of the uvea and especially of the iris causes an increase in the viscosity of the aqueous, mainly due to leakage of fibrin and cellular components from the blood vessels. This hinders the outflow of the aqueous. There can also be adhesions in and around the irido-corneal angle. Since uveitis is a frequently occurring disorder, especially in pups after being scratched by a cat, secondary glaucoma is also seen frequently.

As a result of uveitis, adhesions can develop between the iris and the anterior lens capsule (posterior synechia) or the pupil can become completely closed (pupil occlusion). This can occasionally lead to blockade of the pupil. Because of the difference in pressure between the posterior and anterior chambers, the iris is then displaced anteriorly and an iris bombé occurs. This narrows or closes the irido-corneal angle and results in a shallow anterior chamber.

Therapy: Treatment of glaucoma due to uveitis can utilize the same medications as in primary glaucoma, with the exception of the miotics. Miotics are contraindicated as they can increase the uveitis. It is better to use timolol or epinephrine. Since corticosteroids may increase IOP, they should be used with caution in uveitis complicated by glaucoma. Iris bombé and occlusion of the pupil can be freed surgically, but usually this manipulation leads again to severe uveitis and recurrence of the glaucoma or even phthisis bulbi. Patients with such complicated problems should be referred, despite the fact that the prognosis must be reserved.

11.4.2.2 Iris atrophy/iridoschisis
Degeneration of the anterior face of the iris, especially at its base, can lead to narrowing of the irido-corneal angle of the anterior chamber and thus to a chronic elevation of the IOP. However, this cause of glaucoma occurs only sporadically in animals.

11.4.3 Secondary glaucoma associated with trauma

Blunt as well as perforating trauma can induce glaucoma via, for example, the release of exudate, blood, or lens proteins, or breakage of the zonules and a subsequent luxation of the lens (see 4).

11.4.4 Secondary glaucoma associated with intraocular neoplasia

Intraocular neoplasia (for example, located at the base of the iris or in the ciliary body, especially if around the entire circumference) may block the drainage and can thus cause glaucoma by pressure on or by invasion of the drainage angle, or by inducing inflammatory exudate (see 12). If there is an obvious glaucoma and there are indications of neoplasia or, vice versa, or if there is a tumor with glaucoma as a side effect, then enucleation of the globe is the only advisable therapy. It should also be noted that in dogs affected by absolute glaucoma (in which the cause could not be determined clinically without ultrasound), the pathologic examination revealed that intraocular neoplasia was the cause in 10–15% of the cases.

11.4.5 Secondary glaucoma associated with medication

Glaucoma can be caused by the use of parasympatholytic mydriatics, such as atropine, and possibly by the prolonged use of corticosteroids in eyes predisposed to glaucoma.

11.4.6 Secondary glaucoma associated with ocular surgery

11.4.6.1 Extracapsular lens extraction

In this procedure, the anterior capsule and contents of the lens are removed. It is unavoidable that a certain amount of lens protein will be released into the anterior chamber and this can result in anterior uveitis. This reaction can occasionally (in about 1% of such cases in the dog) lead to the development of glaucoma. If the posterior capsule is unavoidably perforated, or if it must be removed because of posterior capsular cataract, then the vitreous is also released (see 11.4.1.1 and 13.4), which can block the drainage of the aqueous.

11.4.6.2 Intracapsular lens extraction

In this procedure, the lens, with its capsule intact, is removed from the eye. The procedure is nowadays almost exclusively indicated in lens luxation. During the procedure, but also during the first days after the operation, the vitreous can prolapse anteriorly and thereby hinder or block the transport of aqueous via the pupil or in the drainage angle (see 13.4).

11.5 Phthisis bulbi

Phthisis bulbi is defined as a shriveled, collapsed, atrophied eye resulting from a decrease in the production of aqueous (pressure usually lower than 15 mmHg). The fall in the IOP can, for example, be the result of damage to the ciliary body by trauma, uveitis (e.g. in equine recurrent uveitis), etc. (see 12.10.7 and 13.5.3).

Therapy: see 9.8.

Literature

1. BLOGG, J.R. & COLES, E.H.: Clinicopathological aspects of canine aqueous humor proteins. Res. Vet. Sci. **12**: 95, 1971.

2. BILL, A.: Formation and drainage of aqueous humor in cats. Exp. Eye Res. **5**: 185, 1966.

3. HEYWOOD, R & STREET, A.E.: Biochemical studies on the aqueous humor of Beagle dogs. Res. Vet. Sci. **17**: 401, 1974.

4. SAMUELSON, D.A., GUM, G.G., GELATT, K.N. et al.: Aqueous outflow in the beagle: Unconventional outflow, using different-sized microspheres. Am. J. Vet. Res. **46**: 242, 1985.

5. BARRIE, K.P. et al.: Quantitation of uveoscleral outflow in normotensive and glaucomatous beagles by ^{3}H-labeled dextran. Am. J. Vet. Res. **46**: 84, 1985.

6. MARTIN, C.L.: Development of the pectinate ligament structure of the dog: study by scanning electron microscopy. Am. J. Vet. Res. **35**: 1433, 1974.

7. WYMAN, M.: Applied anatomy and physiology of the anterior chamber angle. Vet. Clin. North. Am. **3**: 439, 1973.

8. SMITH, R.I.E., PEIFFER, R.L. & WILCOCK, B.P.: Some aspects of the pathology of canine glaucoma. Prog. Vet. Comp. Ophthalmol. **3**: 16, 1993.

9. Presumed inherited eye diseases. Procedure Notes of the Genetics Committee. Trans. Europ. Coll. Vet. Ophthalmol. Bologna, 1998.

10. BROOKS, D.E., GARCIA, G.A., DREYER, E.B. et al.: Vitreous body glutamate concentration in dogs with glaucoma. Am. J. Vet. Res. **59**: 864–867, 1997.

11. BOEVÉ, M.H. & STADES, F.C.: Glaucoom bij hond en kat. Overzicht en retrospectieve evaluatie van 421 patiënten. I. Pathobiologische achtergronden, indeling en raspredisposities. II Klinische aspecten. Tijdschr. Diergeneesk. **110**: 219, 1985.

12. BEDFORD, P.G.C.: A gonioscopic study of the iridocorneal angel in the English and American Breeds of Cocker Spaniel and the Basset Hound. J. Small Anim. Pract. **18:** 631, 1977.

13. LINDE-SIPMAN, J.S. VAN DER: Dysplasia of the pectinate ligament and primary glaucoma in the Bouvier des Flanders dog. Vet. Path. **24:** 201, 1987.

14. WYMAN, M. & KETRING, K.: Congenital glaucoma in the Basset Hound: A biologic model. Trans. Am. Acad. Ophthalmol. Otolaryngol. **81:** 645, 1976.

15. READ, R.A., WOOD, J.L.N. & LAKHANI, K.H.: Pectinate ligament dysplasia (PLD) in Flat-Coated Retrievers I: objectives and techniques for PLD survey. Vet. Ophthalmol. **1:** 85, 1998.

16. WOOD, J.L.N., LAKHANI, K.H. *et al.*: Relationship of the degree of goniodysgenesis and other ocular measurements to glaucoma in the Great Dane. Am. J. Vet. Res. **62:** 1493, 2000.

17. EKESTEN, B.: Correlation of intraocular distances to the iridocorneal angle in Samoyeds with special reference to angle closure glaucoma. Prog. Vet. Ophthalmol. **3:** 67, 1993

18. BOEVÉ, M.H. & STADES, F.C.: Glaucoom bij hond en kat. Overzicht en retrospectieve evaluatie van 421 patiënten. I. Pathobiologische achtergronden, indeling en raspredisposities. II Klinische aspecten. Tijdschr. Diergeneesk. **110:** 219, 1985.

19. GELATT, K.N. *et al.*: Ocular hypotensive effects of carbonic anhydrase inhibitors in normotensive and glaucomatous Beagles. Am. J. Vet. Res. **40:** 334, 1979.

20. LIU, H.K., CHIOU, C.Y. & GARG, L.C.: Ocular hypotensive effects of timolol in cat's eyes. Arch. Ophthalmol. **98:** 1467, 1980.

21. MERIDETH, R.E. & GELATT, K.N.: Cryotherapy in veterinary ophthalmology. Vet. Clin. North. Am. **10:** 873, 1980.

22. FRAUENFELDER, H.C. & VESTRE, W.A.: Cryosurgical treatment of glaucoma in a horse. Vet. Med. **76:** 183, 1981.

23. NASISSE, M.P. *et al.*: Treatment of glaucoma by use of transcleral neodymium:yttrium aluminum garnet laser cyclocoagulation in dogs. JAVMA **197:** 350, 1990.

24. CULLEN, C.L.: Cullen frontal sinus valved glaucoma shunt: preliminary findings in dogs with primary glaucoma. Vet. Ophthalmol. **7(5):** 311, 2004.

25. WOOD, J.L.N., LAKHANI, K.H. & READ, R.A.: Pectinate ligament dysplasia (PLD) in Flat-Coated Retrievers II: Association with glaucoma, heritability and prevention. Vet. Ophthalmol. **1:** 91, 1998.

12 Uvea

12.1 Introduction

The uvea is the heavily pigmented vascular tunica of the eye. It consists of three main components: the iris, the ciliary body, and the choroid.[1,2] The main function of the uvea is to provide for the metabolic needs of the eye. In addition, the iris regulates the amount of light that falls on the retina, and the ciliary body produces the aqueous humor and regulates the accommodation (very low in dog, cat and horse) process of the lens. The choroid portion of the uvea lies between the protective fibrous sclera on the outer side and the friable neural tunica, the retina, on the inner side (Fig. 12.1).

12.1.1 Iris

The iris, the base of which is located at the level of the limbus, forms the variable diaphragm of the eye. The plane in which the iris is situated is perpendicular to the visual axis of the eye. The iris also divides the space anterior to the lens into the anterior and posterior chambers. The pupil in the center of the iris is round in dogs, pigs, and primates. It forms a vertical slit in miosis and is round in mydriasis in domestic cats, and is horizontally oval in herbivores such as horses and cattle.

The anterior face of the iris consists of an epithelial layer that passes from the corneal endothelium, via the drainage angle, to the pupil. In the pupil, this layer merges with the double-layered epithelium from the posterior face of the iris. Between the anterior and posterior layers of the iris is the highly vascularized iris stroma. Directly under the epithelium, just within the base of the iris, there is a tortuous arterial circle, particularly prominent in cats, and supplied by the two long posterior ciliary arteries at the 9- and 3-o'clock positions. Trauma, inflammation (also of the cornea), or surgery in this area will particularly result in hyperemia or hemorrhage. The sphincter muscle of the pupil, which has parasympathetic (CN III) innervation, lies directly adjacent to the edge of the pupil. In cats, the fibers of this muscle are in a woven pattern dorsally and ventrally, as a result of which a slit-shaped pupil occurs in

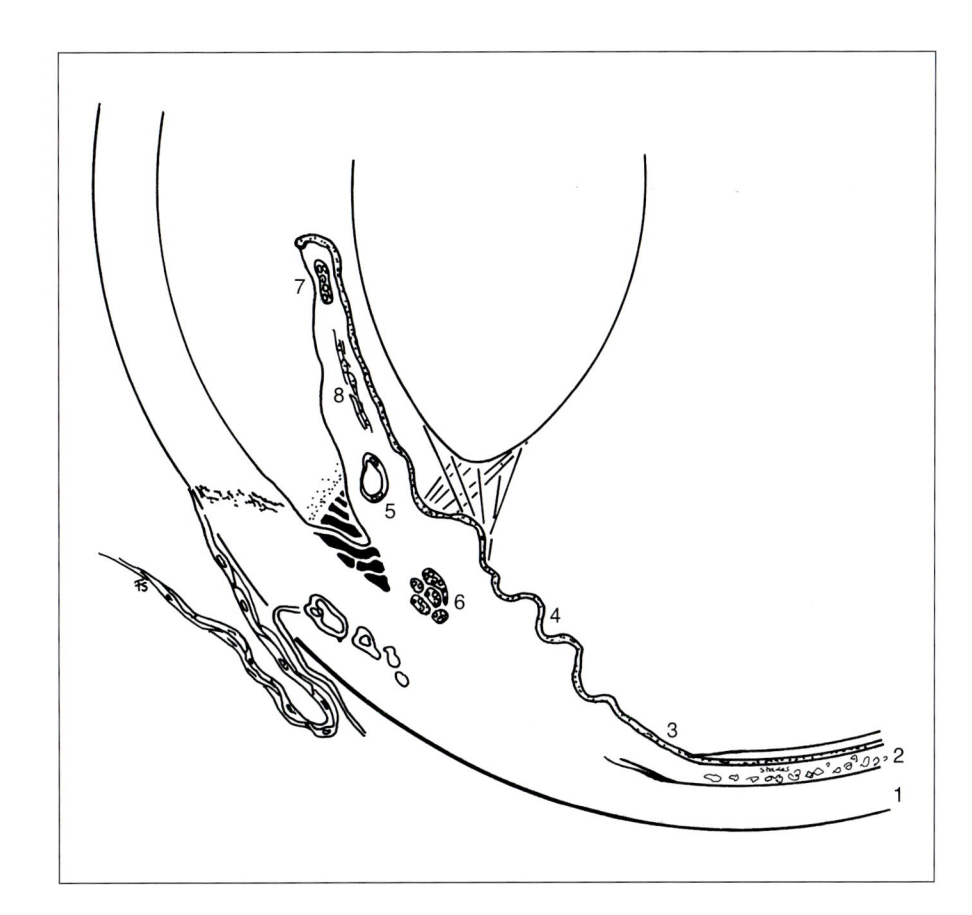

Fig. 12.1:
Uvea structures.
(1) Sclera,
(2) choroid,
(3) retinal pigment epithelium,
(4) ciliary body,
(5) iris,
(6) ciliary muscle,
(7) pupillary sphincter muscle,
(8) pupillary dilator muscle.

miosis. In these places, there are very few fibers of the radially oriented dilator muscle of the pupil. The dilator muscle has sympathetic innervation.

The color of the iris (for most owners the color "of the eye") varies from brown to golden yellow to green and blue (in exceptional cases white or red), depending on the amount of pigment in its anterior face and posterior pigment epithelium. Occasionally, the pigmented epithelium of the posterior surface of the iris everts over the edge of the pupil and then over the anterior surface of the iris, so that a dark pigmented edge is visible. In herbivores, heavily pigmented, cauliflower-like masses can be found on the upper pupil margin and smaller ones on the lower pupil margin (granula iridis), as a continuation of the pigment epithelium (Plate 2.13). If pigment is absent from the anterior side but present on the posterior side, the iris appears blue. If the ability to produce melanin is absent (tyrosinase deficiency), the melanocytes remain non-pigmented and the iris is red (true albino). Siamese cats are said to be partial albinos; they produce inadequate pigment and thus have a blue iris. In white cats with blue eyes, melanocytes are missing from the anterior surface of the iris.

12.1.2 Ciliary body

The ciliary body begins behind the iris and continues to the ora ciliaris retinae (serrata). It is divided into two portions, the caudal flat portion (pars plana) and the anterior thickened portion (pars plicata). It is roughly triangular with the thickened portion facing rostrally. The plicata has many (70–80) villus-like projections known as ciliary processes, and functions as the suspension apparatus for the lens. The ciliary processes are the secretory organs for aqueous production. The two layers of its epithelium are tightly joined and contain tight junctions, which comprise the blood-aqueous barrier. These layers surround a very vascular stroma from which is derived the blood for the nourishment of the anterior segment and its contents via the aqueous. Anteriorly, the ciliary body merges into the iris at the level of the scleral venous plexus. At its base are the fibers of the ciliary muscle. In domestic animals, these muscles are weakly developed and thus their accommodation ability is very limited. Irritation of these muscles (e.g. as a result of uveitis or from an injured cornea) can result in a very painful ciliary muscle spasm (photophobia).

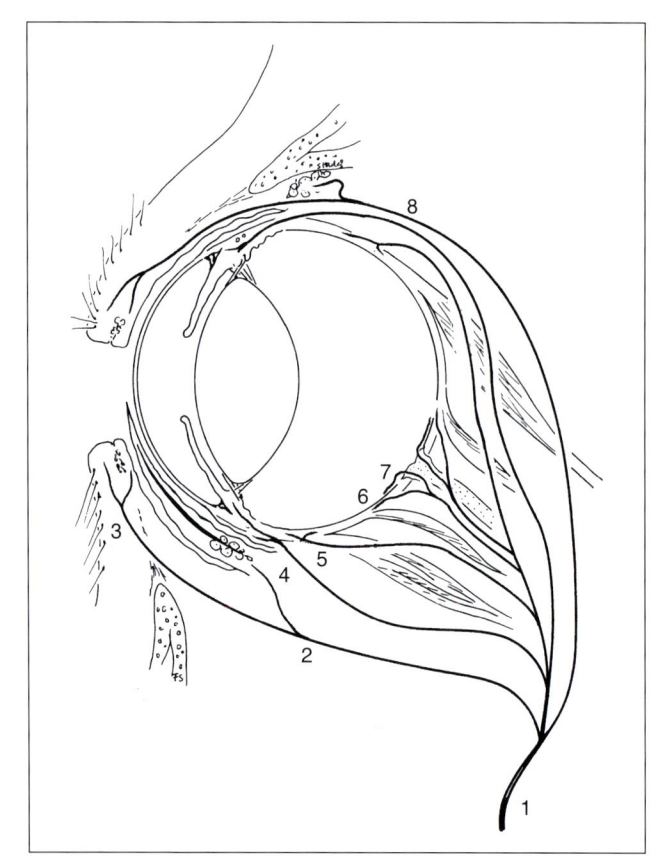

Fig. 12.2:
Vascularization of the eye. (1) ext. ophthalmic artery (a.), (2) malaris a., (3) palpebral a.; (4) ant. ciliary a., (5) post. long. ciliary a., (6) post. brev. ciliary a., (7) retinal arterioles, (8) lacrimal a.

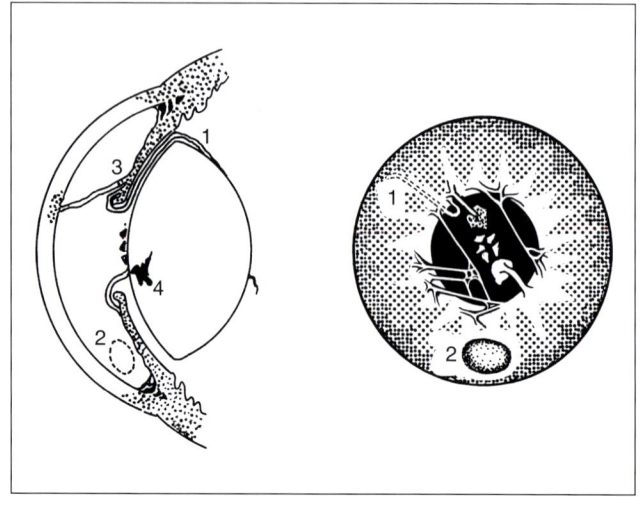

Fig. 12.3:
Abnormalities to be found in the anterior chamber. (1) Persistent ant. vascular tunic of the lens; (2) iris cyst; (3) persistent pupillary membrane (PPM), different forms; (4) congenital cataract, behind a PPM-contact point.

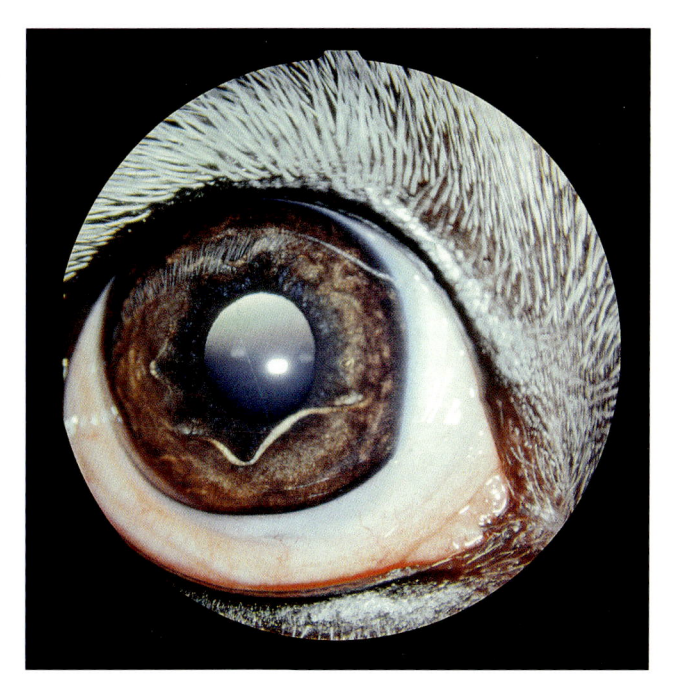

Plate 12.1:
Persistent pupillary membranes of the "iris-to-iris" type (OD, dog).

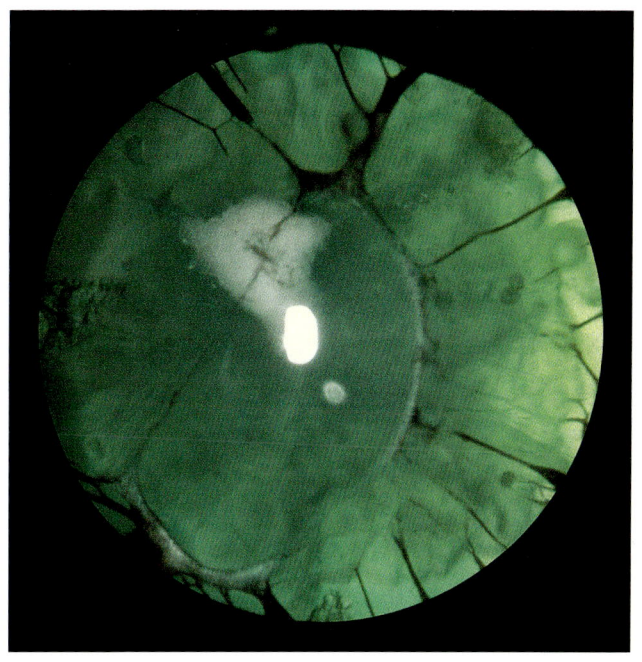

Plate 12.2:
Persistent pupillary membrane of the "iris-to-lens" type (OS, dog). The clouding behind the PPM is cataract. The dense white of some of the lumps, with the aspect of boiled egg white, is typical for *congenital* cataract.

12.1.3 Choroid

The choroid is the layer of vessels that extends between the papilla and the ora ciliaris retinae, which is the junction between the pars nervosa retina and the pars plana. The choroid is responsible for the metabolic support of the rods and cones. The remaining cell layers of the neural retina (interconnecting and ganglion cells, and nerve fibers) are mainly supplied by the short posterior ciliary arteries (Fig. 12.2). The anterior parts (iris and ciliary body) are supplied by the long posterior arteries, explaining the difference in appearance of anterior and posterior uveitis. Venous drainage is via the vortex veins which have large emissaries through the sclera. Normally, the interstices of the choroid are richly endowed with dense pigment which, together with the overlying pigment epithelium of the retina, results in the heavily pigmented structure viewed ophthalmoscopically, that also belongs to the choroid. Most of the background of the eye has this characteristic which functions to absorb scattered light (Plate 2.14). This is the tapetum nigrum (or just nigrum) but in Anglo-American countries the preferred terms is the non-tapetal fundus. In the back of the globe is a brilliantly reflective structure which can be roughly triangular, oval, or rounded in domestic animals and extends dorsally. It varies in size and color but is usually less than one-third of the background of the eye. This structure is referred to as the tapetum lucidum (or just lucidum), but in Anglo-American countries is referred to as the tapetum. It is composed of 1–15 or more layers of cells located between the large choroidal vessels and the choriocapillaris (which is not visible during funduscopy). The pigment epithelium (of the retina) in front of the lucidum, is not pigmented, thus allowing this area to be seen. The cells of the lucidum selectively absorb or reflect specific wavelengths of light, resulting in the color observed, ranging from greenish to reddish orange. The tapetum lucidum is cellular in carnivores and fibrous in herbivores. The pigmentation of the fundus is sometimes less dense or is partially or completely absent as in color-diluted animals, blue merles and eyes with white irises. The more or less radially oriented large vessels of the choroid can be recognized in these areas as can, sometimes, even the sclera lying between the choroidal and vortex vessels.

12.2 Persistent (epi)pupillary membrane

The pupillary/epipupillary membrane (PM) is formed by vascular loops (which grow out during ontogeny over the anterior surface of the embryological lens) rising from the arterial circle in the area which will become the base of the iris (Fig. 13.1). This vascular membrane should completely disappear between the second and fourth week after birth. Non-absorbed rests are called persistent PM (PPM) (Fig. 12.3). In some breeds of dogs (e.g. Basenji, Petit Basset Griffon Vendéen), this abnormality is hereditary, presumably recessive.[3,4]

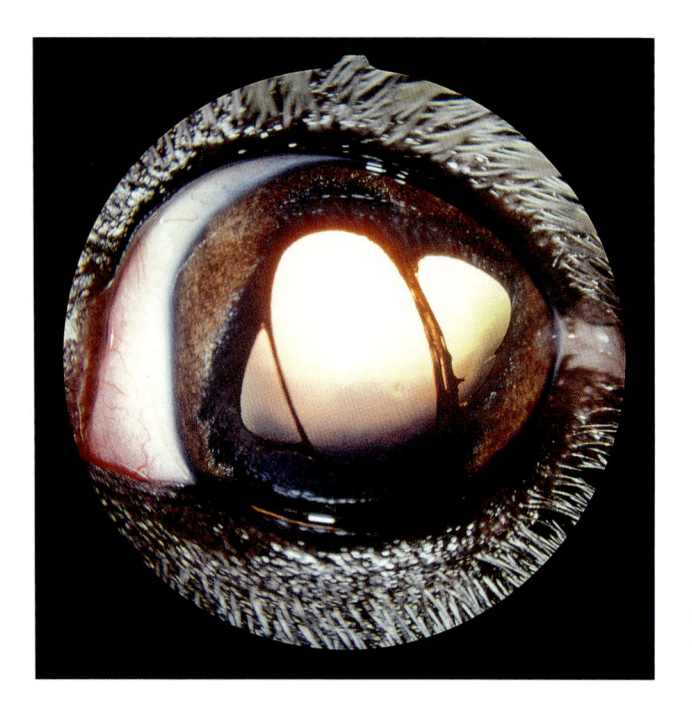

Plate 12.3:
Atypical iris coloboma in the 3- and 9-o'clock position (6 o'clock would be more typical; OS, dog).

The abnormality is seen infrequently except in the above breeds, often in combination with other congenital abnormalities such as cataract, microphthalmia, or palpebral aplasia.

PPM is chiefly recognizable as one or more pigmented threads in the anterior chamber. These are not connected to the edge of the pupil but to the surface of the iris, 1–3 mm peripheral to the pupil (Plates 12.1, 12.2). This circular region is referred to as the collarette of the iris and can be used to distinguish between acquired inflammatory strands (synechia) and PPMs. One end can be attached a short distance from the other. This type of PPM is usually scarcely visible against the background of the identically colored surface of the iris. Also, small particles of pigment or pieces of membrane can remain on the central part of the anterior lens capsule or against the corneal endothelium. Thread-like remnants can traverse the pupil, where they may appear to be white, or they can be adhered to the anterior capsule of the lens and/or to the corneal endothelium. Sometimes, they closely resemble a spider's web. If PPMs adhere to the capsule of the lens, they can cause local congenital cataract (Plate 12.2). If PPMs are adhered to the corneal endothelium, they cause a scar and a variable amount of corneal opacity. The history is then often very suggestive of corneal trauma during the nursing period. Usually, a PPM can be differentiated from a synechia when the surface of the iris is viewed from the side. A solitary thread extending between the cornea and the surface of the iris is sometimes noted by the owner much later in the animal's life and is then often thought to be a thorn (Plate 4.18). However, in contrast to a foreign body, this causes no pain nor signs of uveitis, the cornea is not stained by fluorescein, and there is no scar in the overlying stroma.

Therapy: Treatment is rarely necessary. If the patient is definitely blind and handicapped by this abnormality, because it affects the central part of the cornea, only a corneal transplant can be expected to bring about improvement.

Prevention: As a preventive measure, it is advisable to examine the immediate family members and to exclude affected individuals of the predisposed breeds and other severely affected animals from breeding (see also 13.2 and 15).

12.3 Coloboma

Colobomas are congenital defects in closure. Most are slit-shaped (e.g. cleft palate), but in the eye they are usually round to triangular (Plate 12.3). Their etiology is poorly understood but they are presumed to be inherited developmental defects. In the iris, such defects are usually in or adjacent to the edge of the pupil, and because of the embryological development (fetal fissure), they lie typically at the six-o'-clock position. Multiple defects (polycoria or more then one pupil) also occur. Since the pupillary sphincter muscle fibers are no longer attached, the defect usually becomes wider in the direction of the edge of the pupil. Colobomas can also occur in combination with other dysplastic abnormalities of the eye, such as Van Waardenburg's syndrome, microphthalmia, or cataract. The defects are present from early life, remain constant in size, and appear to cause no problems.

In the differential diagnosis, this abnormality could be mistaken for iris atrophy, but the latter occurs in older animals and is progressive. In addition, the pupil is not deformed and continues to function normally.

Prognosis: The prognosis is favorable, unless there are other dysplastic abnormalities present, in which case the prognosis is determined by the latter.

12.4 Acorea / aniridia

Acorea is a congenital absence of the pupil; aniridia is a congenital partial or complete absence of the iris. The etiology is poorly understood, but presumably these are inherited developmental defects. They occur infrequently. Usually, they are a component of a number of other dysplastic abnormalities of the eye. Acorea and aniridia can be unilateral or bilateral. In acorea, the iris is usually a flat surface and there is no recognizable pupil. In aniridia (in the Rottweiler, among other dog breeds, and horses),[5] the iris tissue along the pupil is very thin and transparent or it is completely missing. There can also be abnormalities in the drainage angle and, hence, glaucoma can develop. Because the pupil cannot be narrowed in higher light intensities, secondary retinal degeneration can develop as a result of excessive exposure to light.

Therapy / prognosis: There is no known treatment (besides sun glasses or colored contact lenses) for aniridia. Acorea can be corrected by surgical creation of a pupil, but both this and the prognosis may be determined by the presence of other abnormalities.

12.5 Heterochromia of the iris

Heterochromia is defined as different colored irides or parts of the iris. The term is generally used only for congenital differences. In dogs, these are mainly seen in the blue merle syndrome, while in cats the abnormality has only been seen as a solitary developmental abnormality. The iris, or just a part of it, is dark brown or blue, white, or red. There are no known complications.

12.6 Blue iris / white coat

In white cats with one or two "blue eyes" (odd eyes), the melanocytes are absent. This can be the result of an autosomal genetic defect. Such cats can also have other congenital abnormalities (e.g. deafness).

12.6.1 Oculocutaneous albinism and deafness

Color differences can be the result of a hereditary syndrome (Van Waardenburg's syndrome in humans). Such color-diluted animals have a whitish coat, lack pigment in the iris and choroid in one or both eyes, may be night blind, are deaf in one or both ears, and are often less fertile.

12.6.2 Partial oculocutaneous albinism

In Aleutian mink and occasionally in other animals, there is a syndrome of partial oculocutaneous albinism with an increased sensitivity to infectious disease and a prolonged coagulation time (Chédiak-Higashi syndrome).[6,7] This is an autosomal recessive defect. In addition to the lack of pigmentation of the iris and tapetum nigrum, there can be nystagmus, cataract, and photophobia. Diagnosis is made on the basis of enlarged granules in the leukocytes and enlarged melanin granules in the hairs.

Therapy / prevention: There is no known treatment. The breeding of affected individuals or their immediate relatives should be discouraged as strongly as possible (see also 15).

12.7 Acquired color differences in the iris

Pigment charges in the surface of the iris occur infrequently, usually in the form of spots. However, they occur regularly in cats. The iris tissue appears to be unaffected and affected cats usually appear to have no problems related to these changes.

Pigment changes in the iris can, however, also be an indication of the development of uveitis or neoplasia. In animals with pigment changes, additional diagnostic investigations should be pursued. The surface of the iris should be examined regularly with a slit-lamp biomicroscope to detect exudate or an increase in tissue mass.

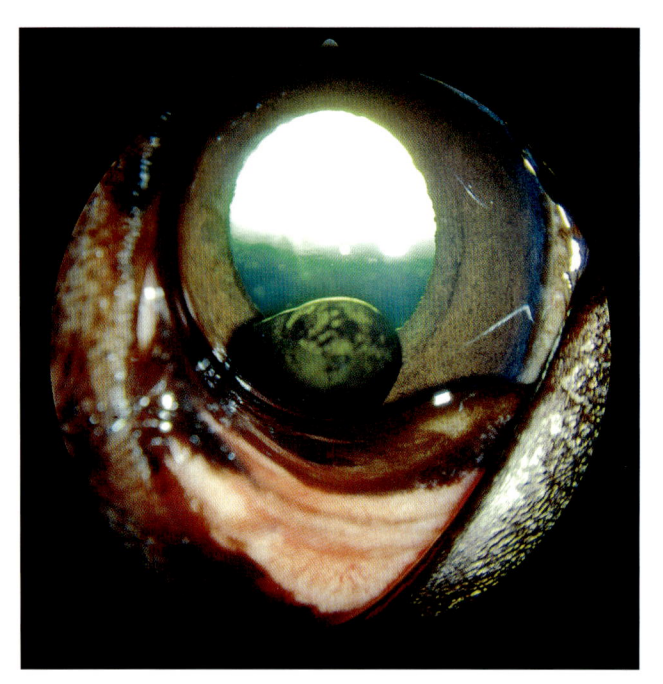

Plate 12.4:
Iris cyst in the anterior chamber (OS, dog). The transillumination shown here is an important criterion in the differentiation of neoplasia.

12.8 Iris cysts

Iris cysts are very fragile, pigmented (but sometimes almost colorless), more or less egg-shaped cysts in the anterior or posterior chamber of the eye (Fig. 12.3; Plate 12.4). They can arise from the iris base or the ciliary body. Their etiology is not well understood. If the cysts are located just behind the edge of the pupil, the iris is pushed anteriorly away from the surface of the lens. Cysts in the anterior chamber are usually more pigmented and hang or drift in the ventral part of the chamber. Iris cysts rarely cause clinical problems. With time, they may enlarge and finding more space between the lens and the center of the cornea, will move upwards into the pupil area. There they may burst, resulting in a pigmented sheet hanging on the corneal endothelium in the visual axis. They must be differentiated from neoplasia arising from the iris or the ciliary body, but such neoplasms consist of solid tissue in or on the iris or ciliary body.

In the horse iris cysts must also be differentiated from loosened "corpora nigra", hanging in the lower anterior chamber. These may damage the corneal endothelium.

Therapy: Iris cysts rarely cause clinical problems. If iris cysts are located in the pupil they may hinder vision, but these patients can be referred for surgical removal of the cysts (i.e. aspiration via paracentesis or laser destruction).

12.9 Hyphema

Hyphema is the presence of blood in the anterior chamber (Plates 4.7, 4.8). Since the aqueous is a physiologic environment to blood cells, the blood does not coagulate, but the cells sediment horizontally. This results in a progressively sinking horizontal layer of blood cells in the anterior chamber. The anterior chamber becomes clear above the cells and the iris becomes visible again, so that the eye again appears "dark". The blood cells should be absorbed within 1–3 days. Persistent problems are usually related to the cause of the bleeding. Causes of hyphema include:

12.9.1 Dysplastic abnormalities

Dysplastic abnormalities of the eye, in which vessel walls of the hyaloid system or other structures are deformed, can lead to bleeding into the anterior chamber.

12.9.2 Trauma

Blunt or perforating trauma can rupture vessels of the iris or the ciliary body. Blind eyes (for example, due to retinal atrophy or glaucoma) are particularly vulnerable to trauma.

During intraocular surgery, the accidental brushing against or grasping of or cutting into iris tissue almost immediately results in bleeding and hence hyphema. There is also a slightly increased likelihood of hyphema following surgery.

12.9.3 Leaking of vessels

Weak vessel walls, increased blood pressure, and retinal detachment can lead to loss of blood in the anterior chamber.

12.9.4 Coagulation disorders

Coagulation disorders, caused by intoxications (e.g. anticoagulants), autoimmune diseases, or neoplasia (lymphoma), can lead to the formation of unilateral or bilateral hyphema.

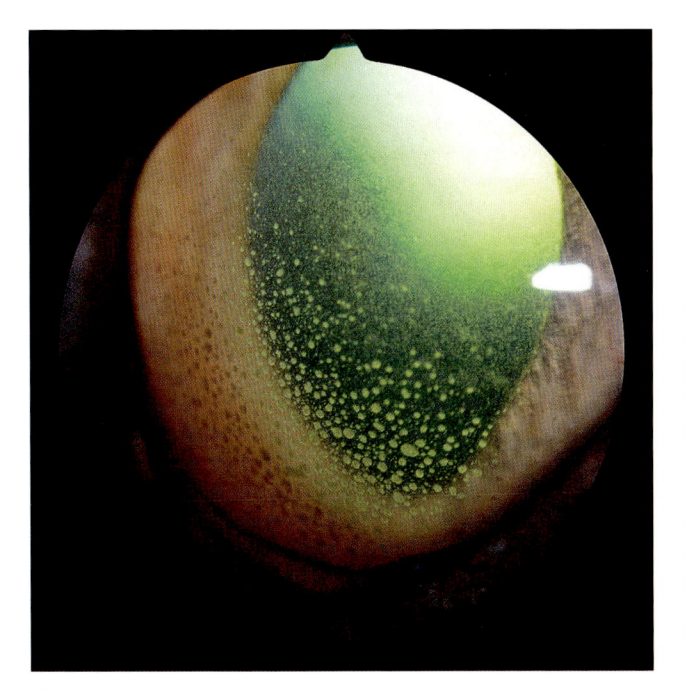

Plate 12.5:
Endothelial precipitates induced by anterior uveitis in a cat (OS).

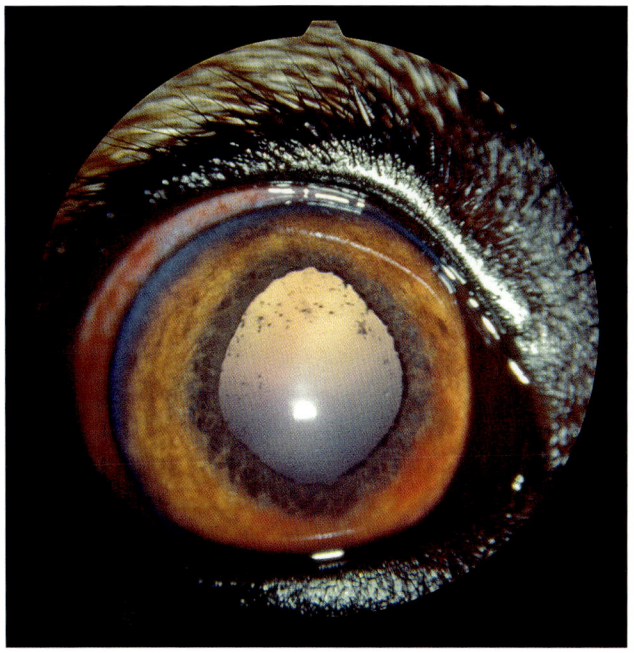

Plate 12.6:
Precipitates on the anterior capsule of the lens and rubeosis iridis due to anterior uveitis (OD, dog). There are also adhesions between the posterior side of the iris and the anterior capsule of the lens. Due to this, the pupil cannot open in a circle and so is pear-shaped.

12.9.5 Uveitis (Uveitis posterior: see 14.14)

Inflammation of the uvea can cause hyphema, swelling, and vascular lesions. In uveitis, there is usually exudate in which blood cells are mixed, leading to a cloud of hemorrhagic material in the anterior chamber.

Note: Bilateral hyphema is rarely caused by trauma. The examination should thus be directed towards the other causes listed above.

Therapy / prognosis: Treatment and prognosis in hyphema depend upon the cause. An obviously traumatic hyphema requires little if any initial treatment (see 4.4.2.3).

12.9.6 Neoplasms

Neoplasms can cause not only coagulation disorders (e.g. in lymphoma) but also directly damage vessels via pressure or invasion. The history and examination should be concerned primarily with these causes. A general physical examination is thus essential and a careful examination of the apparently unaffected eye, including funduscopy, must not be neglected.

12.10 Uveitis (anterior)

Uveitis is an inflammation of part or all of the uvea (Plates 12.5–12.12). Usually, all parts of the uvea are involved, but iritis, iridocyclitis (anterior uveitis), choroiditis, or chorioretinitis (posterior uveitis) can occur separately. Uveitis can also be classified according to the type of inflammation (such as exudative or granulomatous), the manner in which it has developed (exogenous or endogenous), or the stage (acute or chronic). With regard to treatment and prognosis, it is more useful to classify uveitis according to its etiology, as follows:
1. Traumatic uveitis
2. Metabolic uveitis
3. Infections
4. Immune reactions
5. Idiopathic uveitis
6. Pseudo-uveitis caused by neoplasia
7. Equine recurrent (chronic) uveitis (ERU)
8. Anterior uveitis in the rabbit

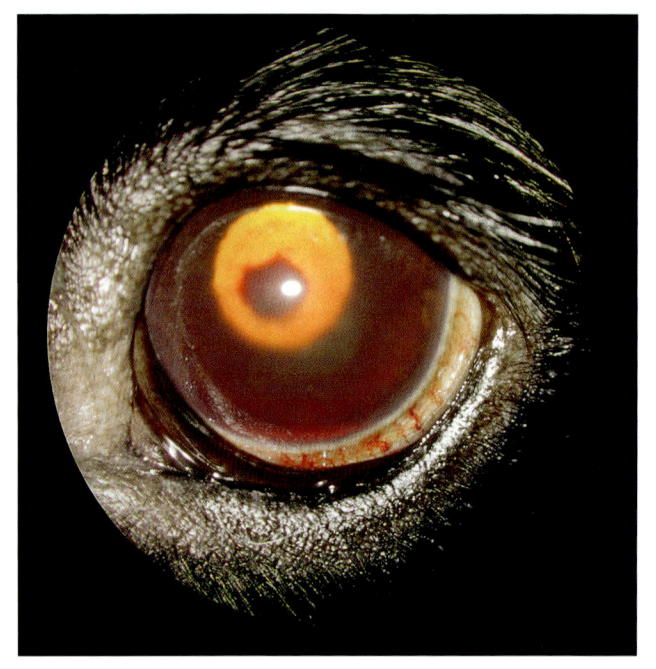

Plate 12.7:
Hypopyon containing much blood, due to anterior uveitis (OS, dog).

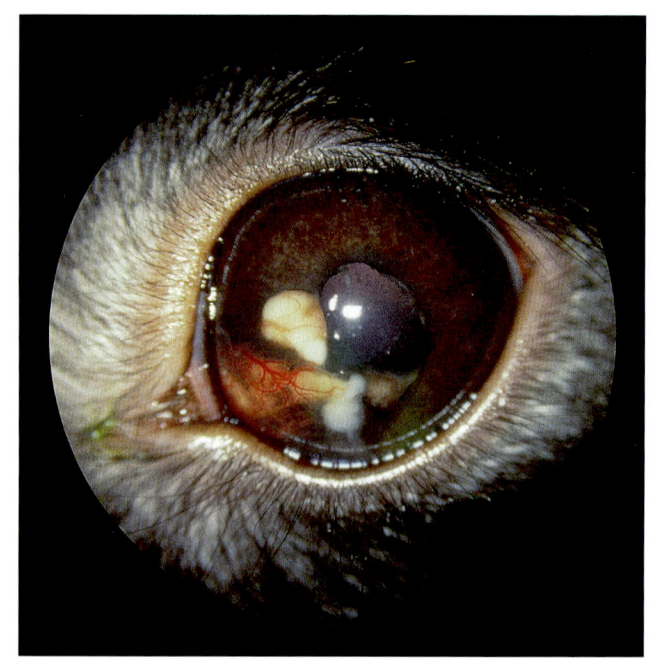

Plate 12.8:
Anterior uveitis with white exudate having the appearance of cheese, in the anterior chamber and iris of a rabbit (OS).

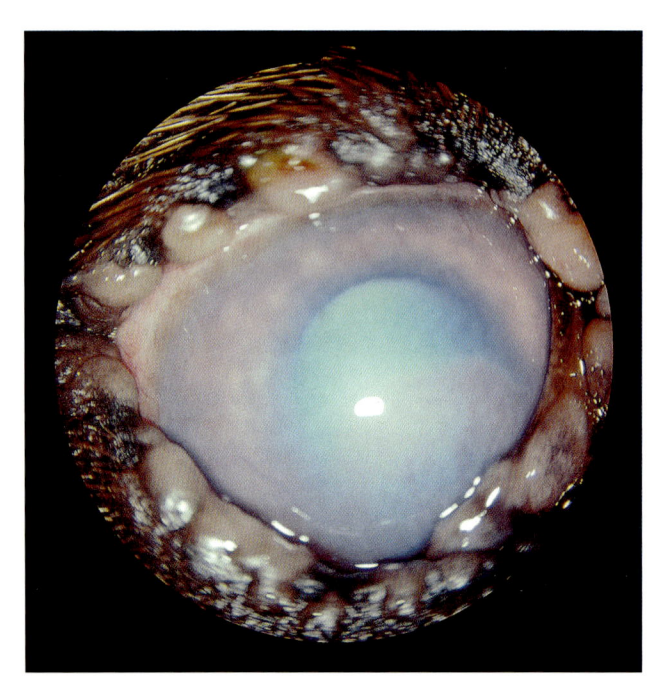

Plate 12.9:
Anterior uveitis with multiple granulomas of the lid margins due to a Leishmania infection (OD, dog). The granulomas were found to be full of Leishmania parasites.

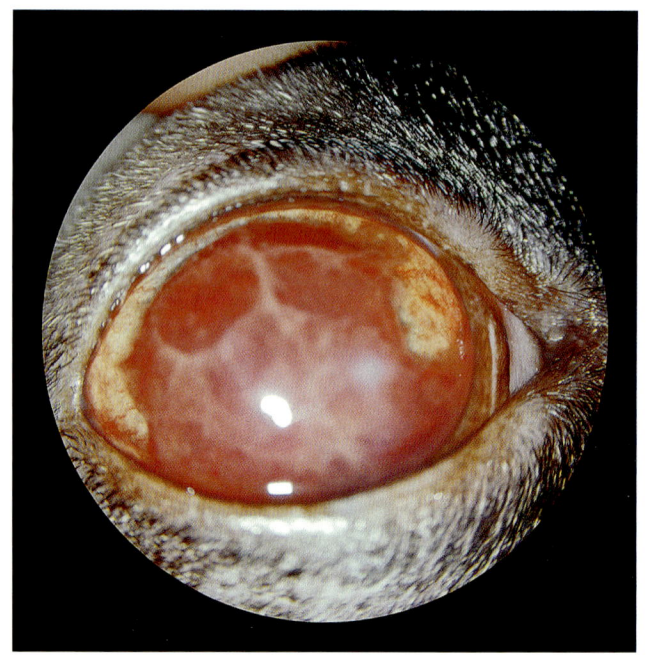

Plate 12.10:
Red, flocculent exudate in the anterior chamber (hypopyon) in a cat, due to anterior uveitis caused by a FeLV infection (OD).

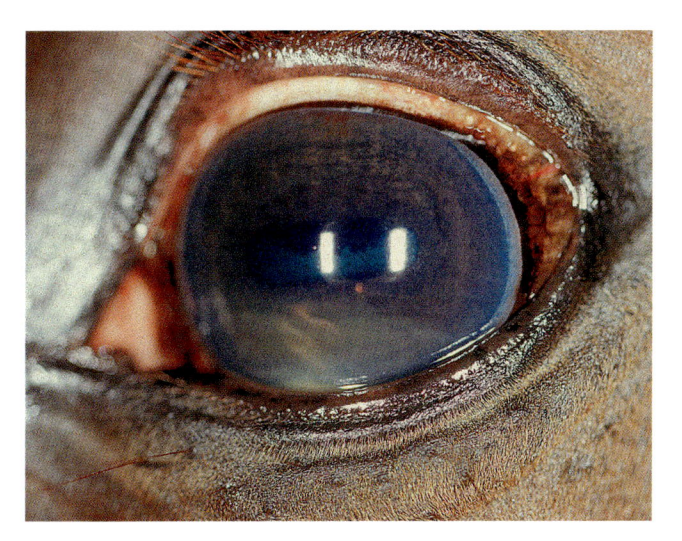

Plate 12.11:
Equine (chronic) recurrent uveitis in a horse; acute phase, with strong miosis (OS).

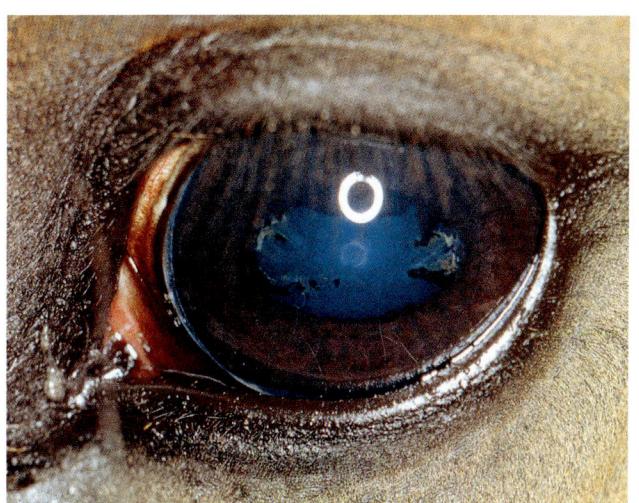

Plate 12.12:
Posterior synechia due to equine recurrent uveitis in a 6-year-old horse (OS).

12.10.1 Traumatic uveitis

Blunt trauma, if severe (e.g. in an automobile accident), can cause uveitis by deformation and the ensuing shock wave, and partly as a reflex via the corneal nerve fibers. Globe-penetrating trauma by a thorn or scratch or due to intraocular surgery leads almost without exception to uveitis. The severity of the inflammation depends on the amount of trauma involved and the type and amount of infectious material that is introduced. The abnormalities can be such that drainage of aqueous is blocked, leading to secondary glaucoma, or the production of aqueous stops, leading to phthisis bulbi. Trauma caused by cat scratches is notorious in this regard. The much feared sympathetic ophthalmia (transfer to the other eye) in humans is not recognized in domestic animals.

12.10.2 Metabolic uveitis

Uveitis may occur sporadically as a result of hyperlipoproteinemia. It is not completely clear whether the lipid leaks as a result of damage to the blood-aqueous barrier (BAB), or the excessive lipoproteins in the blood cause the damage to the BAB.[8] In addition to appropriate treatment of the uveitis, dietary intake of saturated fats should be reduced.

12.10.3 Infections[9]

12.10.3.1 Viral

Viral infections form an important group of causes of uveitis. In dogs, canine adenovirus (CAV-1), which causes infectious canine hepatitis, and the earlier modified virus vaccine against this disease are the most notorious causes of anterior uveitis. The antigen attaches to the endothelium of the cornea and the leukocytes which are attracted can release lysozymes that induce an acute, unilateral, dense corneal edema. Such an eye is referred to as a "blue eye". As a result of the use of improved vaccine antigen, this vaccination reaction is now a rarity. In cats, infectious peritonitis virus (FIP; corona virus) and feline leukemia virus (FeLV; oncorna virus) are quite capable of penetrating into the uvea.[10] There are often none or only few other notable abnormalities, such as weight loss. Therefore, in cats with signs of uveitis, especially hyphema and hemorrhagic or cloudy exudate, it is highly advisable to test for FIP, FeLV, and FIV before treatment is started. In addition, the patient should be isolated until the results of the tests are found to be negative (even negative results do not completely exclude these diseases).

In birds (mainly chicken), avian encephalomyelitis and herpes virus (Mareks disease) may cause anterior uveitis.

12.10.3.2 Rickettsia

In addition to fever, lymphadenitis, and thrombocytopenia, the tick borne diseases *Ehrlichia canis* (ehrlichiosis) and *Rickettsia rickettsii* (Rocky Mountain spotted fever) can also cause anterior and/or posterior uveitis. Diagnosis can be made on serology.

Therapy: Ehrlichiosis is not only treated with systemic "specific choice" antibiotics such as tetracyclines but also the manifested clinical symptoms should be treated, too. Because of recurrences, prognosis is less favorable.

12.10.3.3 Bacterial

Bacterial infections are rarely spread to the uvea by the hematogenous route (e.g. tuberculosis). In the majority of cases, bacteria can only penetrate into the globe via a primary perforation (trauma including surgery, corneal ulcer, etc.). The bacteria which are most alarming in this regard are *Pseudomonas* spp. and proteolytic *Staphylococci* and *Streptococci*. Usually, there is an obviously purulent exudate in the anterior chamber (hypopyon).

Leptospira interrogans has an important role in the horse causing equine recurrent uveitis (see 12.10.7).

Pasteurella multocida (bird cholera) and *Mycoplasma gallisepticum* may cause anterior uveitis and panophthalmitis in birds (mainly chicken).

12.10.3.4 Mycotic

Mycotic agents or yeasts can penetrate even an intact globe and cause uveitis, often extending into the choroid, sometimes with secondary exudative retinal ablation. The appearance of the exudate is variable, though mycotic uveitis can be predominantly granulomatous with little exudate. Extension throughout the entire globe (panuveitis/endophthalmitis) or into the brain and meninges can also occur (e.g. aspergillosis, blastomycosis, candidiasis, coccidiomycosis, cryptococcosis, histoplasmosis, paecilomycosis, etc.).[11,12,13] These forms of uveitis are commonly seen in areas in which the organisms are endemic (Southern Europe and the USA). Diagnosis of such infections can be confirmed by aspiration of the aqueous, vitreous or subretinal fluid, etc.

12.10.3.5 Algae

Algae (e.g. prototheacosis) can cause exudative uveitis.

12.10.3.6 Protozoa

Protozoa such as *Leishmania* spp. (Plate 12.9) and *Toxoplasma gondii* (also in canary) can cause anterior uveitis. Uveitis caused by *Leishmania* spp. (transmitted by a sandfly), is endemic in the Mediterranean region, up to 70 km from the coast. Also animals "found out of compassion" by tourists, or taken with northern people to their "winter" homes or on vacation in the Mediterranean have a high infection risk. Nowadays, they are also a risk factor for infection in the northern European countries. Leishmania are rarely found in the active phase of the disease. Secondary uveitis usually starts following treatment of the disease, possibly due to an increasing reactivity of the immune system to remaining antigen. The appearance of the exudate is variable and Leishmania uveitis can be predominantly granulomatous with little exudate. Extensions throughout the globe to the conjunctiva and lid edges are possible. Diagnosis can be made on serology, repeated serology (toxoplasmosis) or by a PCR test. The *Leishmania* spp. parasites can be found in bone marrow, lymph node material, or directly from granulomatous eruptions, if present.

In the rabbit, *Encephalitozoon cuniculi* can cause a phacoclastic uveitis (Plate 12.8).

Prognosis: Prognosis is less favorable for the long term.

12.10.3.7 Parasites

Parasites such as *Dirofilaria immitis* (transmitted by mosquitoes) can penetrate into the uvea and even into the anterior chamber (Plate 2.10) and thus cause uveitis.[14] Migrating *Toxocara* spp. larvae can cause nodules of chorioretinitis (Plate 14.25).

During the treatment of these types of infestation in the dog and horse with drugs such as ivermectin, anaphylactic reactions, caused by a massive death of microfilaria, may occur.

12.10.4 Immune reactions

Direct or delayed hypersensitivity reactions as well as autoimmune uveitis can occur in all companion animals. Well-known examples are the possible reactions after sensitization by lens proteins[15] and equine recurrent uveitis.

12.10.4.1 Uveo-dermatologic syndrome (UDS)

UDS is an immune-mediated disease, very similar to the Vogt-Koyanagi-Harada syndrome in humans.[16] Melanocytes are the target cells for the disturbed immune system. Some breeds, mainly the large polar dogs such as Akitas, Shibas, Samoyeds, and Siberian Huskies, and other breeds like the Irish Setter, Sheltie, and Rottweiler, seem particularly predisposed to this condition. The disease is mainly found in young adult to middle-aged dogs, and the ocular symptoms seem to start before the dermatologic problems. The ocular abnormalities usually begin with uveal depigmentation, anterior uveitis (primarily granulomatous) and cataract, secondary glaucoma and posterior uveitis. The dermatologic abnormalities include vitiligo and possible alopecia of the lids, nasal planum, lips and footpads, and, less frequently, mild alopecia. There can be generalized or facial poliosis.

Prognosis: Prognosis for the long term is guarded because many dogs die from chronic liver and kidney damage, even though therapy has been started early in the disease.

12.10.4.2 Lupus erythematosus (LE)

LE can also be an immunologic cause of uveitis.

12.10.5 Idiopathic uveitis

The cause remains unknown in many cases of uveitis, even after histologic or microbiologic examination.

12.10.6 Pseudo-uveitis caused by neoplasia

Rapidly growing neoplasms that occupy significant intraocular space, or are generalized, occasionally stimulate the uvea and thus cause secondary signs of uveitis. However, redness, hemorrhagic exudate, and hyphema usually occur without the blepharospasm and photophobia that are notable in uveitis.

Symptoms of uveitis: Uveitis (Plates 12.5–12.12) can be unilateral or bilateral. Bilateral uveitis is more likely to be caused by an infectious disease (e.g. leishmaniasis, mycosis, FeLV, FIP, FIV) or systemic neoplasm. The aqueous becomes cloudy as a result of the release of proteins, cellular debris, pigment cells, blood (cellular elements and fibrin; Plates 12.6–12.9), and inflammatory cells (hypopyon; Plates 12.7 and 12.10). Especially in the cat, small clumps of precipitate can remain adhered to the corneal endothelium ventromedially (Plate 12.5). These clumps of exudate can also become attached to the anterior capsule of the lens (Plates 12.6, 12.7; pseudocataract [Plates 12.8, 12.12], sometimes also secondary cataract), the surface of the iris (also the posterior side), and the drainage angle. This can easily lead to posterior synechiae (adhesions) between the iris and the lens (Plates 12.6, 12.8, 12.12). The surface and also the edge of the pupil are less sharply outlined because of the attached exudate, and the pupil can become distorted. If a 360° adhesion between the iris and the lens develops, iris bombé can occur. Iris bombé or closure of the drainage angle can lead to secondary glaucoma. In general, aqueous production in uveitis is reduced as a result of inflammation of the ciliary body; hence, in anterior uveitis there is usually hypotonia.

The iris will appear swollen and its surface will be tenser. The swelling of the iris can become so severe that the anterior chamber becomes filled. In uveitis there is a definite miosis (except with synechia). Because of hyperemia, the iris vessels are more readily recognized and the surface of the iris becomes reddened (Plates 12.6–12.10). Released prostaglandins, antibodies, lysozymes, and fibrinogen amplify this process further. The prostaglandins cause a breakdown of the BAB, leading to an increase in permeability of blood components into the anterior chamber. Microorganisms, leukocytes, and also antibiotics, can thus penetrate more easily into the anterior chamber.[17,18]

Inflammation and, possibly, an antigen can affect the corneal endothelium so that corneal edema develops. Leukocytes, which attempt to remove the antigen from the endothelium, can release lysozymes when damaged and these also cause irreversible damage to the endothelium. This can lead to a persistent, deep, dense, sometimes bullous edema. The corneal edema can be so dense that the contour of the pupil can only be made visible by retrograde illumination (miosis, deformed, irregularly contoured). Very thin vascular buds can infiltrate the cornea from the limbus. These vessels usually have a more or less broom-like branching pattern. They lie deep in the corneal stroma and so disappear under the sclera at the limbus.

Inflammation also strongly stimulates the ciliary body and the ciliary musculature, which will be brought into spasm (cyclospasm). This is very painful and results in photophobia, enophthalmos, and blepharospasm. The conjunctiva can also be severely affected by the process. Conjunctival vascular injection can develop as well as chemosis and a severe, more diffuse redness. As long as the sclera is still visible, increased vascular activity of the scleral venous plexus can often be seen a few millimeters from the limbus.

Diagnosis: Diagnosis is made on the basis of the clinical symptoms. In cats it is advisable to test every case of uveitis for FeLV, FIP, and FIV. Measurement of the Toxoplasma titer can also be considered, especially if the female owner is pregnant. Patients with severe uveitis or uveitis that responds poorly to treatment should be referred for further investigation, such as ultrasonography and the removal of material from the anterior chamber. Because of the risk of making the process worse by aspiration, this should only be done as a last resort and then only by clinicians experienced in this technique.

Differential diagnosis: Differentiation from glaucoma is important. In glaucoma there is increased ocular tension (IOP), a clear anterior chamber, mydriasis, reduced light perception, and a less painful eye. When keratitis occurs alone (except in cases of fluorescein-positive corneal defects), there should be little or no involvement of the deeper parts of the eye, although there can be a certain degree of reflex miosis.

Therapy: The objectives of therapy in uveitis consist of depressing the inflammation and eventually the underlying cause, the relief of pain and photophobia, and the prevention of synechiae. These objectives are achieved by administration of, respectively, anti-inflammatory agents, antibiotics or chemotherapeutic drugs, and mydriatics. In addition, a reduction in photophobia can be achieved by using a cycloplegic drug and keeping the animal out of strong light.

Corticosteroids can be administered locally in eye drops. Depending on the severity of the uveitis, dexamethasone or prednisolone acetate may be administered 4–8 times daily. Subconjunctival administration is also possible, but when the eye is painful this is not easy without anesthesia. In severe inflammation, prednisolone is given orally (2 mg/kg, once daily, in the morning for 4–5 days, then at the same dose on alternate days for 10 days, and then at a dose of 1 mg/kg on alternate days for 20 days).

The development of antiprostaglandins is currently advancing.[19,20] These drugs should not be given for longer than 3–5 days because the risk of gastrointestinal or renal complications is then significantly increased. They are especially dangerous in combination with parenteral corticosteroids.

Indomethacin, flurbiprofen, diclofenac and ketorolac can be administered locally or parenterally; e.g. carprofen (tablets; dog 2 mg/kg, 2 × daily), ketoprofen (tablets; dog 1 mg/kg/day; cat ¼–½ mg/kg/day; 1 × daily), or meloxicam (suspension; 0.1 mg/kg/day, 1 × daily) over 3–5 days.

Phenylbutazone and flunixin meglumine can be used in the horse.

If there are indications of an infection for which an effective antimicrobial drug is known, this should be administered. If this is not yet certain, administration of an "initial choice" antibiotic can be considered. If distinct exudate (large molecular proteins) is found in the anterior chamber, indicating that the BAB has broken down, one does not have to be concerned about this barrier and adequate concentrations of any systemic antibiotic will penetrate within the eye. If the situation is unclear with respect to the BAB, chloramphenicol is the antibiotic with the highest penetration into the eye because of its small molecular size (tablets; 25 mg/kg, 4 times daily).

To achieve mydriasis and relaxation of the ciliary musculature (cycloplegia), 1% atropine ointment, (especially in cat) or drops are administered 4 times daily. Although 10% phenylephrine can be added as a mydriatic, it gives little or no relief of the spasm of the ciliary musculature.

The animal should be kept in dimmed light in order to suppress the photophobia.

Prognosis: In mild forms of uveitis, the prognosis with adequate therapy is fairly good, although scars, especially in the form of synechiae, often occur. Severe uveitis should be treated promptly or referred immediately; even then the prognosis for vision is guarded. When treatment is delayed or the response to treatment is poor, the chance of secondary phthisis bulbi or glaucoma is very high. When uveitis is caused by one of the infectious diseases mentioned above, the prognosis is usually unfavorable to poor. Alas, cats with uveitis caused by FeLV can respond exceptionally well to treatment initially (Plates 12.15, 12.16), but may die a few months later from the underlying disease.

Prevention: Patients should be isolated until blood results have been obtained. Contact with a contaminated environment should be avoided. Breeders should be advised to use only animals that have tested negative for FeLV, FIP, and FIV.

12.10.7 Equine recurrent (chronic) uveitis (ERU)

ERU is the economically most important eye disease in equines (Plates 12.11, 12.12, 13.15). It is most likely an autoimmune disease, in which *Leptospira interrogans* plays an important role.[21,22,23,24] However, viruses (influenza/adenovirus), bacteria (other *Leptospira* spp.,[25] *Brucella* spp., *Streptococcus* spp.), parasites (*Onchocerca* spp./*Toxoplasma* spp.)[26] can also induce ERU. The first attacks usually develop between 3 and 7 years of age. The general symptoms, are the same as previously described in 12.10 (Plates 12.11, 12.12 and 13.15). The attacks are very painful (epiphora, mucopurulent discharge, conjunctival redness and congestion, diffuse corneal edema, and severe blepharospasm) and acute, thus resembling ocular trauma. The attack can continue for 2 weeks to 6 months or longer. During the illness, lens changes frequently develop. Consequently, the most important cause of cataract (Plate 12.12) and lens luxation (Plate 13.15) in equines is ERU. Also, vitreous floaters, chorioretinitis, and even retinal detachment and phthisis bulbi in equines are frequently due to ERU. The abnormalities can be found in one or both eyes.

Therapy: Due to blepharospasm at the beginning of the attack, it may be almost impossible to administer the local therapy as described above for uveitis. In such cases, the initial therapy can consist of installing a subpalpebral lavage system in the conjunctival sac for topical treatment, and of systemic flunixin meglumine I.V. (2 mg/kg, once daily, followed by 1 mg/kg for 5–7 days; an alternative is phenylbutazone or vedaprofen); thereafter, acetylsalicylic acid (30 mg/kg/24 hours for a period of 1–3 months). After sedation, subconjunctival atropine (1–2 mg), and/or a depot-corticosteroid (methylprednisolone, 15–20 mg; not over 1 ml total volume) can be administered. Plasminogen activator (20–50 µg) injected into the anterior chamber may be used to dissolve coagula or synechia. The patient should be stalled in a dimly lit stable and should do no work. After the severe signs have subsided, topical therapy can be administered. When the pupil becomes larger (initial vertical size should be noted, or photographed), atropine is given once daily.

More recently partial pars plana vitrectomy has been advocated to decrease relapses of ERU. Vitreous, exudates and inflammatory mediators are removed and replaced by balanced salt solution with gentamycin.[27]

Prognosis: Because recurrences may develop at very irregular intervals, the prognosis is less favorable. Signs of earlier attacks of ERU include clouds in the anterior chamber, synechia, cataract, lens luxation, vitreous floaters, scars from chorioretinitis, retinal detachment, and a low-pressure globe. Precise notation, drawings in an examination protocol, photographs, etc. can prevent problems if the horse is later offered for sale. This also implies, when signs of uveitis are found during a physical examination, that the horse should not be pronounced fit for serious dressage or jumping. Recurrences are likely, and purchase should be discouraged. When in doubt, a second opinion should be obtained.

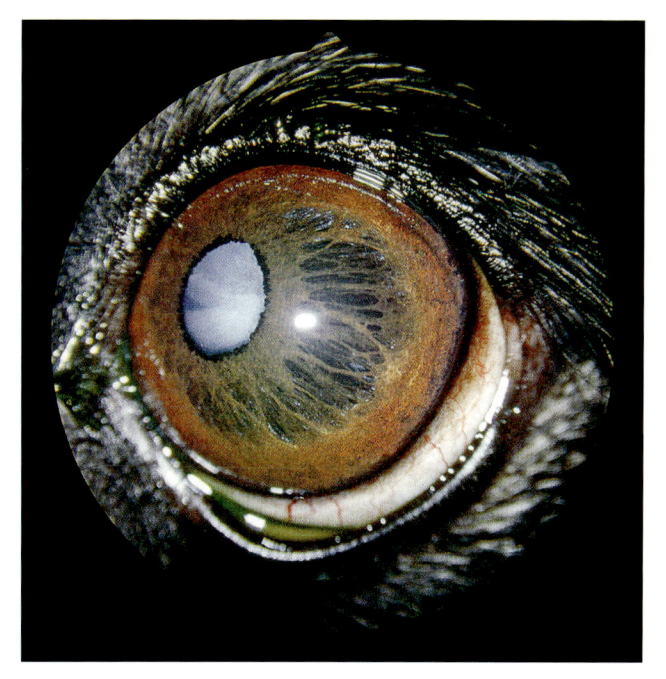

Plate 12.13:
Iris atrophy and mature cataract in a 12-year-old Poodle (OS).

12.10.8 Anterior uveitis in the rabbit

In the rabbit, swellings of the iris can be found with yellow-white, cheese-like material in the center, surrounded by a red-brown ring, resembling neoplasia (Plate 12.8). The lesions are frequently due to chronic, multifocal, uveal abscesses which, unfortunately, respond poorly to the usual uveitis therapy.

12.11 Iris atrophy

Iris atrophy is a disorder in which there is chronic loss of iris tissue (Plate 12.13). In the primary form, crypts and holes develop in the surface of the iris and the fundus reflex can be seen through them. This abnormality rarely leads to glaucoma or other complications.

Secondary iris atrophy can be the result of an earlier trauma, iritis, or glaucoma. The iris tissue degenerates as a result of pressure or overstretching.

Therapy / prognosis / prevention: There is no known treatment. In secondary atrophy, the primary cause must be removed. The prognosis is favorable. There are no known preventive measures.

12.12 Dysautonomia or pupil dilatation syndrome (Key-Gaskell Syndrome)[28]

Dysautonomia can be described as a degenerative dysfunction of the ganglia and neurons of the autonomic nervous system. This rare abnormality may occur more frequently in cats that have just reached adulthood, but the spread in age is great (15 weeks to 11 years). No breed or sex predisposition has been found. A similar, but even rarer syndrome has also been described in a dog.[29] Outside of the United Kingdom, only a few cats have so far been diagnosed with this disease.

Clinical signs usually appear to develop within 1–3 days. The most important signs are depression, anorexia, constipation, dryness of the nose and mouth, lowered tear production, protrusion of the nictitating membrane, megaesophagus (with gagging, vomiting, and dysphagia), mydriasis, low heart rate, loss of the anal reflex, incontinence, and paresis.

Diagnosis: Diagnosis is based on the history and the clinical signs, and radiographs of the thorax and esophagus. Differential diagnoses include intoxication, foreign body, upper respiratory infection, acute disorders of the abdomen, acute blindness, etc.

Therapy: The most hopeful treatment appears to consist of maintaining the fluid, electrolyte, and acid-base balance, together with the use of laxatives and corticosteroids.

Prognosis: The prognosis should be reserved. Only about one-fifth of the reported cases appeared to recover reasonably well. The pupil reflex usually remains absent.

12.13 Horner's syndrome

Horner's syndrome is characterized by unilateral enophthalmos, protrusion of the nictitating membrane, miosis, and a variable degree of ptosis. In horses, warmness and sweating of the ipsilateral part of the neck, ear, and face can occur (for further details, see 5.4.2).

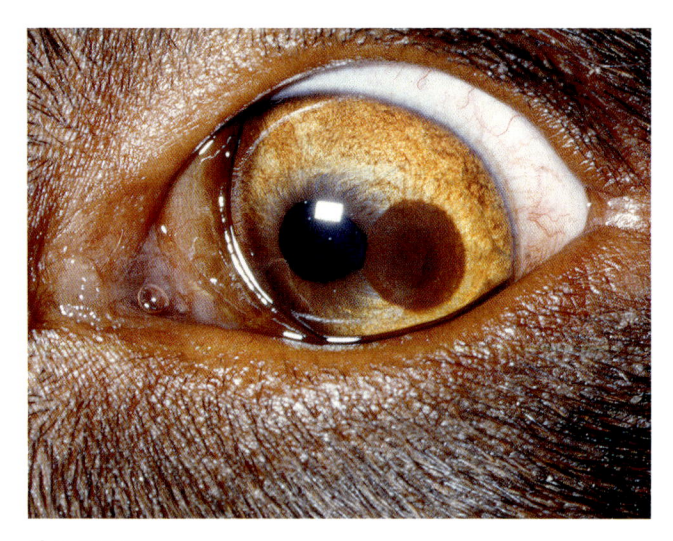

Plate 12.14:
Melanoma of the iris (OS, dog).

12.14 Other pupillary abnormalities

Information about these abnormalities can be obtained in more specialized neurologic literature.

12.15 Neoplasia

Neoplasms of the uvea can be classified as primary, generalized, or metastatic.[30] They can be located in the iris, ciliary body (infrequent), or choroid (very infrequent). Commonly encountered primary neoplasms include melanomas, adenomas (of the ciliary body), adenocarcinomas, and melanosarcomas (Plate 12.14–12.17). Generalized neoplasia, such as malignant lymphomas and histiocytosis, often manifest themselves to owners initially in the eye (in dogs, more often manifested as hyphema). Almost all types of neoplasia can metastasize to the eye, carcinomas in particular (e.g. originating from the kidney, mammary gland, and nasal cavity).

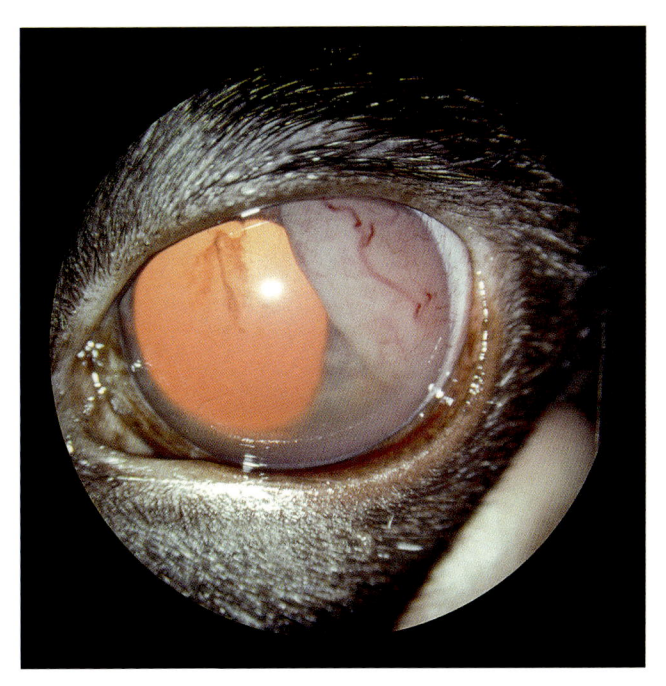

Plate 12.15:
Granulomatous swelling of the iris and exudate in the anterior chamber of a cat due to uveitis caused by a FeLV infection (OS; see also Plate 12.16).

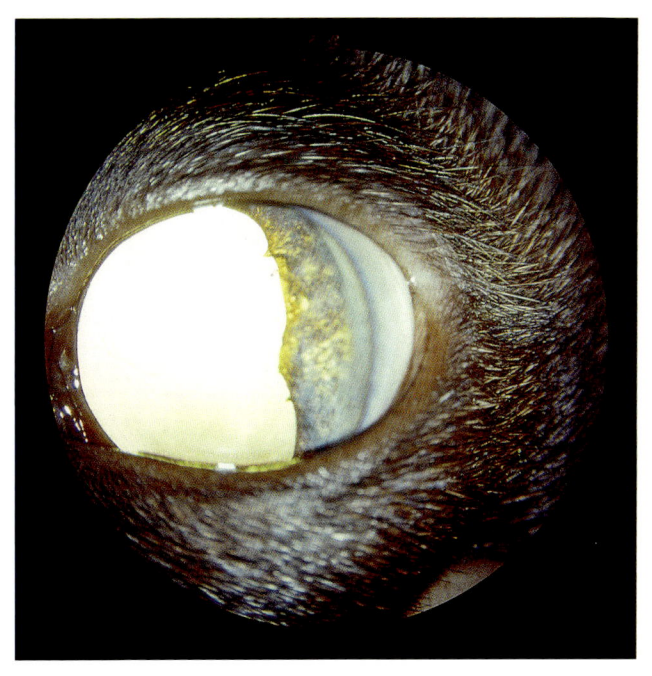

Plate 12.16:
Result of treatment of uveitis with prednisolone on alternate days and in a decreasing dosage (start: 2 mg/kg) and topical atropine after 14 days of treatment (same eye as shown in Plate 12.15).

On the basis of the eye examination alone, it is seldom possible to differentiate between primary and secondary neoplasia, with the exception of early primary neoplasms, which rarely result in inflammatory disease until the mass outgrows its blood supply. In contrast, metastatic neoplasia more frequently results in signs of inflammation. The first signs of a primary uveal neoplasm are focal color change (usually pigmentation) and swelling of the iris tissue without associated signs of uveitis. For example, the surface of the iris and the edge of the pupil can be deformed but remain sharply outlined. If the neoplasm originates from the ciliary body, the base of the iris at that location may protrude into the anterior chamber (Plate 12.17). Eventually, the pinkish-white tissue behind the edge of the pupil will become visible. Basically, the rule is the more extensive the neoplasm, the greater the likelihood of signs of secondary uveitis (exudate, redness). It is also possible that the increase in tissue is more or less uniform and circular. Sometimes, the neoplasm is in the drainage angle, so that the mass is only discovered when it leads to secondary glaucoma or during histologic examination of the eye. Animals with generalized or metastatic neoplasms are usually initially presented with signs of uveitis, seldomly because of a massive increase in tissue. Neoplasms associated with a more diffuse increase in tissue, with more acute signs of uveitis (e.g. hyphema and exudate but no pain), or with tissue resembling "lobes of the liver" in the anterior chamber are mostly caused by generalized neoplasms (Plates 12.15, 12.16).

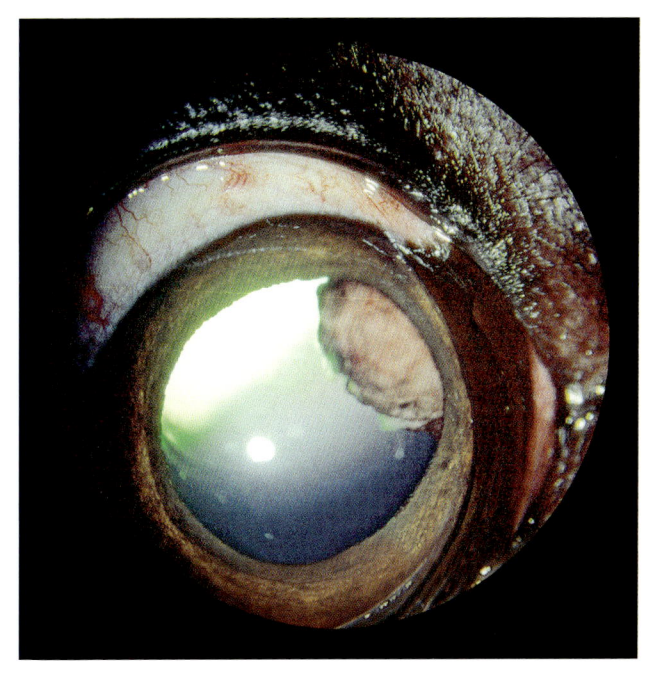

Plate 12.17:
Adenocarcinoma of the ciliary body between the 1- and 3-o'clock positions (OD).

Diagnosis: Diagnosis is made on the basis of the clinical signs and an extensive physical examination. Hematologic examinations, examination and aspiration biopsies of lymph nodes and thoracic radiographs can reveal signs of metastasis. However, primary intraocular neoplasms mostly metastasize late. In case of doubt, referral for such procedures as ultrasonography, CT, MRI, contrast radiography, aqueous fluid cytology, and biopsy should be considered.

Therapy: Small and sharply defined neoplasms in an early stage can sometimes be removed by means of a partial iridocyclectomy. Such patients should be referred without undue delay. Enucleation of the globe is indicated for larger neoplasms where there is no indication of metastasis. When there is evidence of extension through the globe into the orbit, exenteration of the orbit is indicated (see 5.9). Because this procedure is generally a very radical (and definitive) experience for the owner, referral, at least for confirmation of the diagnosis, is usually advisable. Treatment in cases of generalized or metastatic neoplasia is dependent on the prognosis for controlling the primary neoplasm by chemo-, radio-, or thermotherapy.

Prognosis: Prognosis for the eye after iridocyclectomy for small, primary intraocular neoplasms must be guarded. After enucleation of the globe for neoplasms that cannot be removed by iridocyclectomy, the prognosis is favorable as intraocular neoplasms are usually late to metastasize. If there is indication of invasion through the globe (e.g. visible in the sclera or after histologic examination), the prognosis must be more reserved.

Prevention: Affected cats should be isolated until it has been confirmed that it is a primary intraocular neoplasm and not a neoplasm associated with FeLV.

12.16 Posterior Uvea

Abnormalities of the choroid are described in 14.

Literature

1. SHIVELY, J.N. & EPLING, G.P.: Fine structure of the canine eye: Iris. Am. J. Vet. Res. **30:** 13, 1969.

2. MILLER, M.E., CHRISTENSEN, G.E. & EVANS, H.: Anatomy of the dog. Philadelphia, W. B. Saunders, 1964.

3. ROBERTS, S.R. & BISTNER, S.I.: Persistent pupillary membrane in Basenji dogs. JAVMA **153:** 533, 1968.

4. BOEVÉ M.H., STADES, F.C. & SCHERPENHUIJSEN ROM, B.E.M.: Persistent pupillary membrane in the Petit Basset Griffon Vendéen. Book of abstracts. Int. Soc. Vet. Ophthalmol. Vienna, (2. 10. 1991).

5. ERIKSON, R.: Hereditary aniridia with secondary cataract in horses. Nord. Vet. Med. **7:** 773, 1955.

6. COLLIER, L.L., PRIEUR, D.J. & KING, E.J.: Ocular melanin pigmentation anomalies in cats, cattle, mink, and mice with Chédiak-Higashi syndrome: Histologic observations. Curr. Eye Res. **3:** 1241, 1984.

7. KERN, T.J. et al.: Uveitis associated with poliosis and vitiligo in six dogs. JAVMA **187:** 408, 1985.

8. OLIN, D.D., ROGERS, W.A. & MACMILLAN, A.D.: Lipid-laden aqueous humor associated with anterior uveitis and concurrent hyperlipidemia in two dogs. JAVMA **9:** 861, 1976.

9. MARTIN, C.L.: Ocular infections. In: Clinical Microbiology and infectious diseases of the dog and cat. Ed.: C.E. Greene. Philadelphia, W.B. Saunders, 1984.

10. DOHERTY, M.J.: Ocular manifestations of feline infectious peritonitis. JAVMA **159:** 95, 1979.

11. BUYUKMIHCI, N., RUBIN, L.F. & DEPAOLI, A.: Protothecosis with ocular involvement in a dog. JAVMA **167:** 158, 1975.

12. CARLTON, W.W., FEENEY, D.A. & ZIMMERMANN, J.L.: Disseminated cryptococcosis with ocular involvement in a dog. JAAHA **12:** 53, 1976.

13. BUYUKMIHCI, N.C. & MOORE, P.F.: Microscopic lesions of spontaneous ocular blastomycosis in dogs. J. Comp. Pathol. **97:** 321, 1987.

14. DUNBAR, M. et al.: Treatment of canine blastomycosis with ketoconazole. JAVMA **182:** 156, 1983.

15. WILCOCK, B.P. & PEIFFER, R.L.: The pathology of lens-induced uveitis in dogs. Vet. Path. **24:** 549, 1987.

16. MORGAN, R.V.: Vogt-Koyanagi-Harada syndrome in humans and dogs. Comp. Cont. Educ. **11:** 1211, 1989.

17. DZIEZYC, J., MILLICHAMP, N.J., KELLER, C.B. & SMITH, W.B.: Effects of prostaglandin F_{2a} and leukotriene D4 on pupil size, intraocular pressure, and blood-aqueous barrier in dogs. Am J. Vet. Res. **53:** 1302, 1992.

18. WILKIE, D.A.: The background of ocular prostaglandins and their role in ophthalmic physiology and pathology. Trans. Am. Coll. Vet. Ophthalmol. **20:** 3, 1989.

19. YOSHITOMI, T. & ITO, Y.: Effects of indomethacin and prostaglandins on the dog's iris sphincter and dilator muscles. Invest. Ophthalmol. Vis. Sci. **29:** 127, 1988.

20. BRIGHTMAN, A.H., HELPER, L.C. & HOFFMANN, W.E.: Effect of aspirin on aqueous protein values in the dog. JAVMA **178:** 572, 1981.

21. WILLIAMS, R.D.: Equine uveitis: a model system for study of immunologically mediated tissue injury. Ph. D. Thesis, Purdue University, 1971.

22. DEEG, C.A. EHRENHOFER, M. et al.: Immuno-pathology of recurrent uveitis in spontaneously diseased horses. Exp. Eye Res. **75:** 127, 2002.

23. WOLLANKE, B., ROHRBACH, B. & GERHARDS, H.: Serum and vitreous humor antibody titers in, and isolation of *Leptospira interrogans* from horses with recurrent uveitis. JAVMA **219:** 795, 2001.

24. RIMPAU, W.: Leptospirose beim Pferd. Tierärztliche Umschau. **2:** 177, 1947.

25. WILLIAMS, R.D., MORTER, R.L., FREEMAN, M.J. & EN LAVIGNETTE, A.M.: Experimental chronic uveitis – ophthalmic signs following equine leptospirosis. Invest. Ophthalmol. **10:** 948, 1971.

26. SCHMIDT, G.M. et al.: Equine ocular onchocerciasis;: Histopathologic study. Am. J. Vet. Res. **43:** 1371, 1982.

27. FRÜHAUF, B., OHNESORGE, B., DEEGEN, E. & BOEVÉ, M.H.: Surgical management of equine recurrent uveitis with single port pars plana vitrectomy. Vet. Ophthalmol. **1:** 137, 1998.

28. KEY, T.J.A. & GASKELL, C.J.: Puzzling syndrome in cats associated with pupillary dilation. Vet. Rec. **110:** 160, 1982.

29. WISE, L.A. & LAPPIN, M.R.: A syndrome resembling feline dysautonomia (Key-Gaskell syndrome) in a dog. JAVMA **198:** 2103, 1991.

30. SCHERLIE, P.H., SMEDES, S.L. et al.: Ocular manifestation of systemic histocytosis in a dog. JAVMA **201:** 1229, 1992.

13 Lens and Vitreous

13.1 Introduction

13.1.1 Ontogenesis

A lens placode begins to form in the surface ectoderm over the optic cup shortly after conception (Fig. 13.1). The placode invaginates and, about 16–24 days post coitus (dog and cat), the lens vesicle becomes separated into the optic cup.[1] The cells forming the posterior wall of the vesicle elongate in an anterior direction and fill the vesicle in about a week. These primary lens fibers form the embryonic nucleus. The basement membrane of the original cells of the lens vesicle becomes the adult lens capsule. The anterior cuboidal cells are retained and become the germinal epithelium located under the anterior lens capsule.

The germinal epithelial cells migrate to the periphery and elongate at the equatorial zone both anteriorly and posteriorly. This process occurs throughout the life of the animal but slows down as the animal ages. The secondary lens fibers thus formed become longer and laid down in layers around the embryonal nucleus in an onion-skin-like order. Closure or suture lines are formed where the fibers meet (Fig. 13.2). These, ophthalmoscopically discreet, suture lines form a "Y" anteriorly (Plate 13.4) and an inverted "Y" posteriorly. In horses, the posterior pattern is less regularly formed. The fetal nucleus forms around the embryonal nucleus and the adult nucleus is formed around this in turn. The youngest cells that are deposited around the nucleus form the cortex. The central nuclei gradually become sclerotic, especially via a decrease in the amount of water-soluble lens proteins and the percentage of water, and

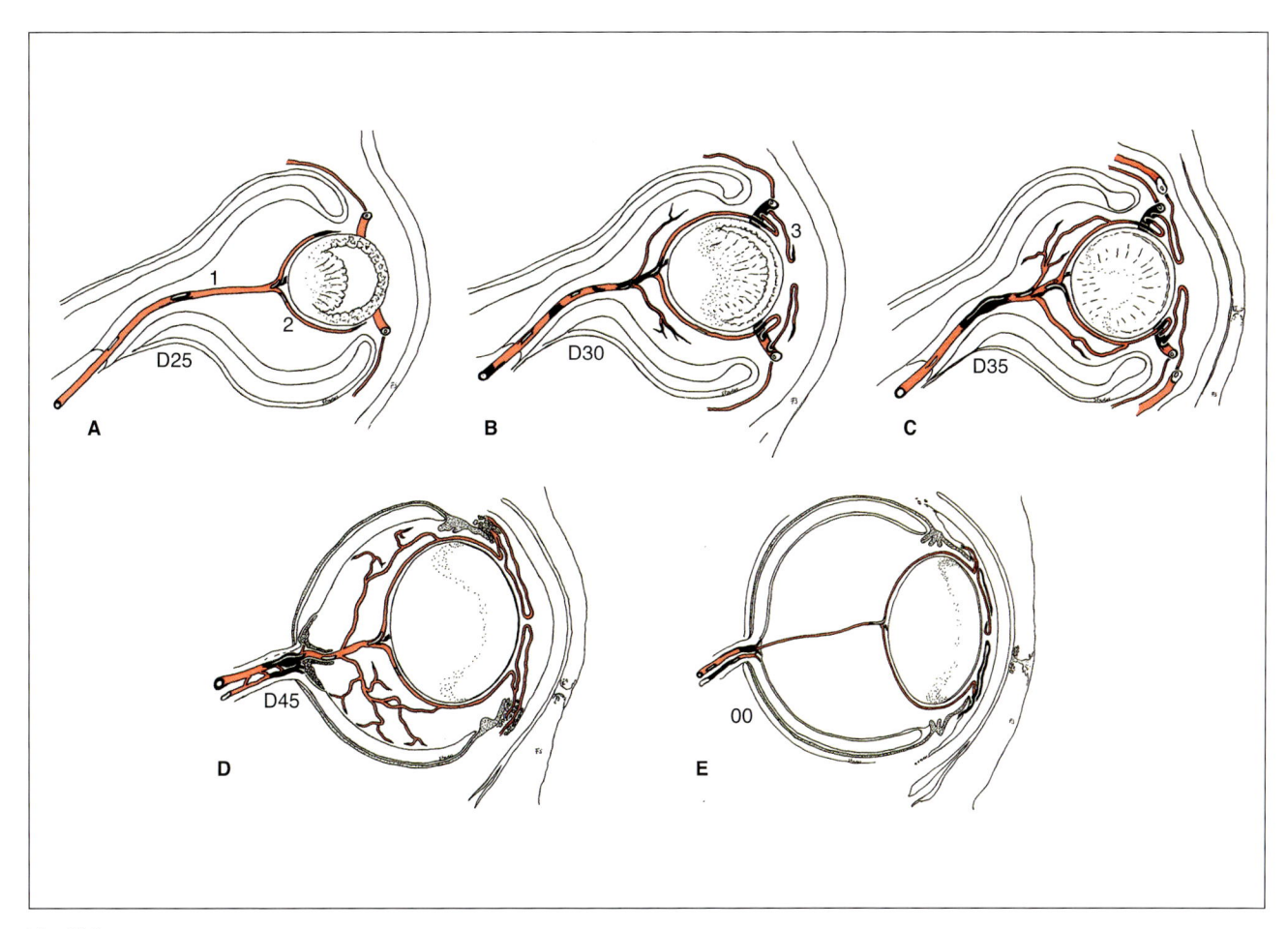

Fig. 13.1:
Hyaloid system. (1) Hyaloid a., (2) tunica vasculosa lentis, (3) pupillary membrane (in the dog on day: 25, 30, 35 and 45 of gestation, and at birth: 00).

a proliferation of fibers of the lens epithelium. This causes the physiologic increase in density of the three nuclei of the lens in 5- to 6-year-old animals. This is called lens sclerosis (Plates 13.1, 13.2), though it is also incorrectly called "senile cataract".

Physiological variations in lens structure may develop in the horse that can be confused with pathological changes, such as visible concentric, onion-skin-like lines; spontaneous, single vacuoles in the cortex; and well visible and more branched suture lines. Nuclear sclerosis in the horse is less distinct, starts approximately at 15 years of age and is more difficult to visualize. In very old horses, the whole lens has often a yellowish discoloration.

As the lens vesicle becomes separated from the surface ectoderm, the hyaloid artery (HA) grows out through the primitive vitreous to the posterior pole of the lens. The HA branches around the lens in a vascular net, the tunica vasculosa lentis (TVL). Anteriorly, there are anastomoses with the annular vessel of the optic cup, where the base of the iris will be formed later. The thickening of the lens capsule proceeds parallel to the outgrowth of the TVL. Vascular loops grow out from the annular vessel over the front side of the lens to form the pupillary membrane (PM). The hyaloid system is developed maximally around the 40th–45th day post coitus; thereafter, the system goes into regression. The entire system is resorbed between the 2nd and 4th week in the cat and dog, and in horse up to 9 months after birth. Only a very small rudimentary string of the HA remains at a small spot (called Mittendorf's dot; only recognizable using a slit-lamp biomicroscope), just under the posterior pole of the lens.[2]

13.1.2 Anatomy and physiology

The adult lens is a fully transparent, elastic, biconvex, intraocular organ. It is a part of the dioptric apparatus that, together with the cornea, brings light into focus on the retina. The accommodation capacity of the lens in companion animals is very limited. The lens has a diameter of 9–12 mm and is 6–8 mm thick (dog and cat).

In the horse, the lens is more strongly curved posteriorly, has a diameter of 20–22 mm, and is 12–14 mm thick.

The lens' composition is about 65% water and 35% protein, with a very small fraction consisting of minerals, carbohydrates, and lipids. The lens is surrounded by a capsule. The anterior lens capsule is thicker and tougher than the posterior capsule, and it becomes thicker and denser with age. The zonular fibers, by which the lens is suspended in the center behind the pupil, are attached to the capsule in the equatorial region, and in small animals they form a very firm attachment with the ciliary body in between the ciliary processes. The zonular fibers are also not so readily dissolved with materials such as alpha-chymotrypsin, which is used in intracapsular lens extraction in humans. The attachment between the posterior capsule and

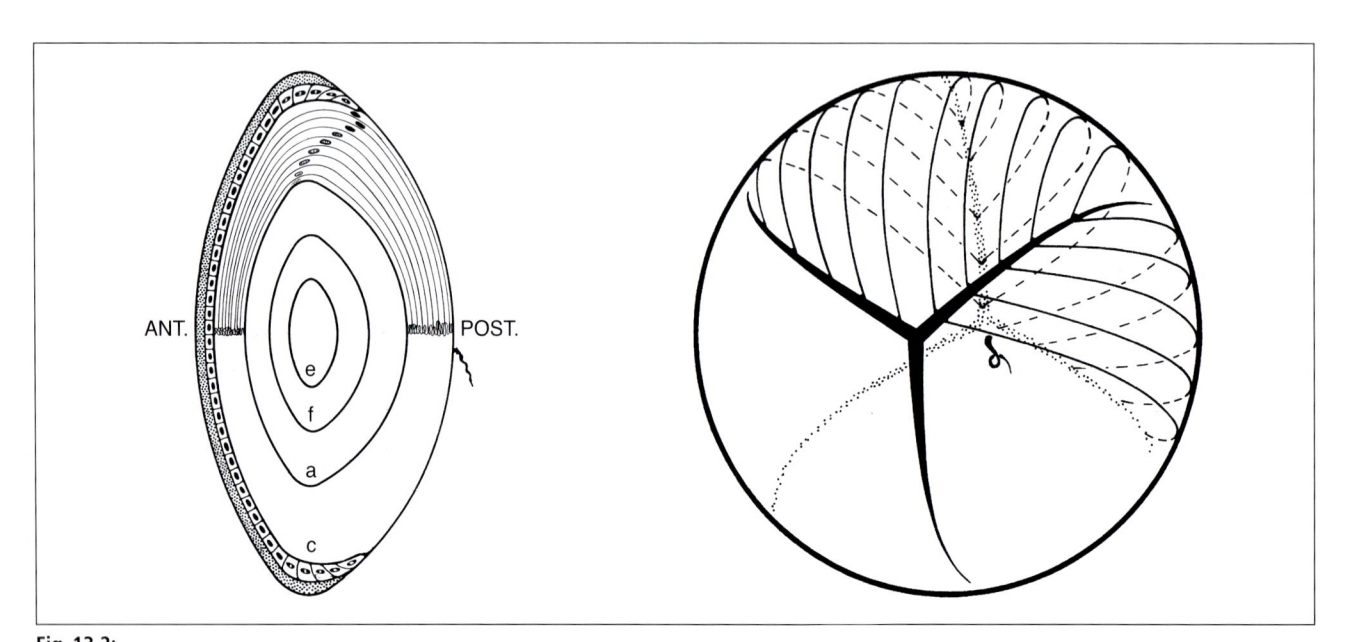

Fig. 13.2:
Section and fiber pattern of an adult lens (nuclei: E. embryonal; F. fetal; A. adult; C. cortex). Y-figure is anterior, inverted Y-figure is posterior, and the "pigtail" is the rest of the hyaloid a. (only visible using a biomicroscope).

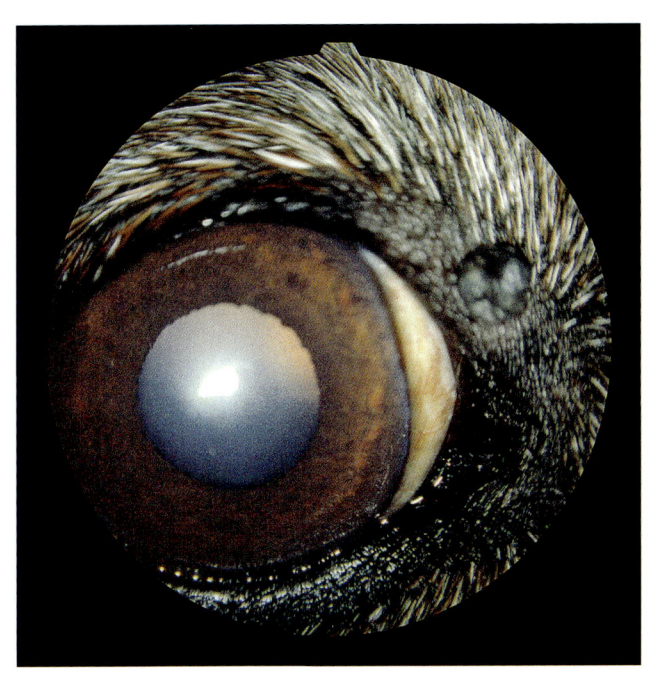

Plate 13.1:
Sclerosis of the lental nucleus (OD) in a 15-year-old dog, in miosis. This is a consequence of the normal aging process. In addition, a papilloma is present at the (superior) lid margin at the 2-o'clock position (see also Plate 13.2).

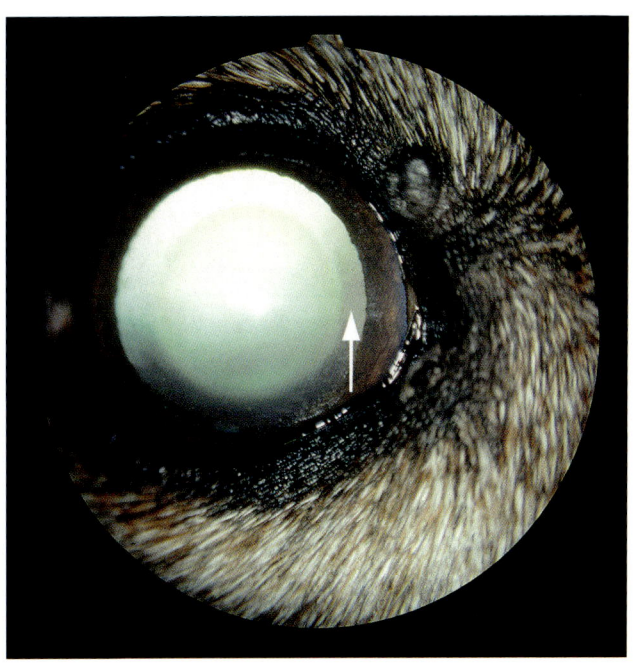

Plate 13.2:
Sclerosis of the lental nucleus (OD) in a 15-year-old dog, in mydriasis (the same dog as in Plate 13.1). A small, triangular opacity is visible at the 3-o'clock position on the pupillary margin (see arrow). This is a small, but non-physiological, senile cataract.

the vitreous is also very strong. Hence, during lens extraction in animals only the central part of the anterior capsule and the contents of the lens are removed. The equatorial and posterior parts of the capsule are thus left intact (*extracapsular* lens extraction; see 13.3.3). Only when there is luxation of the lens, is the lens and its capsule removed completely (*intracapsular* lens extraction; see 13.3.3).

The physiologic state of the lens proteins is of great importance for maintenance of the transparency of the lens. These proteins are already separated from the rest of the body by the capsule at the 20th–25th day post coitus (dog and cat). The lens proteins can later lead to severe anterior uveitis if they escape into the anterior chamber as a result of swelling of the lens, trauma or lens extraction.

In later life, the lens has no blood supply of its own and because lens innervation is also lacking, primary inflammatory lens changes are not possible. All metabolically important substances are delivered or removed via the aqueous and through the capsule. The most important energy source for the lens is glucose, which is metabolized via a number of enzyme systems.

Loss of the lens fibers' transparency leads to formation of cataract, which is usually irreversible apart from, for example, certain types of traumatic cataracts (Plates 13.3–13.10). Changes in the lens proteins, resulting in cataract, can be caused by hereditary defects, metabolic influences (excess of glucose in diabetes mellitus, deficiency diseases), breakdown products, intoxication (e.g. naphthalenes), and physical influences (irradiation, electric or mechanical insults like trauma). Usually, during the denaturation of the lens proteins, there is also an increased water content and thus swelling of the lens.

13.1.3 Vitreous

The vitreous is a very elastic hydrogel. The largest part of the globe is filled and held in form by the vitreous. In addition, it provides the necessary counterpressure to hold the neural part of the retina fixed against the pigment epithelium. About 1% of the vitreous consists of a network of polygonal fibrils of hyaluronic acid and collagen, with an occasional hyalocyte. The remaining 99% is water. The "walls" of the vitreous do not consist of membranes but of condensations of fibrils. These condensations and the colloidal structure provide for the maintenance of its water content and prevent the entrance of cells, such as inflammatory cells and bacteria. During the animal's lifetime, some physiological increase in the density of the vitreous occurs, leading to very fine white fibrous structures which can become visible with the slit lamp. In old age, the stability of the colloid can decrease, leading to liquefaction (synchysis) of the vitreous.[3]

Remainders of the primary vitreous, such as the Cloquet's canal ("tube" around the former hyaloid artery, from the optic disc to the posterior pole of the lens; Fig. 13.1) are much more distinct in the horse than in the dog or cat. Also the different parts of the vitreous (cortical, intermediate and central) can be much better seen in the horse. For this reason, and also due to a post-natal condensation of vitreous fibrils in the horse, these changes may give the impression of vitreous liquefaction, floaters and membranes. However, they generally do not have any pathological significance. Real synchysis is rare and is generally due to inflammatory changes of the posterior segment (see 13.5).

13.2 Developmental disorders of the lens

This is a group of rare abnormalities of the eye. Usually, they are part of other developmental disorders of the eye, such as microphthalmia, anophthalmia, and uveal anomalies. The etiology is not well understood. These abnormalities can be due to a chance error in embryogenesis, but there is also clearly a possibility that the abnormalities have a hereditary background (hereditary cataract). In such cases, it is advisable to follow the advice given in 15. The breeding of affected animals and their immediate family members is discouraged.

13.2.1 Aphakia / coloboma / spherophakia / microphakia / lenticonus / lentiglobus

These are rare congenital developmental abnormalities in the lens.
- Aphakia is the total absence of the lens or the presence of rudimentary parts of the lens.
- Coloboma or possibly better said dysplasia of the lens is a defect in the equator.
- Spherophakia is an excessive roundness of the lens.
- Microphakia is inadequate size of the lens.
- Lenticonus or lentiglobus is a conical malformation of the lens on the anterior or posterior side.

Such abnormalities often occur in combination with persistent parts of the hyaloid system and/or the vitreous, or other congenital dysplastic abnormalities such as microphthalmia, persistent pupillary membrane, etc. (see 9.7; Plates 12.2 and 13.6).[4]

13.2.2 Persistent hyaloid artery (PHA)

PHA is due to a lack of regression of part or all of the HA. The artery can remain present as a string, still containing blood, between the optic disc and the lens, though usually only a small connective tissue string remains adhered to the posterior capsule of the lens. During movements of the eye, this string-like structure lags slightly behind and so can have a waving motion, which is best observed in the beam of a slit lamp. Scars or densities also often occur where the PHA is attached to the capsule of the lens (just under the center of the suture lines of the lens) and in the immediately surrounding area. In more severe cases, these scars can also lead to cataract formation in the connecting lens fibers. The abnormality can be inherited (as in the Sussex Spaniel).

Therapy: Larger cataracts caused by a persisting hyaloid artery can be removed by extra capsular lens extraction, including posterior central capsulorrhexis. However, there is more risk for intra- and post-operative complications, such as vitreous prolapse.

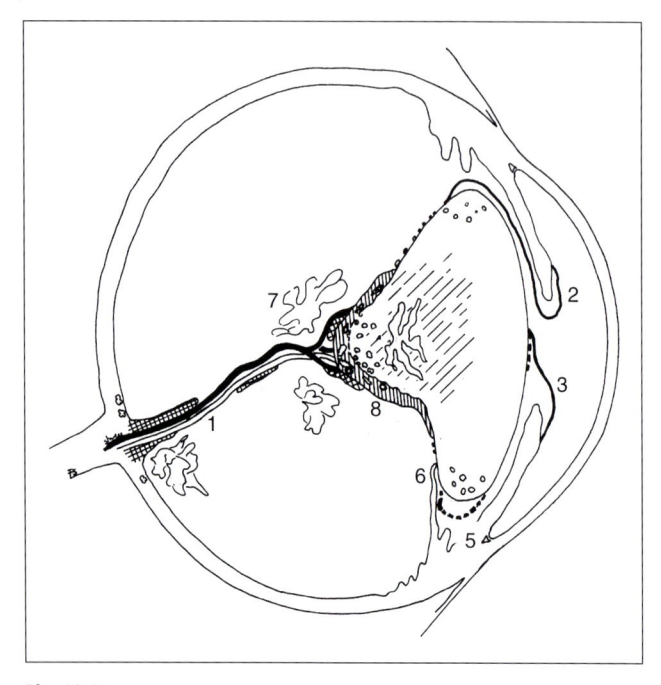

Fig. 13.3:
PHTVL/PHPV. (1) Persistent hyaloid a./v.; (2) persistent anterior TVL; (3) persistent pupillary membrane; (4) lenticonus with cataract; (5) lens, "coloboma/dysplasia"; (6) elongated ciliary process; (7) retrolental blood; (8) fibrovascular, retrolental plaque.

13.2.3 Persistent hyperplastic tunica vasculosa lentis / persistent hyperplastic primary vitreous (PHTVL / PHPV)

In this group of apparently rare (unilateral) disorders,[5] parts of the hyaloid system and primitive vitreous become hyperplastic and remain present postnatally, which may also lead to cataract.[6] In the Doberman and Staffordshire Bull Terrier, this disorder is bilateral, inherited (probably incomplete dominant), and therefore more frequent in occurrence.[7,8,9]

Symptoms: Very small dots of connective tissue from the vascular network can remain retrolental on the posterior capsule of the lens (grade 1; doubtful if unilateral and of minimal degree). These dots do not progress and do not influence the visual capacity of the dog. They are only seen with the aid of a slit-lamp bio-microscope.

The severe forms (grades 2–6; Fig. 13.3) occur bilaterally and lead to visual problems for the dog (Plate 13.7). A plaque of white fibrovascular tissue can remain on the posterior capsule, accompanied by grade 1 retrolental dots. In addition, other parts of the hyaloid system can persist: lenticonus, or even more severe malformations of the lens such as pigment or blood in the lens or behind it; colobomas; spherophakia, etc.; and/or microphthalmia may be present. In the severe forms, cataract develops, usually beginning centrally. This can be present at birth, and the animal may be born blind but not identified until the lids open. The cataract can also slowly increase in severity during the animal's life. The differential diagnosis includes primary cataract or microphthalmia alone, or other dysplastic abnormalities.

Therapy: In severely abnormal eyes (grades 2–6), if blind, intracapsular or extracapsular lens extraction (see 13.3.3) can be performed together with anterior vitrectomy. One must, however, consider whether this is reasonable in a very young dog or whether euthanasia is the better choice. In adult dogs that are already part of the family, the situation is different.

Prognosis / prevention: The prognosis for intracapsular lens extraction operation in severely affected cases is less favorable (60–70%) than with extracapsular lens extraction in uncomplicated cataracts, because of the greater likelihood of complications (postoperative bleeding, retinal detachment). In these cases, implantation of an artificial lens is not well possible.

Examination for PHTVL / PHPV can be carried out in litters of pups, preferably older than 6 weeks of age and after chipping or tattooing, by veterinarians who are appointed to the panels involved in hereditary eye disease schemes. Because the globes are still small at this time and the fine dots may be overlooked, the result of the examination should be considered temporary. On the other hand, early examination prevents buyers from obtaining severely affected puppies.

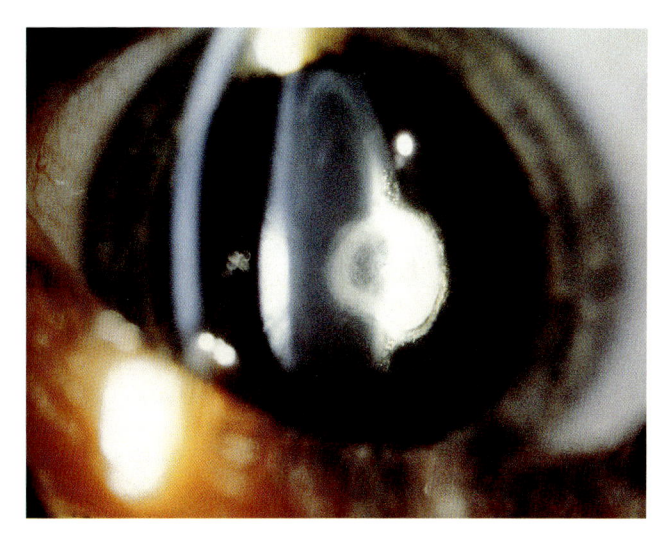

Plate 13.3:
Slit-lamp microscopic view of an eye with anterior and posterior polar cataracts (human eye; OS; by courtesy Dr. A.T.M. van Balen, Amsterdam).

At least obviously affected animals (grades 2–6) should be excluded from breeding. Because of an adequate breeding program (grade 1 are only used when mated to unaffected animals), the number of severely affected Dobermans in the Netherlands and Germany has dropped very significantly over the last years.[10]

13.3 Cataract

Every non-physiologic whitening or other cloudiness of the lens fibers and/or the lens capsule is called cataract. Cataract is generally caused by a reduced oxygen uptake and thus an increased water uptake by the lens (Plates 13.3–13.10). This causes swelling (intumesce) at first and then dehydration, followed by shrinkage and an increased risk of luxation. Cataracts can be classified according to localization (Fig. 13.4), stage, type, and cause. In practice, the type and stage are the most important criteria for judging progression and possibilities for operation. An early cataract, which still allows a good inspection of the fundus, is called immature (Plates 13.3, 13.7, 13.8). If the fundus can no longer be examined and the patient is therefore blind, the cataract is called mature (Plates 13.4, 13.9, 13.10). If the cataract is more or less dissolved, this is a hypermature cataract. In the latter, small amounts of lens protein can be resorbed, leading to shrinkage and wrinkling of the capsule and frequently to uveitis. In exceptional cases, this resorptive process can continue to such an extent that spontaneous clearing (less resorption) occurs.

194 Lens and Vitreous

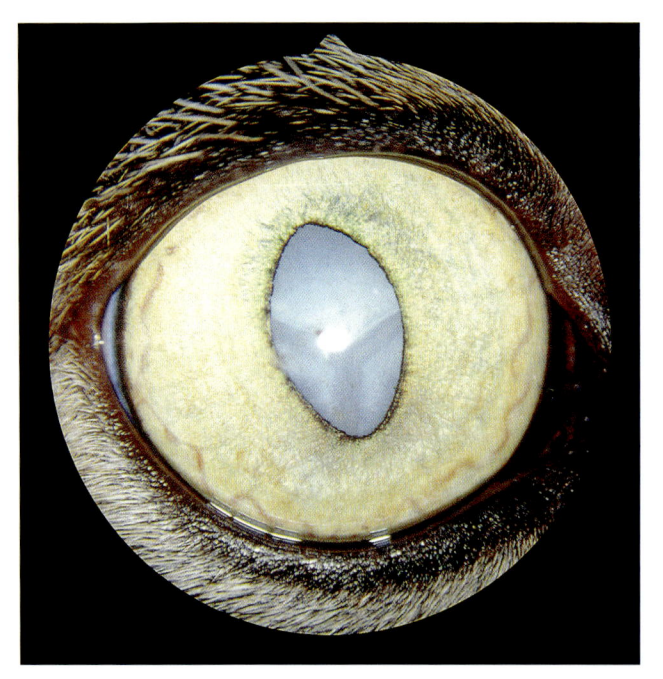

Plate 13.4:
Mature cataract in a cat (OD). The Y-shaped suture lines are due to the course of the interconnections of the lens fibers. This configuration is characteristic of the anterior part of the lens.

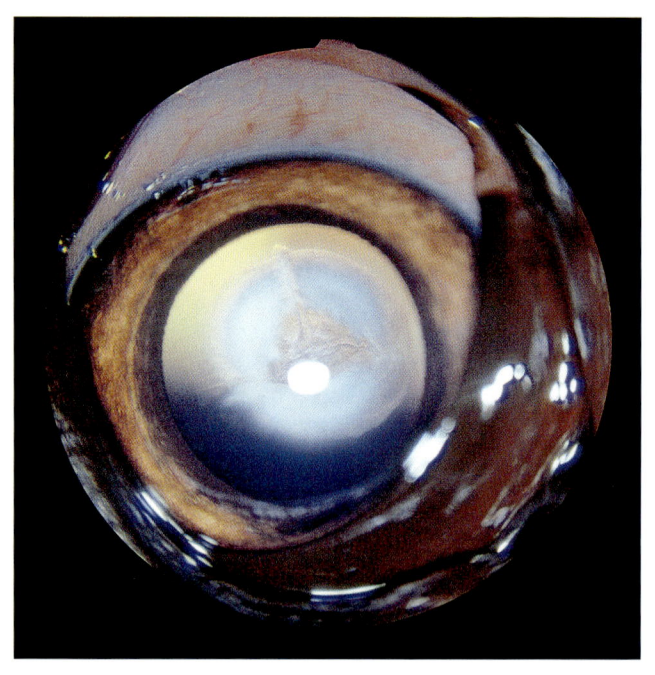

Plate 13.5:
Immature congenital cataract in the posterior pole of the lens, recognizable by the inverted Y-shaped lines and the boiled egg white aspect (OD, dog).

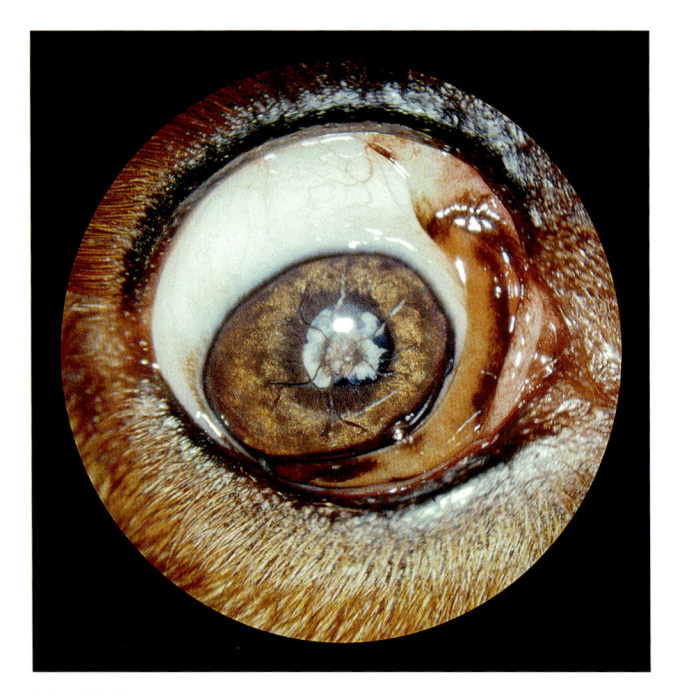

Plate 13.6:
Microphthalmia, persistent pupillary membrane and congenital (with the aspect of boiled egg white) mature cataract in an English Cocker Spaniel puppy at the age of 6 weeks (OD).

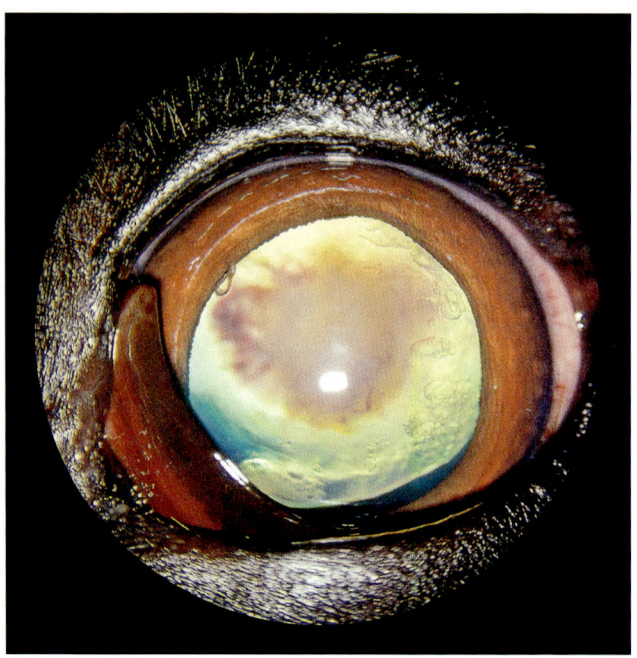

Plate 13.7:
Persistent hyperplastic tunica vasculosa lentis and primary vitreous (PHTVL / PHPV) in a Doberman (OS). A tunica vasculosa lentis anterior persistens can be seen at the pupillary margin at the 10-o'clock position.

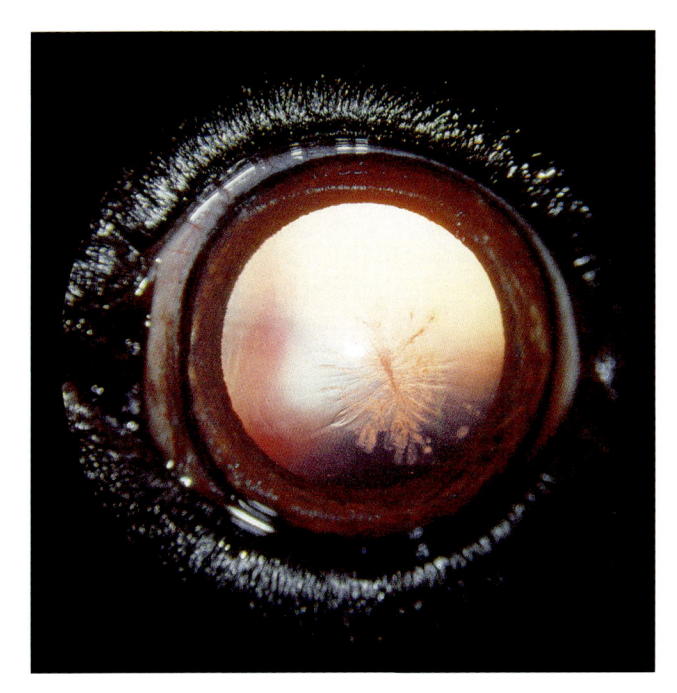

Plate 13.8:
Immature cortical cataract in an American Cocker Spaniel at the age of 3 years (OS).

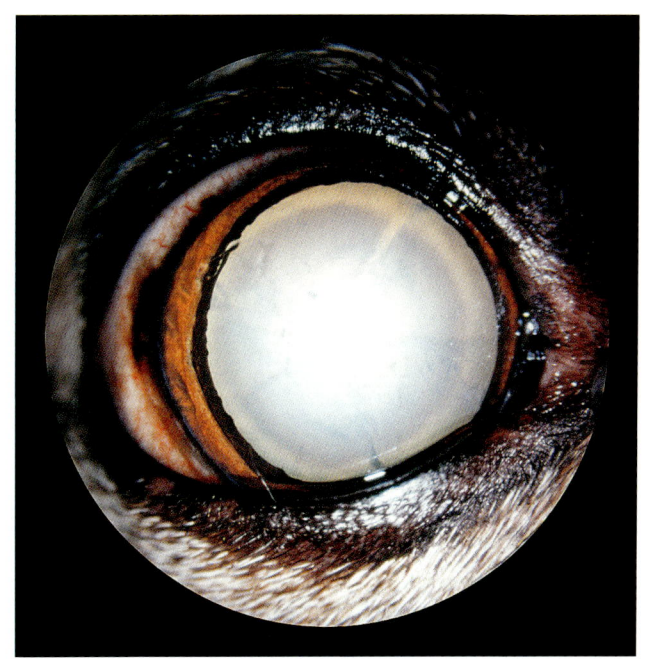

Plate 13.10:
Hypermature cataract associated with hereditary retinal degeneration (PEA; night blindness form) in a Miniature Poodle (OD). From the hyperreflectivity showing in the equatorial part of the lens, the additional presence of retinal atrophy can be suspected.

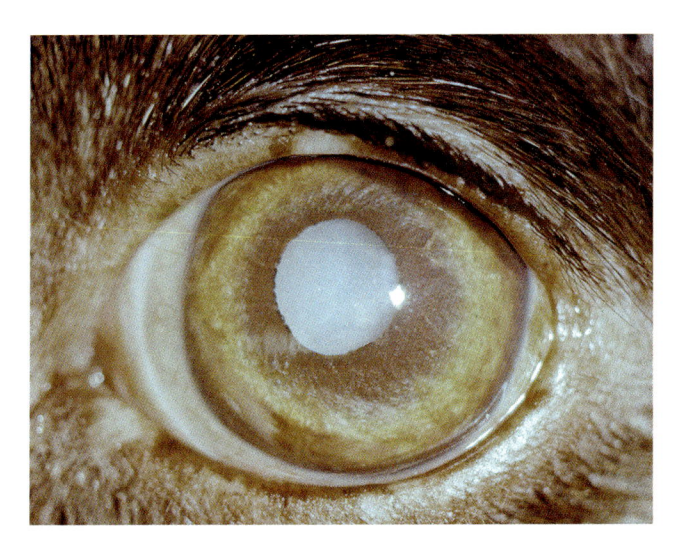

Plate 13.9:
Mature intumescent cataract (OD, dog). The iris shows an extra convex course due to swelling of the lens.

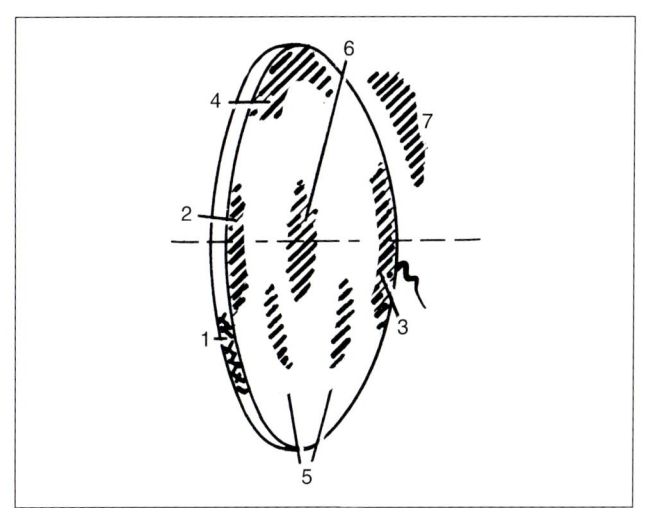

Fig. 13.4:
Location of abnormalities in and around the lens. (1) Capsular; (2) cortical, subcapsular, polar, anterior; (3) *idem*, posterior; (4) equatorial; (5) cortical; (6) nuclear; (7) retrolental.

If cataract is already present before the 6th–8th week of life, it is considered to be congenital (in dog and cat; Plate 13.5). Cataract developing after the 8th week is an acquired cataract and is termed juvenile, and in old age it is termed senile (Plate 13.2).

Inherited cataracts are usually bilateral, more or less in the same stage of maturity, and often begin in the cortex near the posterior pole or in the equatorial area.

In addition to primary cataract, there are many forms of secondary cataracts. They may be due to intraocular or systemic disease (see 13.3.2).

Differentiating primary and secondary cataracts is often difficult, but important for the therapeutic results and breeding.

13.3.1 Types of cataract

Congenital cataract. This cataract is often very dense, white (like boiled egg white), and usually progresses slowly. It often occurs in combination with other congenital abnormalities such as microphthalmia, PPM, PHA, or PHTVL / PHPV.

Juvenile cataract. Juvenile cataract develops usually between the 1st and 8th years of life (or much later, for example, in parrots). If causes such as diabetes mellitus, trauma, intoxication, or radiation are unlikely or can well been excluded, it is possible that the cataract is hereditary. This cataract usually begins in the cortex, and is progressive and bilateral.

Senile cataract. This is a local cloudiness of the lens that almost always develops in the elderly animal. This cataract must not be confused with the physiologic central increase of density of the lens nuclei in sclerosis (Plates 13.1, 13.2).

Radiation cataract. Exposure to infrared, ultraviolet, microwave or x-ray irradiation and radioactive materials can induce cataract.[11,12]

Alimentary / intoxication cataract. Substances such as naphthalene, dinitrophenol, and possibly some substances in food can cause cataract; sometimes this type of cataract is reversible.[13,14,15,16]

In the ferret, too much fat, hypovitaminosis E or low protein diets can be associated with cataract formation.

Traumatic cataract. Traumatic cataract can develop as a result of a deep stab wound by a thorn, splinter, or cat claw. If the capsule heals quickly (sometimes in 2 layers), the damage can remain limited to a local, non-progressive cataract. Perforating trauma in cats and hunting dogs is usually caused by an airgun or shotgun pellet. This usually results in a complete cataract. Lens extraction in these cases is of little value because of secondary string formation in the vitreous and damage to the choroid.

Hereditary cataract. A recessive hereditary defect (sometimes simple) is the most frequent cause of cataract in dogs. Hereditary cataract, in the end, is usually bilateral und generally begins at the posterior pole, in the cortex. It is usually progressive. In several breeds (e.g. Golden and Labrador Retrievers), a more or less stationary, triangular cataract in the posterior pole also occurs fairly often. Hereditary cataract can be congenital or juvenile. The predisposed breeds are:
- **Congenital:** Cavalier King Charles[17] and English Cokker[18] Spaniels, Old English Sheepdog[19], Golden and Labrador Retrievers[20], Miniature Schnauzer[21], and West Highland White Terrier.[22]
- **Juvenile:** Afghan Hound, American and English Cocker Spaniels[23], Bedlington, Boston[24], West Highland White, and Jack Russell Terriers; Toy Schnauzer; German Shepherd Dog[25]; Chesapeake Bay, Golden and Labrador Retrievers;[26] Great Münsterländer; Poodles[27]; Welsh Springer Spaniel[28]; and canaries.

Hereditary cataracts have not been recognized in the horse, except in the Morgan horse. Congenital, nuclear cataracts are one of the most frequent congenital eye anomalies in foals; however, without any other anomalies (e.g. PPM or PHA). They are generally non-progressive, with subsequent minor to moderate visual handicap.

Note: Predisposed breeds and frequencies of these hereditary abnormalities can differ from country to country or region to region. For information about regional incidence rates, the practitioner should contact the local panel members of the hereditary eye disease schemes.

13.3.2 Secondary cataract

Cataract can develop as an associated or secondary abnormality (cataract complicata) in a number of other primary ocular abnormalities such as uveitis (see 12.10.7; Plate 12.12), lens luxation, retinal dysplasia, and hereditary retinal degeneration (PEA; in the dog). Such cataracts may be capsular, cortical or nuclear or in a combination of these locations. Especially with retinal abnormalities, the clinician should not be so distracted by the presence of the cataract as to overlook the primary abnormality that may make surgical removal of the lens pointless (see 14).

13.3.2.1 Diabetic cataract

In diabetes mellitus, the increase in concentration of glucose in the aqueous and the capsule and individual lens cell membranes is insulin-independent, i.e. insulin is not necessary for glucose to pass through the cell wall. The excessive glucose is metabolized via the aldose reductase pathway resulting in increased concentrations of intracellular sorbitol. This is an inert sugar alcohol which cannot pass the lens cell membranes and produces a significant osmotic gradient. Water is drawn into the lens cells and the lens swells. This results in damage to the membranes of the lens fibers and loss of transparency. Diabetes mellitus almost always leads to bilateral cataract after a shorter (sometimes within 14 days) or longer period of time.[29] It is, therefore, advisable to ask the owner of a patient presented with cataracts about the presence of polyuria and polydipsia, and to check plasma and urine glucose concentrations. Furthermore, diabetic patients are also best referred to an ophthalmologist within 1–2 weeks after diagnosis for eye examination, to exclude complicating eye disease for later lens extraction.

13.3.3 Therapeutic possibilities

Attempts to prevent or retard the development of cataracts by medical means have so far been unsuccessful. Some of the "medications" have to be administered intraocularly, which in itself can lead to severe complications, such as post-traumatic uveitis.

Atropine (0.5–1%, 1 drop in the morning) can be worthwhile if the cataract is still small and is in the central visual axis. Atropine dilates the pupil, allowing the animal to see around the cataract. If the cataract is mature, only lens extraction can improve vision.

In evaluating a cataract patient for lens extraction, the following aspects should be considered:

Condition of the patient. The condition of the patient should be such that the patient can withstand the operation or the patient has to be first treated to normalize its condition before surgery. There should also be a sufficiently good life expectancy, so that after the operation the patient can benefit for a significant period of time from the improved vision.

Condition of the eye. If there is corneal dystrophy, uveitis or, especially, bilateral retinal abnormalities (progressive retinal atrophy [PRA], retinal dysplasia, etc.; see 14), lens extraction is not useful and only a burden for the patient and the owner. The pupillary reflex is not a dependable method of evaluating the condition of the retina: a lively pupillary response does not exclude PRA, for example. Only if the pupillary reaction to light is completely absent can it be concluded with some certainty that there is retinal degeneration or another retinal or neurological entity. For these reasons, the referral of a patient with cataract for lens extraction should be done within 1–3 weeks, when a cataract is found in the first eye and preferably when it is in an immature stage. By means of indirect ophthalmoscopy of the other eye, the ophthalmic surgeon can simply determine the condition of the deeper parts of the eye. If the patient is only referred after a mature cataract is present in both eyes, the condition of the retina is uncertain and only an electroretinography (ERG; see 14.1.2) and ultrasonography can provide reliable information about the condition of retina.

Behavior of the animal. Very wild, nervous, or aggressive animals can cause serious problems in postoperative treatment and are more likely to strike their head against objects; hence, there is clearly a greater risk of complications.

Visual handicap. The animal should be clearly handicapped. The owner is usually emotionally affected by the thought of the animal's blindness. In reality, animals are much less dependent on their sight than humans.

Motivation of the owner. The owner must be sufficiently motivated and manually able to perform the after-care. The costs of the operation are relatively high in comparison with other common operations, and the after-care requires considerable time and effort from the owner.

The chance of success in the dog or cat is 80–95% for extracapsular lens extraction.

The success rate in horses depends not only on the type of the cataract (primary or secondary), but also on other factors such as positioning, recovery phase, automutilation. The overall result in cataract surgery in horse has the best prognosis in the foal.

In addition, the owner should be aware that after a successful operation and the after-care period, the animal will remain slightly handicapped (far-sighted). However, after some weeks of adaptation, the legs of tables and chairs, going up and down stairs, making small jumps, etc., will no longer give problems. Horses will even perform a hurdle course smoothly.

Further improvement in vision can be obtained by the use of glasses, contact lenses, or intraocular lenses.[30] The necessity for further improvement in vision in animals is, however, less important as in humans. Glasses or contact lenses are difficult to apply in animals. The implantation of an intraocular lens (40–43 diopters) is technically well possible, and the lens is usually well tolerated[31] by the eye as long as it is implanted in the remaining capsular bag.[32] After-cataract in the posterior capsule, i.e. posterior to an implant lens, is very difficult to remove without disturbing the implant lens. It can be removed by the use of a neodymium-YAG laser, but the apparatus is very expensive.[33] Also, loosening of the implanted lens, uveitis, and glaucoma are possible complications. In addition, lens implantation brings considerable additional costs. The use of an intraocular lens is associated with a similar or slightly decreased chance of complications compared to extracapsular lens extraction without an implant. Still, in case of doubt, a simple extracapsular lens extraction without an implant is to be preferred above a complicated implant procedure.

Lens extraction

Unless the veterinarian has taken a special interest in lens extractions and has performed the operation very frequently, cataract patients should be referred. If there is inadequate equipment, experience, and especially technical ability, there is a great chance of complications. If the anterior chamber is opened for longer than 5–10 minutes, a severe irritation of the iris occurs, leading to exudation.

For this operation to be successful, it is important that the owner is well informed about the pre-operative preparation, the surgery, and the after-care. For this reason, lens extraction will be described in more detail.

Pre-operative treatment and anesthesia. It is recommended that the patient (dog, cat) should become accustomed to wearing a protective collar before the operation. Two to three days before the operation, 0.1% dexamethasone-"specific choice" antibiotic eye drops are administered 4 times daily.

Ketamine anesthesia (which is still frequently used in cats) is more or less suitable for ocular or intraocular surgery. This anesthesia has the great advantage that the eye does not recede into the orbit and turn away. In dogs, and to a lesser extend in cats, however, this form of anesthesia is much less easily controlled. When other forms of anesthesia are used, rotation of the globe and enophthalmos occur. To prevent this, it is necessary to use inhalation anesthesia and a muscle relaxant (such as [cis]atracurium, norcuronium or vecuronium). Since the respiratory muscles are also affected with this type of anesthesia, it is necessary to provide artificial respiration. During manipulations into the eye in animals, there is a strong tendency for inflammatory reactions, mainly resulting in exudation into the anterior chamber (chance for synechia). These inflammatory reactions can be largely prevented by corticosteroids before the operation day and pre-operative dexamethasone intravenously in the dog and cat. In the horse, NSAIDs are administered intravenously preoperatively.[34]

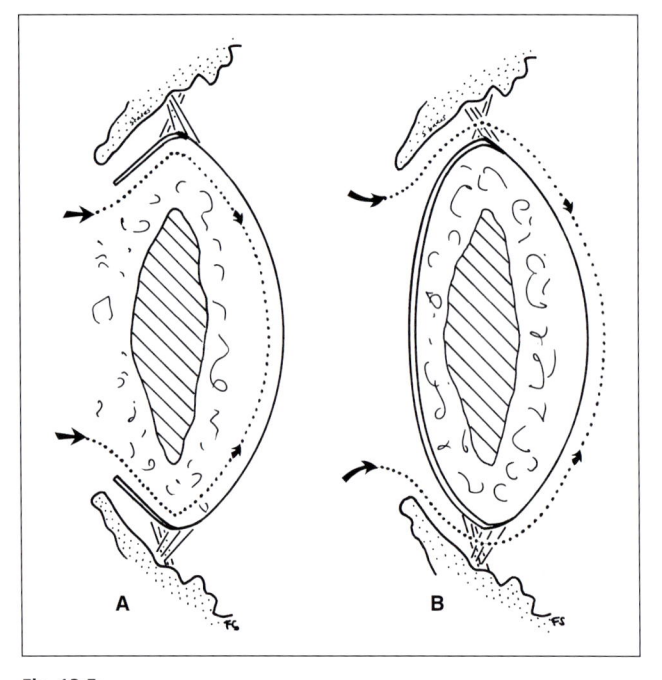

Fig. 13.5:
The removal by extracapsular (A) and intracapsular (B) lens extraction (dotted line).

Surgery. To perform lens extraction, a strong (x5–30 magnification) operating microscope or loupe (x5 only in lens luxation), highly specific instruments, and microsuture material must be used. There are two basic techniques for removal of a cataractous lens, namely intracapsular and extracapsular (Fig. 13.5).

Intracapsular extraction. In this method, the lens is removed *in toto*. For this purpose, the zonular fibers must be broken or dissolved and the lens be loosened from the vitreous. In animals, there is a high risk of complications with this method (bleeding and vitreous prolapse) and hence it is rarely used. An advantage of this method is that no lens protein is released during the extraction. The method is certainly indicated in cases of lens luxation.

Extracapsular extraction (Fig. 13.6). In this method, the central part of the anterior capsule and the cloudy contents of the lens are removed. The operation consists of the following steps: after the globe is opened by a corneal cut at 0.5 mm from and parallel to the limbus (often epinephrine is installed in the anterior chamber to induce mydriasis). The anterior chamber is maintained in shape and the endothelium is protected, using a viscoelasticum. Thereafter, the central part of the anterior capsule is removed circularly by a controlled capsulorrhexis (for example, by a cannula stab, followed by two small scissor cuts and further circular tearing, using special forceps. The nucleus of the lens is washed or pressed out via a half-opened cornea. This procedure is used in foals[35] and in birds, where the contents can be aspirated by use of a blunt needle.

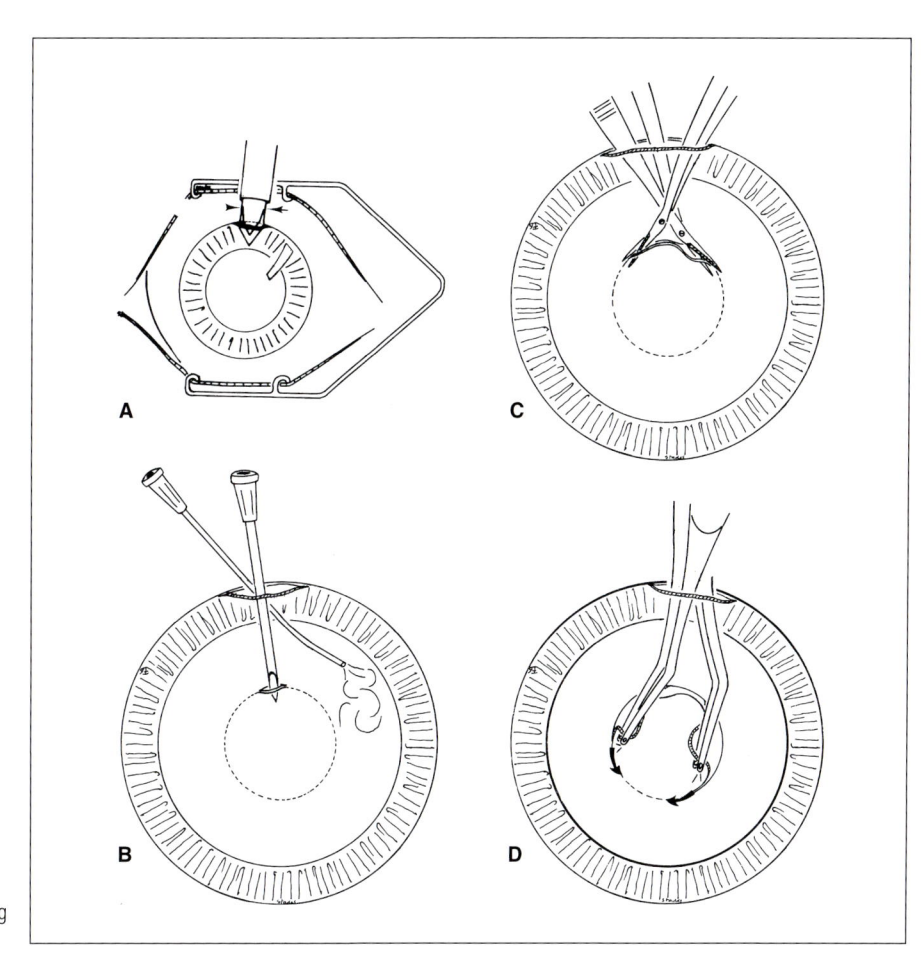

Fig. 13.6:
Extracapsular lens extraction: (A) incision in cornea in/near limbus (12-o'clock position); (B) filling of the anterior chamber with viscoelastic and stab incision in the anterior capsule; (C–D) scissors cuts both sided, and controlled circular tearing of the central part of the ant. capsule (capsulorrhexis). The shaded ring is the iris.

The actual technique in other animals is phacoemulsification (Fig. 13.7). In this procedure, the hard contents (core) of the lens are pulverized (ultrasonically), and the detritus is flushed out and aspirated.[36] This second method requires a much smaller corneal incision (approximately 3 mm) than the first. The apparatus is, however, very expensive and it cannot be used in every type of cataract. Moreover, the technique requires a lot of training to perform the procedure in the necessary short period of time and with using as low a degree of phacoenergy as possible. The remaining mucoid cortical fibers are washed out very carefully (Fig. 13.7 B) using an irrigating-aspirating apparatus. The fragile posterior capsule must not be perforated. If the posterior capsule also appears to be opaque, then its central portion is also removed using a controlled capsulorrhexis, and if necessary an anterior vitrectomy is performed.

Thereafter an intra-ocular lens (IOL) can be placed into the remaining capsular bag (Fig. 13.8). If a hard (e.g. polymethylmetacrylate [PMMA]) IOL is used (optic part 6–7 mm diameter, 1–2 mm thick) the corneal incision has to be enlarged up to approximately 8 mm. The haptics of the IOL are introduced in the remaining capsular bag and the IOL is rotated until it is centered (Fig. 13.8 AB). Alternatively, a foldable (e.g. acrylic) IOL can be injected through the 3-mm corneal incision, directly into the capsular bag, where it will unfold and center itself spontaneously (Fig. 13.8 CD). The foldable IOLs are at the moment 2–3 times more expensive then the hard ones, but the small corneal incision is an advantage.

The corneal incision, if longer than 2 mm, is closed with simple interrupted sutures 1–2 mm apart (monofilament resorbable [more reactive], or nylon, 8-0 to 10-0, 3/8 circle, spatula-shaped needle). The wound is closed in such a way to make it both watertight and resistant to the effects of struggling or barking. If there are no complications during surgery on the first eye, there are advantages in operating on both eyes in one sitting. This avoids the possibility of a reaction to the lens proteins following a later second operation. However it makes the procedure more expensive, time-consuming, and the first operated eye may be damaged during the surgery of the second eye and the animal can see very well with only one eye.

After-care: Immediately after the operation, 2–3 deposits of a water-soluble depot-corticosteroid preparation (10–15 mg, subconjunctivally) are administered.

After surgery, the following eye drops are administered: a "specific choice" antibiotic (combination) 4–6 times daily for 3–4 weeks, and 0.1% dexamethasone (4–6 times daily) for 2–4 months. If the posterior capsule has been removed or intracapsular lens extraction performed, the pupil is held at a diameter of 2–5 mm by the use of 1–2% pilocarpine. The sutures are either removed 16–20 days after surgery (depending on the tissue bridging) or resorbable sutures are left in place, but they will resorb only slowly. The patient should still wear a protective collar for about 5 days more and only be taken out on the leash (cats should be kept indoors).

Prognosis: The success rate for an extracapsular extraction varies from 80–95%, depending on the type of cataract, the skill of the surgeon, the method used, and the cooperation (partly related to age) of the patient and the owner. Frequent complications are adhesions and after-cataract.

In the horse, complications such as massive uveitis, hyphema, synechia and secondary glaucoma are more frequent.

In a low percentage of cases, these complications may result in a recurrence of blindness. Severe complications such as glaucoma, endophthalmitis, and phthisis bulbi are rare (~ 1%).

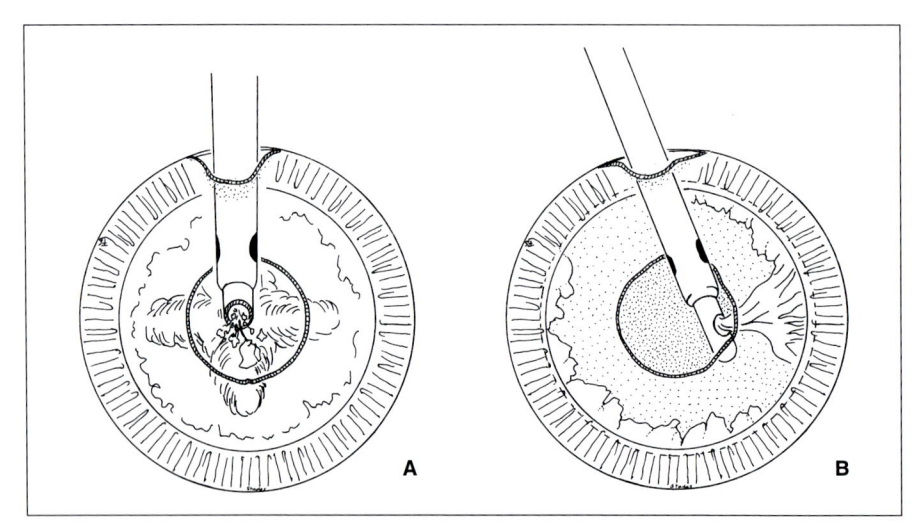

Fig. 13.7:
Extracapsular lens extraction: phacoemulsification technique. (A) The hard lens nucleus is emulsified, flushed and aspirated; (B) further cortex cells are aspirated. The shaded ring is the iris.

13.3.4 Prevention of cataract

Affected animals should be excluded from breeding. If the number of animals available for breeding allows it, parents or siblings of affected animals should also be excluded from breeding, because they have a significantly higher chance of being a carrier of the disease. Recently, a DNA Test for the detection of juvenile cataract in the Staffordshire Bull und Boston Terriers has become available (for further information see: *www.aht.org.uk*).

13.4 Lens luxation or ectopic lens

The lens can become loose by rupture of the zonular fibers (Fig. 13.9–13.11). The fibers can be abnormally developed, degenerate, or, in exceptional situations, they can rupture directly. The abnormality occurs much more frequently in dogs than in cats (about 9:1). In several small terrier breeds,[37,38,39] lens luxation is a hereditary (recessive) disease.[40] These breeds are: Dandie Dinmont Terrier, Fox Terrier, German Hunting Terrier, Jack Russell Terrier, Tibetan Terrier, and Welsh Terrier. The Border Collie and Shar Pei are also affected. There is no definite breed predisposition for lens luxation in cats, but in our experience, lens luxation is the most frequent cause of glaucoma in this species. In horses and cats, primary lens luxation is rare, while secondary lens luxation in these two species can often be caused by chronic (recurrent) uveitis.

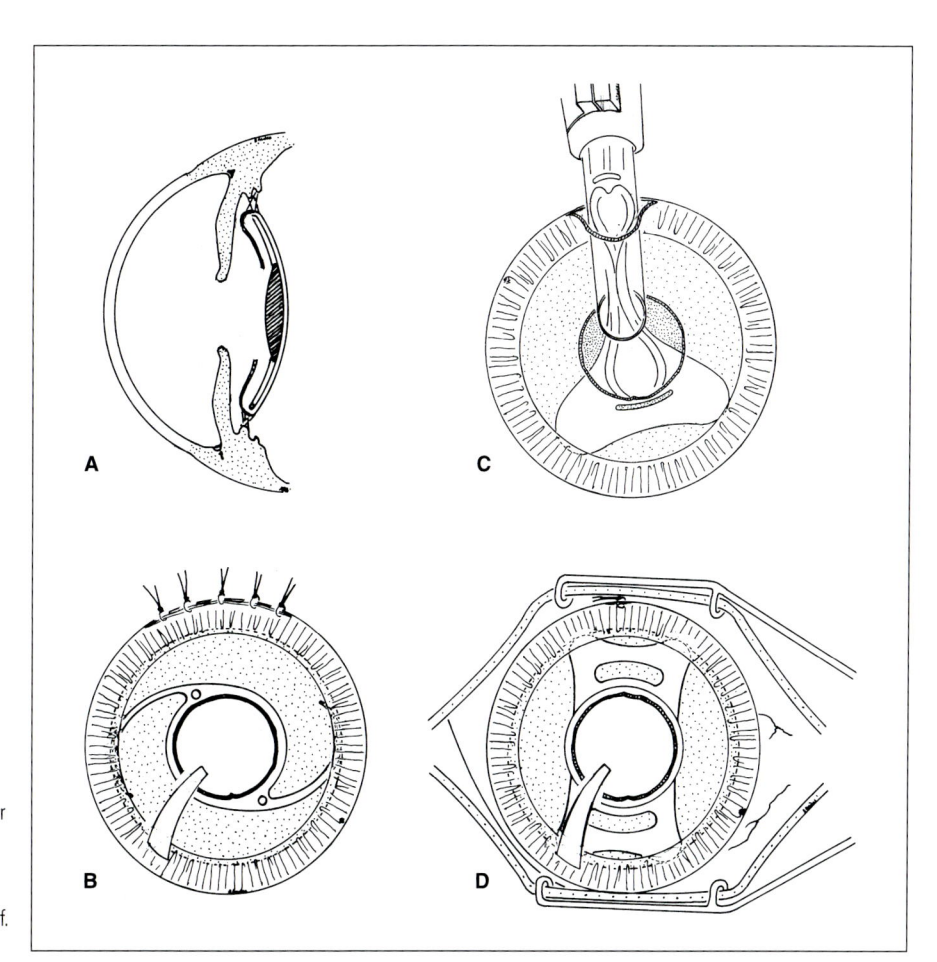

Fig. 13.8:
Intraocular lens (IOL) implantation, in the remaining, cleared capsular bag. (A) In section; (B) hard PMMA-IOL (optic 6–7 mm diameter, section 1–2 mm thick) positioned in the capsular bag by rotation, frontal view. (C) A foldable, acrylic IOL is injected through the 3- to 4-mm corneal incision, into the capsular bag; (D) The IOL unfolds in the capsular bag and centers itself. The shaded ring is the iris.

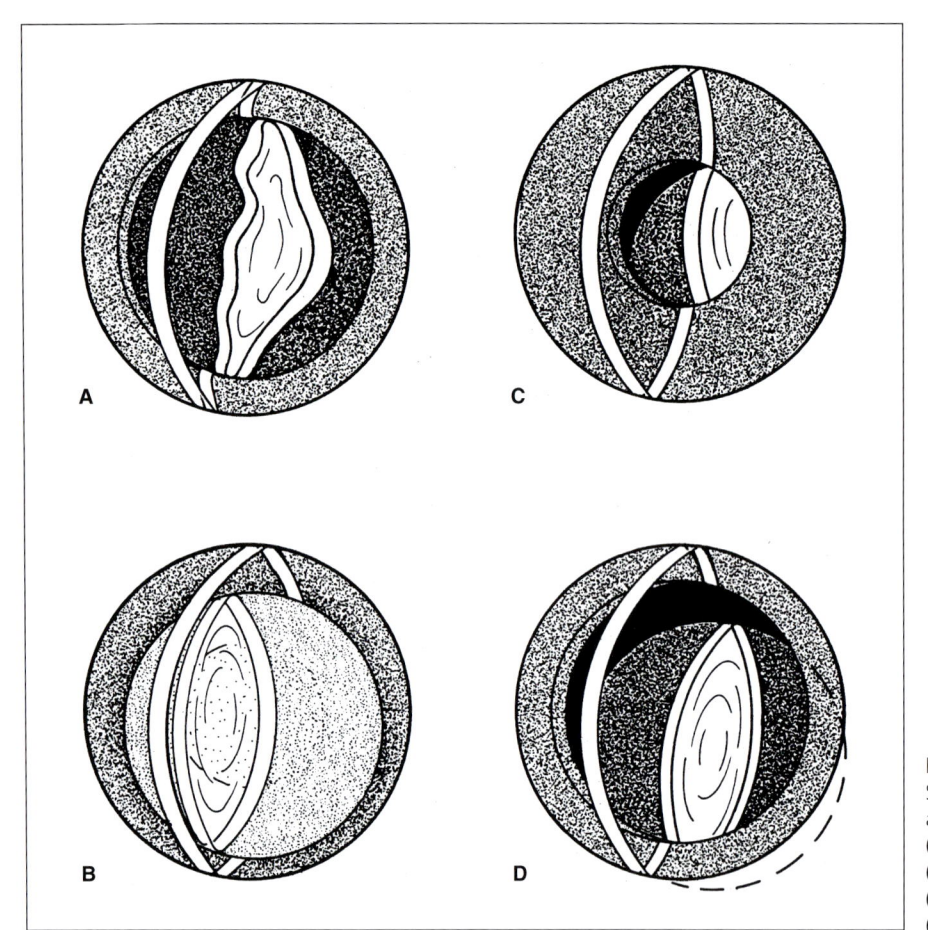

Fig. 13.9:
Slit-lamp picture of form and location abnormalities of the lens.
(A) Folded anterior capsule,
(B) lens luxation to the anterior chamber,
(C) posterior lens luxation in miosis, and
(D) mydriasis.

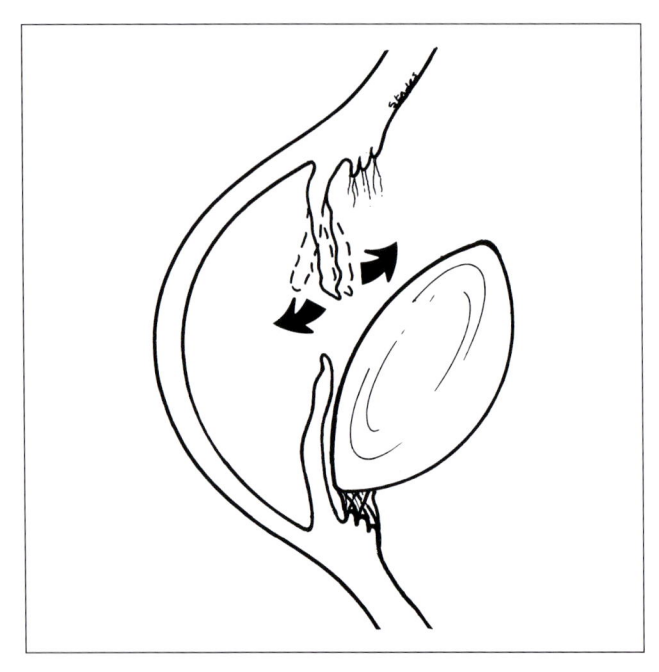

Fig. 13.10:
Lens subluxation/dislocation posterior with partly ruptured zonula resulting in loss of support of the iris (iridodonesis).

If multiple fibers are ruptured, vitreous can leak via the posterior chamber over the edge of the pupil into the anterior chamber (Fig. 13.11). If the fibers are ruptured over a greater area, subluxation will occur. If the lens becomes completely loose, it can remain more or less in its normal position or it can be displaced anteriorly or posteriorly. The lens and/or the vitreous can thus block the drainage of the aqueous in the pupil or at the level of the drainage angle, resulting in secondary glaucoma. Secondary glaucoma occurs usually less acutely and less rapidly in cats than in dogs. Cats can have a lens luxation for a longer time without developing glaucoma.

Symptoms: The earliest recognizable sign of lens subluxation is leakage of vitreous, which hangs over the edge of the pupil and into the anterior chamber like very thin white clouds (Fig. 13.11; Plate 13.11). If the lens is displaced, an aphakic crescent (Plate 13.12) will develop between the edge of the pupil and the lens equator, and light penetrating this opening can reflect the color of the tapetum lucidum. If the lens is displaced anteriorly (Plates 13.12–13.15), the iris is pressed anteriorly, the anterior chamber becomes shallow, and the angle of the chamber becomes narrower. If the lens is displaced posteriorly, the anterior chamber is deeper and the

Lens luxation or ectopic lens **203**

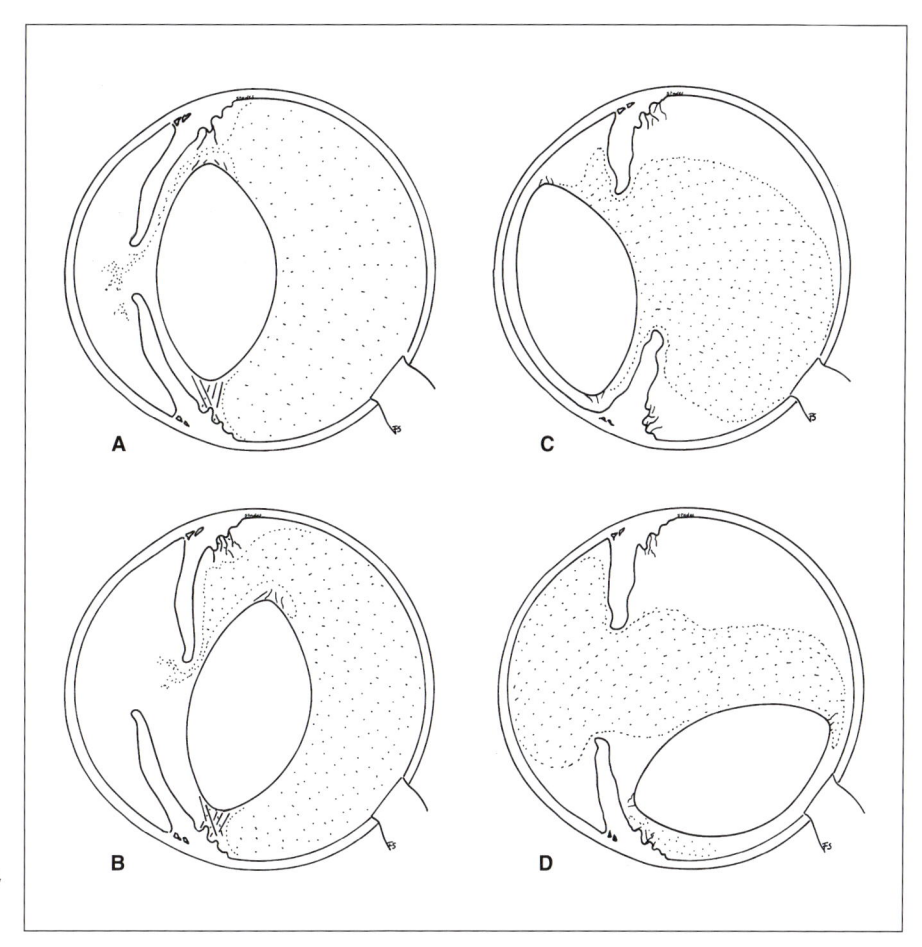

Fig. 13.11:
Lens luxation. (A) Rupture of a number of zonular fibers, allowing leakage of vitreous into the anterior chamber. (B) Rupture of the upper part of the zonules and subsequent posterior displacement of the upper part of the lens. (C) Dislocation of the lens into the anterior chamber, pulling vitreous into the anterior chamber also. (D) Luxation of the lens posteriorly, allowing leakage of vitreous into the anterior chamber.

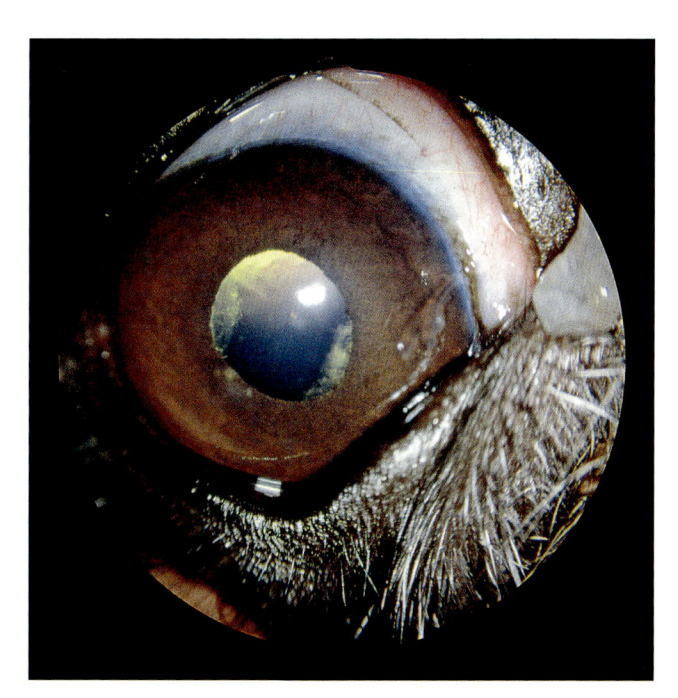

Plate 13.11:
Beginning lens luxation in a Tibetan Terrier (OD). Thin white clouds of vitreous can be seen at the edge of the pupil.

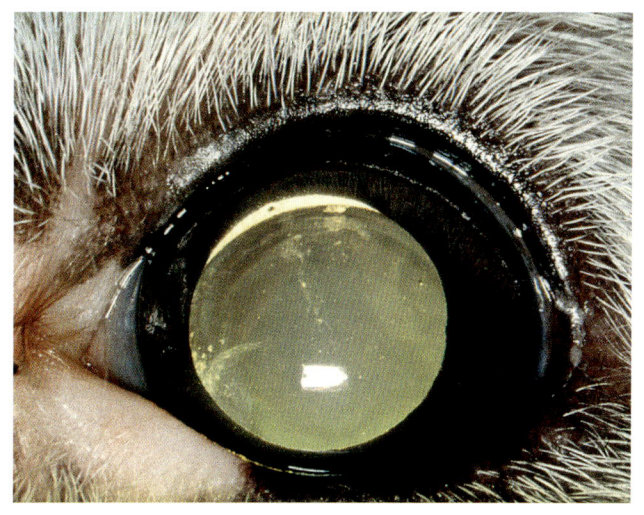

Plate 13.12:
Developing lens luxation in a Wire-haired Fox Terrier (OS). The lens has become displaced some millimeters ventrolaterally. This causes a crescent bordered by the lental equator and the pupillary margin, recognizable from the 10- to 1-o'clock positions, through which the fundus reflection has become visible.

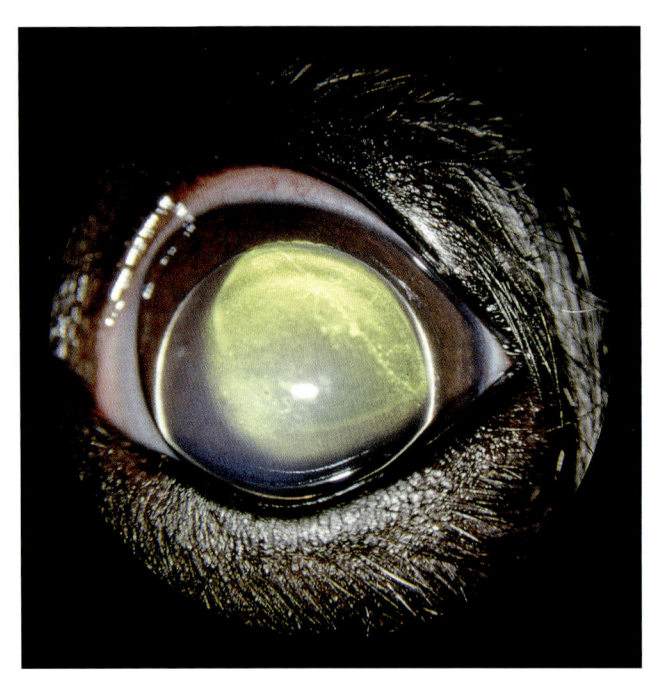

Plate 13.13:
Anterior lens luxation in a German Hunting Terrier. The lens is in the anterior chamber (OS).

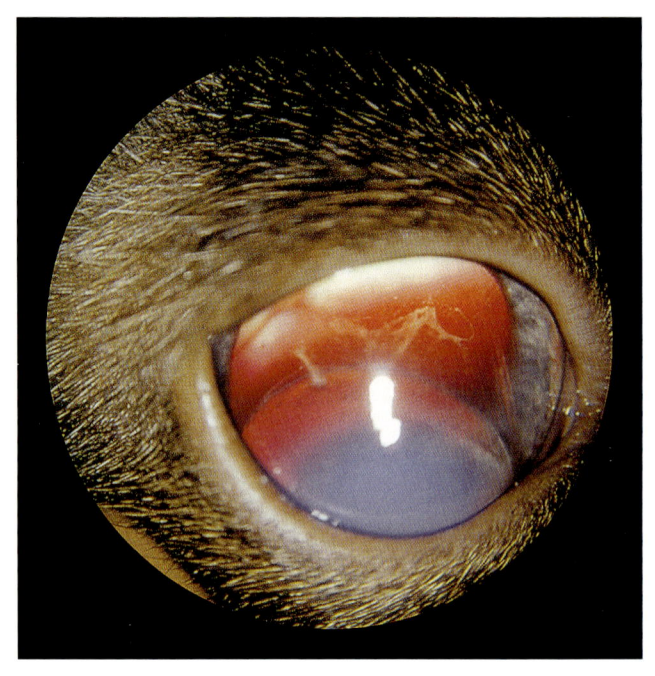

Plate 13.14:
Lens luxation in a 10-year-old Siamese cat (OD). The dislocated lens hovers on the pupillary margin. Dorsal to the lens, vitreous strands that have been pulled into the anterior chamber, are discernable. In the depths, the fundus and even the optic disc are visible to the naked eye.

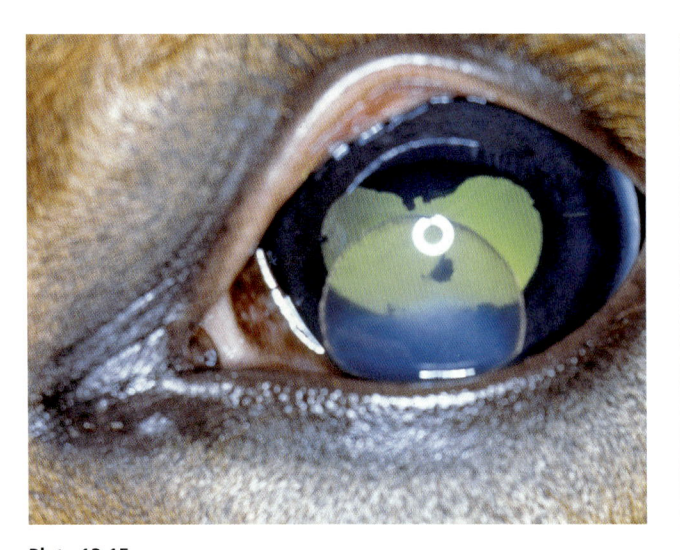

Plate 13.15:
Lens luxation as a complication of an equine (chronic) recurrent uveitis (OS). The lens is luxated totally to the anterior chamber. There are remainders of iris to lens synechia posterior, hanging from the edge of the iris.

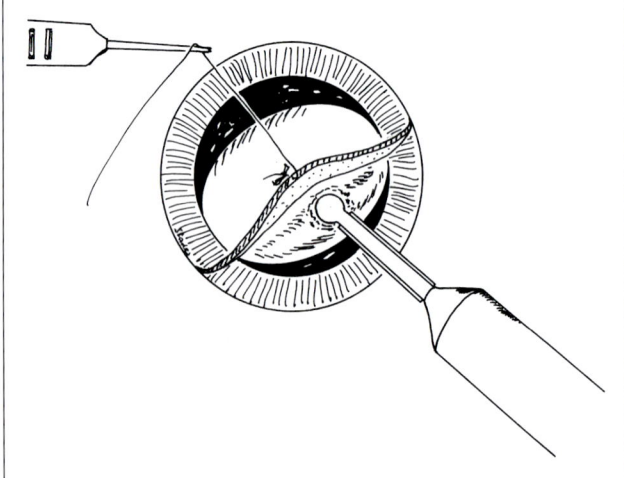

Fig. 13.12:
Intracapsular extraction of a luxated lens with cryoextractor. The extractor is frozen to the capsule and the cortex of the lens.

angle of the chamber is noticeably wider. Because the iris loses its support, it forms a flat disc instead of curving with the rounded form of the lens. The slit-lamp light line of the iris is then straight or even bent posteriorly. The loss of support for the iris can also result in an iridodonesis. This phenomenon is usually visible on the edge of the pupil at the end of or following a movement of the eye. Because the lens is lying loose, it can also lag behind in the movement of the eye and waggle (lentodonesis; Fig. 13.10). If the lens is completely displaced ventroposteriorly, the fundus can be seen with the naked eye (Plate 13.14). If the lens is completely in the anterior chamber, it is recognizable as a glassy disc lying directly behind the cornea (Plates 13.13–13.15); the iris and pupil are then more difficult recognizable. Contact with the lens can damage the corneal endothelium, via which central corneal edema can develop, eventually with growth of deep vessels. If secondary glaucoma has already developed, a diffuse and dense corneal edema will occur. The luxated lens is then often hardly recognizable; ultrasonography will then be very useful.

Primary glaucoma must be considered in the differential diagnosis, with or without the complication of secondary luxation of the lens. If there is already a definite buphthalmos, it will be no longer possible to determine what the primary cause was. Gonioscopy of the normal eye (if available) can be conclusive if it is a primary (i.e. occlusion of the pectinate ligament) or secondary (normal drainage angle) glaucoma.

Therapy: Therapy consists of complete removal of the lens (intracapsular). In dogs and horses, this should be performed within a week, and if there is glaucoma, within 1–3 days. Because secondary glaucoma occurs less rapidly in cats, removal of the lens is less urgent. In the intervening period, the patient should be treated medically. If the lens is behind the iris, the pupil is held closed with the help of 1–4% pilocarpine 4 times daily, or the more powerful latanoprost (1 drop once daily). If the lens is in the anterior chamber, the use of such a powerful miotic should be avoided and dichlorphenamide should be used instead (1–2.5 mg/kg, 4 times daily orally) or brinzolamide drops (3–4 times daily; see 11.3.3). The patient with a lens luxated into the anterior chamber should be referred immediately; otherwise damage to the corneal endothelium by the lens or adhesion of the lens to the endothelium is unavoidable. More seriously, it is also impossible to predict when secondary glaucoma will develop. Only if the condition of the patient does not permit immediate referral for lens extraction should lens luxation continue to be treated medically.

Intracapsular lens extraction

The intracapsular lens extraction for lens luxation is in general similar to extracapsular extraction for cataract (see 13.3.3). The most important differences are as follows:
1. Pre-operative administration of atropine is always contraindicated. Topical 1% dexamethasone 4 times daily should be given for only 1–4 days in advance.
2. During the operation, the anterior chamber should be perforated with great care so that aqueous, which is usually under increased pressure, has time to flow out gently. If the escape is too rapid, there is a greatly increased risk of prolapse of the vitreous and, more seriously, of retinal detachment. There also may be a miosis, which is not wanted in posterior lens luxation.

The lens should be removed from the eye in the intact capsule. Therefore, the capsule should not be grasped with forceps. The lens should also not be pressed out of the eye because of the risk of retinal detachment. A reliable method is to freeze the capsule, together with the underlying lens fibers, to a cryoprobe so that the lens can be completely lifted out (intracapsular cryoextraction; Fig. 13.12). The phaecoemulsification of the luxated lens is an alternative. In cases of emergency, a suction cup (erisiphake) can be used, but the likelihood of tearing the capsule just behind the equator is greater. During cryoextraction, the iris or corneal endothelium must not be touched. The lens is lifted slightly and rotated. Then the vitreous is loosened from the posterior capsule. Vitreous that has prolapsed into the anterior chamber is lifted up and cut off or is removed using a vitrectome. After the first sutures have been placed, an air bubble is introduced into the anterior chamber as quickly as possible in order to blow the vitreous behind the pupil and thus place pressure against the retina again. The pupil should be in miosis or forced to míosis, using 1% acetylcholine intraoculary.

As part of the postoperative treatment, pilocarpine 1–2% (4 times daily) is used in order to prevent as far as is possible a rise in IOP and vitreous prolapse.

Prevention: Affected animals should be excluded from breeding. If the number of animals available for breeding allows it, parents and siblings of affected animals should also be excluded from breeding, because they have a significantly higher chance of being a carrier of this disease.

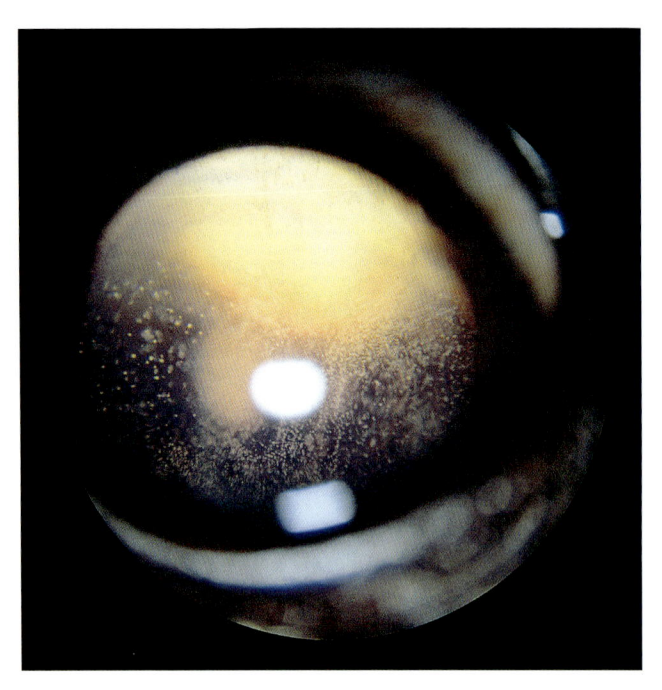

Plate 13.16:
Asteroid hyalosis (OS, dog). The dorsally recognizable orange-yellow hyperreflection is caused by the associated retinal atrophy.

13.5 Vitreous floaters, asteroid hyalosis, and synchysis scintillans

Small or large densities can develop in the vitreous (Plate 13.16) from conglomerates of calcium-lipid complexes, condensations of vitreous fibrils, groups of erythrocytes or pigment cells (including remnants of the hyaloid system). These move with the movements of the eye. In older animals, degeneration of the vitreous can lead to liquefaction (syneresis), in which case the densities lag behind eye movements or whirl up. These changes are rare in the dog and cat and generally do not need any treatment.

In horses, such physiological densities and membrane-like structures (due to remnants of Cloquet's canal and post-natal condensation of vitreous fibrils) may give the impression of vitreous liquefaction, floaters and membranes. They have to be differentiated from the rare, pathological synchysis and densities of the vitreous.

13.5.1 Vitreous floaters

Vitreous floaters, mouche volantes, muscae volitantes, or flitting flies are larger flakes or streaks in the vitreous that may or may not move. If they are very moveable, and especially if viewed against bright light, they can give the impression that something resembling a fly is passing by. In humans, they can be a sign of tear-induced retinal detachment or chorioretinitis. These abnormalities rarely occur in animals, and seldomly require treatment, though they may induce misbehavior (jittery horses).

13.5.2 Asteroid hyalosis

In this condition (Plate 13.16), there are many small (<1 mm), possibly slightly pigmented, particles in the vitreous of one or both eyes. These move during and after movement of the eye, but return to their original place. They seldom influence vision.

13.5.3 Synchysis scintillans

In this condition, there are many (cholesterol) particles floating in a more or less liquefied vitreous. Especially after movement of an eye, they can resemble a snow flurry behind the lens. They can sometimes cause dazzling when viewed against bright light. The abnormality is rare and also seldom causes problems. It may be associated with retinal atrophy.

13.6 Hemorrhages and/or exudates in the vitreous

13.6.1 Blood

Blood rarely occurs in the vitreous. Spontaneous bleeding can be the result of congenital anomalies, such as in Collie eye anomaly (see 14.7), as well as being due to intoxication, trauma, or neoplasia (malignant lymphoma). Penetrating trauma such as caused by airgun or shotgun pellets can easily cause floaters of blood in the vitreous. The penetration tunnel is often marked by prolapsed lens material, blood residue, traction threads, and other scars. Blunt trauma seldom causes blood in the vitreous. Cats and dogs that have been away from home for a few days and/or in the area of hunters, and which have signs of trauma including blood in the vitreous, should be examined by radiography or ultrasonography for the presence of metal particles.

Therapy: Therapy consists of atropine drops 4 times daily, dexamethasone and "initial choice" or, when indicated, "specific choice" antibiotics (see 4). If there are indications of glaucoma, the pressure should be lowered with dichlorphenamide (see 11.3.3). The surgery on the vitreous that is carried out in such cases in humans has still found little place in veterinary medicine.

13.6.2 Hemorrhagic or other exudate in the vitreous

Floaters of hemorrhagic or other exudates in the vitreous, especially if diffuse and certainly if bilateral, are usually produced by exudative uveitis. Inflammation of the vitreous (hyalitis) is also almost always a secondary process (the vitreous has no intrinsic vascular system or nerve supply). In principle, this type of abnormality can be caused by severe trauma (bullet, shot, intraocular surgery), chorioretinitis, retinal detachment, and intraocular neoplasia. In cats such abnormalities are usually caused by systemic diseases (for example, FIP, FIV, and FeLV). They can also be caused by lymphoma in dogs. The history and further examination in such cases should thus be directed towards these disorders. If FIP, FeLV, or lymphoma cannot be demonstrated, it is worth referring such patients immediately. Treatment and prognosis depend on the cause (see also 12.10).

These abnormalities are most frequently due to recurrent uveitis in the horse (see 12.10.7). Because of the different anatomy of the horse vitreous, secondary peripheral fibrosis and retinal detachment are more frequent.

13.7 Retinal detachment and intraocular neoplasms

Retinal detachment and intraocular neoplasms can occupy part or almost all of the vitreous space. In retinal detachment (for example, due to traction bands, exudative chorioretinitis, or an elevated blood pressure), the retina can come to lie against the lens. Grayish, ballooning membranes containing thin vessels are recognizable directly behind the posterior capsule of the lens (slit lamp). Retrolental space-occupying processes which do not fit this picture are strongly suspicious of intraocular neoplasia. Such patients should be referred immediately for slit-lamp examination, ultrasonography, arterial blood pressure measurement, etc. Treatment and prognosis are dependent upon the initial cause of the disease (see also 12 and 14).

Literature

1. BOEVÉ, M.H., LINDE-SIPMAN, J.S. VAN DER & STADES, F.C.: Early morphogenesis of the canine lens, hyaloid system and vitreous body. Anatom. Rec. **220**: 435, 1988.

2. GLOOR, B.: The vitreous. In: Adler's Physiology of the Eye. Eds.: R.A. Moses and W.M. Hart. St. Louis, C.V. Mosby, 1987.

3. EISNER, G. & BACHMANN, E.: Vergleichend morphologische Spaltlampenuntersuchung des Glaskörpers von Schaf, Schwein, Hund, Affen und Kaninchen. Graefe's Arch. Klin. Ophthalmol. **192**: 9, 1974.

4. AGUIRRE, G. & BISTNER, S. I.: Posterior lenticonus in the dog. Cornell. Vet. **63**: 455, 1973.

5. GRIMES, T.D. & MULLANEY, J.: Persistent hyperplastic primary vitreous in a Greyhound. Vet. Rec. **85**: 607, 1969.

6. BOEVÉ M.H., LINDE-SIPMAN, J.S.VAN DER & STADES, F.C.: Early morphogenesis of persistent hyperplastic tunica vasculosa lentis and primary vitreous. The dog as an ontogenetic model. Invest. Ophthalmol.Vis. Sci. **29**: 1076, 1988.

7. STADES, F.C.: Persistent hyperplastic trunica vasculosa lentis and persistent hyperplastic primary vitreous (PHTVL / PHPV) in 90 closely related Doberman Pinchers: Clinical aspects. JAAHA **16**: 739, 1980.

8. STADES, F.C.: Persistent hyperplastic tunica vasculosa lentis and persistent hyperplatic primary vitreous in Doberman Pinchers: Genetic aspects. JAAHA **19**: 957, 1983.

9. CURTIS, R., BARNETT, K.C. & LEON, A.: Persistent hyperplastic primary vitreous in the Staffordshire Bull Terrier. Vet. Rec. **115**: 385, 1984.

10. STADES, F.C., BOEVÉ M.H., BROM, W.E.VAN DEN & LINDE-SIPMAN, J.S.VAN DER: The incidence of PHTVL / PHPV in Doberman and the results of breeding rules. Vet. Quart. **13**: 24, 1994.

11. MICHAELSON, S.M., HOWARD, J.W. & DEICHMANN, W.B.: Response of the dog to 24,000 and 1285 MHZ, microwave exposure. Indust. Med. **40**: 18, 1971.

12. ROBERTS, S.M. et al.: Ophthalmic complications following megavoltage irradiation of the nasal and paranasal cavities in dogs. JAAHA **190**: 43, 1987.

13. MARTIN, C.L.: The formation of cataracts in dogs with disophenol: Age susceptibility and production with chemical grade 2, 6-diiodo-4-nitrophenol. Can. Vet. J. **16**: 228, 1975.

14. GUO-TONG WU, ZIGLER, J. & LOU, M. F.: Establishment of a naphthalene cataract model in vitro. Exp. Eye Res. **54**: 73, 1992.

15. MARTIN, C.L. & CHAMBREAU, T.: Cataract production in experimentally orphaned puppies fed a commercial replacement for bitch's milk. JAAHA **18**: 115, 1982.

16. GLAZE, B. & BLANCHARD, G.L.: Nutritional cataracts in a Samoyed litter. JAAHA **19**: 951, 1983.

17. NARFSTRÖM, K. & DUBIELZIG, R.: Posterior lenticonus, cataracts and microphthalmia; congenital ocular defects in the Cavalier King Charles Spaniel. J. Small Anim. Pract. **25:** 669, 1984.

18. OLESEN, H.P., JENSEN, O.A. & NORN, M.S.: Congenital hereditary cataract in Cocker Spaniel. J. Small Anim. Pract. **15:** 741, 1974.

19. KOCH, S.A.: Cataracts in inter-related Old English Sheepdogs. JAVMA **160:** 299, 1972.

20. GELATT, K.N.: Cataracts in the Golden Retriever dog. Vet. Med. Small Anim. Clin. **67:** 1113, 1972.

21. GELATT, K.N., SAMUELSEN, D.A., BARRIE, K.P. et al.: Biometry and clinical characteristics of congenital cataracts and microphthalmia in the Miniature Schnauzer. JAVMA **183:** 99, 1983.

22. NARFSTRÖM, K.: Cataract in the West Hightland White Terrier. J. Small Anim. Pract. **22:** 476, 1981.

23. YAKELY, W.L.: A study of hereditary cataracts in the American Cocker Spaniel. JAVMA **172:** 814, 1978.

24. CURTIS, R.: Late-onset cataract in the Boston Terrier. Vet. Rec. **115:** 577, 1984.

25. BARNETT, K.C.: Hereditary cataract in the German Shepherd dog. J. Small Anim. Pract. **27:** 387, 1968.

26. CURTIS, R.: Late-onset cataract in the Boston Terrier. Vet. Rec. **115:** 577, 1984.

27. RUBIN, L.F. & FLOWERS, R.D.: Inherited cataract in a family of Standard poodles. JAVMA **161:** 207, 1972.

28. BARNETT, K.C.: Hereditary cataract in the Welsh Springer Spaniel. J. Small Anim. Pract. **21:** 621, 1980.

29. SATO, S., TAKAHASHI, Y; WYMAN, M. & KADOR, P.: Progression of sugar cataract in the dog. Invest. Opthalmol. Vis. Sci. **32:** 1925, 1991.

30. POLLET, L.: Refraction of normal and aphakic canine eyes. JAAHA **18:** 323, 1982.

31. NEUMANN, W.: Chirurgische Behandlung der Katarakt beim Kleintier. Kleintierpraxis **36:** 17, 1991.

32. GILGER, B.C., WHITLEY, D., MCLAUGHLIN, S.A. et al.: Scanning electron microscopy of intraocular lenses that had been implanted in dogs. Am. J. Vet. Res. **54:** 1183, 1993.

33. NASISSE, M.P. et al.: Neodymium:YAG laser treatment of lens extraction-induced pupillary opacification in dogs. JAAHA **26:** 275, 1990.

34. KROHNE, S.D. & VESTRE, W.A.: Effects of flunixin meglumine and dexamethasone on aqueous protein values after intraocular surgery in the dog. J. Am. Vet. Res. **48:** 420, 1987.

35. GELATT, K.N., MYERS, V.S. & MCCLURE, J.R.: Aspiration of congenital and soft cataracts on foals and young horses. JAVMA **165:** 611, 1974.

36. GWIN, R.M., WARREN, J.K. & SAMUELSON, D.A.: Effects of phacoemulsification and extracapsular lens removal on corneal thickness and endothelial cell density in the dog. Invest. Opthalmol. Vis. Sci. **24:** 227, 1983.

37. MARTIN, C.I.: Zonular defects in the dog: A clinical and scanning electron microscopic study. JAAHA **14:** 571, 1978.

38. CURTIS, R.: Lens luxation in the dog and cat. Vet. Clin. North Am. (Small Anim. Pract.) **20:** 755, 1990.

39. GELATT, K.N.: Glaucoma and lens luxation in a foal. Vet. Med. **68:** 261, 1973.

40. WILLIS, M.B., CURTIS, R. & BARNETT, K.C.: Genetic aspects of lens luxation in the Tibetan Terrier. Vet. Rec. **104:** 409, 1979.

14 Fundus and Optic nerve

14.1 Introduction

The fundus of the eye is considered to be the posterior aspect of the inner eye as seen ophthalmoscopically (Fig. 14.1; Plates 14.1, 14.3–14.9). Many abnormalities in this area reside in the tunica nervosa (interna or retina) and the tunica vasculosa (choroid) or the optic nerve, but seldom in the tunica fibrosa (sclera).

14.1.1 Ontogenesis

The development of the eye begins with an outgrowth of the neuroectodermal tissue of the neural tube and the surrounding mesoderm to just beneath the surface ectoderm. The retina and optic nerve develop from this neuroectoderm. Infolding of the optic vesicle results in a double-walled ocular cup. This invagination in the start is incomplete ventrally and hence closure defects (colobomas) are usually in the 6-o'clock-position. The inner wall of the ocular cup increases in thickness in the fundus region and from this develops the sensory retina. The pigment epithelium arises from the outer wall. Anteriorly, the retina (pigment epithelium) continues as the epithelium of the ciliary body and posterior epithelium of the iris. The space between the sensory retina and the pigment epithelium disappears, but the layers do not become fused. Extensions (axons) of the ganglion cells converge as they grow out to the inner covering of the closing central eye stalk and make contact with the brain as the optic nerves. The mesenchymal tissue around the ocular cup fuses with the uvea and the surrounding sclera. The tapetum lucidum (or non-tapetal area) is formed in the choroid between the 5th and 8th week after birth (dog and cat) (Plates 14.3, 14.4).

14.1.2 Retina

The retina consists of an inner and an outer layer (Fig. 14.2).
The inner or neuroretina can be subdivided into three major and nine sublayers. The three major layers are: ganglion cell layer, second order neurons or transmitter cells, and the photoreceptors.
More precisely, the neuroretina consists from vitreous to choroid of the following layers:
1. Inner limiting membrane
2. Nerve fiber layer (ganglion cell axons)
3. Ganglion cell layer
4. Inner plexiform layer (synapses between cells of the inner nuclear layer and the ganglion cell layer)

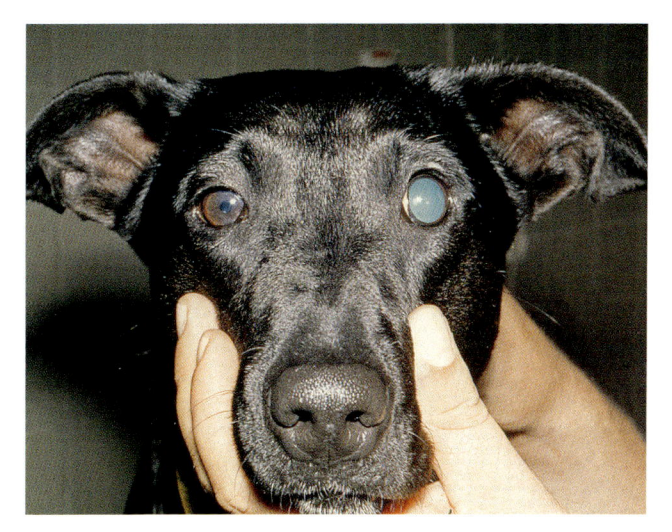

Plate 14.1:
Differences in fundus reflection caused by a light bundle directed dorsoposteriorly in a dog in which one pupil (OD) is miotic and the other pupil (OS) is mydriatic. In the left eye, the light bundle can pass the wide-open pupil undisturbed. Subsequently, the light rays are reflected from the tapetum lucidum. This phenomenon may disturb the owner after the administration of a mydriatic to the animal or in the dark.

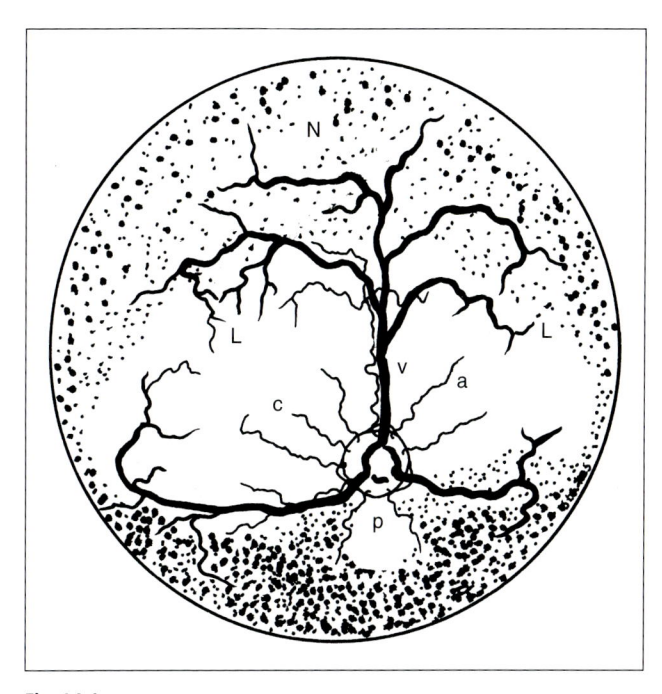

Fig. 14.1:
Fundus picture of the canine right eye. Tapetum nigrum (N); tapetum lucidum (L); papilla (p); retinal a./v. (a, v); area centralis (c).

5. Inner nuclear layer (bipolar cells, horizontal cells, amacrine cells)
6. Outer plexiform layer (synapses between photoreceptors and second order neurons)
7. Outer nuclear layer (cell nuclei of the photoreceptors)
8. Outer limiting membrane
9. Photoreceptor outer segments (rods and cones)

The inner layer of the retina is the neural or sensory part (pars optica) of the retina. This extends out from the junction of the ciliary body (ora ciliaris retinae) to the optic papilla (or optic disc, although papilla is more accurate because it is not flat) and continues as the optic nerve. The outer segments of the photoreceptors lie embedded in the pigment epithelium but are not attached to it. The retina is held in place by the pressure of the vitreous and the aqueous fluid. Retinal detachment (ablatio retinae) may occur when the counterpressure becomes inadequate. Examples of diseases that can predispose to detachment include: high blood pressure, when the counter pressure decreases; as a result of vitreal traction bands on the retina; holes in the retina; or as a result of exudation or transudation in the space between the photoreceptors and the pigment epithelium, due to high blood pressure or inflammation.

The outer layer (pars ceca) is formed by the retinal pigment epithelium (RPE). This extends out from the papilla, over the ciliary body and the posterior surface of the iris to the edge of the pupil and sometimes even over the pupil margin onto the anterior face of the iris. The RPE is bound to the choroid by means of the membrane of Bruch.

Because of the inverse structure of the retina, incoming light has to pass through all the retinal layers to finally stimulate the photoreceptors. The retinal thickness is approximately 225 μm in the central retina and is reduced to 100 μm in the far periphery.

The number of ganglion cells is low compared to the number of the photoreceptors. In the cat, for example, 130 photoreceptors project to one single ganglion cell. The resulting large receptive fields account for the cat's high light sensitivity, but low resolution. The photoreceptors can be divided into rods (thin) and cones (plump). The rods are more sensitive to light and movement. They are mainly of importance for seeing in dim light (scotopic vision; the maximal vision is only reached after 30–40 minutes in dim light). The cones are less sensitive to light and are responsible for the differentiation of details and colors (photopic vision). The highest concentration of cones is in the area centralis, just temporal to the optic disc.[1,2] The ability to see colors has been confirmed in dogs (Toy Poodle, Italian Greyhound), horse and pigs; and it has been shown to be highly probable in cats and birds. Dogs appear to have dichromatic color vision with two photopigments (spectral peaks of 429 nm [violet] and 555 nm [green]).[3,4,5] Three pigments (blue, green, and red) have only been shown in primates.

Dogs and cats possess a much higher density of rods than primates (approximately x2.5 more), and therefore they see very well in dim light. The distribution of rods and cones over the retina is not uniform. The greatest concentration of rods is just outside the area centralis (macula or yellow patch in primates), where they can be reached by light when the pupil is wide open in dim light.

The rods and cones are composed of outer segments, inner segments, the nucleus, and the synaptic terminals. The inner segments are considered to be the source of energy. They pro-

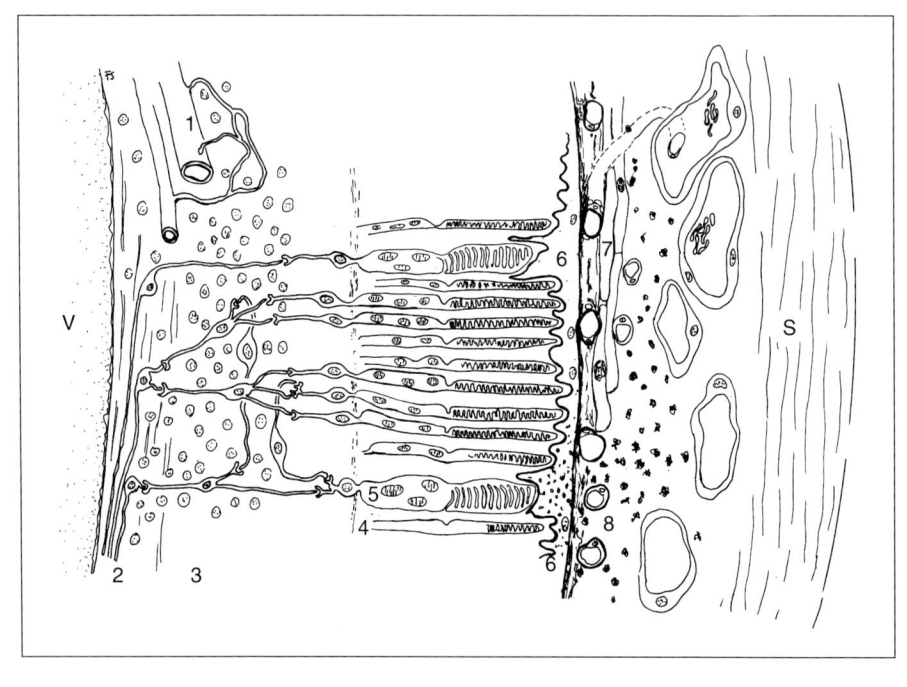

Fig. 14.2:
Section of the fundus:
(1) retinal a./v.,
(2) ganglion and nerve fiber layers,
(3) transmitter cell layer (photoreceptors),
(4) rod,
(5) cone,
(6) pigment epithelium,
(7) tapetum lucidum,
(8) choriocapillaris. S: sclera; V: vitreous.

vide rhodopsin and other visual pigments, via the rhodopsin-retinine-vitamin-A cycle, to the discs in the outer segments.[6] These discs, located with the light pigments, grow out in the direction of the pigment epithelium. The outer segments, especially of the rods, lie embedded in the RPE, from and via which the expended plates are dissolved and resorbed.[7] Energy is provided from the choriocapillaris of the choroid. In retinal detachment, the photoreceptors can initially still be reasonably functional and hence the pupillary reflexes may also be present, but in time they degenerate because of the lack of metabolites and oxygen.

Light stimulation of the retina results in a series of photochemical reactions accompanied by changes in potentials. In light-stimulated photoreceptors, the photopigment of the lipid membranes of the rods and cones is activated and later regenerated. The degree of activation of the visual pigments depends on the intensity, duration and wave length of the light stimulus.

Visual pigments are substances capable of absorbing light within the visible spectrum. The rod visual pigments (e.g. rhodopsin) are composed of a carotenoid part, the 11-cis retinal, and a protein part, the opsin. Different visual pigments can be distinguished by their absorption spectrum. The best studied visual pigment is rhodopsin, the rod pigment. Light stimulation of all photoreceptors results in hyperpolarisation. This change in potential is passed on to the second-order neurons.

The changes in potential can be recorded with suitable recording equipment, such as in electroretinography.[8] The normal electroretinogram (ERG) consists of an initial negative a-wave generated by the photoreceptor outer segments. The following positive b-wave is generated by second-order neurons in the inner nuclear layer, especially by bipolar cells. With long visual stimuli, a third positive deflection – the c-wave – can be recorded, which is generated within the RPE.

Superimposed on the b-wave of dark-adapted retinas are somewhat smaller wavelets, the oscillatory potentials (Plate 14.2).[9] The ERG is the mass response of all retinal cells with the exception of the ganglion cells. Thus, it is a test for outer retinal function, not for vision. Examination of vision requires the recording of visual evoked potentials (VEP) from the occipital region.[10]

In addition to information about the function of the retina, VEPs also provide information about the optic tract and the processing of signals within the brain.

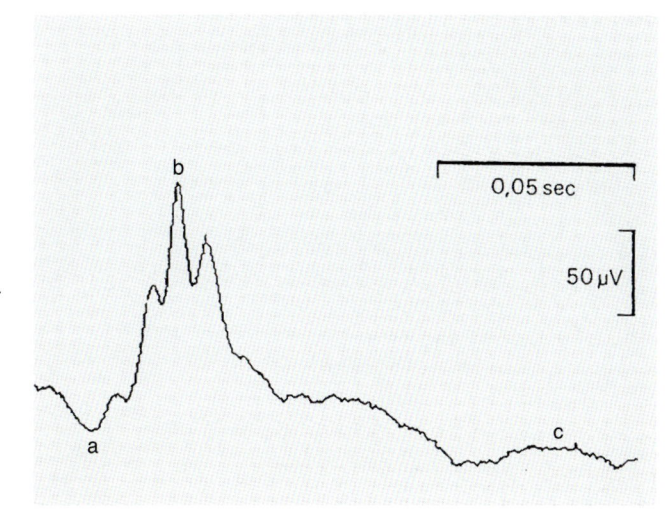

Plate 14.2:
Normal electroretinogram or ERG. There is a negative a-wave generated by the photoreceptors. The positive b-wave comes from the inner nuclear layer (bipolar cells). Prolonged light stimuli may induce a positive c-wave in the pigment epithelium.

14.1.3 Optic nerve or tract

Signals from the photoreceptors are transmitted via the transmitter cells to the ganglion cells. Their axons join together ventrolateral to the caudal pole of the globe in the papilla or optic disc (Plates 14.3–14.6, 14.8), which protrudes slightly into the vitreous and continues as the optic nerve or tract.[11] In cats, the fibers only become myelinated after passing through the scleral tissue (lamina cribrosa).[12] This means that the papilla in cats is fairly round. In contrast, in dogs, horses, and ruminants, myelinization also occurs within the globe and thus more triangular and irregular white, myelin-sheathed papilla shapes occur. Around the optic nerve is a connective tissue sheath which is an extension of the dura mater and which continues around the eye as the sclera.

The visual information is transported via both optic nerves and the optic chiasm (50 to as much as 95% crossing over) to the lateral geniculate bodies in the thalamus, and from there to the caudal cerebral cortex (area 17 or striata).[13,14]

The optic disc is overshadowed by the pecten in birds (Plate 14.9). This ventrolaterally localized, heavily pigmented choroidal structure extends into the vitreous like a rock into the sea. The function of the pecten has not been fully identified, but it is a vascular structure which has been interpreted as the nutrient source to the inner layers of the retina.[15]

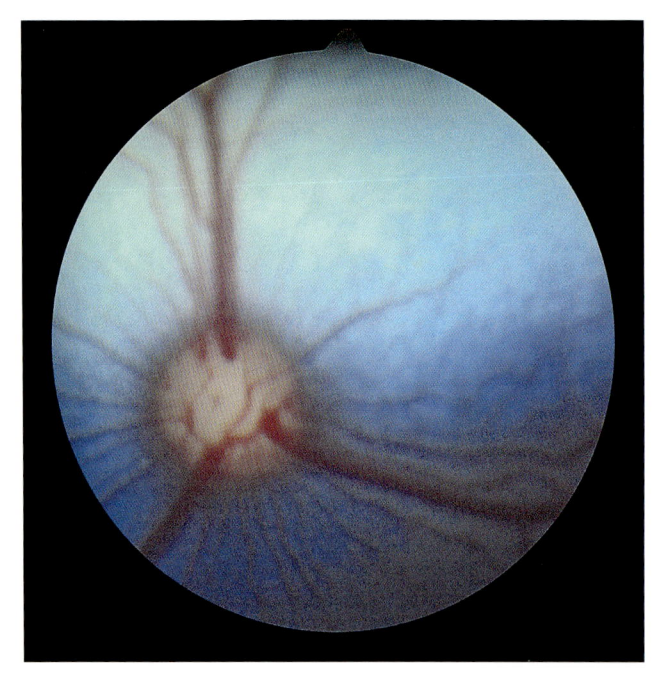

Plate 14.3:
Normal fundus of the left eye of a Doberman puppy at 6 weeks of age.

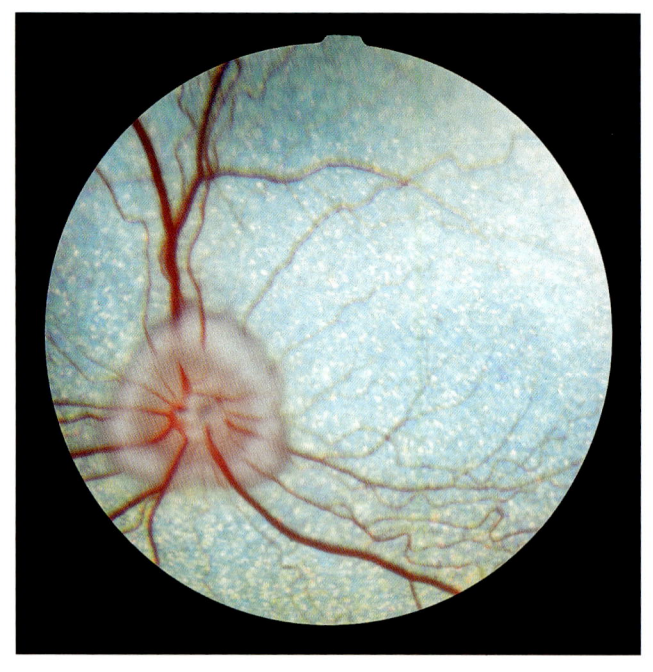

Plate 14.4:
Normal fundus of an adult Dutch Hunting Dog (OS).

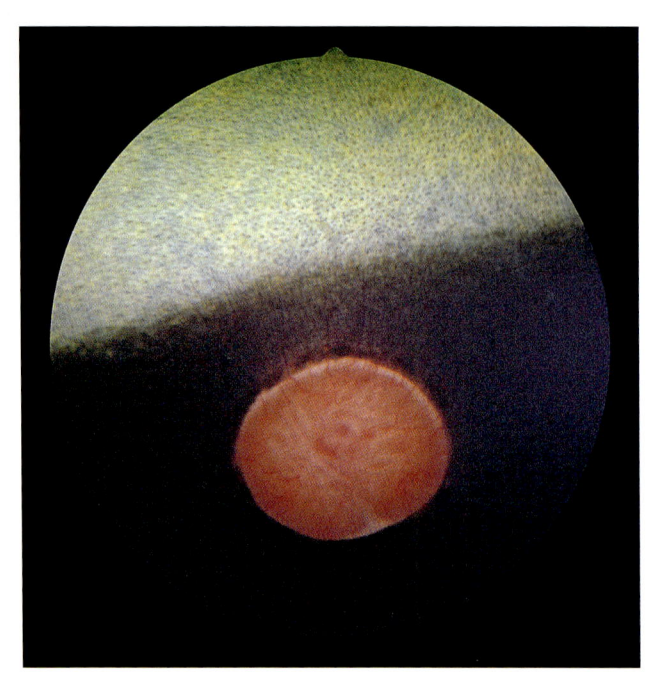

Plate 14.5:
Normal fundus of an adult horse (OD).

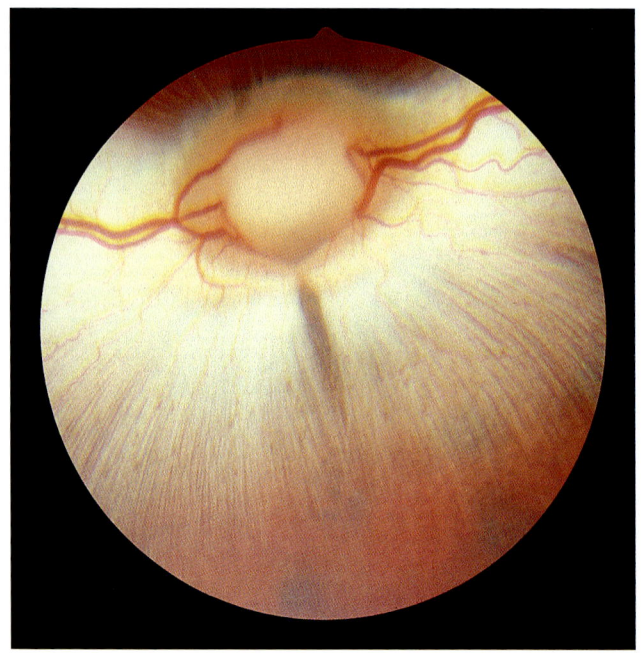

Plate 14.6:
Normal fundus of a rabbit.

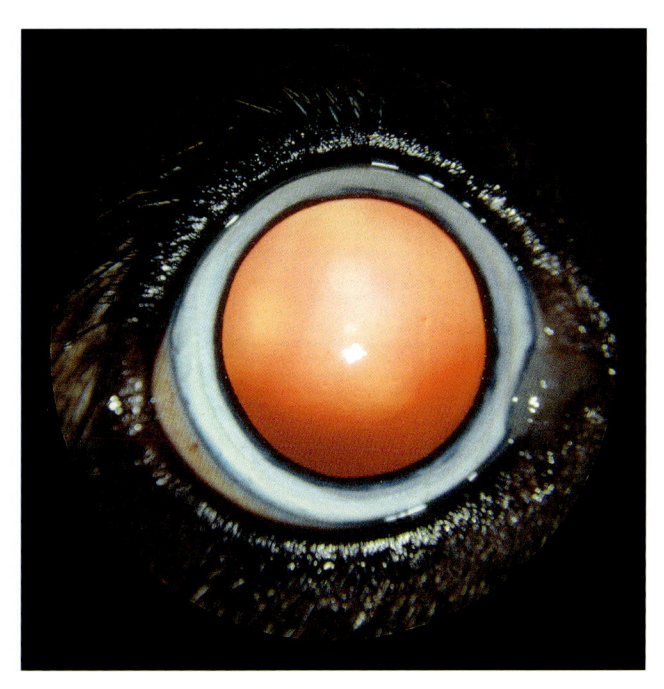

Plate 14.7:
Fundus reflection in a dog with a pale blue iris in full mydriasis (OD). This dog's unpigmented fundus provides the red reflection (see also Plate 14.8).

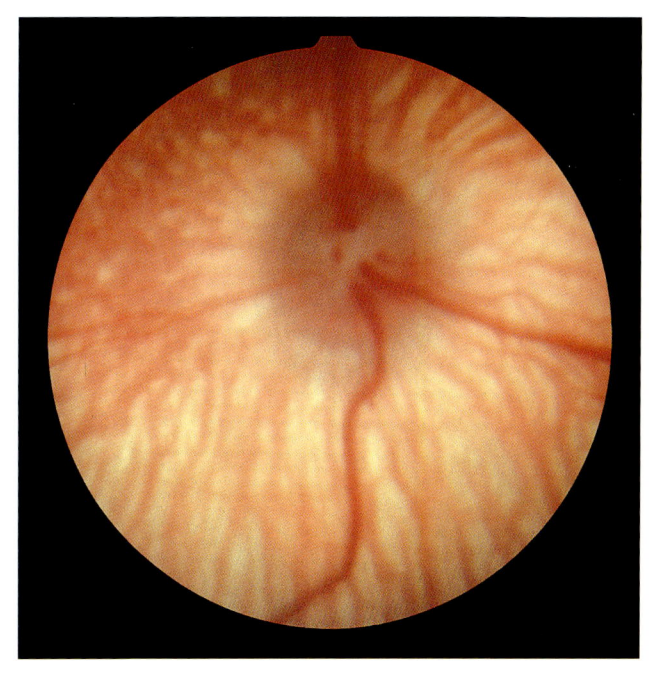

Plate 14.8:
Fundus in a dog with a pale blue iris (the same eye as in Plate 14.7). The large choroidal vessels are now also visible due to the absence of choroidal pigment and a tapetum lucidum.

14.1.4 Vascular supply

In the center of the papilla there is a small impression where the hyaloid artery was located. Dogs and cats do not have a central retinal artery but a number of cilioretinal arterioles. These are end arteries and supply the anterior layers of the retina.[16] In cats, the arteries and veins spread from the edge of the papilla. In dogs, the arteries also spread out from the edge of the papilla, while the veins pass clearly more to the center where they may partly anastomose. The main vessels of the retina in cats and dogs spread more or less to the 3-, 12- and 9-o'-clock positions in a 'T' form. In cats, the leg of the T passes medially to the papilla, approximately in the direction of the temporally located central area. In dogs, in comparison, the leg of the T points vertically upwards. The other vessels embrace the central area. In horses, the very thin retinal vessels spread roughly like the rays of the sun from the papilla. They are visible over approximately the length of one optic disc diameter.

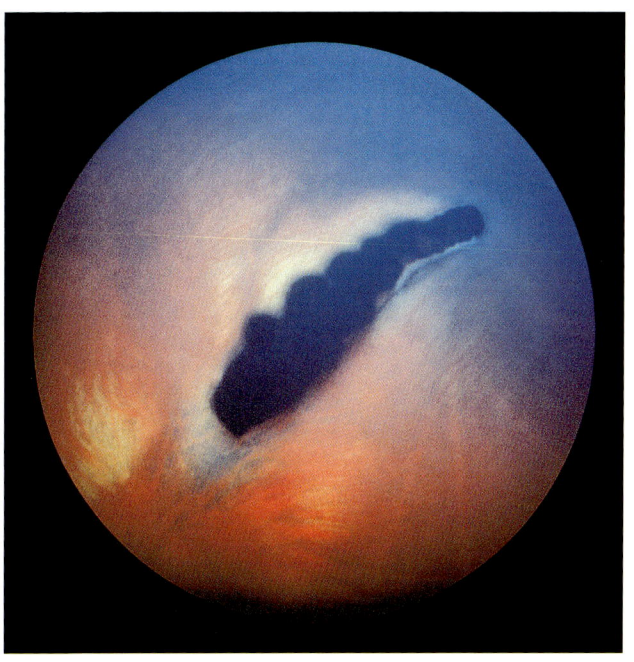

Plate 14.9:
Pecten in the fundus of a bird's eye.

14.1.5 Choroid (vascular membranes)

The choroid is the vascular layer which extends between the papilla and the ora ciliaris retinae. The outer layer is formed by the suprachoroidea, which joins the vascular tunic to the fibrous tunic (sclera). Inside this lies the vessel layer which progresses inwardly to the capillaries. This choriocapillaris provides the metabolic needs of the rods and cones through the pigment epithelium. The interstitial tissue is usually heavily pigmented and it, together with the retinal pigment epithelium, contributes to the color of the tapetum nigrum (Gr.: tapétion = covering or carpet; nigrum: L. = black).

These together provide the dark pigmentation of the inner covering of the eye, which absorbs direct and scattered light directed into the eye. In animals which are amelanotic, the fundus pigmentation is often less dense or partly or even completely absent. In the non-pigmented areas, the radially arranged large choroidal arteries and veins (vortex system) and streaks of the sclera can be observed during ophthalmoscopic examination (Plates 14.7, 14.8).

The choroidal tapetum lucidum (Lucidum: L. = clear), a more or less triangular, sometimes half circular area, is usually situated in the dorsal area of the posterior pole of the eye (Plates 14.1, 14.3–14.6). In Anglo-American literature the terms "tapetal area" for the tapetum lucidum and "non-tapetal" area or fundus for the tapetum nigrum are often used. The tapetum lucidum contains reflecting crystals (cellulosum) in carnivores and is composed of regularly arranged collagenous fibers (fibrosum) in herbivores. The tapetum lucidum (cellulosum) reportedly consists of 1–15 cell layers containing crystalline structures that act as prisms and selectively absorb, scatter, or reflect light so that colors ranging from yellow to greenish-blue are produced. In this region, the pigmented epithelium of the retina contains no melanin granules and hence is "non-pigmented", which allows the tapetal structure to be uninhibitedly reflective. The photoreceptors of the retina receive a second stimulation via the light reflected from this structure. The separation between the retina and the choroid is formed by the membrane of Bruch.

14.2 Symptoms, pathologic changes, and reaction patterns of the fundus (Plates 14.10–14.30)

Vision disorders: Pathologic changes can develop in the fundus resulting in unilateral or bilateral blindness. In order to determine the cause of the abnormalities, it is important to inquire how long the blindness has been present, whether its onset was acute or gradual, and whether the vision disorder was noticeable in dim or in bright light. One must take account of the fact that an owner may suddenly become aware of a loss of vision which has been developing gradually and thus, in good faith, interprets it as acute. This is also a consequence of the fact that abnormalities of the fundus seldom cause pain. If the anterior media of the eye are not abnormal (no corneal opacities, anterior chamber flare, cataract, glaucoma, lens luxation, etc.), consideration must be given to virtually all of the acute and chronic disorders of the retina, choroid, optic nerve, and brain which are associated with vision. These include congenital anomalies, hemorrhage, inflammation, degeneration, retinal detachment, vascular occlusions, and neoplasms.

Night blindness / day blindness: Night blindness occurs when the rods are abnormally developed (dysplastic) and/or are atrophied or degenerated. Day blindness occurs when there is primary damage to the cones. In most European literature, the term hemeralopia is used for night blindness and the term nyctalopia for day blindness (Gr: nyx, nyktos = night; hemera = day; e.g. nyktalopia was used by Hippocrates [400 BCE] as day blindness, and defined by Galenos [200 CE] as night blindness).[17] In the Anglo-American literature both terms are used but for the opposite meaning. The use of these terms should thus be avoided until international agreement on their meaning has been reached.

Pupillary reaction. Unfortunately, the pupillary reflex is not a reliable indicator of functional vision. The presence of lively pupillary reflexes decreases the probability that there is a generalized disorder of the fundus, but even in diffuse retinal degeneration in an advanced stage the pupillary reaction can remain present for a long time. A non-responsive and wide pupil is usually an indication that there is something wrong with the function of the fundus, CN II, CN III, or the brain. However, slowed pupillary reflexes can be an indication of a disorder of the fundus, but they can also be caused by the animal's anxiety or aggression via an elevated epinephrine level in the blood ("flight-fright-fight reactions").

Abnormalities such as glaucoma, lens luxation, dysautonomia (see 12), cerebral contusion, hypertension, neoplasia of the brain or pituitary must also be considered in the differential diagnosis.

Retinal vessels: The absence of retinal vessels indicates aplasia (except in anangiotic fundus animals). If the vessels are very thin or are only visible as shadowy outlines, this may be indicative of advanced retinal degeneration. If retinal vessels are not visible in the fundus but are recognizable in gray blue ballooning structures in the vitreous, retinal detachment is probable.

Dark, thin, or locally widened vessels can be an indication of ischemia or possibly embolism. Pale, grayish-white filling of the vessels can indicate hyperlipoproteinemia. Excessive twisting and turning of the vessels on an apparently sound structure usually indicates a congenital abnormality (for example, Collie eye anomaly). Very abnormal vascular structures, often associated with vague contours, are usually an indication of posterior uveitis and neoplasia (Plate 14.30).

Hemorrhages: (Plates 14.10, 14.19, 14.27, 14.30) Blood can leak from the vessels as a result of congenital abnormalities of the vessels (persistent hyaloid artery, Collie eye anomaly, etc.),

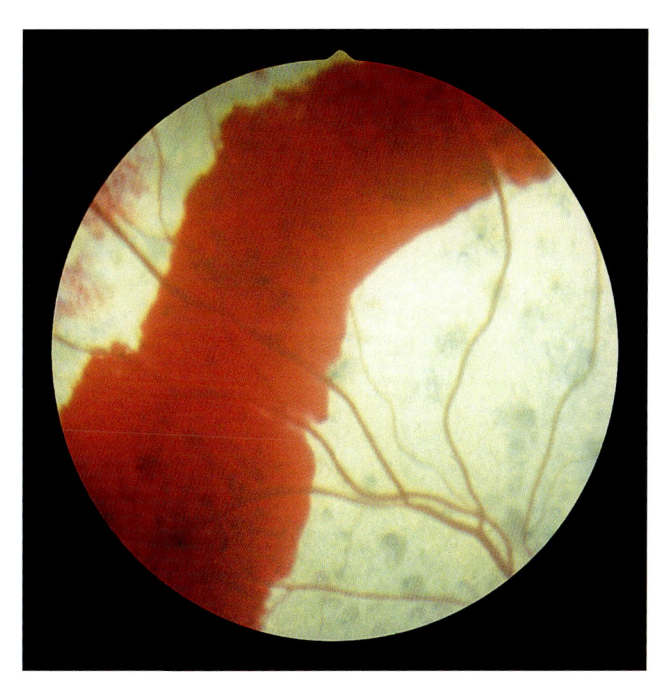

Symptoms, pathologic changes, and reaction patterns of the fundus **215**

Plate 14.10:
Band-shaped subretinal hemorrhage (OD, dog).

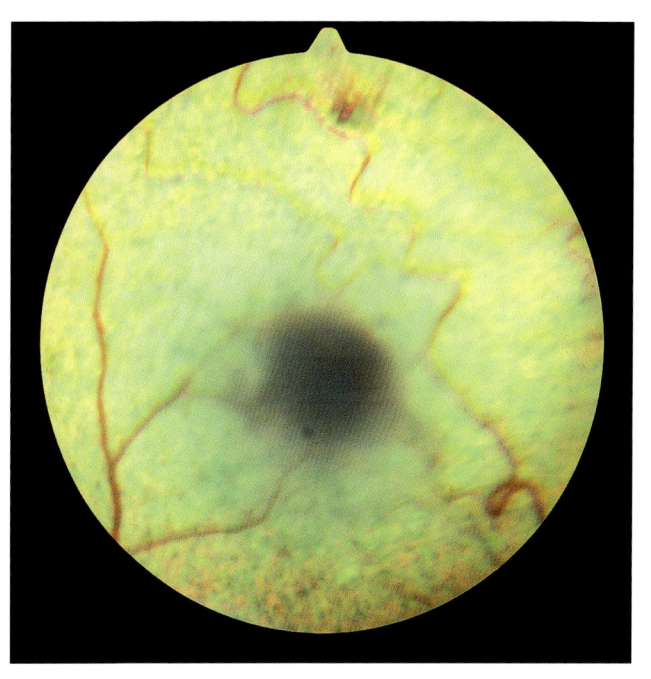

Plate 14.11:
Preretinal flake of exudate due to a local chorioretinitis in a dog (OS; see also Plate 14.12.).

trauma, or intoxication, as well as inflammation, hypertension, coagulation defects, or neoplasia. If a retinal vessel disappears behind the hemorrhage, it can be assumed that there is preretinal hemorrhage from a retinal vessel. If the hemorrhage lies behind an apparently sound retinal vessel, then it can be assumed that there has been deep retinal or subretinal hemorrhage from the choriocapillaris. The appearance of the hemorrhage is also helpful in locating the position of the hemorrhage within the retina. The nerve fiber layer of the retina has essentially parallel fibers, and blood in this layer will appear linear or "flame shaped". Hemorrhage within the deeper structures are restricted by the supporting fibers of Müller and appear as small round lesions, which then places these hemorrhages within the deeper layers of the retina but above the external limiting membrane. For a more exact diagnosis of the localization of the vascular leakage, the patient can be referred for fluorescent angiography.

Pigmented spots: Spots occurring in the tapetum lucidum (tapetal area) with the same color as the surrounding tapetum nigrum (non-tapetal area) are usually not abnormal, especially if they are located near the transition between the two zones (Plate 14.21). If the pigment spot has a hyperreflecting area, usually with a very thin vessel to the pigmented spot, it is most probably a scar of a previous focal chorioretinitis (Plates 14.12, 14.13).

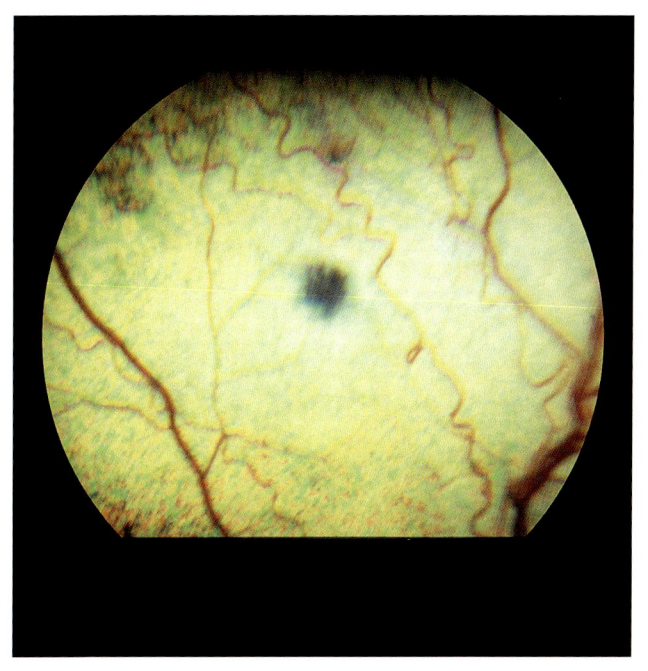

Plate 14.12:
Scar of a previous chorioretinitis (OS, dog; same eye as shown in Plate 14.11; half of the magnification; 3 months later).

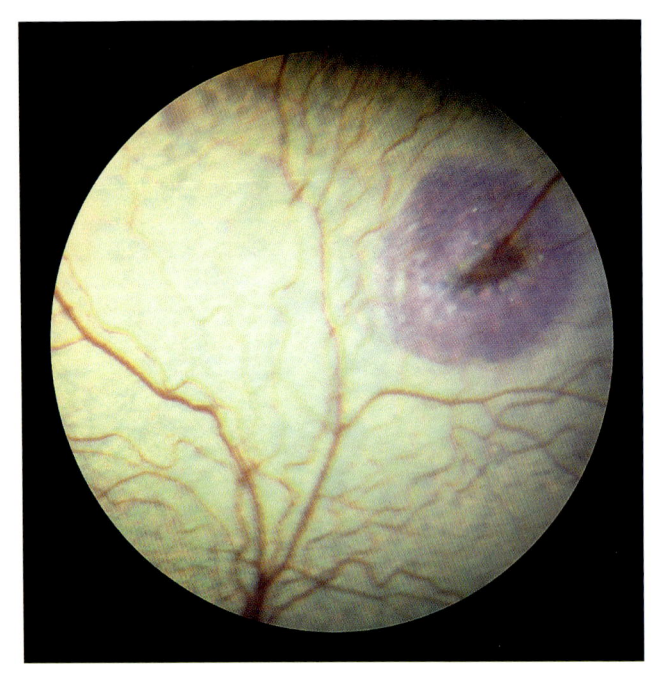

Plate 14.13:
Chorioretinitis scar with central pigmentation, surrounded by the typical purple hyperreflective area of retinal atrophy (OD, dog).

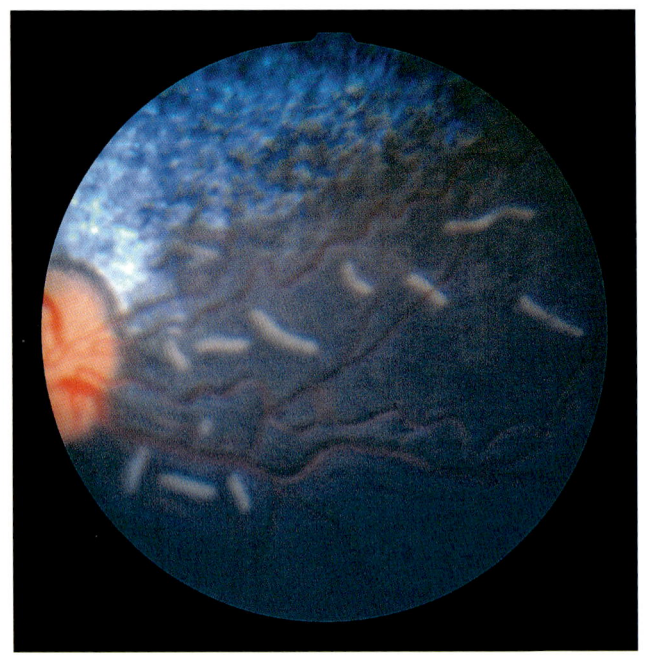

Plate 14.14:
Retinal folds in front of the tapetum nigrum, as a mild manifestation of retinal dysplasia (multifocal form) in a Rough Collie (OD).

Brownish-yellow spots: Spots of this color, with a diameter of 1–2 vessel diameters, more or less diffusely spread over the tapetum lucidum (tapetal area; Plate 14.22), are usually accumulations of detritus of atrophied outer segments of the cones. This is seen in pigment epithelial dystrophy, among other conditions. In retinal dysplasia, larger brown spots can occasionally be found.

"Oil-drop-like" spots: Sharply outlined blisters or spots may indicate retinal dysplasia or chorioretinitis.

Sharply outlined but centrally hazy/less sharp spots: Such spots (Plates 14.17, 14.18) in the fundus can indicate a closure defect (coloboma). The bottom of the defect lies further away from the examiner's eye and is therefore less sharp.

Hazy spots: (Plates 14.11, 14.24, 14.27) These generally indicate swelling and exudation and therefore retinitis, posterior uveitis, or processes associated with inflammation, such as hypertension or neoplasia (malignant lymphoma).

Highlights or hyperreflection: (Fig. 14.3) This can be focal or diffuse, and in the latter case it often resembles lamp light from behind colored glass.

- **Focal hyperreflection** indicates a circumscribed complete atrophy of the retina. No light can be absorbed and it is thus completely reflected. If there is a pigment spot in the center of such an area, it is the scar of a previous chorioretinitis. An oval area of hyperreflection at the level of the area centralis, having a diameter approximately equal to that of the papilla or slightly larger and more in the form of a disc, or even larger and extending above the papilla, indicates retinal degeneration, beginning mainly with the cones. When this is bilateral, the cause can be taurine deficiency (see 14.13.3) or feline central retinal degeneration.
- **Diffuse hyperreflection** originating mainly in the periphery of the retina, usually at the edges of the tapetum lucidum (tapetal area) or a horizontal band, is primarily an indication of generalized retinal atrophy beginning with the rods (night-blindness form). Ultimately, both forms end in total atrophy, whereby the entire fundus is diffusely reflective, often with some radial striping.

Pale spots of clearing over the tapetum nigrum (non-tapetal area), can be found in advanced stages of retinal degeneration, indicating a loss of pigment in the pigment epithelium.

Grayish-white streaks, folds, blisters (Plates 14.14, 14.15, 14.19, 14.28) indicate focal dysplasia or acquired exudation with focal retinal detachment.

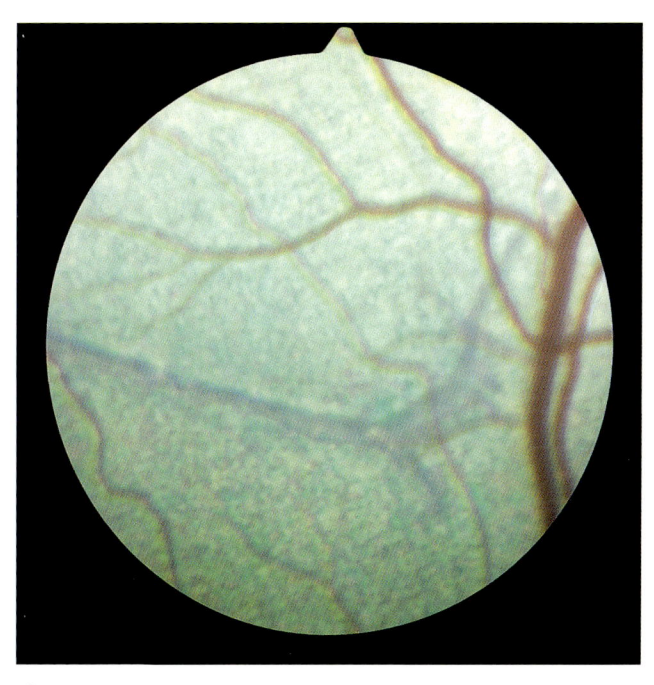

Plate 14.15:
Retinal folds in front of the tapetum lucidum, as a mild manifestation of retinal dysplasia (multifocal form) in an English Springer Spaniel (OS).

Membranous or vesicle-like structures indicate retinal detachment. The retinal vessels are often still recognizable in the balloon, and the papilla shines through the retina when it is totally loose and hanging over it.

Grayish-white structures around the papilla, generally of the same color as the papilla and reasonably sharply bordered, usually indicate ectopic glial tissue or extra myelin. If they are mainly glassy or cystic, they can be difficult to differentiate from edema.

Darker zone around the papilla can be a physiological variation, but also indicates degenerated tissue around the papilla as a result of excavation due to glaucoma. There can be flame-shaped spots of hyperreflection consisting of degenerated retina around the darker zone, also as a result of glaucoma.

Swelling of the papilla is often visible only with the help of binocular indirect ophthalmoscopy or fundus contact glass examination. The swelling can develop:
- **Without** further signs of inflammation. The papilla becomes pinker, there is a reasonably sharp border, the vessels can show a bend at the edge, and they can be slightly swollen. This papilledema can be caused by vascular obstruction in the papilla.

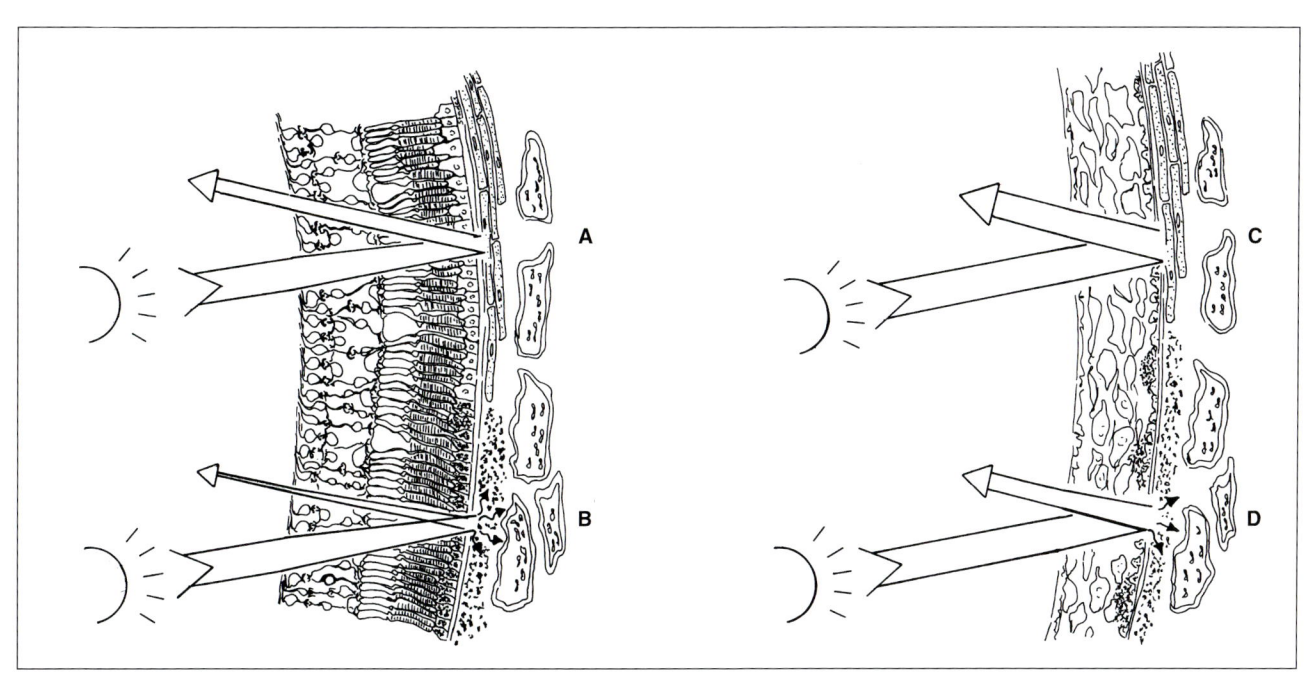

Fig. 14.3:
Normal and abnormal fundus reflection. (A) Normal tapetum lucidum reflection, and (B) reflection on the tapetum nigrum (non-tapetal area); hyperreflection on totally degenerated retina on the tapetum lucidum (C) and the tapetum nigrum (non-tapetal area; D).

- **With** other signs of inflammation. These include hyperemia; glassy, cloudy swelling; the lack of a sharp outline; flaky infiltration; and hemorrhages. The inflammation can also spread out into the retina. These signs indicate a papillitis (i.e. an inflammation of the papilla), but they can also be caused by neoplasia in this area.

Papilledema is often difficult to differentiate from papillitis. Additional diagnostic procedures can include fluorescence angiography, ultrasonography, optical thecography, CT, or MRI, etc.

Odd structures (Plates 14.29, 14.30), in which few or no normal fundus structures are still recognizable, strongly indicate neoplasia.

No visible ophthalmoscopic abnormalities may be found in spite of definite visual disturbances. This is referred to as amblyopia. If there is no vision at all, the condition is called amaurosis.

14.3 Aplasia

Complete absence of the retina and/or deeper parts of the fundus or the optic nerve occurs only sporadically. Usually there are also other, more severe, developmental disorders such as microphthalmia.[18]

14.4 Micropapilla and hypoplastic papilla

In micropapilla (too small) or hypoplasia (non-functional) of the papilla, the optic nerve is underdeveloped and, therefore, the condition is a manifestation of an absence of axons and histologically can be correlated to a decreased concentration of ganglion cells.[19] The cross-sectional diameter of the papilla is usually less than half the normal diameter. If the abnormality occurs bilaterally, comparison must be made with the papilla of a normal animal of the same breed and age. The vascular pattern is usually unremarkable. The hypoplastic papilla is known to be a fairly rare, recessively inherited abnormality in Toy Poodles. The abnormality can also occur in combination with other dysplastic abnormalities (see also 14.7). In hypoplastic papilla, vision is either handicapped or totally lacking. Blindness is the presenting sign in an animal with bilateral hypoplastic papilla. Because the ganglion cells do not contribute to the ERG, it may be totally normal in these cases.[20] A unilateral micro- or hypoplastic papilla is usually found by chance or during screening programs.

Therapy / prevention: There is no treatment. Affected animals and, if the number of animals available for breeding allows it, members of their immediate family should be excluded from breeding.

14.5 Coloboma

A fundus coloboma is a defect in the closure of the posterior wall of the eye (Fig. 14.4). With the outgrowth of neural tissue around the hyaloid artery, the seam of closure is located ventromedial to the papilla (6-o'clock position); therefore, a typical coloboma is usually located ventromedial in or below the papilla (Plates 14.17, 14.18). However, atypical colobomas occur elsewhere. Colobomas are usually round to oval and can vary in diameter from one quarter to as much as 4 times the diameter of the normal papilla. Although the coloboma area itself has no functional receptors, the vision of the affected eye is seldom detectably disturbed. The abnormality is rarely a solitary abnormality but when it is, it is then found only by chance. Colobomas are regularly found as part of the Collie eye anomaly complex (see 14.7) during screening programs.

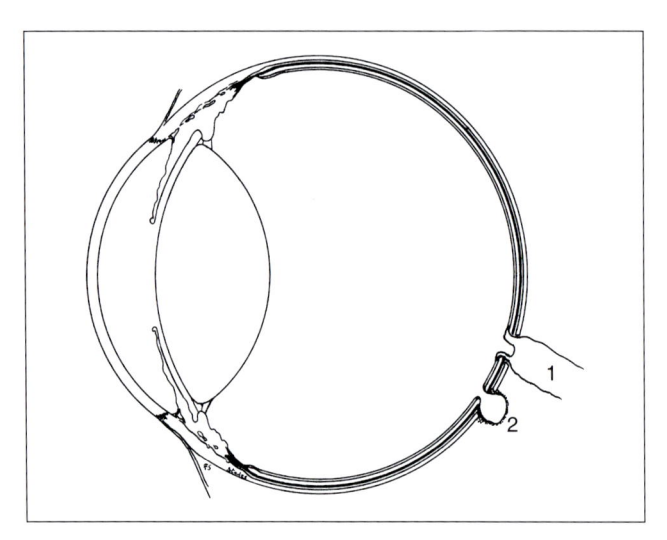

Fig. 14.4:
Coloboma in the papilla (1); coloboma below the papilla (2).

Therapy / prevention: There is no treatment. Affected animals and immediate family members should be excluded from breeding.

14.6 Retinal dysplasia (RD)

In this condition, parts of the retina and usually also the choroid are underdeveloped or abnormally developed (differential growth rates) (Plates 14.14–14.16). The retina has folds or becomes detached over larger areas. RD occurs in the dog, cat, horse and birds of prey. The abnormality is thought to be inherited recessively.

Mild or (multi) focal forms of RD result in the formation of folds or rosettes in the inner layer of the retina (Plates 14.14, 14.15). Small folds can sometimes flatten out in the first months of life, especially in Collies. The mild forms have no evident influence on vision. The abnormality is known to occur in several dog breeds, such as the American Cocker Spaniel,[21] Collie, Rottweiler,[22] Beagle,[23] and Labrador Retriever.

The **intermediate or geographic** (Plate 14.16) form occurs in the English Springer Spaniel, mainly in the tapetum lucidum, in which the folded parts can later become degenerated and hence hyperreflective.[24]

The **severe or total** form can occur in Bedlington,[25] Sealyham, and Yorkshire Terriers;[26] the English Springer Spaniel; and in the Labrador Retriever[27,28] (sometimes in combination with chondrodystrophic skeletal abnormalities). In this form, there are usually large to complete detachments bilaterally, sometimes in combination with cataract. Vision is thus severely impaired.

Prevention: In the mild form, some authorities do not recommend against breeding and for the time being only affected animals are registered. Unanimity is lacking throughout the world in this regard; however, if there is evidence of an inherited predisposition, regardless of the severity within an animal, it seems prudent to recommend not using these animals in a breeding program. Affected animals showing the intermediate forms of RD, and in particular those with the severe forms, should definitely be excluded from breeding. Also, it would be better if their immediate family is excluded from breeding, too (see also 15).

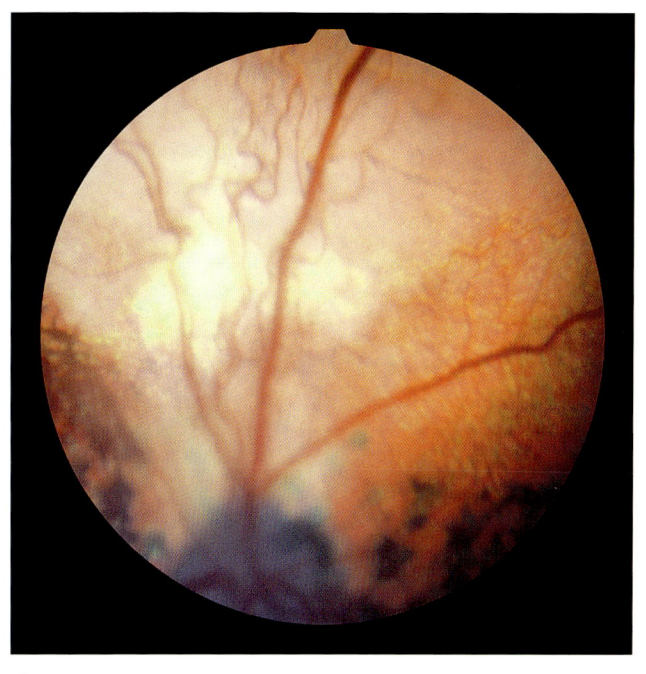

Plate 14.16:
Localized retinal atrophy (hyperreflective area dorsal to the optic disc) due to retinal dysplasia (geographic form) in an English Springer Spaniel (OS).

14.7 Collie eye anomaly (CEA)

Collie eye anomaly is the collective name for a group of developmental defects resulting in a lack of normal ingrowth of the mesodermal layers of the developing eye, with subsequent focal hypoplasia or dysplasia of the choroidal vessels, and/or in larger defects of scleral development with subsequent colobomas adjacent to or in the optic nerve.[29] Retinal detachment and hemorrhage in CEA is secondary to the above-described lesions.[30] The abnormality occurs mainly in the Long-haired Collie and Shetland Sheepdog (in the Netherlands, 40–50% of the population), but it also occurs in Short-haired, Bearded, and Border Collies. The most accepted hypothesis is that the abnormality is inherited as a simple autosomal recessive, though polygenetic inheritance and differences in penetrance may be possible. Choroidal hypoplasia and colobomas are likely to be inherited separately.[31,32]

Symptoms: The most frequently observed CEA lesions are choroidal hypoplasia and, to a lesser extent, dysplasia of the retina and/or hypoplasia (C[R]H or CRD), just lateral (temporal) to the papilla (Plates 14.17–14.19).

Distended, deformed, or wildly deformed and/or structured choroidal vessels are present with parts of the white sclera visible between them. In the mildest forms, these areas can be covered by the developing tapetum lucidum (tapetal area; 7th–8th week post partum) and therefore not be visible

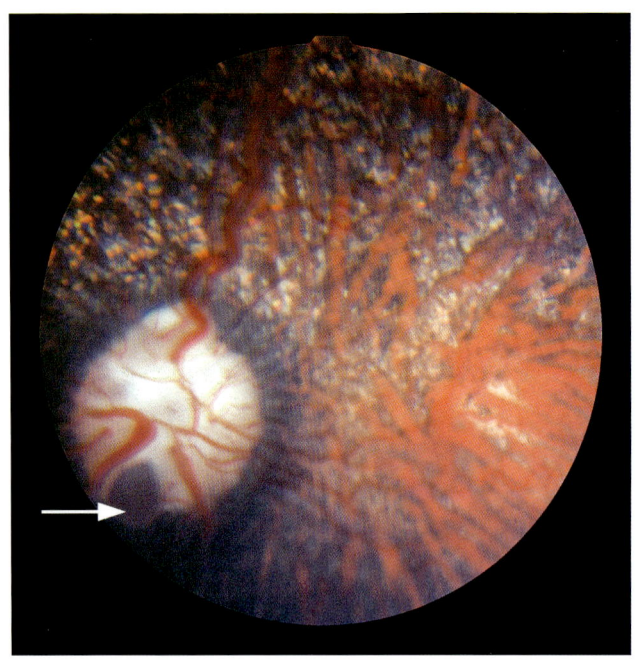

Plate 14.17:
Collie Eye Anomaly (CEA). Choroidal hypoplasia (lateral to the optic disc) and a coloboma of the optic disc at the typical 6-o'clock position (see arrow) in a Rough Collie (OS).

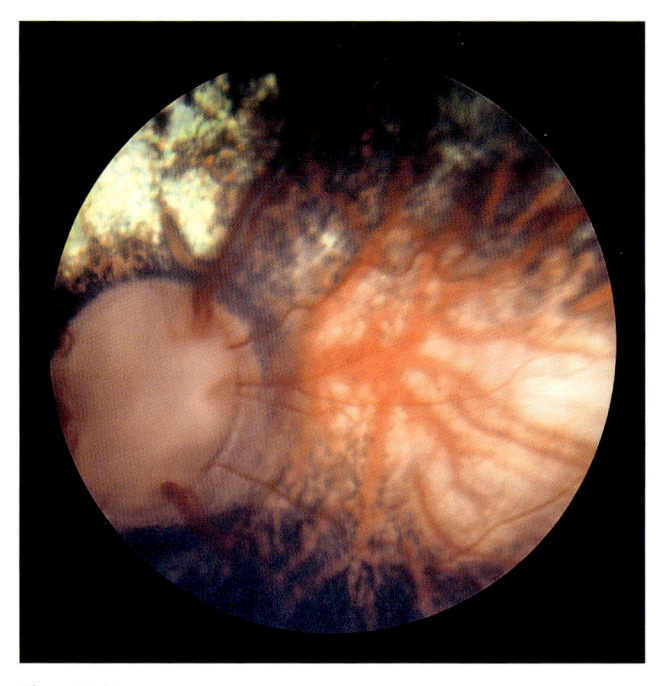

Plate 14.18:
Collie Eye Anomaly (CEA). Severe choroidal hypoplasia (OS; lateral to the optic disc) and an enormous coloboma of the optic disc itself.

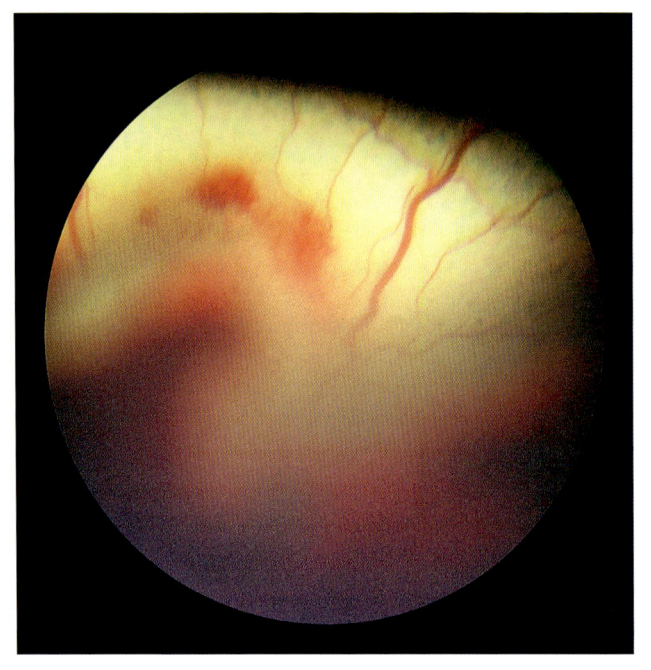

Plate 14.19:
Collie Eye Anomaly (CEA). Intraocular hemorrhage and a partial retinal detachment in a Rough Collie (OS).

when the animal is examined at a later date ("go normals"). The other mild form of expression of this disorder is excessive tortuosity of the retinal vessels (tortuositias vasorum retinae). There is some difference of opinion as to whether this form really is part of the anomaly. Especially in blue merle dogs, both of these abnormalities can occur in such transitional forms and combinations that even the experienced ophthalmologist may not immediately recognize these dogs as being affected by CEA. Such dogs should be recorded as being "undetermined". In such animals, it is only possible to confirm the disease by DNA-testing or test breeding.

A more severe expression of CEA is the group of colobomas and ectasias. These occur mostly peripapillar.[33] They can vary from small depressions to large cystic defects. None of the above-mentioned abnormalities cause blindness in the affected eye. The severe clinical manifestations of CEA (about 5% of dogs with CEA) are intraocular hemorrhages, retinal detachment, and possibly also hypoplasia of the optic disc. Severely affected eyes usually are or will become blind.

CEA can be unilateral or bilateral (CH or CRD is usually bilateral), can occur in different forms and degrees, and is usually not progressive. The intraocular hemorrhages and retinal detachment can result in a progressive loss of vision via further retinal detachment or increase in hemorrhage.

Therapy / prevention: There is no treatment. Breeders and owners should be encouraged to have their animals examined for CEA and other inherited eye abnormalities in screening programs. Examination for CEA provides most information if it takes place in the nursing period (6th week post partum, but after chipping or tattooing). Compared to other abnormalities, breeding measures can be more effective in cases of CEA: this is because CEA can be diagnosed early and in this way there is direct information available about the hereditary properties of the parents. In addition, the percentage of affected animals that are bilaterally blind is low. Thus test crossings are possible without the production of puppies with severe problems. Carriers can be detected by crossing a phenotypically free dog to a CEA-affected dog (see 15.1).

Since the end of 2004, a DNA test for the detection of choroidal hypoplasia in Rough und Smooth Collies, Sheltie, Border Collie, Australian Shepherd und Lancashire Heeler is available. Carriers can also be recognized, thus providing breeders a better tool for reducing CEA in the population. They now can also use the carriers without risk, as long as also all their progeny is tested (for further information, see e.g. *www.optigen.com*).

CEA-affected animals should be excluded from breeding. However, they make acceptable pets, in particular because the illness is usually stationary, and there is a low percentage of bilaterally blind animals. If the total number of dogs available for breeding is sufficient, parents and siblings of an affected animal should also be excluded from breeding. Preventive breeding measures have been shown to be effective. In the Lake District in the USA, good information and breeding measures reduced the percentage of CEA-affected animals from 97 to 59% in 3 years. Moreover, better show results were also obtained using progeny testing than with breeding by just looking at the parents.

14.8 Inherited enzyme deficiencies

Examples of these rare abnormalities are GM1 gangliosidosis, mucopolysaccharidosis, and galactosidase and ornithine (d-A) transferase deficiencies in cats, and neural ceroid lipofuscinosis in dogs.[34,35] As a result of such inherited inborn errors of metabolism, abnormal accumulations of metabolites in the reaction chain (e.g. amino acids, polysaccharides, or glycolipids) can occur in the body (storage disease). The first two examples mentioned above have been described as autosomal recessive disorders in Siamese cats. They cause a progressive degeneration of the central nervous system. Ocular abnormalities can occur via accumulation of the materials not only in the cornea (see 10.7) but also in the retinal ganglion cells. These are recognized as well-circumscribed, small, pale gray spots in the retina. Blindness and signs of increasing loss of neurons can occur later. In hyperornithinemia due to ornithine transferase deficiency, progressive retinal atrophy is found.

Neural ceroid lipofuscinosis is an inborn error disease in which an abnormal accumulation of lipid pigment can occur in the brain and retina. This abnormality has thus far been described in the English Setter, Collie, Dalmatian, and it possibly also occurs in the Tibetan Terrier.

14.9 Hereditary (progressive) retinal dysplasias / atrophy / degeneration (PRA)

The term PRA is used for the entire group of inherited primary dysplasias with secondary degeneration / atrophy and primary degeneration / atrophy of the retina. The most important types of PRA are characterized by progressive irreversible abnormalities of the other retinal components (with the exception of the pigment epithelial dystrophy). A number of main groups can be differentiated:

Photoreceptor dysplasia:
- rod / cone dysplasia and subsequent degeneration
- rod dysplasia: stationary night blindness
- cone dysplasia: stationary day blindness

Photoreceptor degeneration
- rod / cone degeneration

Because strong evidence has been presented recently that pigment epithelial dystrophy (PED) is primarily alimentary, with a familial predisposition, this disease is discussed later (see 14.9.4).

14.9.1 Hereditary progressive retinal degeneration / progressive retinal atrophy

Hereditary retinal degeneration can be divided into many forms, but mainly in photoreceptor dysplasia and photoreceptor atrophy. In dysplasia the photoreceptor never develops normally, whereas in photoreceptor atrophy they do develop normally and then degenerate later in life. This is mainly of importance in connection with the age at which signs of night blindness first appear. If the rods and cones are abnormally developed (dysplastic), they will also degenerate early in life. Night blindness then occurs within the first 6 months of life and the animals are completely blind by 1–2 years of age. This occurs in breeds such as the Irish and Gordon Setters,[36,37] Collies, Rough-haired Dachshund, Shetland Sheepdog, Norwegian Elkhound,[38] and the Abyssinian and Persian cats. In the late onset photoreceptor atrophy forms, the rods and cones are developed normally and degeneration begins later (night blindness by 3–5 years of age, blind by 6–9 years). The affected breeds include under many: Poodles,[39] Dutch Pointer, Schapendoes,[40] and English[41] and American Cocker Spaniels, Labrador Retriever and Entlebuch Cattle Dog. There are also intermediate forms (night blindness by 1–2 years, blind by 3–5 years) and the affected breeds include the Miniature Schnauzer, Tibetan Terrier,[42] Labrador Retriever,[43] and Abyssinian cat.[44,45] There are also breeds in which at least two forms occur: Norwegian Elkhound, Irish Setter, Rough-haired Dachshund, and the Abyssinian cat.[46]

All of these forms, in the breeds reported, appear to be transmitted as a simple autosomal recessive trait and the signs are nearly identical. This is with the exception of the Siberian Husky and Samoyed, in which the gene is bound to the X-chromosome, resulting in males being affected.[47,48]

In a number of forms and/or breeds much more is known about the cause and pathogenesis. Examples are:

1. Rod-cone dysplasia, later followed by atrophy, in the Irish Setter. There is a delayed (postnatal, as early as the 18th day) development of the photoreceptors. There is an abnormality in the cyclic guanosine-3-5-monophosphate (cGMP) phosphodiesterase activity and hence accumulation of cGMP in the retina.[49]
2. Rod-cone dysplasia, later followed by atrophy, in the Collie, clinically identical to the form in the Irish Setter. However, test breeding has revealed that mating of affected individuals from the two breeds (Collie x Setter) results in no affected offspring, implying that a separate gene is involved.
3. Rod dysplasia, cones initially normal, followed by atrophy and without cGMP accumulation, in the Norwegian Elkhound and Miniature Schnauzer.
4. Early retinal degeneration in the Norwegian Elkhound, which can be differentiated from the previous form with the help of an ERG.
5. Rod-cone dysplasia in the Abyssinian cat. Night blindness begins at 8–12 weeks, and as an exception, this disease has a possible incomplete dominant inheritance.[50]
6. Rod-cone degeneration in the Toy and Miniature Poodles and possibly also in the English and American Cocker Spaniels. There is presumed to be a disturbance in the renewal of the membrane of the outer segments of the photoreceptors.[51] Test matings between Miniature Poodles and English and American Cocker Spaniels with PRA have produced affected offspring.
7. Rod-cone degeneration in the Abyssinian cat, beginning with morphologic disintegration of the plates in the outer segments of the rods.[52]

Symptoms: Except for the etiology and the age of onset, all symptoms in the affected dog and cat breeds are similar. The signs of PRA night blindness (Plates 14.20, 14.21) are mydriasis, slow or absent pupillary reflexes, and reduced vision in low light, and they may begin, depending on the form, while the puppy is still nursing or not until 3–4 years of age. A very observant owner will sometimes notice the animal's slightly anxious, more careful behavior in dim light. At this stage, an experienced examiner will be able to observe by ophthalmoscopic examination the very light, diffuse color changes and an increased reflectivity, especially in the periphery of the tapetum lucidum (tapetal area). The reflectivity increases gradually and the retinal vessels become attenuated. Eventually, the atrophy is complete. A rule of thumb can be: the arterioles should branch three times, if less, attenuation is likely. In the end stage, the retinal vessels are only shadows, there is a diffuse hyperreflection in the area of the tapetum lucidum (tapetal area), and in the tapetum nigrum (non-tapetal area) there are circumscribed, pale clear spots with a size of one-fifth to 1 papilla diameter. The papilla is pale and atrophic. The animals are then completely blind. The abnormalities are always bilateral with approximately the same degree of progression. Frequently, cataracts develop in the final state of PRA so that the fundus can no longer be examined with an ophthalmoscope. There is a lack of consensus with regard to the association of cataracts and PRA; one school believes there is a direct association, while the other believes they are separate entities occurring in the same animal.

Diagnosis: Diagnosis is based on clinical signs and can be confirmed by an ERG or DNA testing. In the differential diagnosis, the disease could be confused with non-inherited, bilateral, diffuse forms of progressive retinal degeneration (retinopathy), such as taurine deficiency in the cat. The differentiation is difficult especially in the final stages. Usually, however, the very gradual progression is clear and there is no evidence for nutritional errors or previous inflammation.

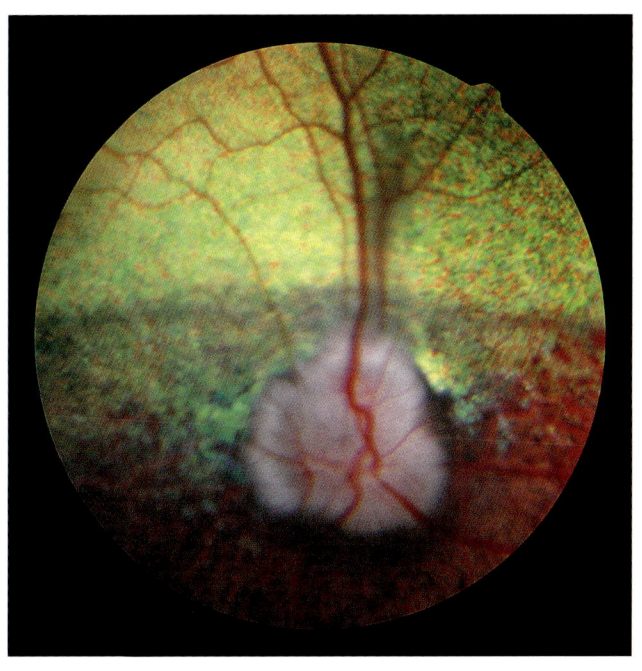

Plate 14.20:
Hereditary retinal degeneration or progressive retinal atrophy (PRA) in a 5-year-old English Cocker Spaniel (OD). The retinal vasculature is attenuated and the area ventral to the horizontal demarcation line just above the optic disc shows an increased reflectivity. In this stage, this dog only had difficulty with the obstacle test in the dark.

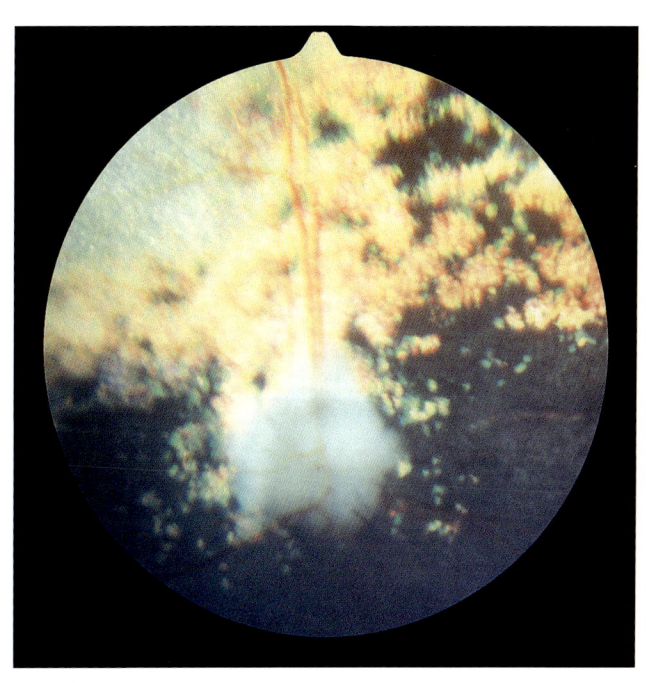

Plate 14.21:
Hereditary retinal degeneration or progressive retinal atrophy (PRA) in a 6-year-old Toy Poodle (OD). There is a strong hyperreflection, the retinal vasculature is severely atrophied, and the optic disc is pale. The dog was completely blind at this stage.

Therapy / prognosis: There is no available therapy as yet. The prognosis for vision is hopeless. Blind animals can, however, manage quite well in their familiar environment. Playing with a ball or stick, or catching mice, or jumping over low fences or hurdles of a known location, can still be done. Euthanasia would seem to be the responsible choice only if the animal is severely handicapped and has a very anxious (aggressive) behavior.

Recently, new gene-therapy methods have produced encouraging results.[53] In homozygote RPE65-defective blind dogs, an artificial RPE65 was injected subretinally. In all treated dogs, the improved clinical vision and ERG parameters lasted for up to a period of 9 months.

Prevention: Animals with signs of generalized, bilateral retinal degeneration should be considered as having PRA until proven otherwise. It is also of great importance that the diagnosis is confirmed by someone experienced in this area and officially designated for this purpose. At the same time, the owner must be convinced of the importance of allowing the information about the animal to be conveyed to the breed association and the breeder(s) of its parents. It is also recommended that members of the animal's immediate family be examined, even if there have been no plans to breed any of them. Because of the, in most cases, simple recessive pattern of inheritance, breeders should be made aware that both parents are at least carriers of the gene and that brothers and sisters of an affected animals have a more than 50% chance of carrying the PRA gene. Breeding affected animals or their immediate family members should be most strongly discouraged (see 15.1).

Nowadays DNA tests for hereditary retinal degenerations are available for a long list of breeds (see 15.4). Further information can be found under e.g. www.optigen.com. Mutation tests allow reliable recognition of affected animals and carriers of the disease. Using marker tests, the proof is less precise and carriers may not be recognized at all.

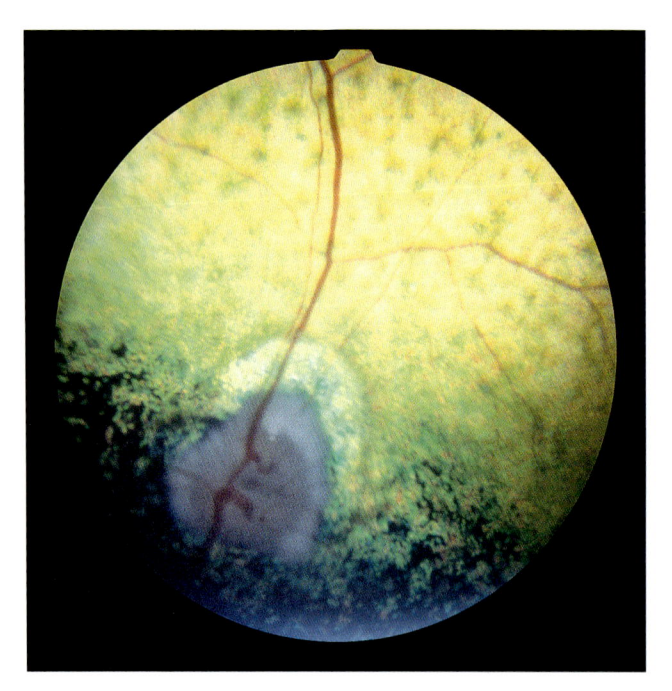

Plate 14.22:
Pigment epithelial dystrophy (PED) in a 4-year-old, day-blind English Cocker Spaniel (OS).

14.9.2 Hereditary (stationary) night blindness

In these diseases, the affected animals (Briards, Appaloosa horse) are night blind though in general most day vision remains. In congenital night blindness, there are no ophthalmoscopic abnormalities, but the ERG, after dark adaptation, is flat.[54]

14.9.3 Hereditary day blindness

In hereditary day blindness, the cones degenerate after an initial normal development. This disorder is found in the Alaskan Malamute (beginning at 8 weeks to 6 months of age) as a simple recessive hereditary disease.[55] The abnormality is usually recognized only by the behavior of the dog; there are no definite abnormalities on ophthalmoscopy. The diagnosis can be confirmed by an ERG.

14.9.4 Pigment epithelial dystrophy (PED)

In this disorder (Plate 14.22), the targeted tissue is the RPE. As a result there is an accumulation of lipid pigments in the RPE and, later, elsewhere in the retina. It is possible that this is caused by an inadequate phagocytosis of the outer segment material of the photoreceptors. Degeneration of the photoreceptors then develops, beginning with the cones. Ultimately, there is degeneration of the entire retina. The abnormality has been diagnosed in many breeds and predominantly in Great Britain. The abnormality has been confirmed in the Briard,[56] Golden and Labrador Retrievers, Collies, Shetland Sheepdog, English Cocker and Springer Spaniels, and the Cardigan Welsh Corgi. Apart from this, PED seldom occurs. Recently, strong evidence was presented showing that vitamin E and taurine are involved in the etiology of PED, with a familial predisposition.[57] The abnormality had been hitherto thought to be transmitted as an autosomal recessive (possibly dominant in the Labrador Retriever).

Symptoms: The symptoms consist of reduced vision (at 3–5 years of age) in "full" light. Movements can be recognized but non-moving objects are seen less well. There are small brown-beige foci in the tapetum lucidum (tapetal area) in the fundus and there is a light hyperreflection over the entire lucidum. In the course of the disease, the foci become larger, the remaining areas become more hyperreflective, and vascular atrophy develops. Finally, the animals may become blind at 5–9 years of age, though PED does not always lead to complete blindness.

14.10 Hemorrhages and other vascular abnormalities

Petechiae or larger hemorrhages, vascular tortuosities, and aneurism-like vascular dilations in the fundus can, apart from congenital vascular abnormalities, be caused by trauma, intoxication, blood coagulation disorders, hypertension, diabetes mellitus, arteriosclerosis, inflammation, degenerative processes, lupus erythematosus, thrombocytopenia, autoimmune hemolytic anemia, or neoplasia. Larger subretinal hemorrhages can cause retinal detachment (see 14.15). The diagnostic steps should be guided by these possible causes, and the therapy and prognosis will be dependent on the cause that is found.

14.10.1 Vascular occlusion

Rarely, one or more of the retinal end arteries can be occluded, for example, by sclerosis or occluding emboli. An acutely non-functioning retina occurs in the resulting area of infarction. Initially, ophthalmoscopic examination reveals few visible abnormalities. The vessels may be darker or have wider and narrower segments. With time, a diffuse atrophy occurs in the area that was supplied by the infarcted vessel. Diagnosis can be confirmed by use of fluorescein angiography.

Prognosis: The prognosis for vision is usually hopeless. Treatment with anticoagulants does not appear to be therapeutically useful. Lytic agents, such as streptokinase or actilyse, may prove to be useful in the future.

14.10.2 Hyperlipoproteinemia

An excess of lipids in the blood can cause a grayish filling of the vessels. Sometimes the abnormality can cause a decrease in vision. A low-fat diet should bring about improvement.[58]

14.11 Trauma

Gross blunt or perforating trauma and luxation of the globe can lead to small or large hemorrhages, inflammation, or in very exceptional cases, to tearing and retinal detachment. In most cases, administering anti-inflammatory medications (see 12.10) and prescribing rest is all that can be done therapeutically. Foreign bodies in the immediate surroundings of the retina, but outside the globe, usually become encapsulated. The surgical removal of such foreign bodies usually causes more problems than is resolved by the trauma of the foreign body itself (see also 4).

14.12 Intoxications

Intoxications (for example, by cumarine derivatives, but also many other compounds) can cause petechiae, larger hemorrhages, or inflammation. The fundus is the only place in the body where vessels and nervous tissue can be evaluated directly (by ophthalmoscopy). Accordingly when an intoxication is suspected, ophthalmoscopy can provide valuable additional information. For this reason, ophthalmoscopy is almost always a required procedure in the evaluation of new drugs.

For further information about diagnosis and treatment, the literature on intoxications should be consulted.

14.12.1 Iatrogenic intoxications

Acute and diffuse retinal degeneration in cats, resulting in temporary or definitive blindness, may be caused by the parenteral use of fluoroquinolones, including enrofloxacin.

Therapy: Care should be taken to follow closely the manufacturer's current dosage scheme for such compounds and the feline patient should be kept under continual clinical observation.[59,60]

14.13 Abnormalities of nutritional origin

It has become apparent that cats are more dependent on certain elements in their food (especially from the group of animal proteins) than are dogs. In the dog, however, it is likely that vitamin E and taurine are involved in the etiology of PED (see 14.9.4), although the disease is associated with a familial predisposition.

14.13.1 Vitamin A and vitamin E deficiencies

Vitamins A and E are fat-soluble vitamins found in animal fats and especially in the liver. Experience from developing countries in particular has shown that vitamin A deficiency in humans causes KCS and night blindness. Especially in cats, there is a possibility of the development of these abnormalities in vitamin A deficiency, as they cannot convert carotene to vitamin A. However, this has been not thoroughly investigated. Furthermore, the spontaneous development of this abnormality in cats is not very likely because adequate vitamin A is present in almost all commercially manufactured foods (also in dog foods). There is also enough vitamin A in animal and vegetable fats. In addition, many cats supplement their diets with animal fats in the form of mice and birds.[61]

In cattle, hypovitaminosis A may result in blindness.[62] Vitamin E deficiency can also result in a retinopathy that resembles the picture of PED.[63]

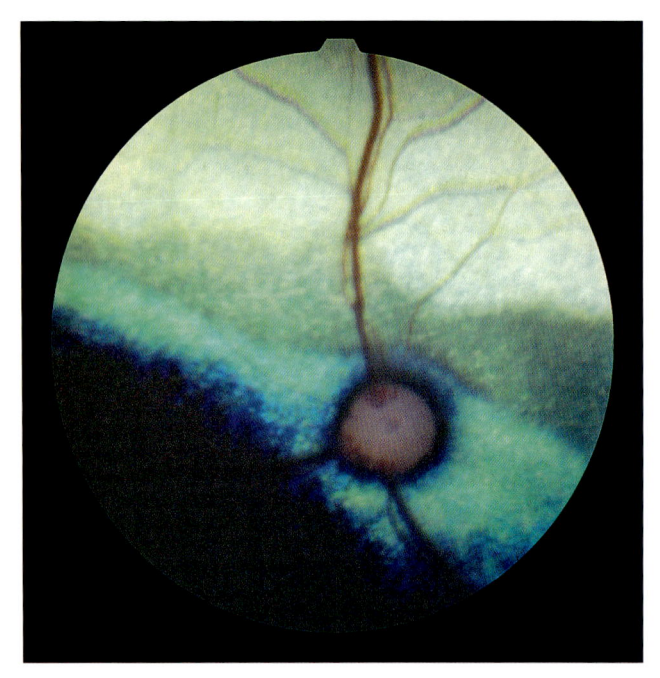

Plate 14.23:
Typically shaped zone of retinal atrophy dorsal to the optic disc (OS), due to taurine deficiency in a 2-year-old cat which had been fed a vegetarian diet (also excluding milk) from kittenhood.

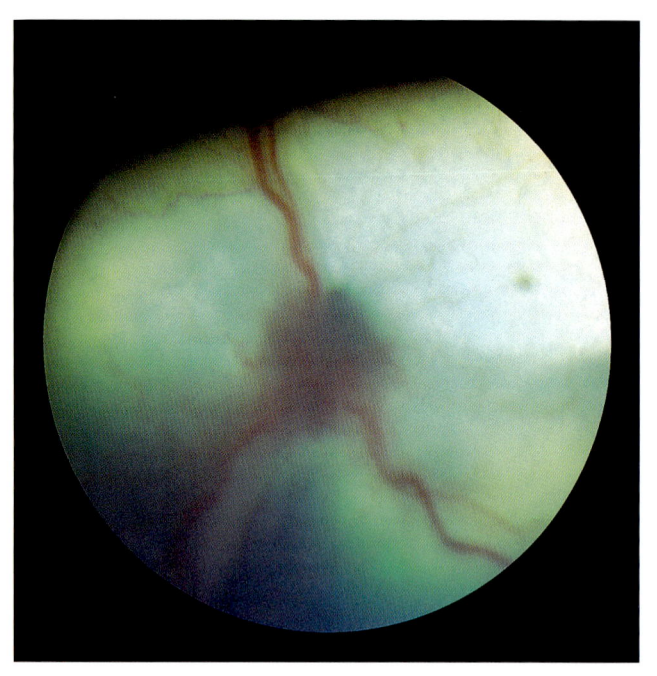

Plate 14.24:
Chorioretinitis in a cat with infectious peritonitis (OD).

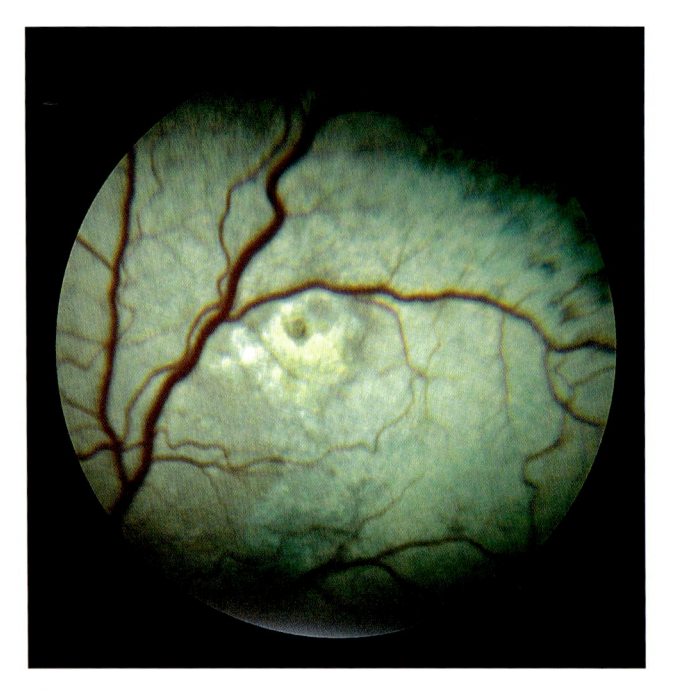

Plate 14.25:
Chorioretinitis in a dog, due to a migrating larva. The larva has the appearance of a figure six and did move. Two months later, the larva had disappeared without a trace of scarring (Photo by courtesy of Dr. A. Hein, Oisterwijk).

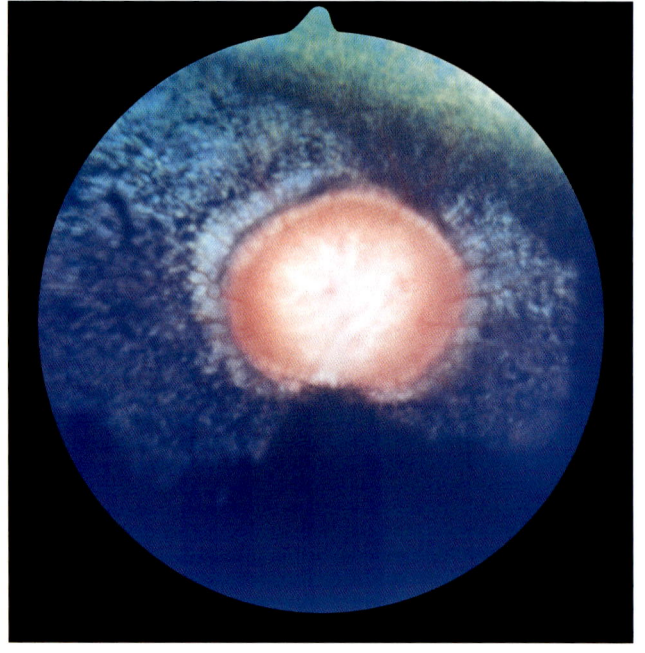

Plate 14.26:
Horse showing an old peripapillar chorioretinitis in a "butterfly lesion" pattern. There was no visual deficit and there where no symptoms of ERU.

14.13.2 Thiamine (aneurine) or vitamin B₁ deficiency

Thiamine is a water-soluble vitamin from the B-vitamin group. Thiamine deficiency in humans results in beriberi. The deficiency causes inadequate production of acetylcholine and thus disturbance in the impulse transfer across the synapse. There is adequate thiamine in animal and vegetable foodstuffs. However, a number of types of fish (particularly freshwater ones) contain the enzyme thiaminase. This abnormality can be expected in cats that eat almost exclusively raw fish.

In cats, thiamine deficiency can possibly initially cause abnormalities similar to those of taurine deficiency. This finally results in a generalized diffuse retinal degeneration that can no longer be differentiated from other forms of retinal degeneration in their final stage.

14.13.3 Taurine deficiency (Plate 14.23)

Taurine is an acid amine but not an amino acid. In most animal species, it is not an essential nutritional element, but cats cannot produce sufficient taurine themselves. High concentrations of taurine are found in the retina, brain, liver, and heart. Considerable taurine is also present in other animal "products" such as milk, meat, fish, and shellfish.

Taurine is especially important in neurotransmission and for the cell membranes and photoreceptors, but it also has a function as a bile acid conjugator and in energy transport.

Taurine deficiency can be expected in cats that are fed an exclusively vegetarian diet or only dog food (often containing much less meat than the label suggests).[64,65]

Symptoms: Disturbances in the ERG occur after only 5 weeks on a taurine-free diet. After about 20 weeks, granulation develops in the central area, which is the area with the highest concentration of cones. Hyperreflection in this area then occurs and spreads out dorsally along the papilla in a more or less discus or stripe form (feline central retinal degeneration or FCRD; see 14.17.1). Finally, there is generalized hyperreflection and vessel atrophy, usually after more than a year of deficient taurine intake, and the cat is completely blind.

Diagnosis: Diagnosis can be made on the basis of the history and can eventually be confirmed by measuring the concentration of taurine in the animal's plasma. This costly measurement is seldom performed. The reference values are of the order of 15–150 µmol/l, therefore blood from healthy reference animals should also be included. In the differential diagnosis, consideration must be given to such abnormalities as PRA and, in the end stage, all abnormalities associated with bilateral generalized, diffuse retinal atrophy.

Therapy: Treatment consists of changing the diet and, if necessary, adding meat, fish, shellfish, or taurine in powder form. The degeneration already present is irreversible but the process will, however, be stopped.

Prevention: To prevent the disease, owners should be made to realize that cats are emphatically carnivorous and should therefore be fed an appropriate diet.

14.14 Posterior uveitis / chorioretinitis / retinitis

Posterior uveitis is an inflammation in the uvea of the posterior segment (choroid) of the eye (Plates 14.11–14.13, 14.24–14.28). The inflammation can also be part of a generalized inflammation of the entire uvea as in equine recurrent uveitis (Plate 14.28). Because the choroid and retina are very closely related both anatomically and functionally, inflammation of the choroid without involvement of the retina, or vice versa, is exceptional. Classification of posterior uveitis is similar to that given for anterior uveitis (see 12.10). The most important causes of chorioretinitis come from the group of infectious diseases. In northern Europe these are FIP, FeLV, and FIV, toxoplasmosis, ehrlichiosis, migrating larvae (Plate 14.25), etc. In southern countries, cryptococcosis, histoplasmosis, anaplasmosis, and blastomycosis are also regularly found as causes.[68,69] Chorioretinitis is, therefore, almost always a manifestation of systemic disease that is associated with anterior uveitis and which usually occurs bilaterally.[66,67]

Symptoms: Affected animals are usually presented because of the development, sudden or otherwise, of bilateral blindness and unresponsive pupils in mydriasis, swelling, and exudate in the fundus. Increased tortuosity or dilation of the vessels can develop in the fundus. Ophthalmoscopically, swelling or exudate in the fundus results in haziness or lack of sharpness of the image. The cloudiness can extend into the vitreous making examination of the fundus impossible. If there is exudate between the photoreceptors and the pigment epithelium, retinal detachment can occur (see 14.15). If the process is limited to a small area, it may have the appearance of a drop of oil or have a cottony appearance (for example, inflammation due to larva migrans; Plates 14.11, 14.12, 14.25). The fundus can also have a granulomatous aspect, especially in mycotic processes.

The signs observed ophthalmoscopically are usually not very specific. A general physical examination is necessary and laboratory tests for infectious disease (e.g. FIP, FeLV, FIV, and toxoplasmosis) are recommended. The patient can eventually be referred for additional diagnostic procedures such as ultrasonography or vitreous paracentesis. In Europe, the latter is certainly not a routine procedure, in view of the high risks. In countries where ocular mycoses are endemic and frequent (e.g. Florida in the USA), these tests are performed routinely by the local ophthalmologists.

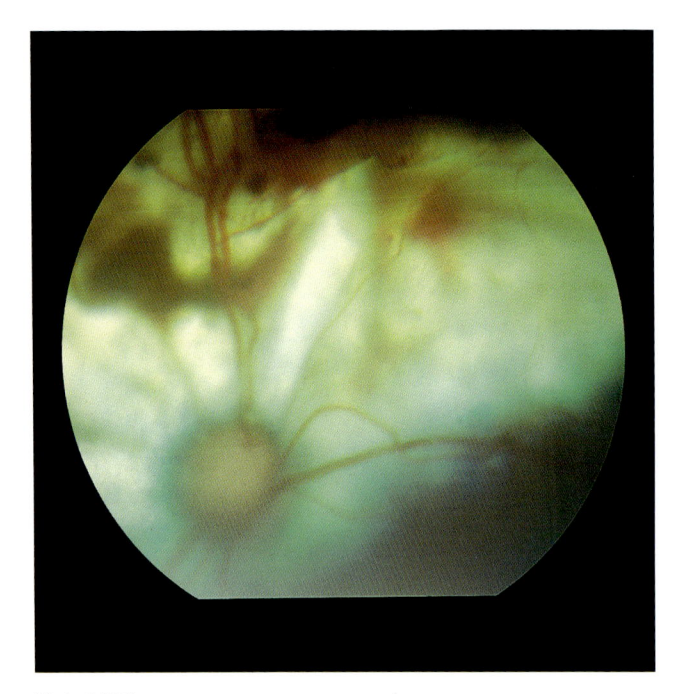

Plate 14.27:
Retinal hemorrhages and retinal detachment in an old cat with hypertension.

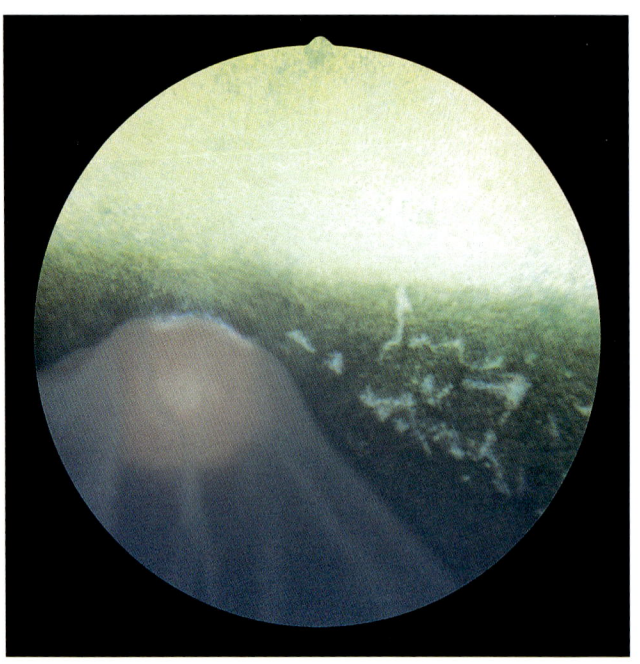

Plate 14.28:
Retinal detachment in a horse (OS).

Therapy: Medical therapy consists of "specific choice" systemic antibiotics and, after studies into the cause have been completed, corticosteroids if not contraindicated. In mycotic processes, amphotericin B or other antifungal agents are usually indicated (see also 12.10). The patient should be isolated until the cause of the retinitis is known. During the healing of chorioretinitis, it is usually noticed first that the haziness recedes and the components of the fundus again become more sharply outlined. The visual disturbances can disappear quickly. Scars from local inflammation usually result in small pigment accumulations at the end of a very thin vessel and surrounded by a hyperreflective zone of retinal atrophy.

The prognosis must take into account the underlying cause of the abnormalities. In idiopathic chorioretinitis, the prognosis can usually be cautiously optimistic.

14.15 Retinal detachment

In retinal detachment or ablatio retinae, there is a separation between the inner layer of the retina and its outer layer, the RPE (Fig. 14.5; Plates 14.19, 14.27, 14.28). Separation is also possible between the layers of the neuroretina itself, called retinoschisis, but this is very rare in animals. In retinal detachment, the photoreceptors are left without any nutrient supply, without which their functional ability decreases. If this condition persists, degeneration of the photoreceptors occurs and irreversible blindness results. The separation can develop via accumulation of exudate or transudate, or outgrowth of tissue (massive retinal detachment) posterior to the neuroretina, or traction (for example, after perforating trauma or lens luxation), via leakage through a hole or tear in the retina, or via dissolution of the vitreous. Exudative retinal detachment occurs most frequently. The most important causes are chorioretinitis (see 14.14) and transudate hypertension, and the latter mainly in the cat (Plate 14.27). Small local detachments are only seen sporadically. This is not only because they seldom lead to signs of illness, but they are also rarely found in screening examinations in large groups of animals.

A small retinal detachment is seen as a not very sharp, grayish-blue "cyst" in the retina. Large detachments look more like grayish-blue to red parachute-shaped balloons, in which retinal vessels are recognizable and through which the papilla may gleam.

Diagnosis: Diagnosis is made on the basis of the appearance of the fundus and can be confirmed by ultrasonography (in particular to exclude neoplasia behind the detachment). Measurement of blood pressure, etc. (see also 14.16), and laboratory tests for FIP, FeLV, FIV, toxoplasmosis, malignant lymphoma, etc. are recommended. If there is systemic hypertension (usually secondary to renal, adrenal, or thyroid diseases), systolic pressures (measured directly) far above about 200 mmHg can be expected. The demonstration of a mycotic agent is usually only possible by cytologic or histologic examination of material from the anterior chamber or, preferably, from the vitreous. The intraocular collection of material does, however, carry great risks and should be carried out only in specific cases. They are mainly done in countries where these infections are frequent and then only by experienced ophthalmologists.

Therapy: An attempt is made to hasten the absorption of the exudate by means of prednisolone (1–2 mg/kg, once daily) and dichlorphenamide (0.5–2.5 mg/kg, 4 times daily). The prednisolone is reduced and given on alternate days (beginning with 1–2 mg/kg orally in the morning for 4–5 days, then every other day for 8–10 days, and there after half the dosage every other day and so on). If there are indications of recovery (improvement in vision and ophthalmoscopic findings) treatment is continued over a long period. If there is no improvement within 1–2 weeks, prognosis for recovery of vision is usually hopeless and treatment can be reduced within a short period. For hypertension therapy, see 14.16.

If there are indications of a treatable infectious disease, a specific antibiotic is administered (see 14.14).

Surgically, in theory, all methods employed in human ophthalmology to deal with retinal detachments can also be applied in veterinary ophthalmology.[70] However, cases in which surgical correction of retinal detachments is possible and promising are comparatively rare. The most common methods of retinopexy employ cold or heat. Heat- or cold-induced focal inflammation is used to cause adhesions between the RPE and neuroretina. A recurrence of the detachment is successfully prevented in the treated area. Laser energy can be applied directly through the optic media by way of a laser ophthalmoscope, or can be applied transsclerally. Cryopexy or diathermy can only be applied transsclerally.[71] Nowadays, even complete retinal detachments with disinsertion of the retina at the ora ciliaris, e.g. giant tears, can be treated successfully. The retina can be reattached with the aid of silicone oil or gas.[72] Scleral buckles are very rarely used in veterinary ophthalmology.[73,74]

Prognosis: In case of an acute exudative idiopathic detachment, the prognosis for reattachment and restoration of vision is relatively favorable. In all other cases, the prognosis is usually grave.

14.16 Hypertensive Retinopathy

Physiologic systolic blood pressure in dogs and cats does not exceed 160 to 180 mmHg (depending also on the resistance of the animal). Systolic pressures in excess of this upper limit of normal values are termed systemic hypertension. Systemic hypertension may be the result of chronic renal insufficiency or hyperthyroidism.[75] Systemic hypertension leads to alterations in blood vessel walls leading to changes in permeability and hemorrhage. In the eye, high blood pressure manifests as hypertensive oculopathy or hypertensive retinopathy.[76]

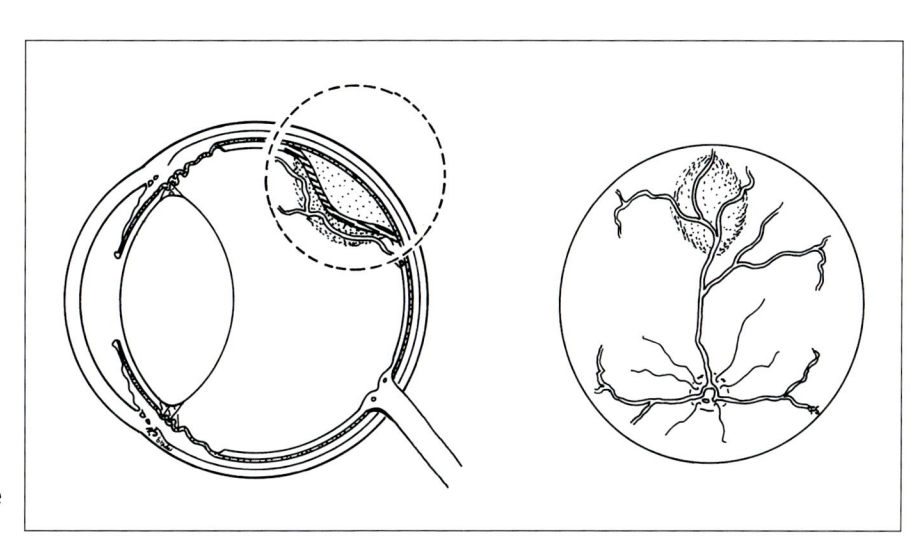

Fig. 14.5:
Retinal detachment (local) can be seen as a more anterior displaced structure containing vessels.

Hypertension is more often diagnosed in cats than in dogs. The underlying cause is in most cases a chronic renal insufficiency.[77] Affected cats are presented for acute vision loss with fixed and dilated pupils. Older animals with a history of PU/PD, weight loss, intermittent vomition, etc. are over-represented. The anterior segment is usually normal, although hyphema and iris hemorrhages may be a presenting complaint. There are retinal hemorrhages and detachments, which are difficult to distinguish from inflammatory lesions based on ophthalmoscopy alone.

The diagnosis is based on fundus lesions (Plate 14.27) accompanied by elevated blood pressure. The systolic pressure in typical cases is usually in excess of 200 mmHg.

Serum chemistry profiles and urinalysis will reveal whether there is renal disease or hyperthyroidism.

Therapy: Besides the management of the underlying systemic disease, reduction of blood pressure is of importance. Good results are achieved with calcium antagonists, such as amlodipine at the dosage of 0.625–1.25 mg per cat daily, and 0.1–0.2 mg/kg daily in dogs. If the pressure reduction is insufficient, amlodipine can be combined with angiotensin converting enzyme (ACE) inhibitors, such as benazepril, enalpril, or captopril at a dosage of 0.5 mg/kg daily. Alternatively, amlodipine may be combined with a β-blocker, such as atenolol at a dosage of 0.5 mg per cat daily.

Prognosis: With this treatment strategy, the animal's blood pressure can be maintained within physiologic values in most cases. The retina eventually reattaches, however, the prognosis for return of vision is usually poor.

14.17 Non-hereditary degenerative abnormalities

Local or generalized retinal degeneration can also occur without a hereditary factor or an exogenous agent playing an apparent role. The generalized forms can have the appearance of a degeneration: (1) beginning in the central area with the cones (see, for example, taurine deficiency: 14.13.3), or (2) a more diffuse picture of rod or rod-cone dysplasia and/or atrophy (see 14.9).

14.17.1 Feline central retinal degeneration (FCRD)

The clinical picture of this abnormality is almost identical to that of taurine deficiency with the exception of the progression. FCRD should progress less rapidly; however, one can question whether FCRD is really another (idiopathic) abnormality or whether it is a non-recognized form of taurine deficiency. If this is indeed the case, some of the commercial cat foods must be deficient in taurine or there must be cats that have an inadequate ability to metabolize taurine.[78]

In the differential diagnosis, the clinician must yet again elicit the cause of the observed degeneration and must try to confirm the diagnosis by means of a directed anamnesis and additional examinations (including genetic ones).

14.18 Papilledema

Papilledema is a sporadically occurring edematous swelling of the papilla without symptoms of a preceding inflammation of the optic nerve or parts of the rest of the fundus. The abnormality is probably caused by lymphatic obstruction in the papilla or by brain lesions such as pituitary or other central nervous system neoplasms.

Symptoms: The papilla is swollen, pinker than usual, and bulges out more into the vitreous (visible by binocular indirect ophthalmoscopy and by examination with a fundus contact lens). The vessels can be bent at the edge of the papilla and be swollen and wrinkled. The pupillary reflexes are disturbed, there may be mydriasis, and sometimes there are visual disturbances. Affected animals are, however, usually presented in connection with neurological deficits and balance disturbances. These signs can be bilateral, especially in processes close to the optic chiasm.

In the differential diagnosis, it is often difficult to differentiate papilledema from papillitis. With papilledema, however, there are no indications of inflammation such as peripapillary exudate, cellular infiltration, and bleeding. These patients will usually be referred for additional examinations such as ultrasonography, optic thecography, brain scintigraphy, CT, or MRI.

Therapy / prognosis: Therapy and prognosis both depend on the underlying cause. If no cause can be confirmed, general anti-inflammatory treatment can be considered (see 14.19).

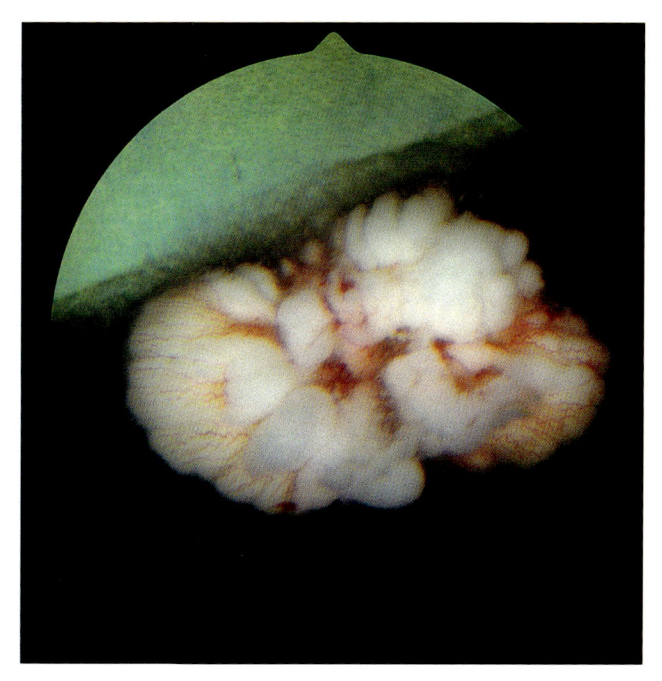

Plate 14.29:
Severely changed optic disc in a horse with bilateral proliferative opticus neuropathy (OD). The horse was completely blind.

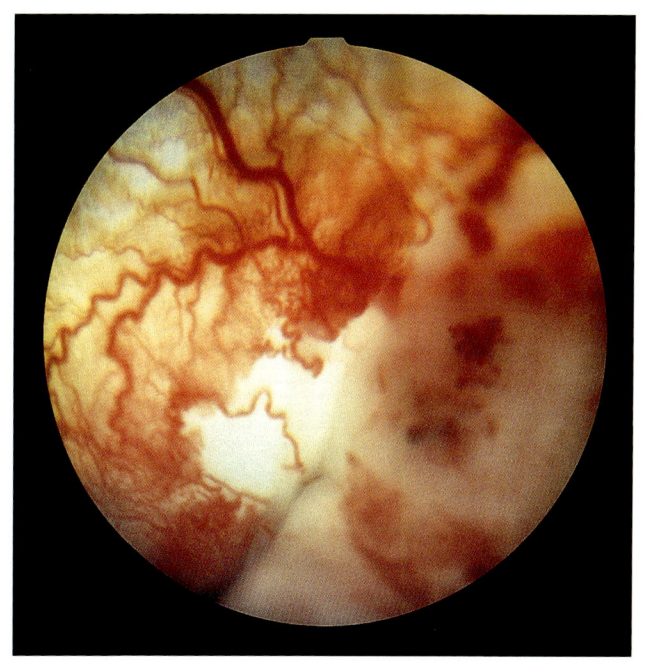

Plate 14.30:
Totally abnormal fundus. Highly abnormal optic papilla and abnormal vessels, retinal detachment and a large pink lesion peripheral to the papilla in a dog (see also Plate 14.31).

14.19 Papillitis, optic neuritis

This is an inflammation of the papilla and/or the optic nerve. It can be due to local infectious or non-infectious causes (see 12.10 and 14.14), but it can also be a sign of brain abnormalities associated with increased pressure (tissue or cerebrospinal fluid).

Papillitis/optic neuritis is almost always associated with a severe decrease in vision or complete blindness in the affected eye and a dilated pupil that is insensitive to light. The papilla is edematous, swollen, bulges out into the vitreous (sometimes several diopters), is hazy, not sharply outlined, glassy or pinkish-red, or hyperemic. Flecks of cellular infiltrates or hemorrhages can be seen in or around the papilla. The inflammation can easily extend to the retina in the area around the papilla (see 14.14). Unfortunately, the abnormalities can also be located in the optic nerve just behind the papilla. These patients must usually be referred for additional examinations (see 14.21). An ERG can be helpful to differentiate between a retinopathy and a retrobulbar neuritis of the optic nerve.

Therapy: Treatment consists of immediate administration of large doses of prednisolone (2–5 mg/kg, once daily, P.O. or, if necessary, I.V. dexamethasone), followed by decreasing dosages. If there are indications of an infectious cause, chloramphenicol (110 mg/kg/daily I.V./P.O.) or a "specific choice" antibiotic at the recommended therapeutic dose should be administered. If there is a positive response to treatment (disappearance of signs within 2–7 days), the corticosteroids should be continued and monitored for a prolonged period (months).

Prognosis: The prognosis is reasonably favorable if there is a response to treatment, although the occurrence of a brain neoplasm as an underlying cause still cannot be excluded with certainty. If there is no improvement, the medications can be decreased and withdrawn more quickly. The prognosis for vision is then usually hopeless and the likelihood of a life-threatening cause is clearly increased.

14.20 Neoplasia

Primary neoplasms (Plates 14.29–31) in the fundus are very rare, but malignant lymphoma/leukemia occurs regularly and there are exceptional cases of metastasis of neoplasms (for example, adenocarcinomas) from other locations. The fundus changes in leukemia/FeLV are usually limited to signs of severe inflammation, such as exudates, hemorrhage, and retinal detachment. Clearly delineated neoplastic growths in these cases are exceptional.[79] In contrast to human, melanomas in the fundus are very rare in animals.[80-84]

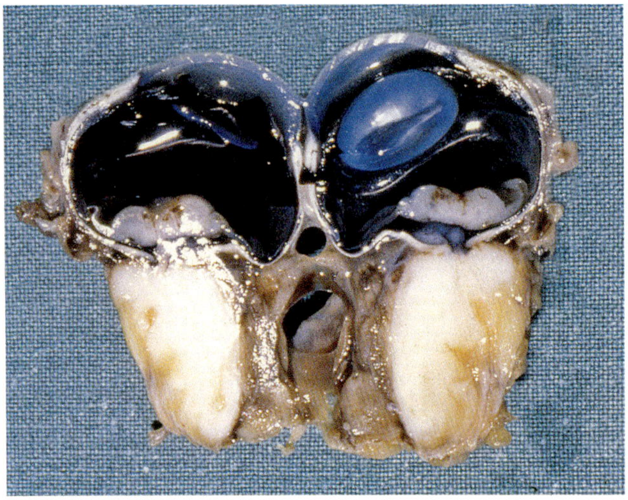

Plate 14.31:
Same eye as in Plate 14.30, after exenteration of the orbit. Neurofibroma in and behind the bulbus.

When there are unexplained retinal hemorrhages, inflammation, or absolute glaucoma, neoplastic causes should be considered (including metastasis from other sites). Such patients should usually be referred for additional examinations such as ultrasonography, optic thecography, brain scintigraphy, CT, or MRI. Unfortunately, the final diagnosis can often be only confirmed on pathologic examination.

14.21 Amblyopia / amaurosis

Amblyopia can be described as poor vision, amaurosis as blindness, without abnormalities being found on ophthalmoscopic examination. Amblyopia/amaurosis can, for example, be due to temporary occlusion of vessels near the eye and/or the brain, or cranial nerve (CN II), or brain abnormalities associated with loss of function.

Sudden onset, total blindness is almost always recognized by the owner. Amblyopia is often recognized only as a slight change in behavior. The clinician sometimes finds dilated, light-insensitive pupils. The animal may have a staring expression and a confused and anxious behavior.

Diagnosis: Diagnosis can sometimes be confirmed by ERG, VEPs, angiography, or other brain examinations.

In particular, the differential diagnosis must include abnormalities such as SARD (14.21.1) emboli, dysautonomia (see 12.12), hepatoencephalopathy, or other brain abnormalities.

Therapy: Treatment as for papillitis/optic neuritis can be considered.

Prognosis: The prognosis for recovery depends on the response to treatment of the underlying abnormalities.

14.21.1 Sudden acquired retinal degeneration (SARD).

SARD, or toxic neuroretinopathy, is a rare abnormality that is characterized by mydriasis and a sudden loss of vision without direct indication of fundus abnormalities (amaurosis).[85] Eventually after one to several months, retinal degeneration occurs. The ERG is completely flat in this disorder. There are indications that subclinical liver abnormalities and hyperadrenocorticism can play a role in this disorder.[86–88]

Literature

1. KOCH, S.A. & RUBIN, L.F.: Distribution of cones in retina of the normal dog. Am. J. Vet. Res. **33**: 361, 1972.

2. STEINBERG, R.H., REID, M. & LACY, P.L.: The distribution of rods and cones in the retina of the cat (*Felis domesticus*). J. Comp. Neurol. **148**: 229, 1973.

3. NEITZ, Y., GEIST, T. & JACOBS, G.H.: Color vision in the dog. Vis. Neurosci. **3**: 119–125, 1989.

4. LOOP, M.S., BRUCE, L.L. & PETUCHOWSKI, L.: Cat color vision: effects of stimulus size, shape and viewing distance. Vision Res. **19**: 507, 1979.

5. MARTIN, G.R., GORDON, I.E., & CADLE, D.R.: Electroretinographically determined spectral sensitivity in the tawny owl (*Strix aluco*). J. Comp. Physiol. Psychol. **89**: 72, 1975.

6. KOLB, H. & FAMIGLIETTI, E.V.: Rod and cone pathways in the inner plexiform layer of cat retina. Science. **186**: 47, 1974.

7. BRIDGES, C.D.B.: Retinoids in photosensitive systems. In: The retinoids, 5th ed. Eds.: M.B. Sporn, A.B. Roberts & D. Goodman. New York, Academic Press, 1984.

8. AGUIRRE, G.D. & RUBIN, L.F.: The electroretinogram in dogs with inherited cone degeneration. Invest. Ophthalmol. Vis. Sci. **14**: 840, 1975.

9. SPIESS, B.: Elektrophysiologische Untersuchungen des Auges bei Hund und Katze. Stuttgart: Enke Copythek. 351, 1994.

10. SIMS, M.H. & LAREATTA, L.J.: Visual-evoked potentials in cats, using a light-emitting diode stimulator. Am. J. Vet. Res. **49**: 1876, 1988.

11. LECOUTEUR, R.A. et al.: Indirect imaging of the canine optic nerve, using metrizamide (optic thecography). Am. J. Vet. Res. **43**: 142, 1982.

12. ROBERTSON, T.W., HICKEY, T.L. & GUILLERY, R.W.: Development of the dorsal lateral geniculate nucleus in normal and visually deprived Siamese cats. J. Comp. Neurol. **191**: 573, 1980.

13. ROBERTSON, T.W., HICKEY, T.L. & GUILLERY, R.W.: Development of the dorsal lateral geniculate nucleus in normal and visually deprived Siamese cats. J. Comp. Neurol. **191**: 573, 1980.

14. KALILK, R.E., JHAVERI, S.R. & RICHARDS, W.: Anomalous retinal pathways in the Siamese cat: An inadequate substrate for normal binocular vision. Science **174**: 302, 1971.

15. ISKANDAR, L.A., SAMUELSON, D.A. & WHITLEY, R.D.: The pecten and the posterior circulation in the avian eye. Invest. Ophthalmol. Vis. Sci. (Suppl.) **29**: 381, 1988.

16. ENGERMANN, R.L., MOLITOR, D.L. & BLOODWORTH, J.M.B.: Vascular system of the dog retina: Light and electron microscopic studies. Exp. Eye Res. **5**: 296, 1966.

17. PSCHYREMBEL, W.: Klinisches Wörterbuch. 254th ed. Berlin, W. de Gruyter, 1982.

18. GELATT, K.N. & VEITH, L.A.: Heredity multiple ocular anomalies in Australian Shepherd dogs. Vet. Small Anim. Clin. **65**: 39, 1970.

19. KERN, T.J. & RIIS, R.L.: Optic nerve hypoplasia in three Miniature Poodles. JAVMA **178**: 49, 1981.

20. SPIESS, B., LITSCHI, B., LEBER-ZÜRCHER, A.C. & STELZER, S.: Bilaterale Hypoplasie der Nervi optici bei einem Pudelwelpen. Kleintierpraxis **36**: 173, 1991.

21. MACMILLAN, A.D. & LIPTON, D.E.: Heritability of multifocal retinal dysplasia in American Cocker Spaniels. JAVMA **172**: 568, 1978.

22. BEDFORD, P.G.C.: Multifocal retinal dysplasia in the Rottweiler. Vet. Rec. **111**: 304, 1982.

23. HEYWOOD, R. & WELLS, G.A.H.: A retinal dysplasia in the Beagle dog. Vet. Rec. **87**: 178, 1970.

24. LAVACH J.D., MURPHY, J.M. & SEVERIN, G.A.: Retinal dysplasia in the English Springer Spaniel. JAAHA **14**: 192, 1978.

25. RUBIN, L.F.: Heredity of retinal dysplasia in Bedlington Terriers. JAVMA **152**: 260, 1968.

26. STADES, F.C.: Hereditary retinal dysplasia (RD) in a family of Yorkshire Terriers. Tijdschr. Diergeneek. **103**: 1087, 1979.

27. BARNETT, K.C., BJORCK, G.R. & KOCK, E.: Hereditary retinal dysplasia in the Labrador Retriever in England and Sweden. J. Small Anim. Pract. **10**: 755, 1970

28. CARRIG, C.B., SPONENBERG, D.P., SCHMIDT, G.M. & TVEDTEN, H.W.: Retinal dysplasia associated with skeletal abnormalities in Labrador Retrievers. JAVMA **170**: 49, 1977.

29. DONOVAN, E.F. & WYMAN, M.: Ocular fundus anomaly in the Collie. JAVMA **148**: 1465, 1965.

30. FREEMAN, H.M., DONOVAN, R.H. & SCHEPENS, C.L.: Retinal detachment, chorioretinal changes and staphyloma in the Collie. I. Ophthalmoscopic findings. Arch. Ophthalmol. **76**: 412, 1966.

31. BARNETT, K.C. & STADES, F.C.: Collie eye anomaly in the Shetland Sheepdog in The Netherlands. J. Small Anim. Pract. **20**: 321, 1979.

32. WALLIN-HAKANSON, B., WALLIN-HAKANSON, N. & HEDHAMMER, A.: Collie eye anomaly in the Rough Collie in Sweden: genetic transmission and influence on offspring vitality. J. Small Anim. Pract. **41**: 254, 2003.

33. STADES, F.C. & BARNETT, K.C.: Collie eye anomaly in the Netherlands. Vet. Quart. **3**: 66, 1981.

34. KOPPANG, N.: Neuronal ceroid lipofuscinosis in English Setters. J. Small Anim. Pract. **10**: 639, 1970.

35. AGUIRRE, G.D., STRAMM, L. & HASKINS, M.: Animal models of metabolic eye diseases. *In*: Goldberg's genetic and metabolic eye diseases, 2nd ed. Ed.: W.A. Renie. Boston, Little Brown, 1986.

36. MAGNUSSON, H.: Über Retinitis Pigmentosa und Konsanquinita beim Hunde. Arch. Verg. Ophthalmol. **2**: 147, 1911.

37. AGUIRRE, G.D. & RUBIN, L.F.: Rod-cone dysplasia (progressive retinal atrophy) in Irish Setters, JAVMA **166**: 157, 1975.

38. AGUIRRE, G.D. & RUBIN, L.F.: The early diagnosis of rod dysplasia in the Norwegian Elkhound. JAVMA **159**: 429, 1971.

39. AGUIRRE, G.D. & RUBIN, L.F.: Progressive retinal atrophy in the Miniature Poodle: An electrophysiologic study. JAVMA **160**: 191, 1972.

40. STADES, F.C., BOEVÉ, M.H. et al.: Praktijkgerichte oogheelkunde voor de dierenarts. Hannover, Schlütersche Verlag, pp. 181, 1996

41. AGUIRRE, G.D. & ACLAND, G.: Progressive retinal atrophy in the English Cocker Spaniel. Trans. Am. Coll. Vet. Ophthalmol. **14**: 104, 1983.

42. BARNETT, K.C. & CURTIS, R.: Lens luxation and progressive retinal atrophy in the Tibetan Terrier. Vet. Rec. **103**: 160, 1978.

43. AGUIRRE, G.D. & ACLAND, G.: Progressive retinal atrophy in the Labrador Retriever is a progressive rod-cone degeneration (PRCD). Trans. Coll. Vet. Ophthalmol. **20**: 150, 1989.

44. NARFSTRÖM, K.: Progressive retinal atrophy in the Abyssinian cat: Clinical characteristics. Invest. Ophthalmol. Vis. Sci. **26**: 193, 1985.

45. CURTIS, R., BARNETT, K.C. & LEON, A.: An early-onset retinal dystrophy with dominant inheritance in the Abyssinian cat. Invest. Ophthalmol. Vis. Sci. **28**: 131, 1987.

46. DJAJADININGRAT-LAANEN, S.C., BOEVÉ, M.H., STADES, F.C. & OOST, B.A. VAN: Familial non-*rcd1* generalised retinal degeneration in Irish setter dogs. J. Small Anim. Pract. **44**: 113, 2003.

47. ACLAND, G.M., BLANTON S.H. et al.: XLPRA: a canine retinal degeneration inherited as an X-linked trait. Am. J. Med. Gen. **52**(1): 27, 1994.

48. ZEISS, C.J., RAY K. *et al.*: Mapping of X-linked progressive retinal atrophy (XLPRA), the canine homolog of retinitis pigmentosa 3 (RP3). Human Mol. Gen. **9**(4): 531, 2000.

49. AGUIRRE, G.D. *et al.*: Rod-cone dysplasia in Irish setters: A cyclic GMP metabolic defect of visual cells. Science **201**: 1133, 1978.

50. NARFSTROM, K.: Progressive retinal atrophy in the Abyssinian cat. Clinical characteristics. Invest. Ophthalmol. Vis. Sci. **26**(2): 193, 1985.

51. AGUIRRE, G., ALLIGOOD, J. *et al.*: Pathogenesis of progressive rod-cone degeneration in miniature poodles. Invest. Ophthalmol. Vis. Sci. **23**(5): 610, 1982.

52. NARFSTROM, K. & NILSSON S.E.: Progressive retinal atrophy in the Abyssinian cat. Electron microscopy. Invest. Ophthalmol. Vis. Sci. **27**(11): 1569, 1986.

53. NARFSTROM, K., KATZ, M.L. *et al.*: In vivo gene therapy in young and adult RPE65-/- dogs produces long-term visual improvement. J. Heredity **94**(1): 31, 2003.

54. NARFSTRÖM, K. WRIGSTAD, A. & NILSON, S.E.: The Briard dog: A new animal model of congenital stationary night blindness. Br. J. Ophthalmol. **73**: 750, 1989.

55. AGUIRRE, G.D. & RUBIN, L.F.: Pathology of hemeralopia in the Alaskan malamute dog. Invest. Ophthalmol. Vis. Sci. **13**: 231, 1974.

56. BEDFORD, P.G.C.: Retinal pigment epithelial dystrophy (CPRA): A study of the disease in the Briard. J. Small Anim. Pract. **25**: 129, 1984.

57. WATSON, P. & BEDFORD, P.G.C.: Retinal pigment epithelial dystrophy: histological and biochemical aspects. Symposium on retinal degenerations in dogs with focus on PRA und CPRA. Transactions Eur. Soc. Vet. Ophthalmol., Uppsala, 1993.

58. WYMAN, M. & MCKISSICK, G.E.: Lipemia retinalis in a dog and a cat: Case reports. JAAHA **9**: 288, 1973.

59. GELATT, K.N., WOERDT, A. VAN DER *et al.*: Enrofloxacin-associated retinal degeneration in cats. Vet. Ophthalmol. **4**: 99, 2001.

60. WIEBE, V. & HAMILTON, P.: Fluoroquinolone-induced retinal degeneration in cats. JAVMA. **221**: 1568, 2002.

61. HAYES, K.C., ROUSSEAU, J.E. & HEGSTED, D.M.: Plasma tocopherol concentration and vitamin E deficiency in dogs. JAAHA **157**: 64, 1970.

62. PAULSEN, M.E., JOHNSON L. *et al.*: Blindness and sexual dimorphism associated with vitamin A deficiency in feedlot cattle. JAVMA. **194**(7): 933, 1989.

63. RIIS, R.C., SHEFFY, B.E., LOEW, E., KERN, T.J. & SMITH, J.S.: Vitamin E deficiency retinopathy in dogs. Am. J. Vet. Res. **42**: 74, 1981.

64. HAYES, K.C., CAREY, R.E. & SCHMIDT, Y.: Retinal degeneration associated with taurine deficiency in the cat. Science **188**: 949, 1975.

65. AGUIRRE, G.D.: Retinal degeneration associated with the feeding of dog foods to cats. JAVMA **172**: 791, 1978.

66. PARRY, H.B.: Degenerations of the dog retina. IV. Retinopathies associated with dog distemper-complex virus infections. Br. J. Ophthalmol. **38**: 295, 1954.

67. CELLO, R.M. & HUTCHERSON, D.: Ocular changes in malignant lymphoma of dogs. Cornell Vet. **55**: 492, 1962.

68. KURTZ, H.J. & FINCO, D.R.: Granulomatous chorioretinitis caused by *Cryptococcus neoformans* in a dog. JAVMA **157**: 934, 1970.

69. GEISER, C.A., THIEL, J. & CASHELL, I.G.: Visceral leishmaniasis in a dog imported into the United States. Am. J. Trop. Med. Hyg. **6**: 227, 1957.

70. DZIEZYC, J., WOLF, E.D. & BARRIE, K.P.: Surgical repair of rhegmatogenous retinal detachments in dogs. JAVMA **188**: 902, 1986.

71. PIZZIRANI, S., DAVIDSON M.G. & GILGER B.C.: Transpupillary diode laser retinopexy in dogs: ophthalmoscopic, fluorescein angiographic and histopathologic study. Vet. Ophthalmol. **6**(3): 227, 2003.

72. VAINISI, S.J. & PACKO, K.H.: Management of giant retinal tears in dogs. JAVMA **206**(4): 491, 1995.

73. SULLIVAN, T.C.: Surgery for retinal detachment. Vet. Clin. North Am. Small Anim. Pract. **27**(5): 1193, 1997.

74. DZIEZYC, J., WOLF, E.D. & BARRIE, K.P.: Surgical repair of rhegmatogenous retinal detachments in dogs. JAVMA **189**(8): 902, 1986.

75. STILES, J., POLZIN, D.J. & BISTNER, S.I.: The prevalence of retinopathy in cats with systemic hypertension and chronic renal failure or hyperthyroidism. JAAHA **30**(6): 564, 1994.

76. CRISPIN, S.M. & MOULD, J.R.: Systemic hypertensive disease and the feline fundus. Vet. Ophthalmol. **4**(2): 131, 2001.

77. STILES, J.: Ocular manifestations of systemic disease. Part 2: The cat. *In:* Veterinary Ophthalmology, Ed.: K.N., Gelatt. Philadelphia, Lippincott Williams & Wilkins, 1999.

78. BELLHORN, R.W. & FISCHER, C.A.: Feline central retinal degeneration. JAVMA **157**: 842, 1970.

79. SAUNDERS, L.Z., BISTNER, S.I. & RUBIN, L.F.: Proliferative optic neuropathy in horses. Vet. Pathol. **9**: 368, 1972.

80. HYMAN, J.A., KOCH, S.A. & WILCOCK, B.P.: Canine choroidal melanoma with metastases. Vet. Ophthalmol. **5**(2): 113, 2002.

81. MORGAN, R.V. & PATTON, C.S.: Choroidal melanoma in a dog. Cornell Vet. **83**(3): 211–7, 1993.

82. SCHOSTER, J.V., DUBIELZIG, R.R. & SULLIVAN, L.: Choroidal melanoma in a dog. JAVMA **203**(1): 89, 1993.

83. RICHTER, M. *et al.*: Myxosarcoma in the eye and brain in a dog. Vet. Ophthalmol. **6**(3): 183–9, 2003.

84. ALLGOEWER, I., FRIELING, E., FRITSCHE, J., SCHEMMEL, U. & SCHÄFFER, E.H.: Canine choroidal melanoma. Kleintierpraxis **45**(5): 361, 2000.

85. ACLAND, G.M. *et al.*: Sudden acquired retinal degeneration in the dog: clinical and morphologic characterization of the "silent retina" syndrome. Trans. Am. Coll. Vet. Ophthalmol. **15:** 86, 1984

86. VENTER, I.J. & PETRICK S.W.: Acute blindness in a dog caused by sudden acquired retinal degeneration. J. S. Afr. Vet. Assoc. **66**(1): 32, 1995.

87. ACLAND, G., IRBY, N.L. & AGUIRRE, G.D.: Sudden acquired retinal degeneration in the dog: clinical and morphologic characterization of the "silent retina" syndrome. Trans. Am. Coll. Vet. Ophthalmol. **15:** 86, 1984.

88. ACLAND, G. & AGUIRRE, G.D.: Sudden acquired retinal degeneration: clinical signs and diagnosis. Trans. Am. Coll. Vet. Ophthalmol. **17:** 58, 1986.

15 Breed Predispositions and Hereditary Eye Diseases

15.1 Introduction

During routine examinations, particularly of young animals, the clinician may be confronted with eye abnormalities which are presumed or are known to have a genetic cause. In addition to the eventual treatment of the patient, it is important for the owner, the breeder, and the breed association to know what the consequences are for the affected animal, its littermates, its parents, and the breed population (prognosis, whether or not to use the animals for breeding, spreading within the population, etc.).

Inherited abnormalities are in general caused by one or more "abnormal" genes (mutations) in the inheritance pattern (genotype) of the animal. These abnormal factors (also called alleles, defined as any alternative form of a gene responsible for a specific phenotype that can occupy a particular homolog chromosomal locus) are often suppressed or influenced by the rest of the genes of the animal (rest genotype). There are also influences from non-inheritable factors in the environment; for example, the food or housing. The genes and the environment together determine the individual's ultimate appearance (phenotype).

Half of the genes of an individual are received from one parent and half from the other. The number of abnormal genes and the manner in which they are transmitted lead to certain patterns of inheritance. Once the pattern of inheritance is known or presumed, most affected animals and also, eventually, the carriers can be detected. Moreover, then it is often possible to determine the means by which the disease can be eradicated.

It also should be noted that a disease which has a simple mode of inheritance (especially dominant) can generally be eliminated more efficiently than a disease that has a multiple mode of transmission.

15.2 Modes of inheritance

15.2.1 Simple inheritance

In this mode of inheritance only one gene plays a role in transmitting the disease. This gene can be expressed in a number of ways.

15.2.1.1 Autosomal dominant (not sex-linked)

In this mode of inheritance, the disease is caused by a gene mutation (D) that suppresses or is dominant over the corresponding gene for the normal characteristic. The gene for the normal characteristic that is suppressed is called the recessive gene (d). If the animal receives the "D" gene from both parents, then it has the genotype "DD" and will show the disease (affected). If the animal receives the "D" gene from one parent (this parent must therefore have the "D" gene itself) and the "d" gene from the other parent, its genotype is "Dd" and it will also show the abnormality. If the animal is "dd", it is normal and does not inherit the abnormality. Diseases with complete simple dominant inheritance occur, unfortunately, only sporadically. Unfortunate, because in these diseases the carriers are also directly recognizable and thus prevention of the disease by means of breeding rules is greatly simplified. These types of diseases will present in every generation, and genotypically affected animals will also be phenotypically affected. Exclusion of all affected animals from breeding will eliminate the disease.

15.2.1.2 Autosomal recessive (not sex-linked)

In this mode of inheritance, the disease is caused by a gene mutation that is only expressed if it is homozygous, that is both parents contribute the same gene so that it is not suppressed by the corresponding dominant gene. An animal free of the inheritance thus has the genotype "RR" and an animal phenotypically affected by the inheritance has the genotype "rr". If an animal has the genotype "Rr", the expression of the disease will be suppressed but the animal is a carrier (see Fig. 15.1). Unfortunately, carriers can seldomly be recognized and usually only become known because they are offspring of an affected animal or because they have affected offspring. However, DNA testing is now becoming more and more available for (eye) diseases. With this type of tool, not only the affected, but also the carriers can be recognized by using blood tests, for example. The best examples of this mode of inheritance are most types of hereditary retinal degeneration or PRA.[1]

15.2.1.3 Sex-linked inheritance

In this rare mode of inheritance, the gene is located on one or both of the X-chromosomes or on the Y-chromosome. In the X-linked, recessive mode of inheritance, only males will be phenotypically affected, because females will only show the illness if they are homozygous for the disease, and homozygosity is less frequent. An example of a disease with such an inheritance is hemophilia in humans. In the X-linked, dominant mode of inheritance, females are also phenotypically affected. Males, however, will pass the gene to their daughters but not to their sons. An example of a disease with such an X-linked inheritance in animals is the X-PRA in the Siberian Husky.[2]

15.2.1.4 Incomplete recessive or dominant, or incomplete penetrance

In these more complex, but far more frequently occurring, modes of inheritance, the disease can be transmitted by a dominant or recessive gene, but the rest genotype causes a suppression of the gene expression or the gene does not penetrate fully.[3] Because of this, the disease cannot be expressed or it is expressed only in a mild form or with variable signs. An example of a disease with such an incomplete dominant penetrance is PHTVL/PHPV.

15.2.2 Multiple (polygenic) transmission

In this mode of inheritance more genes play a role and often the external circumstances (environment) play a role such that the pattern of inheritance is no longer recognizable. Such diseases can often only be eliminated by examining the offspring for the abnormality. For this purpose, it is best to breed parents that have had on average the best offspring. Examples of such a disease are entropion and hip dysplasia in the dog and other species.

15.3 Is the abnormality inherited?[4]

Especially in numerically small breeds, but also in large numbered breeds in which, for example, one champion has been used excessively for breeding, it is of great importance to detect possible hereditary abnormalities at an early stage and to try to prevent these from becoming spread throughout the population. It is difficult to confirm that an abnormality in an individual is hereditary when there are no known offspring with the abnormality. It is sometimes possible to determine whether or not a disease is inheritable by the examination of chromosomes, by means of gene detection at the DNA level, or by means of parts of DNA that are specifically related to the abnormality (markers). In 1994, the first disease-associated gene, the gene for PRA (rod-cone dysplasia), was isolated in the Irish Setter.[5] Since then, a long list of mutations or markers has been identified. Actual lists can be found on the internet, e.g. *www.optigen.com, www.aht.org.uk* etc.

If there is no gene test available, such abnormalities can only be detected by the use of test crossings. Test matings are, however, not always possible, not always necessary, and certainly not always desirable. They can be helpful in abnormalities which can be confirmed at an early age and which, if affected animals are born, do not cause an unethical and unbearable amount of discomfort for the animal (for example, Collie eye anomaly). Test matings are difficult if not impossible to perform if the abnormality only becomes apparent in older animals or if animals with the abnormality are infertile. Test matings should in general only be carried out under the supervision of a geneticist. However, unintentional test matings have sometimes occurred. Such unintentional test matings must be searched for in the genealogic family tree, since they can provide a great deal of information about the possibility of inheritance of the disease and the mode of transmission. In addition, examination of all offspring for the purpose of detecting and preventing the abnormality is of utmost impor-

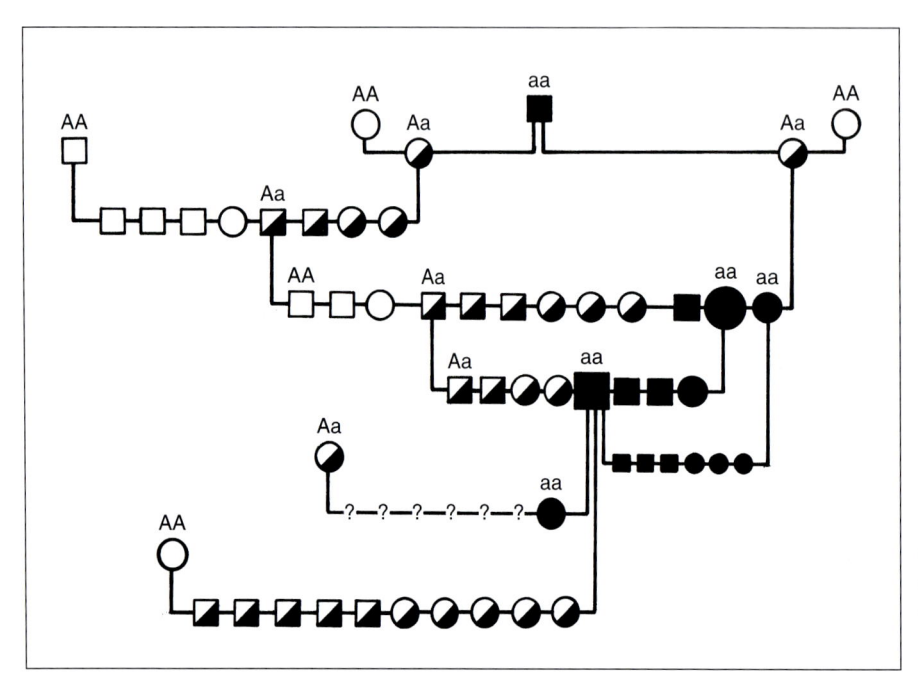

Fig. 15.1:
Genealogic family tree or relation diagram of a family having a simple recessive inherited abnormality (aa; e.g. PRA). Aa are carriers (heterozygotes) and AA hereditarily free (homozygote, dominant) animals.

tance. This is especially true in polygenic inherited abnormalities because the other techniques of detection generally provide less clear information.

If an inherited disease is suspected, the first step is to determine whether anything is known about the occurrence of the abnormality in the species and especially the breed concerned. For this purpose, advice should be sought from publications, such as by RUBIN,[6] or the American College of Veterinary Ophthalmologists (ACVO).[7] An inquiry on the internet may also be very helpful. Moreover, the registration center of the national program for prevention of inherited eye diseases or a member of its research panel can provide invaluable information. In addition, it is necessary to examine closely the parents and littermates for the presence of even mild forms of the abnormality. If one is unable or inadequately equipped to carry out further examinations, efforts should be made at least to motivate the owner or breeder to have the examinations performed and to make arrangements for them. The breeder can help by preparing a genealogic family tree of the affected animal (proband) and its immediate family. This family tree should include at least the brothers and sisters, the parents and their brothers and sisters, and any offspring of the proband.

The affected animals, the unaffected animals that have been examined, and those which have not been examined (living in other countries or dead, with the cause of death if known, etc.) are included in this family tree. In contrast to the type of family tree usually used by breeders, which only gives the direct line from ancestors to the proband, in this type of family tree it is far easier to see if there might be an inherited disorder. It is also much easier to see whether unintentional, but very informative, test matings have taken place.

Most inherited diseases have a recessive or polygenic mode of inheritance. The very slow decrease of the gene frequency for a disease if only the phenotypically affected animals are excluded from breeding, is shown in Fig. 15.2. Furthermore, the identification and the exclusion, or the limited use of carriers from breeding is important. DNA-identified carriers can be bred to DNA-identified unaffected animals, as long as all the resulting progeny is DNA tested. If no DNA test is available, family tree studies have to be used to identify the carriers. In a recessive disease, parents are carriers and siblings have a 66% chance of being a carrier.

Trying to "breed out" an abnormality by crossing the parents with animals from an unaffected line must be discouraged. This does not eliminate an inherited abnormality but instead camouflages it. It then remains concealed until it has been spread through the population and a large number of animals carry the gene. Then the elimination of the abnormality is more difficult, time-consuming, costly, and sometimes even impossible.

It remains, therefore, safer to try to detect monogenic inheritance by means of test matings. When an autosomal recessive mode is expected, the most efficient form of test mating is to cross the suspected carrier with an affected animal from the same breed. At least 5–7 offspring, all free of the disease, are needed to be able to state with 95–97.5% certainty that the tested animal is "hereditarily free" of the disease (note that all of their offspring will at least be carriers). A second possibility is to cross the suspected carrier with a parent or brother or sister. In this case at least 11–12 offspring, none of which are affected, are needed to conclude that the tested animal is "hereditarily free" of the disorder.

If the mode of inheritance is dominant with incomplete penetrance or polygenic, one test mating provides less adequate information. In such cases, more extensive progeny testing or other diagnostic methods must be used.

If adequate information cannot be obtained to indicate or suggest the possible inheritance of an abnormality, the breeder or owner should assume that the abnormality is inherited until confirmation is obtained that it is not. Until then, the animal should not be used for breeding.

Whether or not test matings are carried out or animals are excluded from breeding, it is strongly recommended that the information which has been obtained be reported to the supervising organization and the breed association.

The advantages of DNA testing are enormous. The breeder will be able to identify the status of his animals for the

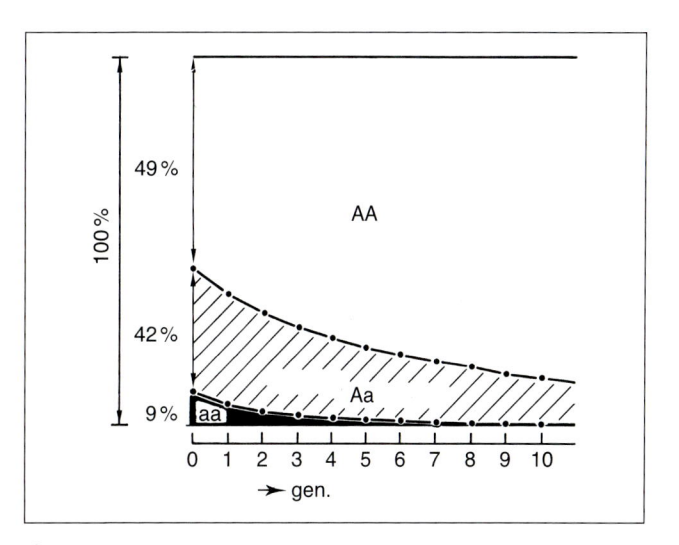

Fig. 15.2:
The theoretical effect (Hardy & Weinberg law, in a closed population and with at random matings) of selection against a simple recessive inherited abnormality, in which the affected animals are excluded from breeding. Started with 9 % affected (aa). Aa: carriers; AA: hereditarily unaffected animals; (gen. = generations).

disease and this also long before the disease becomes clinically apparent. In this way, the breeder can prevent the production of affected offspring from, in other respects, worthwhile (carrier) breeding stock. It may also be possible to eliminate certain diseases within several generations. At the moment, this is only true for the mutation tests. In marker tests, DNA polymorphism is identified near the mutation, which is presumed to be inherited together with the mutation.

The DNA tests are for one specific gene mutation (or marker). If more than one gene is involved in a disease, then all the separate mutations have to be identified individually.

The more dogs are examined, the more data about variations become available. For example, one must be aware that not every retinal degeneration is PRA, that there are different types of PRA even within one breed, and there are breed-specific genes for the same disease. Thus gene testing cannot (yet) replace clinical diagnosis. Moreover, the research in this field and the DNA testing itself is costly. For example, it has taken a very long time and high costs to identify the recently found PRA mutation in the Entlebuch Cattle Dog (*www.optigen.com*).[8]

15.4 Breed predispositions and inherited eye abnormalities

Note: Predisposed breeds and the frequencies of their hereditary abnormalities can differ between countries or regions. For information about their local circumstances, the practitioner should contact local members of the hereditary eye diseases schemes.

Since the end of 2004, a DNA test is also available for CEA choroidal hypoplasia in Rough und Smooth Collies, Shetland Sheepdog, Border Collie, Australian Shepherd and Lancashire Heeler. Now genotypically unaffected, affected and carriers can be identified, thus providing tools for breeders to decrease the frequency of the disease within these breeds. In addition, DNA tests for cataract in the Staffordshire Bull and the Boston Terrier are now available.

Nowadays DNA tests are available for a long list of breeds (see below; for further information see *www.optigen.com* and *www.aht.org.uk,* etc.).

List of DNA tests for hereditary eye diseases (June 2006):

- American Cocker Spaniel: *prcd*-PRA
- American Eskimo Dog: *prcd*-PRA
- Australian (stumpy tail) Cattle Dog: *prcd*-PRA
- Australian Shepherds: CEA/CH
- Border Collie: CEA/CH
- Boston Terrier: *juvenile cataract*
- Briard: CSNB (congenital stationary night blindness)
- Bullmastiff: dominant PRA
- Cardigan Welsh Corgi: rcd3-PRA (rod/cone degeneration Type 3: PDE6A gene)
- Chesapeake Bay Retriever: *prcd*-PRA
- Chinese Crested: *prcd*-PRA
- Collies: CEA/CH
- English Cocker Spaniel: *prcd*-PRA
- Entlebuch Cattle dog: *prcd*-PRA
- Finnish Lapland Hound: *prcd*-PRA
- Irish Setter and Irish Red & White Setter: rcd1-PRA (*rod/cone degeneration Type 1*)
- Labrador Retriever: *prcd*-PRA
- Lancashire Heeler: CEA/CH
- Mastiff: dominant PRA
- Miniature Poodle: *prcd*-PRA
- Miniature Schnauzer: Type A PRA (progressive retinal degeneration Type A)
- Nova Scotia Duck Tolling Retriever: *prcd*-PRA
- Portuguese Water Dog: *prcd*-PRA
- Samoyed: XL PRA (*X-linked PRA*)
- Schapendoes: PRA marker
- Shetland Sheepdog: CEA/CH
- Siberian Husky: XL-PRA (*X-linked PRA*)
- Sloughi: rcd1a-PRA (rod/cone degeneration Type 1a; PED6B gene)
- Staffordshire Bull Terrier: *juvenile cataract*
- Toy Poodle: *prcd*-PRA
- Texelaar sheep: *microphthalmia*

Table 15.1: More frequent and/or important breed predispositions and presumed inherited or familial eye diseases in the dog

Afghan Hound
Cataract: recessive trait

Airedale Terrier
Cataract
Corneal dystrophy (sup): X-linked recessive?
Distichiasis
Entropion

Akita
Cataract
Corneal dystrophy
Distichiasis
Entropion
Uveodermatologic syndrome

Alaskan Malamute
Cataract
Cone dysplasia: autosomal recessive trait
Corneal dystrophy
Glaucoma
Persistent pupillary membranes
Progressive retinal atrophy

American Cocker Spaniel
Cataract: recessive trait
Distichiasis: dominant trait suspected
Ectopic cilium
Glaucoma
Progressive rod-cone degeneration: DNA test
Retinal dysplasia, focal/geographic/total: autosomal recessive trait

American Staffordshire Terrier
Cataract
Distichiasis
Entropion
Persistent hyperplastic primary vitreous

Australian Cattle Dog (Queensland Heeler, Blue Heeler)
Cataract
Lens luxation
Progressive rod-cone degeneration: DNA test

Australian Shepherd Dog
Cataract
Collie eye anomaly: choroidal hypoplasia – DNA test
Distichiasis
Iris changes/coloboma/equatorial staphyloma
    (homozygous merle): autosomal recessive trait

Borzoi
Progressive retinal atrophy

Basenji
Persistent pupillary membranes: inherited trait

Bassets (English, French)
Cataract
Ectropion/macroblepharon
Glaucoma: pectinate ligament abnormality
Trichiasis – entropion – redundant forehead skin

Beagle
Cataract: incomplete dominant trait
Corneal dystrophy: epithelial/stromal
Distichiasis
Primary glaucoma (open- or narrow-angle): autosomal recessive trait
Progressive retinal atrophy

Bedlington Terrier
Cataract
Progressive retinal atrophy
Retinal dysplasia, total: autosomal recessive

Belgian Sheepdog (Belgian Shepherd Dog – Groenendaler)
Cataract
Chronic superficial keratitis (pannus)
Retinopathy (congenital blindness): recessive trait

Bernese Mountain Dog
Cataract
Progressive retinal atrophy

Bichon Frise
Cataract

Bloodhound
Ectropion/macroblepharon
Microphthalmia
Trichiasis – entropion – redundant forehead skin

Bordeaux Dog
Ectropion/macroblepharon

Border Collie
Cataract
Collie eye anomaly: choroidal hypoplasia – DNA test
Lens luxation
Progressive retinal atrophy

Border Terrier
Cataract

Boston Terrier
Cataract, juvenile: DNA test
Endothelial dystrophy

Bouvier des Flandres
Entropion
Glaucoma – pectinate ligament abnormality

Boxer
Distichiasis
Ectropion/macroblepharon
Indolent superficial corneal ulcer (basement membrane dystrophy)

Briard
Cataract
Congenital stationary night blindness: hereditary retinal dystrophy in Briards –
    DNA test
Pigment epithelial dystrophy: familial vitamin E deficiency

Bulldog (English)
Distichiasis
Ectopic cilium
Ectropion/macroblepharon
Entropion
Keratoconjunctivitis sicca
Nasal fold trichiasis
Redundant forehead skin

Bulldog (French)
Exposure keratitis
Corneal ulceration – deep

Table 15.1: More frequent and/or important breed predispositions and presumed inherited or familial eye diseases in the dog (Continue)

Bullmastiff
Distichiasis
Entropion
Glaucoma
Progressive retinal atrophy: dominant – DNA test

Bull Terrier
Entropion
Micropalpebral fissure (blepharophimosis)

Bull Terrier (Miniature)
Lens luxation
Micropalpebral fissure (blepharophimosis)

Cairn Terrier
Pigmentary glaucoma
Progressive retinal atrophy: recessive trait

Cavalier King Charles Spaniel
Cataract
Corneal dystrophy, epithelial/stromal
Distichiasis
Retinal dysplasia, (multi) focal

Chesapeake Bay Retriever
Cataract: dominant trait with incomplete penetrance
Distichiasis
Progressive rod-cone degeneration: DNA test
Retinal dysplasia, focal/geographic/total

Chihuahua
Cataract
Endothelial dystrophy

Chinese crested
Progressive rod-cone degeneration: DNA test

Chow Chow
Cataract
Entropion
Glaucoma
Trichiasis – entropion – redundant forehead skin

Clumber Spaniel
Distichiasis
Ectropion/macroblepharon

Collies
Collie eye anomaly: complex autosomal recessive trait; choroidal hypoplasia – DNA test
Distichiasis
Microphthalmia
Optic nerve hypoplasia/micropapilla
Progressive retinal atrophy (rod-cone dysplasia): autosomal recessive trait

Corgi (Welsh Cardigan)
Progressive rod-cone degeneration: DNA test

Corgi (Welsh Pembroke)
Cataract
Progressive retinal atrophy
Retinal dysplasia, (multi) focal/geographic/total

Coton de Tulear
Cataract
Retinal dysplasia, folds/bullae

Curly Coated Retriever
Cataract
Distichiasis

Dachshund
Cataract
Dermoid: possible inherited trait
Distichiasis
Ectopic cilium
Progressive retinal atrophy, rod cone dysplasia: recessive trait suspected

Doberman
Aphakia
Cataract
Persistent hyperplastic tunica vasculosa lentis/persistent hyperplastic primary vitreous
Persistent pupillary membranes

Drentsche Patrijshond
Progressive retinal degeneration

English Cocker Spaniel
Cataract: recessive trait suspected
Pigment epithelial dystrophy – vitamin E deficiency
Distichiasis: dominant trait suspected
Ectropion/macroblepharon
Progressive retinal atrophy (progressive rod-cone degeneration): autosomal recessive
Trichiasis – entropion – redundant forehead skin

English Springer Spaniel
Distichiasis
Ectropion
Entropion
Glaucoma
Optic nerve hypoplasia/micropapilla
Progressive retinal atrophy
Retinal dysplasia, retinal folds, geographic and total: possible autosomal recessive
Trichiasis – entropion – redundant forehead skin

Entlebuch Cattle Dog
Cataract
Progressive rod-cone degeneration: DNA test

Flat-coated Retriever
Distichiasis
Ectopic cilium
Glaucoma: pectinate ligament abnormality

Field Spaniel
Cataract
Distichiasis
Progressive retinal atrophy
Retinal dysplasia, retinal folds, geographic

Finnish Lapphund
Progressive rod-cone degeneration: DNA test

Fox Terrier
Cataract
Lens luxation

German Shepherd Dog
Chronic superficial keratitis (pannus)
Coloboma

Table 15.1: More frequent and/or important breed predispositions and presumed inherited or familial eye diseases in the dog (Continue)

German Pointer
Cataract
Entropion
Glaucoma

German Hunting Terrier
Lens luxation

Golden Retriever
Cataract
Distichiasis
Retinal dysplasia, multifocal, geographical

Gordon Setter
Progressive retinal atrophy

Great Dane
Ectropion/entropion
Glaucoma – pectinate ligament abnormality
Prolapse of the gland of the third eyelid

Greater Swiss Mountain Dog
Cataract
Distichiasis

Havanese
Cataract
Distichiasis

Irish Setters
Optic nerve hypoplasia/micropapilla
Progressive retinal atrophy (rod-cone dysplasia): autosomal recessive trait – DNA test

Irish Terrier
Cataract
Progressive retinal atrophy

Irish Water Spaniel
Cataract
Progressive retinal atrophy

Irish Wolfhound
Cataract
Distichiasis
Entropion
Retinal dysplasia. multifocal, geographic, total

Italian Greyhound
Cataract
Progressive retinal atrophy

Jack Russell Terrier
Cataract
Lens luxation

Labrador Retriever
Cataract: possible dominant or incomplete dominant trait
Corneal dystrophy, superficial
Distichiasis
Progressive rod-cone degeneration: DNA test
Retinal dysplasia – multi focal/geographical/total – without skeletal dysplasia: presumed autosomal recessive;
Retinal dysplasia – multi focal/geographical/total – with skeletal defects: presumed incomplete dominant trait

Large Münsterländer
Cataract

Leonberger
Cataract
Glaucoma – pectinate ligament abnormality
Ectropion/entropion

Mastiff
Entropion/macroblepharon
Persistent pupillary membrane
Progressive retinal atrophy: dominant – DNA test

Miniature Pinscher
Blepharophimosis

Neapolitan Mastiff
Cataract
Dermoid
Ectropion/macroblepharon
Prolapse of the gland of the third eyelid

Newfoundland
Cataract congenital
Ectropion/macroblepharon

Nova Scotia Duck Tolling Retriever
Cataract
Distichiasis
Progressive rod-cone degeneration: DNA test

Old English Sheepdog
Cataract (congenital): recessive trait suspected

Pekingese
Caruncular trichiasis (ciliated caruncle)
Cataract
Corneal ulceration, deep
Distichiasis: dominant trait suspected
Ectopic cilium
Exposure keratopathy syndrome/macroblepharon
Lagophthalmos/exophthalmos
Nasal fold trichiasis

Petit Basset Griffon Vendéen
Cataract
Corneal dystrophy, endothelial
Persistent pupillary membranes
Retinal dysplasia, retinal folds

Pointer
Cataract: dominant trait
Entropion
Progressive retinal atrophy

Poodle (Miniature and Toy)
Caruncular trichiasis
Cataract, juvenile: autosomal recessive
Distichiasis: dominant trait suspected
Optic nerve hypoplasia/micropapilla
Progressive rod-cone degeneration: DNA test

Poodle (Standard)
Cataract: recessive trait suspected
Congenital night blindness
Distichiasis
Progressive retinal atrophy

Table 15.1: More frequent and/or important breed predispositions and presumed inherited or familial eye diseases in the dog (Continue)

Portuguese Water Dog
Cataract
Distichiasis
Microphthalmia and multiple congenital anomalies
Progressive rod-cone degeneration: DNA test

Pug
Caruncular trichiasis
Corneal ulceration, deep
Entropion (medial lower eyelid)
Exposure keratopathy syndrome / macroblepharon
Lagophthalmos / exophthalmos / macroblepharon
Nasal fold trichiasis

Rottweiler
Aniridia
Cataract, congenital
Entropion
Retinal dysplasia – retinal folds

Saint Bernard
Cataract
Ectropion / entropion / macroblepharon

Samoyed
Cataract
Corneal dystrophy: stromal, epithelial
Distichiasis
Glaucoma – pectinate ligament abnormality
Progressive retinal degeneration: X-linked – DNA test

Schapendoes
Cataract
Distichiasis
Progressive retinal degeneration: DNA-marker test

Schipperke
Blepharophimosis

Schnauzer (Miniature)
Cataract, congenital (microphthalmia, posterior lenticonus): simple autosomal recessive trait
Cataract, juvenile: autosomal recessive trait
Distichiasis
Progressive retinal atrophy (rod-cone dysplasia): autosomal recessive

Shar Pei
Entropion
Glaucoma
Lens luxation
Trichiasis – entropion – redundant forehead skin

Shetland Sheepdog
Collie eye anomaly: complex autosomal recessive trait – choroidal hypoplasia DNA test
Distichiasis
Ectopic cilium
Micropalpebral fissure (blepharophimosis)
Optic nerve coloboma
Optic nerve hypoplasia / micropapilla
Progressive retinal atrophy
Retinal dysplasia – retinal folds

Shiba Inu
Cataract
Distichiasis

Shih Tzu
Caruncular trichiasis (ciliated caruncle)
Cataract
Corneal ulceration, deep
Distichiasis
Ectopic cilium
Exophthalmos / lagophthalmos
Glaucoma
Trichiasis – nasal fold

Siberian Husky
Cataract
Corneal dystrophy, epithelial / stromal: presumed autosomal recessive
Distichiasis
Glaucoma
Progressive retinal degeneration: X-linked – DNA test

Sloughi
Progressive rod-cone degeneration: DNA test

Soft-coated Wheaten Terrier
Distichiasis
Microphthalmia – multiple eye anomalies

Staffordshire Bull Terrier (English)
Cataract, juvenile: DNA test
PHTVL / PHPV

Tatra Shepherd Dog
Glaucoma – pectinate ligament abnormality

Tibetan Terrier
Cataract
Ceroid lipofuscinosis (retinal degeneration)
Distichiasis
Lens luxation: autosomal recessive trait suspected

Tibetan Mastiff
Distichiasis

Weimaraner
Distichiasis
Entropion

Welsh Springer Spaniel
Cataract: autosomal recessive trait
Distichiasis
Glaucoma: autosomal dominant trait

Welsh Terrier
Cataract
Distichiasis
Lens luxation

West Highland White Terrier
Cataract: autosomal recessive trait
Keratoconjunctivitis sicca
Lens luxation
Microphthalmia

Whippet
Progressive retinal atrophy

Yorkshire Terrier
Cataract
Progressive retinal atrophy
Retinal dysplasia, geographic / total: possibly recessive trait

Table 15.2: More frequent and/or important breed predispositions and presumed inherited or familial eye diseases in the cat

Abyssinian
PRA (rod-cone dysplasia)
Progressive rod-cone degeneration

Burmese
Dermoid

Main Coon
Cataract

Manx
Corneal dystrophy

Persian
Cataract
Corneal sequestration
Palpebral aplasia
PRA (rod-cone dysplasia)

Siamese
Strabismus

Table 15.3: More frequent and/or important breed predispositions and presumed inherited or familial eye diseases in the horse

American Saddle
Cataract

Appaloosa
Cataract
Congenital stationary night blindness

Arabian
Cataract

Belgian Draft Horse
Aniridia (iris hypoplasia)
Cataract
Limbal dermoid

Kentucky Mountain Saddle Horse
Anterior segment dysplasia (ADS; cornea globosa)
Cataract: presumed incomplete dominant
Choroidal hypoplasia
Retinal dysplasia: presumed incomplete dominant

Rocky Mountain Horse
Anterior Segment Dysplasia (ADS; cornea globosa)

Table 15.4: More frequent and/or important breed predispositions and presumed inherited or familial eye diseases in ruminants

Cattle

Charolais
Optic nerve coloboma: X-linked recessive

Hereford
Cataract
Coloboma with albinism
Dermoid
Retinal dysplasia

Holstein-Friesian
Cataract – congenital

Jersey
Congenital cataract:: autosomal recessive trait
Convergent strabismus with exophthalmia: recessive trait
Microphthalmia
Multiple ocular anomalies

Shorthorn
Convergent strabismus with exophthalmia
Multiple ocular anomalies
Retinal dysplasia with multiple ocular anomalies

Sheep

Texelaar:
Microphthalmia: DNA-marker test

Data based on:
- Ocular disorders, presumed to be inherited in purebred dogs. ACVO, 1999 and Changes 2000–2002;
- Data Ophthalmology Unit, Dept. Clinical Sciences of Companion Animals, Veterinary Faculty, University Utrecht;
- Data Dutch-ECVO Eye Panel;
- Data Swiss-ECVO Eye Panel (Fonds zur Bekämpfung vererbter Augenkrankheiten FbvA);
- Further information as mentioned in the respective chapters.

Literature

1. AGUIRRE, G.D. & RUBIN, L.F.: Rod-cone dysplasia (progressive retinal atrophy) in Irish Setters. JAVMA **166:** 157, 1975.

2. ACLAND, G., BLANTON, S.H., HERSHFIELD, B. & AGUIRRE, G.D.: XLPRA as a canine model of X-linked retinitis pigmentosa. Supp. Invest. Ophthalmol. Vis. Sci. **31:** 335, 1993.

3. STADES, F.C.: Persistent hyperplastic tunica vasculosa lentis and persistent hyperplastic primary vitreous in Doberman Pinchers: Genetic aspects. JAAHA **19:** 957, 1983.

4. PATTERSON, D.F., AGUIRRE, G.D., FYFE, J.C. *et al.*: Is this a genetic disease? J. Small Anim. Pract. **30:** 127, 1989.

5. RAY, K., BALDWIN, V.J., ACLAND, G.M., BLANTON, S.H. & AGUIRRE, G.D.: Cosegregation of codon 807 mutation of the canine rod cGMP phosphodiesterase β gene and rcd 1. Invest. Ophthalmol. Vis. Sci. **35:** 4291, 1994.

6. RUBIN, L.F.: Inherited diseases in purebred dogs. Baltimore, Williams & Wilkins, 1989.

7. AMERICAN COLLEGE OF VETERINARY OPHTHALMOLOGISTS: Ocular disorders proven or suspected to be hereditary in dogs. 1992.

8. HEITMANN, M.: Untersuchung zur Vererbung von Augenerkrankungen beim Entlebucher Sennenhund. Dissertation Tierärztliche Hochschule Hannover, 2003.

16 Glossary of Terms Relating to the Eye

(vs.: versus or opposite entity)

Accommodation: active bulging or flattening of the lens, to adjust pictures at different distances sharply on the retina.
Acorea: congenital absence of a pupil.
Amblyopia: reduced visual acuity, without clinically detectable defects of the eye.
Amaurosis: blindness, without clinically detectable defects of the eye.
Angle (iridocorneal): (geometric) angle between the base of the iris and the cornea.
Aniridia: congenital absence or partial absence of the iris.
Anisocoria: unequal pupil size.
Ankyloblepharon: delayed or non-spontaneous opening of the lid fissure.
Anophthalmos: absence of a true eyeball.
Aphakia: absence of a true lens.
Aplasia (agenesis): not developed or underdeveloped.
Aqueous humor: watery fluid filling the anterior part of the eye.
Asteroid hyalosis: multiple small white or pigmented foci (>1 mm) in the vitreous. They may move slightly during movement of the globe, but return to their original position.

Blepharitis: inflammation of the lid.
Blepharitis adenomatosa: inflammation of the tarsal glands.
Blepharophimosis: too short lid fissure.
Buphthalmos: secondarily enlarged globe, usually due to glaucoma.

Capsulorrhexis: (anterior) well-controlled circular stab, cut, or tear to remove the central part of the capsule of the lens.
Capsulotomy: incision in the capsule of the lens
Caruncle: small fleshy or pigmented haired eminence in the medial canthal conjunctiva.
Canthus: corner of the lid fissure.
Cataract: every non-physiological opacity of the lens and/or its capsule.
Cataract, immature: partially opaque lens, fundus still visible.
Cataract, intumescent: swollen lens (fibers) due to the osmotic effect of degenerate lens proteins.
Cataract, mature: complete opaque lens, fundus not visible anymore.
Cataract, senile: non-physiologic cataract due to aging (vs. Lens, Sclerosis)
Chalazion: hard, non-painful swelling of a meibomian gland, due to granulomatous overfilling.
Chemosis: conjunctival edema.
Choroid(ea): posterior part of the uvea, between the retina and the sclera.
Ciliary body: middle part of the uvea, containing the pars plicata (ciliary processes) and pars plana (ciliary muscles).
Ciliary processes: 60–80 folds of the ciliary body that produce the aqueous.

Collarette: ring often recognizable on anterior surface of the iris, where the vascular loops of the pupillary membrane arose before birth.
Collie eye anomaly (CEA): group of presumed inherited, congenital, hypoplastic or dysplastic anomalies primarily affecting the choroid and sclera, and indirectly the optic disc (e.g. coloboma).
Coloboma: congenital defect due to a failure in closure of the body halves; in the eye often triangular to rounded.
Conjunctiva: mucous membrane closing the space between the lid margin and the limbus.
Conjunctivitis: non-specific inflammation of the conjunctiva.
Contusion of the globe: blunt trauma to the bulbus.
Cornea: transparent window in the outer layer of the globe, enabling light to enter into the globe.
Corneal dystrophy: possible hereditary, often bilateral, but not always symmetrical, non-inflammatory white to gray crystalline structures in the corneal layers; epithelial-stromal (often cholesterol) or endothelial.
Corneal ulcer: see Ulcer
Cyclodialysis: glaucoma operation to re-establish filtration of aqueous out of the globe by opening the cleft between the ciliary body and the sclera.
Cycloplegia: situation in which the ciliary muscle is put at rest resulting in paralysis of accommodation.

Day blindness: nyctalopia or blindness in high light intensities, starting with dysplasia or degeneration of the cones (vs. hemeralopia). *NB*: in Anglo-American literature, nyctalopia and hemeralopia are used the other way around.
Dacryoadenitis: inflammation of one of the tear glands.
Dacryocystitis: inflammation in the lacrimal sac or nasolacrimal duct.
Dacryorhinostomy: making a passage between the conjunctiva and the nose or nasal sinuses for the drainage of tear fluid.
Dermoid: possibly hereditary ectopic piece of skin in the cornea and/or conjunctiva, and in rare cases continuous to the lid skin.
Descemet's membrane: strong, elastic layer of the cornea in between the stroma and the endothelial inside of the cornea; posterior limiting membrane of the cornea.
Descemet's tear: tear of the Descemet's membrane of the cornea, after enlargement of the globe.
Descemetocele: bulging, uncovered membrane of Descemet.
Distichiasis: presumed inherited, single or multiple hairs arising from the free lid margin. They usually arise from the meibomian duct openings and their hair follicles are located in the lid margin, usually in or near to the base of the meibomian glands.
Drainage angle: circular area, via which aqueous is removed from the globe and returned to the general circulation, including the pectinate ligament and ciliary cleft.

Dysplasia: incorrect, abnormal, or deformed development.
Dystrophia: disorder arising from defective or faulty nutrition.

Ectasia: distension or dilation, e.g. area bulging in or out of the sclera.
Ectopic cilia: presumed inherited, one or more aberrantly located hairs (in general); term mainly used for aberrant hairs growing into the conjunctival sac, towards the cornea.
Ectropion: outwards turning of the margin of the lid; mainly presumed inherited.
Enophthalmos: abnormal deep positioning of the globe into the orbit (vs. exophthalmos).
En(d)ophthalmia(itis): inflammation of all tissues in the globe (vs. panophthalmitis).
Entropion: inwards turning of the margin of the lid; mainly presumed inherited.
Enucleation: surgical removal of the globe.
Epiphora: overflow of tears.
Erosion, corneal: mainly traumatic loss of epithelium of the cornea.
Esotropia: convergent strabismus (squint).
Exotropia: divergent strabismus (squint).
Eversion / inversion of the nictitating membrane: kink-like, bending misgrowth, outwards or inwards respectively, of the distal part of the cartilage of the nictitating membrane.
Evisceration (bulbus): removal of all the contents (of the globe).
Exenteration (orbit): removal of all the contents (of the orbit).
Exophthalmos: abnormal bulging of the globe out of the orbit (vs. enophthalmos).

Fornix: junction of the palpebral and scleral or bulbar conjunctiva.
Fundus (eye): posterior portion of the eye, visible through the ophthalmoscope.

Glaucoma: pathological process of varied etiology, characterized by decreased retinal ganglion cell sensitivity and function, and by ganglion cell death, optic nerve axonal loss, and optic nerve head cup enlargement, incremental reduction in visual fields, and blindness. It is also associated with an increase in IOP.
Glaucoma, primary: presumed inherited glaucoma, not caused by any other eye disease.
Goniodysplasia / Goniodysgenesis: see pectinate ligament abnormality (congenital deformity of the pectinate ligament).
Gonioscopy: technique for examination of the irido-corneal angle including the pectinate ligament.
Hemeralopia: night blindness; blindness in low light intensities (primary abnormality of the rods; vs. nyctalopia; NB: in Anglo-American literature, day blindness).
Heterochromia (iris): different colors (of the iris).

Hordeolum (stye): infectious inflammation of a Zeis, Moll (external), or meibomian gland (internal).
Horner's syndrome: lesion of the sympathetic innervation of the eye, characterized by ptosis, enophthalmos, protrusion of the nictitating membrane, and miosis. Sweating occurs in the horse as well.
Hyalitis: inflammation of the vitreous.
Hyaloid artery: embryologic artery nourishing the lens; growing from the optic papilla to the posterior pole of the lens; regresses before birth.
Hydrophthalmos: enlarged globe, due to chronic rise of the IOP.
Hyphema: free blood in the anterior chamber.
Hypopyon: exudate / pus in the anterior chamber.
Hypoplastic papilla / optic disc: presumed inherited, congenital ocular disorder. In hypoplasia of the papilla, the head of the optic nerve is underdeveloped, and therefore the condition is a manifestation of an absence of axons and histologically can be correlated to a decreased concentration of ganglion cells, resulting in vision impairment. May be difficult / impossible to differentiate from micropapilla.

Intumescent cataract: cataract with swelling of the lens due to inhibition of water.
Iridectomy: excision of a part of the iris.
Iridencleisis: glaucoma operation to re-establish drainage of aqueous out of the globe by an opening in the sclera to the subconjunctival area. Iris is pulled into the wound to prevent closure.
Iridotomy: incision in the iris.
Iris: anterior part of the uvea.
Iris atrophy: degenerative loss of iris tissue.
Iris bombé: anterior bulging of the iris, due to aqueous which cannot drain to the anterior chamber because of a circular synechia of the edge of the pupil to the anterior capsule of the lens.
Iris cyst: usually pigmented balloon-shaped structure hanging from the back of iris over the pupil margin into the anterior chamber, or floating freely in the lower anterior chamber. They originate from the epithelium of the posterior side of the ciliary body or iris.

Juxta: positioned nearby or adjoining.

Keratitis: inflammation of the cornea, without knowing the cause of the entity.
Keratoconjunctivitis sicca: insufficient tear production / tear film and the subsequent secondary inflammatory reactions of the conjunctiva and cornea.
Keratoconus: cone-shaped deformity of a part of or the whole of the cornea.

Lagophthalmos: inability to close the eyelids.
Lens, sclerosis: physiological loss of transparency of the lens nucleus.
Lenticonus: cone-shaped deformity of a part of the lens (anterior or posterior).

Leucocoria: white pupil, e.g. due to cataract.
Limbus: circular demarcation line between the cornea and the sclera.
Luxation, lens: dislocation of the lens; presumed inherited.
Luxation, bulbus: dislocation of the globe through the lid fissure, without it being able to return spontaneously to its normal position (vs. proptosis of the globe).

Macroblepharon: presumed inherited, congenital ocular disorder. Oversized lid fissure; usually in combination with ectropion in the middle and angular entropion, resulting in diamond-shaped 'eyes'. Measures, in stretched condition, over (an arbitrary value of) 40 mm in the dog.
Macrophthalmos: possibly inherited, congenital, enlarged globe.
Microcornea: possibly inherited, congenital, abnormal small diameter cornea.
Micropapilla: possibly inherited, congenital, abnormal small developed optic disc.
Microphakia: possibly inherited, congenital, abnormal small lens.
Microphthalmos: presumed inherited, congenital, abnormal small globe (vs. phthisis).
Mouches volantes: variably sized, usually moving, particles in the vitreous.
Mydriasis: wide-open pupil.
Miosis: constricted pupil.

Night blindness: (hemeralopia) blindness in low-light intensities, primary dysfunction of the rods (vs. nyctalopia). NB: in Anglo-American literature, day blindness.
Nyctalopia: (day blindness) primary dysfunction of the cones (vs. hemeralopia).
Nystagmus: involuntary, rhythmic, horizontal, vertical, or rotating movements of the eye. The nystagmus is named after the direction of the fast movement.

Ora ciliaris retinae: (ora serrata) transition of the retina to the ciliary body.

Palpebral aplasia: congenital underdevelopment of the lid (margin).
Pannus / Keratitis pannosa: fibrovascular tissue infiltration of the surface of the cornea.
Panophthalmia(itis): inflammation of all tissues of the globe (vs. endophthalmitis).
Papilla: optic disc.
Pectinate ligament: fibrous bands radiating from the base of the iris and inserting into the inner surface of the cornea; assists in support of the iris and is the beginning of the outflow system of aqueous from the anterior chamber.
Pectinate ligament abnormality: (goniodysplasia or dysgenesis) presumed inherited, congenital dysplasia of the pectinate ligament. Main types: mildest form – short, broad fibers or fibrae latae; moderate form – sheets or laminae; severe form – more or less closed ligament or occlusion.

Persistent hyaloid artery: a non-regressed part of the hyaloid artery.
Persistent hyperplastic tunica vasculosa lentis / persistent hyperplastic primary vitreous (PHTVL / PHPV): presumed inherited, non-regressed, hyperplastic vascular tunic of the lens and persistent primitive vitreous.
Persistent pupillary membrane: remnant of the embryologic vascular tunic nourishing the anterior part of the lens.
Photophobia: abnormal hypersensitivity to light.
Phthisis bulbi: acquired shrinkage of the globe or small eyeball (vs. microphthalmos).
Pigment epithelial dystrophy retinal (RPED): accumulation of lipid pigments in the pigmented epithelium, possible due to an inadequate phagocytosis of the outer segment material of the photoreceptors, with secondary degeneration of the photoreceptors, beginning with the cones. There is strong evidence that vitamin E and taurine are involved in the etiology of RPED, with a familial predisposition.
Progressive retinal atrophy (PRA): see Retinal degeneration or atrophy.
Proptosis bulbi: frontal displacement of the globe (vs. luxation).
Protrusion (nictitating membrane): forward / frontal displacement (of the nictitating membrane).
Ptosis: drooping of the upper eyelid.
Pupillary membrane: embryologic vascular loops, forming a vessel net, that arise from the annular vessel of the optic cup (where later the collarette of the iris may be recognized), over the front side of the lens, and nourishing the anterior part of the lens. The hyaloid system is maximally developed around the 40th–45th day post conception; thereafter the system goes into regression. The entire system is normally resorbed between the 4th and the 5th week after birth (horse 7–9 months).

Retinal degeneration or atrophy (hereditary; progressive retinal atrophy or PRA): group of presumed inherited photoreceptor diseases (usually referred to as just PRA by breeders and owners). Characterized mainly by either primary photoreceptor dysplasia (early onset) and subsequent degeneration or by primary photoreceptor degeneration (late onset). The diseases are bilateral and most commonly have similar clinical signs such as initial visual impairment at night, followed by night blindness, and later also by day blindness (i.e. complete blindness). The onset and progression vary depending on the pathogenesis.
Retinal detachment: ablation of the inner (neuro)retina from the outer retina or pigment epithelium.
Retinal dysplasia (RD): presumed inherited, congenital ocular disorder. Abnormal development of the retina, characterized by rosettes, neuroretinal folding and retinal detachment. There are three main forms: **(multi) focal** – linear (vermiform), V-, triangular, curvilinear, single or multiple folds of the retina; **geographical** – *confluent* folding and/or irregularly, or horseshoe- or bladder-like shaped dysplastic area of retinal thinning and folding, later usually resulting

also in retinal degeneration in that area; ***total*** – *congenital* separation (ablation) of the neuroretina from the retinal pigment epithelium (outer retina).

Retinal dystrophy / RPE65 null mutation: presumed inherited retinal disease, with a lack of RPE65 protein and therefore no formation of rhodopsin, resulting in congenital night blindness (e.g. Briard dog).

Retinal pigment epithelial dystrophy: see pigment epithelial dystrophy.

Retinopathy: unspecific retinal disease.

Retro: positioned posterior to . . . .

Spherophakia: rounding of the lens into a ball form.

Staphyloma: a protrusion resulting from a bulging area of, or a rupture in, the fibrous tunic of the eye, containing parts of the uvea. *Anterior* staphyloma: located in the cornea or sclera, anteriorly from the ora ciliaris retinae; *posterior* staphyloma: located in the sclera, posterior from the ora ciliaris retinae.

Strabismus: squint, deviation of the visual axes; strabismus convergens (esotropia): inwards squint; strabismus divergens (exotropia) outwards squint.

Striae (of Haab): thin, irregular lines in the cornea, like cracks in ice. They mark (previous) ruptures of the Descemet's membrane and the underlying endothelium. Initially, water enters through the defect, resulting in lines of edema. After normalization of the IOP, the endothelial cells expand and repair the defect, resulting in scar lines.

Suffusion: flat hemorrhage, e.g. between conjunctiva and sclera.

Symblepharon: adhesion between conjunctival layers or conjunctiva and cornea.

Synchysis scintillans: liquefied vitreous containing mainly cholesterol crystals, enabling them to move after a movement of the eye.

Synechia, anterior / posterior: acquired adhesions between parts of the iris and the cornea (anteriorly) or lens (posteriorly).

Syneresis: liquefied vitreous.

Tarsorrhaphy: temporary or permanent closure of the lid fissure.

Tension: IOP plus rigidity of the cornea.

Tenon's capsule: fascia around the globe.

Trichiasis, ocular: abnormally positioned hairs in a normal place around the lid fissure, irritating the conjunctiva and / or the globe; presumed inherited.

Tunica vasculosa lentis (TVL): embryologic vascular tunic around the lens.

Ulcer of the cornea: superficial (epithelial, basal cell membrane degeneration) or deep (most lytic) eroding process in the cornea after loosening or erosion of the superficial layers.

Uveitis: inflammation of the uvea. Usually, all parts of the uvea are more or less involved. Also, other local processes are possible (iritis, iridocyclitis / anterior uveitis, choroiditis, chorioretinitis / posterior uveitis).

Uveodermatologic *syndrome:* immune-mediated syndrome consisting of uveitis, dermal and hair depigmentation. May be complicated by glaucoma and / or retinal detachment (in humans: Vogt-Koyanagi-Harada syndrome).

Zonular fibers: very fine tissue strands which suspend the lens.

Index

A
Abscess
–, corneal 150 ff.
–, retrobulbar 50 ff.
Accommodation 171
Acetazolamide 23
Acetylcholine 23
Acetylcysteine 19, 22, 27
Acorea 175
Acyclovir 25
Adenocarcinoma 184 ff.
Adenoma
–, eyelid 98–100
Adrenaline *cf.* epinephrine
Albinism
–, oculocutaneous 175
– –, partial 175
Algae 180
Alpha-lysine 25
Amaurosis 218, 232
Amblyopia 218, 232
Amlodipine 27
Amphotericin 25
Anamnesis 5
Anesthesia 27 ff.
Aneurine deficiency 227
Angiography 15
Aniridia 175
Ankyloblepharon 74
Anophthalmia 127
Antazoline 22
Antibiotics
–, specific 22, 24
–, standard 22, 24
Antiglaucoma agents 23
Antihistamines 22
Anti-hypertensive agents 27
Antimicrobial agents 24 ff.
Antimycotics 25
Antiphlogistics 25
Antiviral drugs 25
Aphakia 192
Aplasia palpebrae 10, 74 ff., 173
Applanation tonometer 13
Application *cf.* Therapeutics
Apraclonidine 23
Aqueous humor 157, 171
–, drainage
– –, with implant 167
– –, improved capacity 165 ff.
–, outflow 157 ff.
–, production 157

– –, reduction 165
Area
–, centralis 15
–, seventeen 211
–, striata 211
Artery
–, hyaloid 189 ff.
– –, persistent 192
–, retinal 209
Artificial
–, lens 200 ff.
–, tears 26, 63
Atenolol 27
Atrophic globe 10, 127, 170
Atropine 14, 22, 24, 26, 61
Autotransplantation
–, free conjunctival 146

B
Bacitracin 24
Bacteria 180
Basal cell carcinoma 100
BCG = Calmette-Guérin bacillus 100
Belladonna 61
Benoxinate hydrochloride 26
Beta blockers 23
Beta radiation 27
Betamethasone 25
Bimatoprost 23
Bipolar cells 210
Bird pox 98
Blepharitis 95 ff., 99
–, adenomatosa 96
Blepharophimosis 94
Blepharoplasty 85, 101 ff.
–, rotation-flap correction 75
Blepharospasm 62
–, differential diagnosis 16
Blindness
–, differential diagnosis 17
Blood vessel
–, architecture 172
–, occlusion 225
–, walls 176
Blood-aqueous barrier 172
Blue eye 179
Botulism 61
Brachycephalic breeds 8
Breed disposition 237–246
Brimonidine 23

Brinzolamide 23
Brow sling 91
Bruch's membrane 210
Bulbus *cf.* Globe
Buphthalmos 12, 128, 162
Butylcyanoacrylate 27

C
Canthoplasty
–, lateral 95
–, medial 90, 95
Canthotomy
–, lateral 94
Capsulorrhexis 193, 200
Carbonic anhydrase inhibitors 23
Carprofen 25
Caruncle trichiasis 91
Cataract 173, 193–201
–, alimentary 196
–, congenital 173, 196
–, diabetic 197
–, inherited 196
–, juvenile 196
–, radiation 196
–, secondary 197
–, senile 196
–, therapy 197–201
–, traumatic 196
CEA *cf.* Collie eye anomaly
Chalazion 96
Chemical burns 34
Chemical cauterizing agents 27
Cherry eye 110–112
Chloramphenicol 24
Chlorhexidine 24
Chlortetracycline 24
Choriocapillaris 173, 211, 214
Chorioretinitis 214 ff. 226–228
Choroid 2, 173 ff., 214
Cilia
–, ectopic 106 ff.
Ciliary
–, body 2, 171 ff., 210
– –, destruction 166 ff.
–, muscles 22
Ciprofloxacin 24
Clinical diagnosis 5–18
–, aids 5, 8 ff.
–, anamnesis 5
–, differential diagnosis 16 ff.
–, methods 5, 8 ff.

–, restraint 8
–, sedation 8
–, signalment 5
Cloxacillin 24
Coagulation disorders 176
Cocaine 26
Collarette 174
Collars 27
Collie eye anomaly (CEA) 219–221
Collyria 26
Coloboma 174, 192, 218 ff.
Computed tomography 15
Cones 210 ff.
Conjunctiva 2, 105–125
–, adhesions 119
–, autotransplant 146
–, clinical diagnosis 11 ff.
–, lacerations 39
–, neoplasia 122
–, oversuturing methods 142, 144–147
– –, bulbar 145 ff.
– –, strip 144
– –, pedicle flap 144
–, scleral 73 ff.
–, stricture 120 ff.
Conjunctival sac
–, flushing 19 ff.
Conjunctivitis 113–119
–, acute
– –, purulent 114 ff.
–, allergic 119
–, bovine 118
–, catarrhal 114
–, follicular 11, 116
–, granulomatous 117
–, neonatorum 117 ff.
–, nodular 117
–, ovine 118
–, papillary 117
–, plasmacellular 116 ff.
–, purulent 114 ff.
Conjunctivomaxillorhinostomy 69 ff.
Conjunctivorhinostomy 69
Cornea(l) 2, 129–154
–, abscess 150
–, abnormalities 132
–, blue-white
– –, differential diagnosis 17
–, clinical diagnosis 13
–, clouding 130
–, cysts 150
–, degeneration
– –, endothelial 152 ff.
– –, deposits 153
–, diameter 12

–, dystrophy 151–153
– –, endothelial 152 ff.
– –, epithelial/stromal 151 ff.
–, edema 35, 130, 135, 141, 153
–, foreign bodies 40 ff.
–, graft
– –, lamella 147
–, healing 132
–, lacerations 40–44
– –, non-perforating 40–42
– –, perforating 43–44
–, lipidosis 151
–, micro- 133
–, mummification 147–149
–, necrosis 147–149
–, neoplasia 155
–, nigrum 147–149
–, perforation 43 ff., 132, 142
–, reflection 9
–, scarring 130
–, sequestrum 147–149
–, symptoms 129–131
–, transplant
– –, free 147
–, ulcer 106, 137–140, 141, 147
Corticosteroids 25
Cromoglicic acid 22
Cryoepilation 76–77
Cryosurgery 29, 100
Cyclocryodestruction 166 ff.
Cyclopentolate 26
Cyclopia 127
Cycloplegia 22, 24
Cyclosporine 27, 63
Cysts
–, conjunctival 108
–, corneal 150
–, iris 176

D

Dacryoadenitis 64
Dacryocystitis 67–70
Day blindness 214
–, hereditary (stationary) 224
Deafness 175
Demecarium bromide 23
Dermoid 76, 133 ff.
Descemetocele 140
Detomidine 8
Dexamethasone 25
Diagnosis *cf.* Clinical diagnosis
Diagnostics 19–30
Dichlorphenamide 23
Diclofenac 25
Dipivalyl epinephrine 23
Dirofilaria immitis 180

Discharge-dissolving agents 27
Distichiasis 10, 76–78
DNA test 240
DNA-synthesis inhibitors 25
Dorzolamide 23
Duct
–, nasolacrimal 60 ff.
– –, flush 68 ff.
–, parotid 64
– –, transposition (PDT) 64
Dysautonomia syndrome 61
Dysplasia 176
–, of the eyelid 76
–, retinal 219

E

Ecothiophate iodine 23
Ectopic lens 201–205
Ectropion 86–89
–, correction 87–89
– –, surgical 87–89
– –, Kuhnt-Szymanowski 87
– – –, –Blaskovics 87
EDTA solution 26
Ehrlichiosis 180, 227
Electroepilation 76 ff.
Electroretinogram (ERG) 211
Electroretinography 16, 211
Emergencies 31–44
Encephalitozoon cuniculi 180
Endophthalamos 12, 48–49, 125
–, differential diagnosis 16
Endophthalmitis 128
Endothelial degeneration
–, senile 152
Endothelial microscopy 16
Endothelial precipitation 177
Enalapril 27
Entropion 10 ff., 78–86, 90–93
–, angular 83, 85
–, correction 81–86
– –, Celsus-Hotz 81–83
– –, Stades 91–92
– –, surgical 81–85
– –, tacking 81
–, habitual 81
–, iatrogenic 79, 84
–, medial 84
–, mild 81
–, severe 81
– –, partial lateral 84
– –, total 78 ff.
Enucleation of the globe 56
–, including conjunctiva 53–55
Eosinophilic granuloma 96, 119, 136

Epilation
–, electro- 76–78
–, cryo- 76
Epinephrine 22–24
Epiphora 113
–, differential diagnosis 16
Episcleritis cf. Scleritis
Epithelializing agents 26
Equine recurrent (chronic) uveitis (ERU) 182 ff.
ERG cf. Electroretinogram
Ethoxyzolamide 23
ERU cf. Equine recurrent (chronic) uveitis
Etodolac 61
Eversion of the nictitating membrane 108 ff.
–, correction 109
Evisceration of the globe 53, 56
Exeneration of the orbit 53, 56
Exophthalmos 47, 49–53, 125
–, differential diagnosis 16
Exudation flakes
–, preretinal 215
Eye
–, blind cf. Blindness
–, drops 19 ff.
– –, duration of effect 20
–, muscles 2, 125
–, ointments 19 ff.
–, painful cf. Painful eye
–, pigmented cf. Pigmented eye
–, pressure
– –, intraocular cf. Intraocular pressure
– –, retrobulbar 12 ff.
–, red cf. Red eye
–, tear stained cf. Epiphora
Eyelid 2, 10 ff., 73–104
–, adenoma 98–100
–, carcinoma 100
–, clinical diagnosis 10 ff.
– –, colobomas 10, 74 ff., 173
–, dysplasia 76
–, granuloma 96
–, lacerations 36, 37–39, 94
–, margin
– –, granuloma 178
– –, investigation 11
– –, lacerations 37–39
– –, upper
– – –, ectropinizing 10
– –, wounds 38, 39
–, melanoma 99
–, neoplasia 99 ff.
–, third cf. Nictitating membrane

F
Face lifting 91
Famcyclovir 25
FCRD cf. Retinal degeneration, feline central
Feline dysautonomia 184
FeLV 179, 227
Fibrae latae 161
Filtration angle 2
–, abnormalities 161
FIP 179, 227
Fistula methods 168
FIV 179, 227
Fixation 5
–, false 10
Flitting flies cf. Vitreous floaters
Flumethasone 25
Flunixin 25
Fluorescein 26
Fluorometholone 25
Fluostigmine 23
Flurbiprofen 25
Flushing 19
Flushing bottle 19
Fly net 27
Follicle 11, 113
Folliculosis 11, 113
Fornix 73
Fracture
–, orbital 34 ff.
Framycetin 24
Frontal bone 47
Fundus 14 ff., 209–235
–, abnormal 214–235
–, changes 214–218
–, clinical diagnosis 14 ff.
–, ontogenesis 209
–, reaction patterns 214–218
–, reflection 209, 213, 217
–, symptoms 214–218
Funduscopy 14 ff.
Fungi 180
Fusidic acid 24

G
Gamma-interferon 25
Ganglion
–, cell layer 209 ff.
Gentamycin 21, 24
Gland
–, lacrimal 59
–, nictitating membrane 73, 105–112
– –, hyperplasia 110–112
– –, deep 64, 105
– –, superficial 59, 105
–, parotid 64

–, zygomatic 47, 64
Glaucoma 159–170
–, absolute 160
–, acute 161–164
–, chronic 162, 164
–, closed irido-corneal angle 161
–, clinical signs 162–164
–, duration 161 ff.
–, open irido-corneal angle 161
–, open pectinate ligament 161
–, primary cf. Primary glaucoma
–, primary morphologically abnormal pectinate ligament 161
–, secondary 160, 168–170
–, therapy 23, 165–168
– –, cyclocryodestruction 167
– –, fistula methods 168
– –, surgical 167 ff.
Globe 125–128
–, clinical diagnosis 12 ff.
–, contusion 35
–, luxation 31–34
–, position 47 ff.
Glycerol 23
GM1 and GM2 gangliosidosis 154
Goniodysgenesis 161
Goniodysplasia 161
Gonioscopy 15, 159 ff.
Gramicidin 24
Granuloma
–, eosinophilic 96, 118 ff., 137
–, eyelid 96 ff.

H
Hemorrhage
–, retinal 214 ff.
–, subconjunctival 113
–, subretinal
– –, band-shaped 215
–, vitreous 206 ff.
Hemostasis 29
Hereditary eye diseases 237–246
Heterochromia of the iris 175
Homatropine 26
Hordeolum 96 ff.
Horner's syndrome 49, 184
Hyaloid
–, artery cf. Artery, hyaloid
–, system 189 ff.
Hyaloidosis
–, asteroid 206
Hydrophthalmia 128, 162
Hyperlipoproteinemia 225
Hyphema 13, 35 ff., 176
Hypophysectomy 61
Hypoplasia

–, choroid 219 ff.
Hypoprolose 26
Hypopyon 13, 178
Hyposphagma 35

I
Idoxuridine 25
i-drops® 64
Immune reactions 180 ff.
Indentation tonometry 13
Indomethacin 25
Infectious canine hepatitis 179
Infiltrates 114
Injection
–, conjunctival 19–21
–, intraocular 21 ff.
–, retrobulbar 21
–, subconjunctival 21
–, subpalpebral system 20
Injuries cf. Lacerations
Intoxications 225
Intraocular
–, pressure 12 ff., 157–170
– –, antiglaucoma agents 23
– –, reference values 12
–, volume
– –, reduction 166 ff.
Inversion of the nictitating membrane 108
Iodine tincture 27
Iridic granules 14
Irido-corneal angle 158
–, malformation 161
Iridodonesis 13
Iris 2, 171 ff.
–, acquired color differences 175
–, atrophy 183
–, blue
– –, /white coat 175
–, clinical diagnosis 14
–, cyst 13, 176
–, granulomatous swelling 185
–, infections 179 ff.
–, melanoma 184
Iritis
–, traumatic 179
Isosorbide 23

J
Juxtapalpebral changes 96

K
KCS cf. Keratoconjunctivitis sicca
Keratitis 134–150

–, deep
–, eosinophilic 136
–, herpetica 150
–, interstitial 136
–, pannosa 134–136
–, photoallergic 135 ff.
–, punctate 149
–, superficial 134–136
–, ulcerative 137–147
–, vascular and pigmentary 135 ff.
Keratoconjunctivitis
–, infectious bovine/ovine 150
–, sicca (KCS) 61–64
– –, ipsilateral 63
Ketoprofen 25
Ketorolac 25
Key-Gaskell syndrome 184

L
Lacerations
–, conjunctival 39 ff.
–, corneal 40–44
–, eyelid 37–39
– –, margin 37–39
–, perforating 37
Lacrimal
–, apparatus 59–71
–, duct 59 ff.
– –, catheterization 69 ff.
–, gland 2, 59
– –, accessory 59
–, punctum 60 ff.
– –, atresia 66
– –, opening 67
– –, secondary closure 66
– –, stenosis 65
–, sac 61
Lagophthalmos 95
Lamina 161
Larvae
–, migrating 227
Laser techniques 29
Latanoprost 23
Lateral geniculate bodies 211
Lavage system
–, subpalpebral 20–21
Leishmania 180
Lens 2, 189–205
–, artificial 200
–, clinical diagnosis 14
–, extraction 198–200
– –, extracapsular 199 ff.
– –, intracapsular 169, 199, 205
–, hard 200
–, luxation 13, 163, 201–205

–, nucleus sclerosis 191
–, ontogenesis 189 ff.
–, perforation 41
–, soft 200
Lenticonus 192
Lentiglobus 192
Leptospira interrogans 180
Lidocaine 26
Ligament
–, palpebral
– –, lateral 73
– –, medial 73
–, pectinate 159
– –, abnormalities 161
– –, open 161
Limbus melanoma 155
Local anesthesia 8
Local anesthetics 22, 26
Locoweed 61
Luxation
–, globe 31–34
–, lens 13, 163, 201–205

M
Macroblepharon 86–89
Macrophthalmia 12, 128
Magnetic resonance imaging (MRI) 15
Magnification equipment 28
Mandibular lymph nodes 8
Mannitol 23
Medetomidine 8
Meglumine 25
Meibomian glands 10, 73 ff.
Melanoma
–, eyelid 99
–, iris 184
–, limbus 155
Meloxicam 25
Membrane
–, persistent (epi)pupillary 173–174
–, nictitating cf. Nictitating membrane
–, pupillary (PM) 190
– –, persistent (PPM) 130, 133, 173–174, 194
Metazolamide 23
Methylprednisolone 25
Miconazole 25
Microcornea 133
Micropapilla 218
Microphakia 192
Microphthalmia 12, 127, 173, 194
Micropunctum 65
Miotics 23
Moll glands 73

MRI cf. Magnetic resonance imaging
Mucopolysaccharidosis 154
Mucus cells 73
Muscae volantes cf. Vitreous floaters
Muscle
–, ciliary 171
–, levator
– –, anguli oculi medialis 73
– –, palpebrae 73
–, malaris 73
–, orbicularis oculi 73
–, pupillary
– –, dilator 171
– –, sphincter 171
–, retractor anguli 73
Mydriatics 23–24

N
Nafazoline 29
Nasal folds
–, resection 89 ff.
–, trichiasis 89 ff.
Nasopharynx 61
Natamycin 25
Neomycin 24
Neoplasia
–, conjunctival 122
–, corneal 155
–, eyelid 99 ff.
–, intraocular 207
–, orbital 51 ff.
–, retinal 231 ff.
–, retrobulbar 51 ff.
–, uveal 177, 181 ff., 184–186
Nerve
–, facial 64
–, optic 2, 209–235
Nictitating membrane 2, 105–112
–, flaps/oversuturing techniques
– –, attached to dorsolateral conjunctiva 144
– –, attached to upper lid 142–144
–, gland 2, 110–112
–, margin
– –, non-pigmented 106
–, protrusion 12, 47
– –, differential diagnosis 16
Night blindness 214
–, hereditary (stationary) 224
Non-tapetal area cf. Tapetum nigrum
Norfloxacin 24
Nystagmus 12, 126 ff.

O
Occlusion 161
Ocular
–, capsule 199 ff.
–, chambers 2, 157 ff., 171
– –, changes 172
– –, clinical diagnosis 13
– –, drainage area 157 ff.
– –, osmotic agents 22
–, therapeutic agents 22–27
Oculocutaneous syndrome 175
Ofloxacin 24
Operating table
–, positioning of patient 28
Ophthalmoscopy 15
Optic
–, chiasm 211
–, nerve 14
–, neuritis 231
–, papilla cf. Papilla
Orbit cf. Periorbita
–, fracture 34
–, neoplasia 51 ff.
– –, primary 52
Orbitomy 56
Osmotic agents 23
Oxybuprocaine 26

P
Painful eye
–, differential diagnosis 16
Palpebra cf. Eyelid
Palpebral
–, aplasia 10, 74 ff., 173
–, fissure 73
– –, length 10
Pannus 131, 135–136
Panophthalmitis 128
Papilla 15, 210
–, coloboma 218 ff.
–, edema 230
–, hypoplastic 218
–, micro- 218
Papillitis 231
Parasites 180
Parasympatholytics 22 ff.
Parasympathomimetics 23
Pasteurella multocida 180
Pecten 211, 213
PED cf. Pigment epithelial dystrophy
Pedicle graft 75
Perforating injuries 37
Periorbita 45–57
PermaTweez® 76–77
Persistent hyaloid artery cf. Artery, hyaloid, persistent

Persistent hyperplastic primary vitreous (PHPV) 193–194
Persistent hyperplastic tunica vasculosa lentis (PHTVL) 193–194
Pharmacoemulsification 200
Phenazopyridine 61
Phenol 27
Phenylephrine 22, 24
Photophobia 172
Photoreceptors 210 ff.
–, degeneration 221–224
–, dysplasia 221–224
PHPV cf. Persistent hyperplastic primary vitreous
Phthisis bulbi 12, 127, 170
PHTVL cf. Persistent hyperplastic tunica vasculosa lentis
Pigment epithelium 210
–, dystrophy (PED) 224
Pigmented eye
–, differential diagnosis 17
Pilocarpine 23, 63
Pimecrolimus 27
Pinocytosis 159
Placing reflex
–, optical 15
PM cf. Membrane, pupillary
Poisoning cf. Intoxications
Polycoria 174
Polymyxin B 24
Posterior synechia 179
Povidone-iodine 24–26
PPM cf. Membrane, persistent pupillary
PRA cf. Retinal degeneration, hereditary (progressive)
Prednisolone 25
Preparation of the operative field 28
Pressure cf. Intraocular pressure
Primary glaucoma 159
–, acute 159
–, chronic 164
Process
–, ciliary 172
–, coronoid 47
Proparacaine 26
Proptosis 31–34
Protozoa 180
Protrusion of the nictitating membrane 107
Pseudo-enophthalmos 125
Pseudo-exophthalmos 125
Pseudomonas 180
Ptosis 94
Pupil 2
–, abnormalities 184
–, clinical diagnosis 14
–, dilatation syndrome 184

Pupillary reaction 214
Radiation cataract 196
Radiotherapy 27
RD cf. Retina, dysplasia
Recurrent uveitis
–, equine 182 ff.
Red eye
–, differential diagnosis 16
Retina(l) 2, 209–211
–, aplasia 218
–, atrophy 219, 221–223, 226
–, degeneration 15
– –, feline central (FCRD) 230
– –, hereditary (progressive (PRA) 221–224
–, detachment 14 ff., 176, 207, 210, 228 ff.
–, dysplasia (RD) 219
– –, geographic 219
– –, multifocal 219
– –, total 219
–, folds 216
–, hemorrhage 215
–, inner layer 209 ff.
–, neoplasia 231 ff.
–, outer layer 210
–, vessels 2, 214
Retinitis 227 ff.
Retinopathy
–, hypertensive 229 ff.
Rickettsia 180
Rods 210
Rose bengal 26
Rotation-flap correction 75
Rubeosis iridis 177

S

Sarcoid 100, 103
SARD cf. Sudden acquired retinal degeneration
Schirmer tear test (STT) 7, 26
Sclera(l) 2, 129–156, 210
–, clinical diagnosis 13
–, venous plexus 159
Scleritis 154
Sebaceous gland 2
Secondary glaucoma 160, 168–170
Sedation 8
Setting sun phenomenon 126
Sialodacryoadenitis cf. Dacryoadenitis
Signalment 5
Sjögren's syndrome 61 ff.
Slit-lamp biomicroscopy 15
Sodium chloride solution 26
Spherophakia 182
Sphinx position 5, 8

Squamous cell carcinoma 100, 122, 155
Staphyloma 141–142
Strabismus 12, 126
STT cf. Schirmer tear test
Subconjunctival hemorrhage 113
Sudden acquired retinal degeneration (SARD) 232
Suffusion 35
Sulfonamides 24, 61
Surgery 27–29
Suture materials 28
Symblepharon 114, 118–120
–, correction 120
Synchysis scintillans 206

T

Tacking cf. Entropion, correction, tacking
Tacrolimus 27, 63
Tapetal area cf. Tapetum lucidum
Tapetum
–, cellulosum 214
–, fibrosum 214
–, lucidum 2, 15, 173, 214
–, nigrum 15, 173, 214
Tarsorrhaphy
–, permanent 33
–, temporary 32–33
Taurine deficiency 227
Tear
–, film 59–61
–, flow 59–61
–, fluid
– –, blockage 61
– –, drainage 61
–, production 9 ff.
–, replacement therapy 26, 63
–, stripe 9, 65
Tears
–, artificial 26, 63
Tension 159
Tetracaine 8, 26
Therapeutics 19–27
–, application
– –, general rules 22
–, injection cf. Injection
Therapy 19–30 cf. Therapeutics
–, cryo- 29, 100
–, laser 29
–, radio- 27
–, surgical 27–29
Thiamine deficiency 227
Timolol 23
Tissue plasmogen activator 27
Tobramycin 24

Tonometer 13
Tonometry 12 ff., 16
Tonopen® 13
TonoVet® 13
Toxoplasma 180
Toxoplasmosis 227
Trabecular system 159
Trauma 41–45, 176, 225,
–, blunt 34–36
–, deep 36–37
–, eyelid 37–39
Travoprost 23
Trichiasis 11, 89–93
–, caruncle 91
–, correction
– –, Stades forced granulation procedure 92
–, nose fold 89 ff.
–, upper eyelid 90 ff.
Trifluorothymidine 25
Tropicamide 14, 24, 26
Tubocurarine 14
Tunica vasculosa lentis 189 ff.
–, persistent hyperplastic (PHTVL) 193

U

UDS cf. Uveo-dermatologic syndrome
Ulceration
–, deep 140
–, superficial 137–139
Ultrafiltration 157
Ultrasonography 16
Uvea 171–187
–, functions 171
–, neoplasia 177, 181 ff., 184–186
–, posterior 186
–, structure 171 ff.
Uveitis 177–179
–, anterior 177–179, 182 ff.
–, chronic relapsing 182 ff., 227
–, idiopathic 181
–, metabolic 179
–, posterior 227 ff.
Uveo-dermatologic syndrome (UDS) 181

V

Van Waardenburg's syndrome 174
Vasoconstrictors 22
Vein
–, facial 64
–, retinal 210
VEP cf. Visual evoked potentials
Vecuronium 14

Visual evoked potentials (VEP) 211
Vitamin
–, A 22, 26
– –, deficiency 225
–, B1 26
– –, deficiency 227
–, C 22, 26
–, E 22, 26
– –, deficiency 225

Vitreous 14, 189–208
–, clinical diagnosis 14
–, floaters 206
–, hemorrhage 206–207
–, ontogenesis 189 ff.
–, persistent hyperplastic primary (PHPV) 193
–, synchysis scintillans 206
Vortex system 214

X
Xerophthalmia 22

Z
Zeis glands 73
Zinc sulfate 26
Zygomatic arch 47

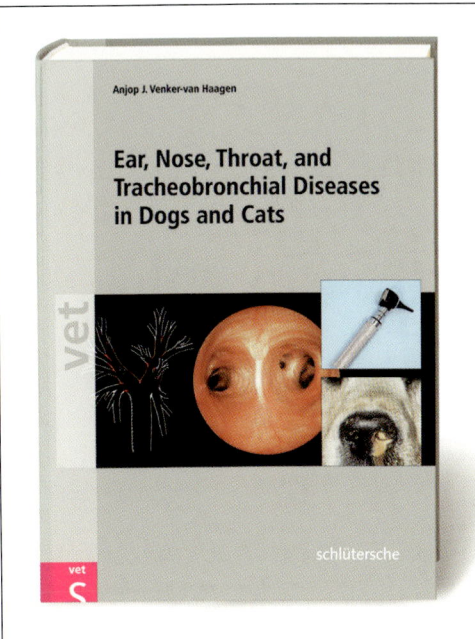

Anjop J. Venker-van Haagen

Ear, Nose, Throat, and Tracheobronchial Diseases in Dogs and Cats

2005. 248 pages, 182 illustrations, 7 1/2 x 10 1/4", hardcover
ISBN 978-3-87706-635-5

Ear, Nose, Throat, and Tracheobronchial Diseases in Dogs and Cats is the first textbook to provide a complete overview of all ENT diseases, both common and rare. It includes such problems as inflammation of the outer ear, deafness, nasal discharge, swallowing disorders, and cough. Detailed and up to date clinical information gives insight into ENT function and dysfunction for teachers and researchers, veterinarians in practice and veterinary students.

Six chapters give key information on functional considerations, aetiology, clinical signs, diagnosis, and therapy of ENT disorders. Special diagnostic and imaging techniques are described in detail.
About 180 top quality illustrations emphasize and supplement the specific features of the diseases and disorders described in the text. A detailed index gives easy access to the content of this book.

This unique textbook will provide a highly useful and informative reference guide to everyday practice, based on the author's 35 years as a specialist in ear, nose, throat, and tracheobronchial diseases in companion animals.

Author

Anjop J. Venker-van Haagen, DVM, PhD, DECVS, is a specialist for ear nose and throat diseases in companion animals. As former Associate Professor of Veterinary Ear, Nose and Throat Diseases at the Faculty of Veterinary Medicine, Utrecht University, she set standards in veterinary ENT medicine.

schlütersche

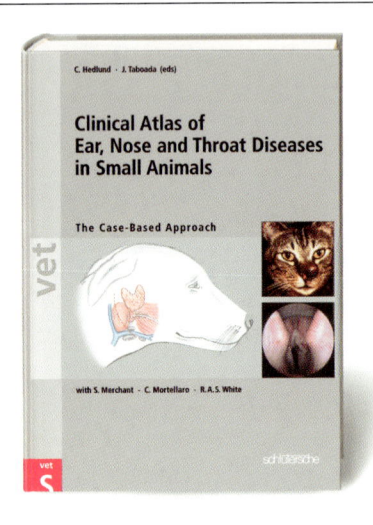

Cheryl Hedlund / Joe Taboada (eds.)

Clinical Atlas of Ear, Nose and Throat Diseases in Small Animals

The Case-Based Approach
With S. Merchant, C. Mortellaro, R.A.S. White

2002. 208 pages, 353 photographs and radiographs,
64 colour drawings, 8 1/2 x 11", hardcover
ISBN 978-3-87706-621-8

"The book has 204 pages packed with 350 truly excellent photographs, X-rays, illustrations and surgical drawings. The text references are very clearly laid out and, facilitate further reading on the topic. The diagrams are very good. This book is a great help. The editors have made an honest attempt to facilitate learning. In my view they have succeed."
Irish Veterinary Journal

"This text combines excellent production values with magnificent reproduction of many colour photographs and radiographs, which complement the text. I would recommend this book to students, both undergraduate and RCVS certificate candidates, as a useful adjunct to the standard textbooks."
The Veterinary Record

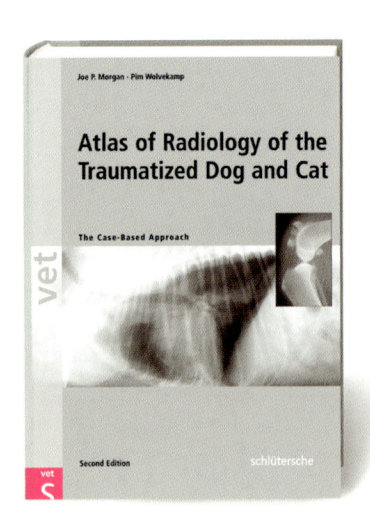

Joe P. Morgan / Pim Wolvekamp

Atlas of Radiology of the Traumatized Dog and Cat

The Case-Based Approach
Second Edition

2004. 568 pages, 790 radiographs, 50 tables, 8 1/2 x 11", hardcover
ISBN 978-3-89993-008-5

The totally revised second edition of this comprehensive atlas describes and explains the uses of diagnostic radiology and provides detailed instructions on how best to apply this technique to the diagnosis of traumatized dogs and cats, including a range of emergency cases. The main focus of the revised concept is the descriptive presentation of clinical cases.

"The images in this text are exemplary and reproduction is of a high quality. There are multiple radiographs and presentations of a single condition, which realistically reflects the various presentations of the traumatised patient. It is a radiography atlas which would be useful tool for any veterinarian who does a lot of emergency work and a useful adjunct to a standard radiology textbook for any veterinary student."
Veterinary Times

schlütersche